Anterior Cruciate Ligament Reconstruction

Rainer Siebold • David Dejour
Stefano Zaffagnini
Editors

Anterior Cruciate Ligament Reconstruction

A Practical Surgical Guide

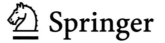

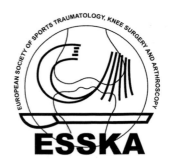

Editors
Rainer Siebold
HKF: Center for Specialised
Hip-Knee-Foot Surgery
ATOS Hospital Heidelberg
Heidelberg
Germany

Institute for Anatomy and Cell
Biology
Ruprecht-Karls
University Heidelberg
Heidelberg
Germany

David Dejour
Lyon Ortho Clinic
Lyon
France

Stefano Zaffagnini
Istituti Ortopedico Rizzoli Clinica
Ortopedica Traumatologica III
Bologna
Italy

ESSKA ASBL
Centre Médical
Fondation Norbert Metz
76, rue d'Eich
1460 Luxembourg
Luxembourg

ISBN 978-3-662-51083-4   ISBN 978-3-642-45349-6   (eBook)
DOI 10.1007/978-3-642-45349-6
Springer Heidelberg New York Dordrecht London

Foreword

The importance of this high-quality work may affect positively health professionals, orthopaedic sports medicine and rehabilitation education. This expectation seems natural and reasonable enough since the authors are also outstanding surgeons. The agenda was built and accomplished by a skillful and laborious team, providing guidance on the best current practice rules of the exciting developments related to anterior cruciate ligament (ACL) reconstruction.

ESSKA would like to gratefully and sincerely thank the authors for their commitment with this book. ESSKA intends to leverage education in the field of orthopaedic sports medicine and degenerative joints in Europe and all around the world. Hopefully it will be in good service for ACL injured patients and for improving people's quality of life.

The state of the art on ACL reconstruction provided here facilitates the access to recent insights concerning some hot topics in a friendly, comprehensive, clear and practical way. Nonetheless, this subject is continuously developing, and this publication brings new knowledge such as how to accurately measure knee laxity before and after reconstruction, prevention of early osteoarthritis, bone morphometrics and lower limb mechanics that can either precipitate ACL tears or prevent them. Therefore, it should be able to impel your extraordinary learning skills and strong motivation. Join the authors and ESSKA in their education mission.

Enjoy your reading, and I am sure you will find the challenge rewarding.

João Espregueira-Mendes
ESSKA President
Clínica Espregueira-Mendes F.C. Porto Stadium
– FIFA Medical Centre of Excellence

Preface

The anterior cruciate ligament (ACL) plays the central role for knee stability, proprioception and protection of internal knee structures.

Rupture often results in giving way, pain and function loss. The risk of secondary meniscal or cartilage injury is high, and chronic instability often ends in early osteoarthritis.

As most patients are young and active it is widely accepted to reconstruct the torn ACL. Also older patients are not willing to compromise their activities and ask for reconstruction.

Thus more and more ACL reconstructions are performed every year.

For many patients today's synonym for a successful surgery is "fast return to play". Especially active patients have very high expectations in our surgery. The highest rerupture rate occurs in patients younger than 20 years (risk 10 %), when returning within 7–9 months (risk 15 %) and when returning to strenuous stop-and-go sports, e.g. soccer (risk 20 %). Only approximately 50 % of our patients are able to return to their previous level of sports. It is our responsibility to make patients and coaches aware of these facts.

Of course surgeons are fascinated by technical details, and thousands of articles on bone tunnel positioning, grafts and surgical steps were published. However, today we have to realize that modern science needs cooperation and exchange of knowledge between surgeons and scientists. Central areas of today's research are ACL anatomy, biomechanics, ACL reconstruction, rehabilitation and prevention of injury and re-injury. All disciplines are of similar importance – and – everywhere there is plenty of room for us to improve.

This illustrative guide book written by world known experts presents the latest exciting news on ACL. Spectacular findings on the flat ACL anatomy are demonstrated. Remnant preservation is discussed along with the classical ACL reconstruction. Bony ACL refixation and reconstruction in kids is explained as is the concept of double bundle. Several chapters deal with the difficult topic of ACL revision and the combination of ACL reconstruction with high tibial osteotomy. Finally there are two chapters on rehabilitation and prevention of (re)-injury.

On behalf of all editors we thank everybody who contributed to the book, and hope that it will be a valuable addendum to your practise.

Heidelberg, Germany   Rainer Siebold
May 2014

Contents

Part III ACL Augmentation

Part IV Single Bundle ACL Reconstruction

Part I
Anatomy

Ribbonlike Anatomy of the Anterior Cruciate Ligament from Its Femoral Insertion to the Midsubstance

1

Robert Śmigielski, Urszula Zdanowicz, Michał Drwięga, Bogdan Ciszek, and Rainer Siebold

Contents

R. Śmigielski (✉) • U. Zdanowicz, MD
M. Drwięga
Head of Orthopaedic and Sports Traumatology
Department, Carolina Medical Center,
Pory 78, Warsaw 02-757, Poland
e-mail: robert.smigielski@carolina.pl

B. Ciszek
Department of Descriptive and Clinical Anatomy,
Medical University of Warsaw,
Chalbinskiego 5, Warsaw 02-004, Poland

R. Siebold
Institute for Anatomy and Cell Biology, Ruprecht-Karls
University Heidelberg, Im Neuenheimer Feld 307,
Heidelberg 69120, Germany

HKF: Center for Specialised Hip-Knee-Foot Surgery,
ATOS Hospital Heidelberg,
Bismarckstr. 9-15, Heidelberg 69115, Germany

1.1 Introduction

A deep understanding of the morphology of the anterior cruciate ligament (ACL) is fundamental for its anatomical reconstruction, and most surgeons would agree that anatomical ACL reconstruction is the "restoration of the ACL to its native dimensions, collagen orientation and insertion sites" [16].

From previous anatomical studies it is well known that the bony femoral ACL insertion is in the shape of a crescent, with the resident's ridge (= lateral intercondylar ridge) as its straight anterior border and the posterior articular margin of the lateral femoral condyle as its convex posterior border [3, 5, 6, 8, 9, 12, 14, 15, 17, 19, 21, 34, 37, 39, 41, 44, 50]. Most ACL fibers are aligned posterior to and directly along the lateral intercondylar ridge. The longitudinal axis is in extension to the posterior femoral cortex and creates an angle to the femoral shaft axis which varies between 0° and 70° [6, 13, 23, 39–41, 44]. The most posterior fibers of the femoral insertion are blending with the posterior cartilage of the lateral femoral condyle and with the periosteum of the posterior femoral shaft [13, 17, 23, 40, 41, 44]. The femoral insertion site area shows big variations in size. According to the literature, the area varies between 46 and 230 mm^2, the length between 12 and 20 mm, and the width between 5 and 13 mm [6, 9, 13, 17, 19, 22, 23, 27, 34, 40, 44]. Girgis et al. [17] described the midsubstance of the ACL to be broad and flat with an average width of 11.1 mm.

R. Siebold et al. (eds.), *Anterior Cruciate Ligament Reconstruction*,
DOI 10.1007/978-3-642-45349-6_1, © ESSKA 2014

Other authors reported the diameter in the range between 7 and 13 mm and the cross-sectional area to be "irregular," "oval," "corded," or "bundled" [2, 4, 6, 12, 17, 25–27, 34, 36, 49].

Recent detailed observations of the femoral insertion site were reported by Mochizuki et al. [29], Iwahashi et al. [23], and Sasaki et al. [40]. Histologically they described the ACL midsubstance fibers to form a narrow "direct" insertion posterior and along to the lateral intercondylar ridge which was continued by a fanlike "indirect" insertion towards the posterior femoral cartilage. Interestingly they found the configuration of the ACL midsubstance to be "rather flat, looking like lasagna" [28].

1.2   Material and Methods

To reconfirm the above findings and to further explore the ACL anatomy, Smigielski et al. performed this cadaveric study. They included 111 fresh frozen cadaveric knees from an international accredited tissue bank. For detailed demographic data see Table 1.1. The key point in the dissections was to very carefully remove the synovial tissue surrounding the collagen fibers of the ACL. Measurements were performed under direct visualization using calipers. In addition, 30 knees were then sent for CT and MRI scans as well as histological examination of the femoral insertion site.

1.3   Results

In all dissected knees, the intraligamentous part of the ACL from close to its femoral insertion to the midsubstance was observed to have a ribbonlike structure (Fig. 1.1a–c). The femoral bony insertion of the ribbon was in exact continuity to the posterior femoral cortex (Fig. 1.2a,

b). A clear separation into bundles was not possible. The morphometric measurements of the ACL were performed with calipers. The results for the width and thickness were as follows (Fig. 1.3a–c):

Mean width 2 mm from femoral insertion, 16.0 mm (range, 12.7–18.1)

Mean thickness 2 mm from femoral insertion, 3.54 mm (range, 2–4.8)

Mean width at midsubstance of ACL, 11.4 mm (range, 9.8–13.8)

Mean thickness at midsubstance of ACL, 3.4 mm (range, 1.8–3.9)

Mean cross-sectional area 2 mm from femoral insertion (calculated), 56.6 mm^2

Mean cross-sectional area at midsubstance of ACL (calculated), 39.8 mm^2

3D CT reconstruction, MRI, and histology reconfirmed the ribbonlike structure of the ACL. The collagen fibers approached to the femoral insertion in an acute angle creating a doubled tidemark at the bone. This may be interpreted as a place within the whole attachment with either greater stress forces or microinjuries. In both interpretations that would be the place where the greatest force is applied (Fig. 1.4a, b).

1.4   Discussion

The most important finding of this cadaveric study was that the ACL formed a flat ribbonlike ligament from its femoral insertion to the midsubstance in all dissected knees.

The ACL fibers were in exact continuity with the posterior femoral cortex and inserted from and posterior to the lateral intercondylar ridge. A clear separation into bundles was not possible. Anatomical observations were based on dissections of 111 cadaveric knees and were reconfirmed on CT, MRI, and histology.

Table 1.1 Detailed demographic data of the study subjects

Sex	Side	Age	Height	BMI	Weight	Races
66 female 45 male	49 right 62 left	Mean 67 years (32–74 years)	Mean 1.70 m (1.50–1.96 m)	Mean 22.6 (12.1–34.7)	Mean 64.3 kg (36–116 kg)	104 Caucasians 6 African Americans 1 Indian American

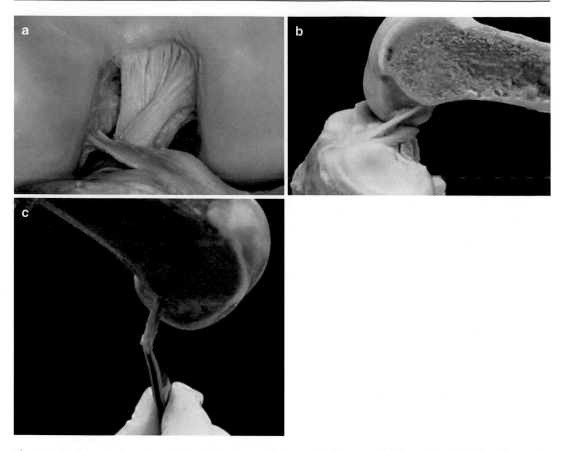

Fig. 1.1 (**a–c**) The ribbon shape of the ACL after careful removal of the synovial tissue: the ACL fibers form a flat ribbon 2 mm from its femoral attachment to the midsubstance

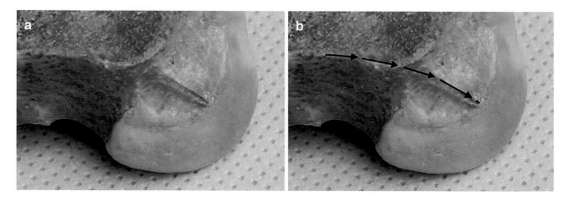

Fig. 1.2 (**a, b**) The direct insertion of the ribbonlike ACL fibers is in continuity of the posterior femoral cortex

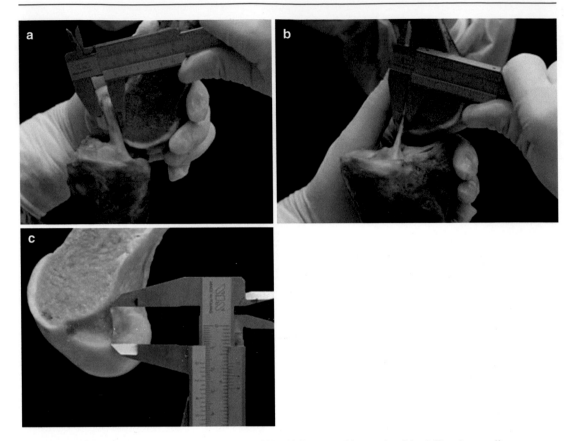

Fig. 1.3 (**a–c**) Measurement of the midsubstance width, thickness, and long axis of the ACL using a caliper

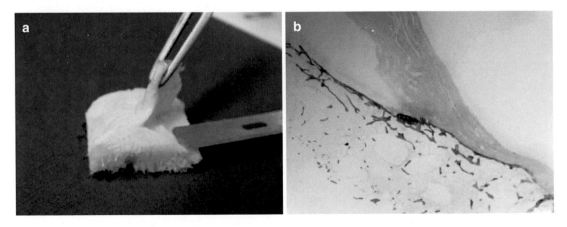

Fig. 1.4 (**a, b**) Histology of the direct femoral insertion of the ACL: macroscopic view (**a**) and microscopic view (**b**) (light microscopy, H&E stain, original magnification ×4). 6b: Note the sharp angle at which the fibers attach to the bone

1.5   Direct and Indirect ACL Femoral Insertion

These findings reconfirm earlier anatomical and histological studies. In 2006 Mochizuki et al. [28] emphasized "that – after removal of the surface membrane – the configuration of the intraligamentous part of the ACL was not oval" "but rather flat, looking like 'lasagna,'" 15.1 mm wide and 4.7 mm thick. Mochizuki et al. [28] also described the femoral insertion of the ACL to be very similar to the midsubstance configuration after the ligament surface membrane was removed from the attachment site. In 2010 Iwahashi et al. [23] reported on the "direct" femoral ACL insertion in which dense collagen fibers were connected to the bone by a fibrocartilaginous layer. This "direct" insertion was located in the depression between the lateral intercondylar ridge and 7–10 mm anterior to the articular cartilage margin. It measured 17.9 mm in length and 8.0 mm in width and covered an area of 128.3 mm². These findings were reconfirmed by Sasaki et al. [40] who observed a narrow "direct" ACL insertion area posterior and along the lateral intercondylar ridge and a "lateral intercondylar posterior ridge." The lengths of the long and short axes of the insertion were 17.7 and 5.3 mm, respectively. Another "indirect" ACL insertion was located just posterior to the direct insertion. The ACL from type I collagen blended into the posterior cartilage on immunohistological observations [40].

In a second report Mochizuki et al. [29] just recently differentiated between the main attachment of the midsubstance ACL fibers and the attachment of the thin fibrous tissue. Later extended from the midsubstance fibers and broadly spread out like a fan on the posterior condyle. The authors termed these fibers "fanlike extension fibers" and described that these two different structures formed a fold at the border between the midsubstance fibers and the fanlike extension fibers in knee flexion.

1.6   MRI Findings

Our MRI measurements as well as MRI reports from the literature also reconfirm the flat ribbonlike midsubstance of the ACL. Staeubli et al. [45]

measured the midsubstance in 53 knees using a 0.23 T MRI and found a width of 6.1 mm in men and 5.2 mm in women; Muneta et al. [31] reported 5.5 and 5.1 mm, respectively, and Pujol et al. [38] 6.1 mm. Cohen et al. [8] scanned the knees of 50 patients using a 1.5 T MRI and measured the dimensions of the AM and PL bundles in the sagittal and coronal plane to be 5.1 mm by 4.2 mm and 4.4 mm by 3.7 mm, respectively.

1.7   Cross-Sectional Area of ACL

The calculated cross-sectional area of the mid substance ACL among our specimen was 52 and 55 mm² for women and men, 2 mm close to its femoral insertion site and 33 and 38 mm² at midsubstance, respectively. This is in agreement with several previous reports. Mochizuki et al. [28] approximated 65 mm² as the femoral attachment area, Harner et al. [19] calculated approximately 40 mm² at midsubstance, Hashemi et al. 46.8 mm² [20], and Iriuchishima et al. 46.9 mm² [22]. Differentiating between gender Anderson et al. [4] calculated a cross-sectional area of 44 mm² for men and 36.1 mm² for women, Dienst et al. [11] of 56.8 mm² for men and 40–50 % less for women on MRI, and Pujol et al. [38] of 29.2 mm² (range 20.0–38.9 mm²).

1.8   Double-Bundle Structure?

From our dissections the intraligamentous collagen fibers of the ACL could not clearly be separated into bundles. This is in agreement with Welsh [47] and Arnoczky [5] and others reporting that the intraligamentous part of the ACL is a collection of individual fascicles that fan out over a broad flattened area with no histological evidence for two separate bundles [5, 10, 12, 24, 34, 47]. However, the recent approach to the ACL is to differentiate between anteromedial and posterolateral bundle [1, 6, 7, 13, 16–19, 27, 32, 44, 48]. Some authors even described three separate ACL bundles [2, 33, 35]. The separation of the ACL into an AM and PL bundle was reconfirmed by Ferretti et al. [15] which found a fine synovial septum in dissected ACLs of fetus.

In any case, the macroscopic anatomical separation of the ACL into two or three bundles remains very difficult and is controversial. According to Arnoczky et al. [5], the bundle anatomy oversimplifies somewhat as the ACL is actually a continuum of fascicles. In 1991 Amis and Dawkins [2] described that it was "sometimes difficult to separate the ACL into three discrete bundles. In these cases the anterior aspect of the ACL was folded itself in flexion suggesting an arrangement of bundles. It was still possible to develop a three-bundle structure corresponding to the folding, but it felt, that the teasing apart was artefactual." In older specimens, however, the separate bundles were often obvious. Amis and Dawkins [2] concluded, "that the ACL wrinkles into the appearance of three bundles as the knee flexes. These bundles are often demonstrably separate structures, twisted together during flexion, but the use of the dissector to separate the fibre bundles can cross the threshold between demonstration of bundles and their creation." From our observation the "double-bundle effect" was created by the twisted flat ribbonlike structure of the ACL from femoral to tibial, which leads to the impression of two or three separate bundles when the knee was flexed. This would reconfirm reports of Amis and Dawkins [2] who made similar observations.

1.9 Consequences for ACL Reconstruction

The ribbonlike shape of the ACL and the flat but long femoral "direct" insertion site would support a rather flat anatomical footprint and midsubstance reconstruction. A double-bundle ACL reconstruction using two 5–6 mm hamstring grafts (see Chap. 29) [23, 28, 30, 40, 42, 43], a flat 5–6 mm patella tendon graft [41], or a flat 5–6 mm quadriceps tendon graft may be a better anatomical option than a large (and too wide)-diameter graft for a single-bundle ACL reconstruction. Sasaki et al. [40] concluded that whereas the indirect insertion plays a role as a dynamic anchorage of soft tissue to bone allowing certain shear movements, the strength

of anchoring is weaker than the direct insertion [46]. Therefore, it would be ideal to make the femoral tunnel on the direct insertion in the native ACL [40]. Mochizuki et al. [29] found that it is very difficult to reconstruct the fanlike indirect extension fibers by a bone tunnel; however, the midsubstance fibers of the ACL can be reconstructed. Of course the most efficient anatomical and biomechanical ACL reconstruction has still to be proven in prospectively designed clinical long-term studies.

> **Memory**
> This is a detailed anatomical study describing the ribbonlike structure of the ACL from its femoral insertion to the midsubstance. A key point was to carefully remove the surface fibrous membrane of the ACL. Two millimeter from its bony direct femoral insertion, the ACL formed a flat ribbonlike ligament without a clear separation between AM and PL bundles. The ribbon was in exact continuity of the posterior femoral cortex. The findings of a flat ligament may change the approach to femoral ACL footprint and midsubstance ACL reconstruction and to graft selection.

References

1. Adachi N, Ochi M, Uchio Y et al (2004) Reconstruction of the anterior cruciate ligament. Single- versus double-bundle multistranded hamstring tendons. J Bone Joint Surg Br 86(4):515–520
2. Amis AA, Dawkins GP (1991) Functional anatomy of the anterior cruciate ligament. Fibre bundle actions related to ligament replacements and injuries. J Bone Joint Surg Br 73(2):260–267
3. Amis AA, Jakob RP (1998) Anterior cruciate ligament graft positioning, tensioning and twisting. Knee Surg Sports Traumatol Arthrosc 6(Suppl 1):S2–S12
4. Anderson AF, Dome DC, Gautam S et al (2001) Correlation of anthropometric measurements, strength, anterior cruciate ligament size, and intercondylar notch characteristics to sex differences in anterior cruciate ligament tear rates. Am J Sports Med 29(1):58–66
5. Arnoczky SP (1983) Anatomy of the anterior cruciate ligament. Clin Orthop Relat Res 172:19–25

6. Baer GS, Ferretti M, Fu FH (2008) Anatomy of the ACL. In: Fu FH, Cohen SB (eds) Current concepts in ACL reconstruction. SLACK, Thorofare, pp 21–32

7. Buoncristiani AM, Tjoumakaris FP, Starman JS et al (2006) Anatomic double-bundle anterior cruciate ligament reconstruction. Arthroscopy 22(9):1000–1006

8. Cohen SB, VanBeek C, Starman JS et al (2009) MRI measurement of the 2 bundles of the normal anterior cruciate ligament. Orthopedics 32(9)

9. Colombet P, Robinson J, Christel P et al (2006) Morphology of anterior cruciate ligament attachments for anatomic reconstruction: a cadaveric dissection and radiographic study. Arthroscopy 22(9):984–992

10. Dargel J, Pohl P, Tzikaras P et al (2006) Morphometric side-to-side differences in human cruciate ligament insertions. Surg Radiol Anat 28(4):398–402

11. Dienst M, Schneider G, Altmeyer K et al (2007) Correlation of intercondylar notch cross sections to the ACL size: a high resolution MR tomographic in vivo analysis. Arch Orthop Trauma Surg 127(4):253–260

12. Duthon VB, Barea C, Abrassart S et al (2006) Anatomy of the anterior cruciate ligament. Knee Surg Sports Traumatol Arthrosc 14(3):204–213

13. Edwards A, Bull AM, Amis AA (2008) The attachments of the anteromedial and posterolateral fibre bundles of the anterior cruciate ligament. Part 2: femoral attachment. Knee Surg Sports Traumatol Arthrosc 16(1):29–36

14. Ferretti M, Ekdahl M, Shen W et al (2007) Osseous landmarks of the femoral attachment of the anterior cruciate ligament: an anatomic study. Arthroscopy 23(11):1218–1225

15. Ferretti M, Levicoff EA, Macpherson TA et al (2007) The fetal anterior cruciate ligament: an anatomic and histologic study. Arthroscopy 23(3):278–283

16. Fu FH, Karlsson J (2010) A long journey to be anatomic. Knee Surg Sports Traumatol Arthrosc 18(9):1151–1153

17. Girgis FG, Marshall JL, Monajem A (1975) The cruciate ligaments of the knee joint. Anatomical, functional and experimental analysis. Clin Orthop Relat Res 106:216–231

18. Hamada M, Shino K, Horibe S et al (2001) Single-versus bi-socket anterior cruciate ligament reconstruction using autogenous multiple-stranded hamstring tendons with endoButton femoral fixation: a prospective study. Arthroscopy 17(8):801–807

19. Harner CD, Baek GH, Vogrin TM et al (1999) Quantitative analysis of human cruciate ligament insertions. Arthroscopy 15(7):741–749

20. Hashemi J, Mansouri H, Chandrashekar N et al (2011) Age, sex, body anthropometry, and ACL size predict the structural properties of the human anterior cruciate ligament. J Orthop Res 29(7):993–1001

21. Hutchinson MR, Ash SA (2003) Resident's ridge: assessing the cortical thickness of the lateral wall and roof of the intercondylar notch. Arthroscopy 19(9):931–935

22. Iriuchishima T, Yorifuji H, Aizawa S et al (2012) Evaluation of ACL mid-substance cross-sectional area for reconstructed autograft selection. Knee Surg Sports Traumatol Arthrosc 22(1):207–213

23. Iwahashi T, Shino K, Nakata K et al (2010) Direct anterior cruciate ligament insertion to the femur assessed by histology and 3-dimensional volume-rendered computed tomography. Arthroscopy 26(9 Suppl):S13–S20

24. Jacobsen K (1977) Osteoarthrosis following insufficiency of the cruciate ligaments in man. A clinical study. Acta Orthop Scand 48(5):520–526

25. Kennedy JC, Weinberg HW, Wilson AS (1974) The anatomy and function of the anterior cruciate ligament. As determined by clinical and morphological studies. J Bone Joint Surg Am 56(2):223–235

26. Kopf S, Musahl V, Tashman S et al (2009) A systematic review of the femoral origin and tibial insertion morphology of the ACL. Knee Surg Sports Traumatol Arthrosc 17(3):213–219

27. Luites JW, Wymenga AB, Blankevoort L et al (2007) Description of the attachment geometry of the anteromedial and posterolateral bundles of the ACL from arthroscopic perspective for anatomical tunnel placement. Knee Surg Sports Traumatol Arthrosc 15(12):1422–1431

28. Mochizuki T, Muneta T, Nagase T et al (2006) Cadaveric knee observation study for describing anatomic femoral tunnel placement for two-bundle anterior cruciate ligament reconstruction. Arthroscopy 22(4):356–361

29. Mochizuki T, Fujishiro H, Nimura A et al (2014) Anatomic and histologic analysis of the midsubstance and fan-like extension fibers of the anterior cruciate ligament during knee motion, with special reference to the femoral attachment. Knee Surg Sports Traumatol Arthrosc 22(2):336–344

30. Mott HW (1983) Semitendinosus anatomic reconstruction for cruciate ligament insufficiency. Clin Orthop Relat Res 172:90–92

31. Muneta T, Takakuda K, Yamamoto H (1997) Intercondylar notch width and its relation to the configuration and cross-sectional area of the anterior cruciate ligament. A cadaveric knee study. Am J Sports Med 25(1):69–72

32. Muneta T, Sekiya I, Yagishita K et al (1999) Two-bundle reconstruction of the anterior cruciate ligament using semitendinosus tendon with endobuttons: operative technique and preliminary results. Arthroscopy 15(6):618–624

33. Norwood LA, Cross MJ (1979) Anterior cruciate ligament: functional anatomy of its bundles in rotatory instabilities. Am J Sports Med 7(1):23–26

34. Odensten M, Gillquist J (1985) Functional anatomy of the anterior cruciate ligament and a rationale for reconstruction. J Bone Joint Surg Am 67(2):257–262

35. Otsubo H, Shino K, Suzuki D et al (2012) The arrangement and the attachment areas of three ACL bundles. Knee Surg Sports Traumatol Arthrosc 20(1):127–134

36. Papachristou G, Sourlas J, Magnissalis E et al (2007) ACL reconstruction and the implication of its tibial

attachment for stability of the joint: anthropometric and biomechanical study. Int Orthop 31(4):465–470

37. Petersen W, Tillmann B (2002) Anatomie und Funktion des vorderen Kreuzbandes. Orthopade 31(8):710–718

38. Pujol N, Queinnec S, Boisrenoult P et al (2013) Anatomy of the anterior cruciate ligament related to hamstring tendon grafts. A cadaveric study. Knee 20(6):511–514

39. Purnell ML, Larson AI, Clancy W (2008) Anterior cruciate ligament insertions on the tibia and femur and their relationships to critical bony landmarks using high-resolution volume-rendering computed tomography. Am J Sports Med 36(11):2083–2090

40. Sasaki N, Ishibashi Y, Tsuda E et al (2012) The femoral insertion of the anterior cruciate ligament: discrepancy between macroscopic and histological observations. Arthroscopy 28(8):1135–1146

41. Shino K, Suzuki T, Iwahashi T et al (2010) The resident's ridge as an arthroscopic landmark for anatomical femoral tunnel drilling in ACL reconstruction. Knee Surg Sports Traumatol Arthrosc 18(9):1164–1168

42. Siebold R (2011) The concept of complete footprint restoration with guidelines for single- and double-bundle ACL reconstruction. Knee Surg Sports Traumatol Arthrosc 19(5):699–706

43. Siebold R, Schuhmacher P (2012) Restoration of the tibial ACL footprint area and geometry using the Modified Insertion Site Table. Knee Surg Sports Traumatol Arthrosc 20(9):1845–1849

44. Siebold R, Ellert T, Metz S et al (2008) Femoral insertions of the anteromedial and posterolateral bundles of the anterior cruciate ligament: morphometry and arthroscopic orientation models for double-bundle bone tunnel placement–a cadaver study. Arthroscopy 24(5):585–592

45. Staeubli HU, Adam O, Becker W et al (1999) Anterior cruciate ligament and intercondylar notch in the coronal oblique plane: anatomy complemented by magnetic resonance imaging in cruciate ligament-intact knees. Arthroscopy 15(4):349–359

46. Weiler A, Hoffmann RF, Bail HJ et al (2002) Tendon healing in a bone tunnel. Part II: Histologic analysis after biodegradable interference fit fixation in a model of anterior cruciate ligament reconstruction in sheep. Arthroscopy 18(2):124–135

47. Welsh RP (1980) Knee joint structure and function. Clin Orthop Relat Res 147:7–14

48. Yasuda K, Kondo E, Ichiyama H et al (2004) Anatomic reconstruction of the anteromedial and posterolateral bundles of the anterior cruciate ligament using hamstring tendon grafts. Arthroscopy 20(10):1015–1025

49. Yasuda K, van Eck CF, Hoshino Y et al (2011) Anatomic single- and double-bundle anterior cruciate ligament reconstruction, part 1: Basic science. Am J Sports Med 39(8):1789–1799

50. Zantop T, Petersen W, Fu FH (2005) Anatomy of the anterior cruciate ligament. Operat Tech Orthop 15(1):20–28

Anatomic and Histological Analysis of the Midsubstance and Fanlike Extension Fibers of the ACL

Tomoyuki Mochizuki, Akimoto Nimura, Kazunori Yasuda, Takeshi Muneta, and Keiichi Akita

Contents

T. Mochizuki, MD, PhD (✉)
Department of Joint Reconstruction,
Graduate School, Tokyo Medical and Dental University,
Tokyo, Japan
e-mail: mochizuki.orj@tmd.ac.jp

A. Nimura, MD, PhD • K. Akita, MD, PhD
Unit of Clinical Anatomy, Graduate School,
Tokyo Medical and Dental University, Tokyo, Japan

K. Yasuda, MD, PhD
Department of Sports Medicine and Joint Surgery,
Hokkaido University Graduate School of Medicine,
Sapporo, Japan

T. Muneta, MD, PhD
Department of Joint Surgery and Sports Medicine,
Graduate School, Tokyo Medical and Dental University,
Tokyo, Japan

2.1 Introduction

There has been some disagreement concerning the size and location of the femoral attachment of ACL. Namely, some original studies reported that ACL is attached to a relatively narrow oval area on the lateral condyle [2, 4, 15, 16]. In contrast, other recent studies have described that ACL is attached to a wide area on the lateral condyle; as a consequence the posterior attachment margin comes into contact with the articular cartilage margin [3, 6, 9, 10, 17]. Therefore, we performed a series of anatomic studies to clarify this discrepancy [5, 8]. In those studies, the femoral attachment of ACL fibers was found to be composed of two different shapes of fibers. One shape is the main attachment of the midsubstance of ACL fibers, and the other is the attachment of the thin fibrous tissue which extends from the midsubstance fibers and broadly spreads out like a fan on the posterior condyle. These fibers were termed "fanlike extension fibers" [8]. In addition, all fascicles which make up the midsubstance of ACL were observed to attach to the relatively narrow oval area on the lateral condyle [5].

2.2 Static and Dynamic Observation of the Fanlike Extension Fibers

At the full extension position, both the midsubstance fibers and the fanlike extension fibers were aligned parallel to the intercondylar roof without curving (Figs. 2.1a and 2.2b). The attachment

R. Siebold et al. (eds.), *Anterior Cruciate Ligament Reconstruction*,
DOI 10.1007/978-3-642-45349-6_2, © ESSKA 2014

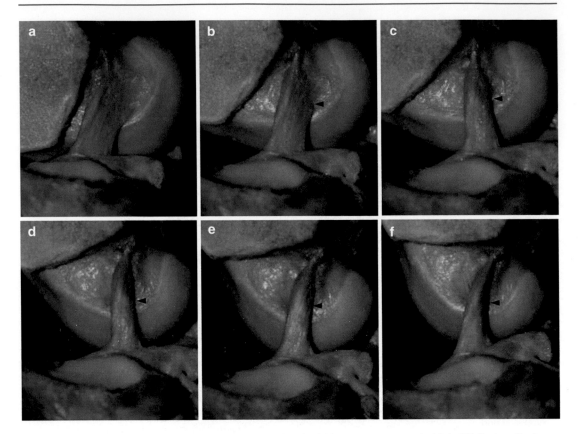

Fig. 2.1 Dynamic observation of the midsubstance and fanlike extension fibers during flexion-extension motion of the knee. (**a**) At full extension, both the midsubstance fibers and the fanlike extension fibers were aligned parallel to the intercondylar roof without curving. (**b**) At 15° flexion, the midsubstance fibers were found to slightly curve (*black arrowheads*) approximately at the postero-proximal edge of the direct attachment of the midsubstance fibers (as judged according to 30° flexion, where the fold was more apparent). (**c**) At 30° flexion, the degree of the curving of the midsubstance fibers was increased. (**d**) At 45° flexion, the curving of the ACL fibers was an obvious fold. (**e**) At 60° flexion, the midsubstance fibers started to become twisted, and the fold became deep specifically at the postero-distal portion. (**f**) At 90° flexion, the whole fold was deeper in the thin space between the midsubstance fibers and the femoral condyle

area of the midsubstance fibers was observed to be slightly protuberant, compared with that of the fanlike extension fibers (Fig. 2.2a). The fanlike extension fibers, which appeared to be thin and coarse compared to the midsubstance fibers, came into contact with the margin of articular cartilage (Fig. 2.2b). When tension was applied to the midsubstance fibers, the tension appeared to be distributed to the fanlike extension fibers. The distinct border between the midsubstance and fanlike extension fibers could not be identified.

At 15° and 30° of knee flexion, the midsubstance fibers were found to be slightly curved anterior to the articular cartilage of the lateral condyle (Fig. 2.1b, c). The border between the midsubstance fibers and the fanlike extension fibers became obvious (Fig. 2.3a). The location and orientation of the fanlike extension fibers could not be changed in relation to the femoral condyle surface because the fibers were adhered to the bone surface (Fig. 2.3b).

At 45° and 60° of knee flexion, the curving of the ACL fibers became an obvious fold (Fig. 2.1d, e). At 90°, the whole fold became deeper, and it was located approximately on the line between the postero-proximal outlet point of the intercondylar edge and the postero-distal edge of the midsubstance attachment of the PL bundle (Fig. 2.1f). When tension was applied to the midsubstance fibers, the tension did not appear to be distributed to the fanlike extension fibers due to the presence of the fold.

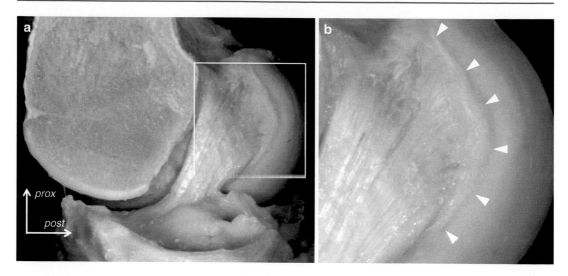

Fig. 2.2 Static observation of the midsubstance and fan-like extension fibers at full extension. (**a**) Both the midsubstance fibers and the fanlike extension fibers were aligned parallel to the intercondylar roof without curving. (**b**) High-magnification view of ACL fibers on the medial wall of lateral condyle. The fanlike extension fibers reached the margin of the articular cartilage (*white arrowheads*) and tended to adhere to the medial wall and became rather sparse as they approached the articular cartilage

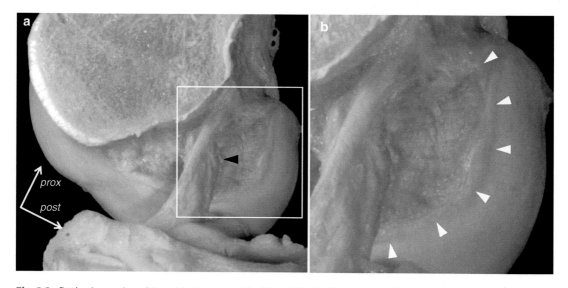

Fig. 2.3 Static observation of the midsubstance and fanlike extension fibers at 30° knee flexion. (**a**) The midsubstance fibers were curved (*black arrowhead*) and changed the direction from the fanlike extension fibers. (**b**) High-magnification view of ACL fibers on the medial wall of the lateral condyle. The fanlike extension fibers were adhered to the bone surface, and the fiber location and orientation in relation to the bone surface did not change, while the orientation of the midsubstance fibers did change with knee flexion. *White arrowheads* indicate the articular margin

2.3   Location of the Fold Within the Whole ACL Attachment

The cutline along the valley of the fold was located approximately parallel to the long axis of the oval-shaped attachment of the midsubstance fibers of ACL (Fig. 2.4). The attachment of the midsubstance fibers was significantly smaller than that of the fanlike extension fibers. The fold ratio (the attachment of midsubstance/whole ACL attachment) was 63.7 % (47.3 ~ 80.2 %). The attachment area of the fanlike extension fibers was on average about twice as large as that of the midsubstance fibers.

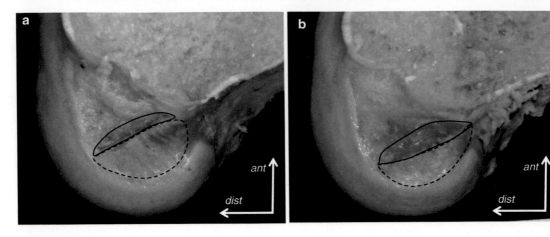

Fig. 2.4 Measurement of location of the fold formed in the ACL attachment. The resected area is delineated by the *black line* and the unresected area by the *black dashed line*. Note that fanlike extension fibers were adhered to the unresected area. The resected area corresponds to the attachment of the midsubstance fibers, and the unresected area corresponds to the attachment of the fanlike extension fibers. Two typical patterns are shown. (**a**) In this specimen the unresected area was much larger than the resected area. (**b**) In a different specimen the unresected area was almost the same size as the resected area

2.4 Histological Observation of the Orientation of Midsubstance and Fanlike Extension Fibers

At the full extension position of the knee, the histological sections in Fig. 2.5a, b demonstrated that the AM bundle of the midsubstance fibers was attached adjacent to the proximal outlet of the intercondylar notch. The postero-proximal edge of the attachment made contact with the margin of the articular cartilage (Fig. 2.5a, b). The sections in Fig. 2.5c, d showed that the thin fanlike extension fibers, which extended from the midsubstance fibers of the PL bundle, were attached to the postero-proximal aspect of the lateral condyle and extended to the articular cartilage of the lateral condyle (Fig. 2.5c, d). In these sections, the surface of midsubstance fibers was slightly concave, but no fold was seen on the surface because of the same direction of these fibers.

At 120° of knee flexion, a fold was observed in the midsubstance fibers several millimeters from the bone surface (Fig. 2.6a–d). The thin fanlike extension fibers were adhered to the bone surface in the same manner as observed in the full extension position (Fig. 2.6a–d). The angle between the direction of the fanlike extension fibers and the direction of the midsubstance fibers was 90° or more.

In this study, histological differences between the fanlike extension fibers and the midsubstance fibers could not be detected. In the structure of the bony insertion, however, a histological difference between the fanlike extension fibers and the midsubstance fibers could be identified. Namely, a cartilaginous zone between the collagen fibers and the bone in the midsubstance fiber insertion could be observed, while almost all collagen fibers directly attached to the bone in the fanlike extension fiber insertion and a cartilaginous tissue were rarely seen between them.

2.5 Discussion

The most important finding of the present study was that, because the fanlike extension fibers were adhered to the bone surface, the fiber location and orientation in relation to the femoral surface did not change, regardless of the knee flexion angle, while orientation of the midsubstance fibers in relation to the femur did change during knee motion. These two different structures formed a fold, observed in knee flexion, at the border between the midsubstance fibers and the fanlike extension. There have been no reports in

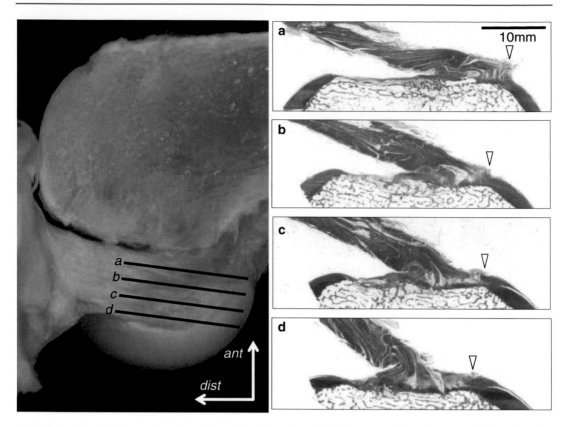

Fig. 2.5 Histological observation of the fiber orientation of the midsubstance and fanlike extension fibers at full extension position. The *left picture* indicates four oblique-axial section planes parallel to the intercondylar roof. The midsubstance fibers of the AM bundle attached adjacent to the proximal outlet of the intercondylar notch (**a**, **b**).

The thin fanlike extension fibers extended from the midsubstance fibers of the PL bundle and adhered to the postero-proximal aspect of the lateral condyle (**c**, **d**). *White arrowheads* indicates the margin of the articular cartilage of the lateral condyle

which fanlike extension fibers were observed in knee flexion positions, although a few anatomic studies histologically have observed fanlike extension fibers only at the full extension position [7, 8, 11]. The histological differences between the fanlike extension fibers and the midsubstance fibers could be observed at the femoral insertion. The insertion of the midsubstance fibers involved the cartilaginous zone, which is regarded as the direct insertion [12]. On the other hand, the fanlike extension fibers directly attached onto the bone without forming transitional cartilaginous zone, which is regarded as the indirect insertion [1]. Recently, Sasaki et al. reported similar observations concerning the femoral attachment of the ACL [11]. This study performed at various flexion positions provided new information, which is important not only to

understand the mechanism of the above-described fold formation but also to consider the function of the fanlike extension fibers.

The results obtained in this study also showed that a deep fold was formed in the postero-proximal aspect of the midsubstance fibers several millimeters from the bone surface as the knee was flexed. No studies have described this phenomenon or considered its functional significance. This is mainly due to the fact that previous studies evaluated ACL fibers in the knee extension position, and the fold formation cannot be observed in this position. Interestingly, the fold formation can be inadvertently noted in a few photographs of ACL, which were taken at a knee flexion position in the previous reports [2, 9, 10, 18], although no discussion of this phenomenon was included in the reports. These above-

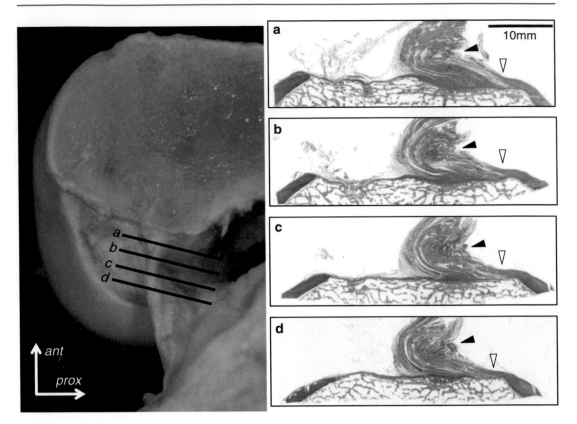

Fig. 2.6 Histological observation of the fiber orientation of the midsubstance and fanlike extension fibers at 120° flexion. The *left picture* indicates four oblique-axial section planes parallel to the intercondylar roof. The fold (*black arrowheads*) was observed at the border between the midsubstance fibers and the fanlike extension fibers several millimeters away from the bone surface (**a–d**). The thin fanlike extension fibers adhered to the bone surface of the lateral condyle. The insertion of the midsubstance fibers (*white arrowheads*, **a–d**) tends to involve cartilaginous zone between collagen fibers and bone surface. The fanlike extension fibers tend to insert into the bone without forming transitional cartilaginous zone

described anatomic results suggested that the load distribution mechanism from the ACL midsubstance to the femur is more complex than the previously thought. At the full extension position, a part of the load is widely distributed to the fanlike extension fibers. As the knee is flexed, midsubstance fibers may play a more important role than the fanlike extension fibers.

This study demonstrated that ACL has two types of attachment margins. One is the relatively narrow oval attachment margin of the midsubstance fibers of ACL, and the other is the broader attachment margin of the fanlike extension fibers. Thus, this study suggested that all of the previous studies have reported correct information on a part of the ACL attachment. Namely, those previous studies might have observed one or both of these two attachment margins.

As for clinical relevance, the present study provides critical information for future clinical studies in the reconstruction of the fanlike extension fibers as well as the midsubstance fibers. The present study also provides important information for future biomechanical studies not only to clarify the biomechanics of the fanlike extension fibers but also to create mathematical models of ACL. Those studies will contribute to the clarification of the precise function of ACL and the injury mechanism. Specifically, concerning the relevance of ACL reconstruction, it is considered to be difficult to reconstruct the natural function of the fanlike extension fibers by creating a tunnel at the femoral and tibial ends of each fiber bundle, although the midsubstance fibers can be reconstructed by creating a tunnel at the femoral and tibial ends of each fiber bundle. Recently, a few studies recommend to create a femoral tunnel in the attachment area of the fanlike extension fibers in order to reconstruct the AM bundle of the ACL [13, 14]. However, we cannot simply say that such surgery can reconstruct the natural fanlike extension fiber function. For such reconstructive surgery, further biomechanical evaluation of the reconstructed bundle function will be needed in the near future.

Memory

The fanlike extension fibers were adhered to the bone surface, and the fiber location and orientation in relation to the femoral surface did not change, regardless of the knee flexion angle, while the orientation of the midsubstance fibers in relation to the femur did change during knee motion. These two different structures form a fold at the border between the midsubstance fibers and the fanlike extension in knee flexion. The attachment of the midsubstance fibers was significantly smaller than the attachment of the fanlike extension fibers.

The present study clarified the anatomic and histological character of the midsubstance fibers and fanlike extension fibers and provided critical information for future clinical and biomechanical studies concerning the two different fibers. Specifically for ACL reconstruction, it is difficult to reconstruct the natural fanlike extension fibers by creating a tunnel at the femoral and tibial ends of each fiber bundle, although the midsubstance fibers can be reconstructed by such procedures.

References

1. Benjamin M, Evans EJ, Copp L (1986) The histology of tendon attachments to bone in man. J Anat 149:89–100
2. Edwards A, Bull AMJ, Amis AA (2008) The attachments of the anteromedial and posterolateral fibre bundles of the anterior cruciate ligament. Knee Surg Sports Traumatol Arthrosc 16:29–36
3. Ferretti M, Ekdahl M, Shen W, Fu FH (2007) Osseous landmarks of the femoral attachment of the anterior cruciate ligament: an anatomic study. Arthroscopy 23:1218–1225
4. Girgis FG, Marshall JL, Monajem A (1975) The cruciate ligaments of the knee joint. Anatomical, functional and experimental analysis. Clin Orthop Relat Res 106:216–231
5. Hara K, Mochizuki T, Sekiya I, Yamaguchi K, Akita K, Muneta T (2009) Anatomy of normal human anterior cruciate ligament attachments evaluated by divided small bundles. Am J Sports Med 37:2386–2391
6. Harner CD, Baek GH, Vogrin TM, Carlin GJ, Kashiwaguchi S, Woo SLY (1999) Quantitative analysis of human cruciate ligament insertions. Arthroscopy 15:741–749
7. Iwahashi T, Shino K, Nakata K et al (2010) Direct anterior cruciate ligament insertion to the femur assessed by histology and 3-dimensional volume-rendered computed tomography. Arthroscopy 26:S13–S20
8. Mochizuki T, Muneta T, Nagase T, Shirasawa S, Akita K, Sekiya I (2006) Cadaveric knee observation study for describing anatomic femoral tunnel placement for two-bundle anterior cruciate ligament reconstruction. Arthroscopy 22:356–361
9. Odensten M, Gillquist J (1985) Functional anatomy of the anterior cruciate ligament and a rationale for reconstruction. J Bone Jt Surg Am 67:257–262
10. Otsubo H, Shino K, Suzuki D et al (2012) The arrangement and the attachment areas of three ACL bundles. Knee Surg Sports Traumatol Arthrosc 20:127–134
11. Sasaki N, Ishibashi Y, Tsuda E et al (2012) The femoral insertion of the anterior cruciate ligament: discrepancy between macroscopic and histological observations. Arthroscopy 28:1135–1146
12. Schneider H (1956) Structure of tendon attachments. Z Anat Entwicklungsgesch 119:431–456 (in German)
13. Shino K, Nakata K, Nakamura N et al (2008) Rectangular tunnel double-bundle anterior cruciate ligament reconstruction with bone-patellar tendon-bone graft to mimic natural fiber arrangement. Arthroscopy 24:1178–1183
14. Suzuki T, Shino K, Nakagawa S et al (2011) Early integration of a bone plug in the femoral tunnel in rectangular tunnel ACL reconstruction with a bone-patellar tendon-bone graft: a prospective computed tomography analysis. Knee Surg Sports Traumatol Arthrosc 19:S29–S35
15. Takahashi M, Doi M, Abe M, Suzuki D, Nagano A (2006) Anatomical study of the femoral and tibial insertions of the anteromedial and posterolateral bundles of human anterior cruciate ligament. Am J Sports Med 34:787–792
16. Yasuda K, Kondo E, Ichiyama H et al (2004) Anatomic reconstruction of the anteromedial and posterolateral bundles of the anterior cruciate ligament using hamstring tendon grafts. Arthroscopy 20:1015–1025
17. Zantop T, Wellmann M, Fu FH, Petersen W (2008) Tunnel positioning of anteromedial and posterolateral bundles in anatomic anterior cruciate ligament reconstruction. Am J Sports Med 36:65–72
18. Ziegler CG, Pietrini SD, Westerhaus BD et al (2011) Arthroscopically pertinent landmarks for tunnel positioning in single-bundle and double-bundle anterior cruciate ligament reconstructions. Am J Sports Med 39:743–752

Tibial C-Shaped Insertion of the Anterior Cruciate Ligament Without Posterolateral Bundle

3

Rainer Siebold, Peter Schuhmacher, Axel Brehmer, Francis Fernadez, Robert Śmigielski, and Joachim Kirsch

Contents

R. Siebold (✉)
Institute for Anatomy and Cell Biology,
Ruprecht-Karls University Heidelberg,
Im Neuenheimer Feld 307, 69120
Heidelberg, Germany

HKF: Center for Specialised Hip-Knee-Foot Surgery,
ATOS Hospital Heidelberg, Bismarckstr. 9-15,
69115 Heidelberg, Germany
e-mail: rainer.siebold@atos.de

P. Schuhmacher • F. Fernadez
HKF: Center for Specialised Hip-Knee-Foot Surgery,
ATOS Hospital Heidelberg, Bismarckstr. 9-15, 69115
Heidelberg, Germany

A. Brehmer
Institute for Anatomy, University of Erlangen – Nürnberg,
Krankenhausstr. 9, 91054 Erlangen, Germany

R. Śmigielski
Orthopaedic and Sports Traumatology Department,
Carolina Medical Center, Pory 78, 02-757
Warsaw, Poland

J. Kirsch
Institute for Anatomy and Cell Biology,
Ruprecht-Karls University Heidelberg,
Im Neuenheimer Feld 307, 69120
Heidelberg, Germany

Previous anatomical studies described the tibial anterior cruciate ligament (ACL) insertion to be oval shaped including the insertions of the antero-medial (AM) and posterolateral (PL) bundles. However, several anatomical and histological cadaveric studies recently reported a flat and "ribbonlike" midsubstance of the ACL with a long but flat direct femoral ACL insertion along the intercondylar ridge. Based on these interesting findings, the purpose of this anatomical cadaveric study was to investigate the macroscopic appearance of the tibial ACL insertion.

3.1   Introduction

The tibial insertion of the anterior cruciate ligament (ACL) was described by many authors in recent years. Cadaveric studies were performed to evaluate its size, shape, and location in the area intercondylaris anterior. Especially the discussion on the "double-bundle (DB) concept" and the position of the tibial anteromedial (AM) and posterolateral (PL) footprints have led to a "renaissance" in anatomical studies. Most authors described the tibial ACL insertion in the fossa of the area intercondylaris anterior to be of oval shape, with the insertion of the AM bundle in the

R. Siebold et al. (eds.), *Anterior Cruciate Ligament Reconstruction*,
DOI 10.1007/978-3-642-45349-6_3, © ESSKA 2014

anteromedial aspect of the ACL footprint and in direct relationship to the medial tibial spine and the insertion of the PL bundle in the posterolateral aspect close to the lateral tibial spine and in front of the posterior root of the lateral meniscus [7, 16, 31]. The size of the tibial ACL insertion was reported to be 136 ± 33 mm^2 with the AM footprint between 35 and 77 mm^2 and the PL footprint between 32 and 64 mm^2 [16], and the tibial attachment was described to be approximately 11 mm wide and 17 mm long in the anteroposterior direction [4, 13, 14]. The ACL "fans out" beneath the transverse meniscal ligament, and a few fascicles of the anterior aspect of the ACL may blend with the anterior attachment of the lateral meniscus as may do some posterior fibers of the ACL with the posterior attachment of the lateral meniscus [4].

According to the above descriptions, the tibial ACL insertion seemed to be well described. However, recent exciting studies reported the femoral direct insertion of the ACL to be long and flat [19, 23, 29] and the midsubstance to be of similar flat shape [22, 23]. In concordance Smigielski et al. [32] recently reconfirmed the above femoral and midsubstance findings and described the ACL to be a "ribbon," and even more exciting the tibial ACL insertion to be "C-shaped" [32] (see Chap. 4).

The purpose of this anatomical cadaveric study was to reconfirm the macroscopic appearance of the distal midsubstance shape of the ACL and its bony tibial "C-shaped" ACL insertion.

3.2   Material and Methods

Fourteen cadaveric knees ($n=6$ fresh frozen, $n=8$ paraffined) were used for this anatomical dissection study. All dissections were performed at the anatomical institutes of the Universities of Erlangen and Heidelberg (Germany) by the first author. The key point in the dissections was to very carefully remove the synovial tissue surrounding the collagen fibers of the ACL using magnifying lenses (Carl Zeiss, Jena, Germany) (Fig. 3.1a–c). Dissections, anatomical observations, and measurements were controlled by all authors. Morphometric measurements were performed using calipers as well as on digital photography. Knees with severe osteoarthritic changes (Grade III and IV according to the Outerbridge classification

[28]) were excluded from the study. Demographic data of the donors are presented in Table 3.1.

3.3   Tibial ACL Anatomy

Five millimeter from its bony tibial insertion, the appearance of the midsubstance of the ACL was flat and thin. It resembled a "ribbonlike" ligament with an average width of 12.2 mm (range 10.4–14.0 mm) and an average thickness of only 3.5 mm (range 1.8–4.8 mm) (Fig. 3.2a–c).

The flat ACL midsubstance formed a narrow C-shaped bony insertion from along the medial tibial spine to the anterior aspect of the anterior root of the lateral meniscus in the area intercondylaris anterior (Fig. 3.2a–c). There were no tibial posterolateral inserting ACL fibers.

> The posterior ACL fibers of the "C" inserted medially along the medial tibial spine and were named posteromedial fibers (PM fibers) by the authors (Fig. 3.2a–c) (see also Chaps. 5 and 29).

Fibers of the anterior and posterior horn of the lateral meniscus blended with the "C"-shaped ACL insertion (Fig. 3.2a–c). Together with the lateral meniscus, the "C"-shaped ACL insertion formed a complete "raindrop-like" ring structure (Fig. 3.2a–c). The "C"-shaped ACL insertion had an average length of 13.7 mm (range 11.5–16.1 mm) and an average width of 3.3 mm (range 2.3–3.9 mm). The most anterior part of the "C" was an average length of 8.7 mm (range 7.8–10.5 mm) in the mediolateral direction, and the medial part of the "C" along the medial tibial spine was an average length of 10.8 mm (range 7.6–14.5 mm) in the anteroposterior direction. The most posterior fibers of the "C" along the medial tibial spine were an average of 2.8 mm (range 1.8–3.8 mm) anterior to the medial intercondylar tubercle (Table 3.2).

3.4   Lateral Meniscus

The flat ACL midsubstance formed a narrow C-shaped insertion from along the medial tibial spine to the anterior aspect of the anterior root of

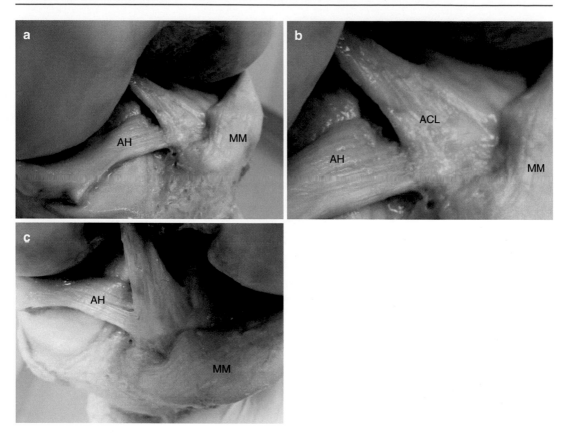

Fig. 3.1 (**a–c**) Anterior horn of the lateral meniscus inserting underneath the ACL; medial meniscus inserting right in front of the ACL; *AH* anterior horn of the lateral meniscus, *MM* anterior horn of the medial meniscus

Table 3.1 Detailed demographic data of the donors

Sex	Side	Age	Height	BMI	Weight	Origin
6 females	11 right	Mean 75 years	Mean 1.66 m	Mean 22.8	Mean 63 kg	14 Caucasians
6 males	3 left	(62–90 years)	(1.55–1.75 m)	(16.3–28.2)	(50–75 kg)	$n=14$
2 unknown	$n=14$	$n=12$	$n=10$	$n=9$	$n=9$	
$n=14$						

the lateral meniscus around a central and postero-lateral area (Fig. 3.2a–c). The outer fibers of the anterior and posterior horn of the lateral meniscus blended with the "C"-shaped ACL insertion like a belt (Fig. 3.3b, c). Together with the lateral meniscus, the "C"-shaped ACL insertion formed a complete "raindrop-like" ring structure (Fig. 3.3b, c).

There were no ACL fibers inserting in the center of the "C"-shaped insertion side and in the posterolateral aspect of the area intercondylaris anterior. There was no posterolateral tibial ACL insertion. The center of the "C" was the place of the wide bony insertion of the anterior root of the lateral meniscus (Fig. 3.3a–c).

The root of the lateral meniscus was covered by fat and overpassed by the flat ACL ligament anteriorly (Figs. 3.1a–c and 3.2b). The average AP length of the tibial ACL insertion along the medial tibial spine was 10.8 mm (range 7.6–14.5 mm) and was in the same AP level as the width of the anterior horn of the lateral meniscus.

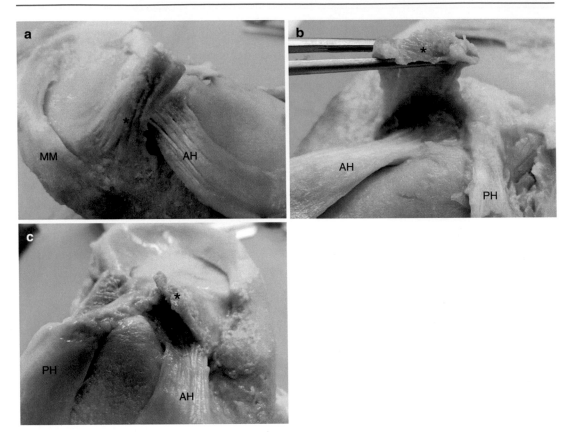

Fig. 3.2 (**a–b**) ACL removed from all surrounding soft tissue and cut off at midsubstance. In this specimen the anterior horn of the lateral meniscus did not blend into the ACL but inserted completely posterior to the anterior "C"-shaped part of the ACL insertion. (**c**) Different speci-men with anterior fibers of the lateral meniscus blend in the anterior "C"-shaped part of the ACL insertion (more common). *AH* anterior horn of the lateral meniscus, *MM* anterior horn of the medial meniscus, *PH* posterior horn of the lateral meniscus, * for ACL

Table 3.2 Measurements of the ACL dimensions at the level of the femoral insertion, midsubstance, and tibial insertion according to literature

	Author	Width (average)	Length (average)	Insertion area
Femoral	Śmigielski [32]	3.5 mm	16.0 mm	Direct female 52 mm^2; male 55 mm^2
	Mochizuki et al. [22]	4.7 mm	15.2 mm	Direct 65 mm^2
	Iriuchishima et al. [18]			Direct 60.1 mm^2
	Mochizuki et al. [23]			Direct 50.8 mm^2; indirect 91.4 mm^2; complete 142.2 mm^2
	Sasaki et al. [29]	5.0 mm	17.7 mm	Direct 88 mm^2
Midsubstance	Smigielski et al. [32]	3.4 mm	11.4 mm	Female 33 mm^2; male 38 mm^2
	Siebold et al. (pending)	3.5 mm	12.2 mm	42.7 mm^2
	Harner et al. [16]			40 mm^2
	Hashemi et al. [17]			46.8 mm^2
	Iriuchishima et al. [18]			46.9 mm^2
	Anderson et al. [3]			Female 36.1 mm^2; male 44 mm^2
Tibial	Siebold et al. (pending)	3.3 mm	13.7 mm	Direct 34.6 mm^2; indirect 78.7 mm^2; complete 113 mm^2
	Iriuchishima et al. [18]			Complete 123.5 mm^2

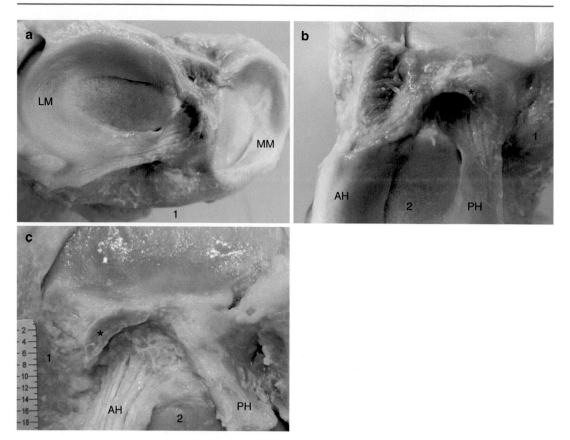

Fig. 3.3 (**a–c**) ACL cut just above the tibial insertion showing its "C"-shaped ACL insertion. The lateral meniscus formed a "raindrop-like" ring with the ACL insertion. (*1*) anterior, (*2*) lateral. *AH* anterior horn of the lateral meniscus, *MM* anterior horn of the medial meniscus, *PH* posterior horn of the lateral meniscus, * for ACL

3.5 Direct and Indirect Tibial ACL Insertion

Macroscopically the tibial insertion could be divided into a "direct" and "indirect" part. The "direct" insertion was the narrow but long C-shaped attachment of the midsubstance fibers, and the "indirect" part was the anterior and broader attachment of the "fanlike extension" fibers (Figs. 3.4 and 3.3c).

The "indirect" fibers extended from the midsubstance fibers and broadly spread underneath the transverse ligament toward the anterior rim of the tibial plateau. The average area of the direct part was 34.61 mm² (range 22.7–45.0 mm²) and the area of the indirect insertion was 78.7 mm² (range 64.5–94.5 mm²). Both insertions together formed a "duckfoot-like" bony ACL footprint with a combined area of 113.03 mm² (range 85.7–130.7 mm²).

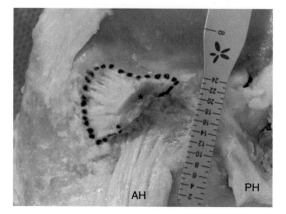

Fig. 3.4 Tibial ACL footprint with its direct "C"-shaped and "ribbonlike" insertion site and its indirect fibers which fan out anteriorly forming a "duckfoot" (*red dots*), (*) ACL

3.6 ACL Fiber Bundles

The distal flat part of the ACL midsubstance consisted of several small fiber bundles (Fig. 3.5a, b). It was impossible to macroscopically clearly

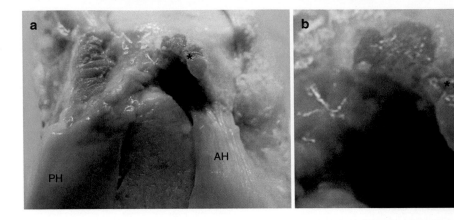

Fig. 3.5 (**a**, **b**) No separate anteromedial and posterolateral bundles could be distinguished during preparation of the ACL and its midsubstance; however, several fiber bundles were identified in most knees. *AH* anterior horn of the lateral meniscus, *PH* posterior horn of the lateral meniscus, * for ACL

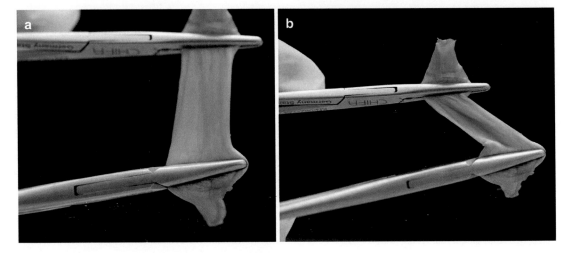

Fig. 3.6 (**a**, **b**) Tendon model of "ribbonlike" ligament: (**a**) flat, (**b**) twisted with bundle "effect"

separate them into bundles. From our observations the appearance of macroscopic "bundles" may be artificial, being created by the twisted, flat, ribbonlike structure of the ACL from femoral to tibial as well as the different alignment of both insertion sites during flexion (Fig. 3.6a, b).

3.7 Discussion

The most important finding of this study was that the distal ACL midsubstance was a flat and ribbon-shaped ligament with a "C"-shaped direct tibial ACL insertion. This direct "C"-shaped insertion ran from along the medial tibial spine to the anterior aspect of the anterior root of the lateral meniscus.

Many previous investigators divided the tibial insertion site into the footprints of the anteromedial (AM) and posterolateral (PL) bundles [9, 16, 21, 31, 33]. In contrast to these reports, we could not observe any central nor posterolateral bony insertion of the tibial ACL fibers which is the place of the bony insertion of the anterior root of the lateral meniscus. Instead of a PL bundle, there were posteromedial (PM) fibers along the medial tibial spine. In contrast to previous studies describing an "oval" midsubstance, we observed a flat and thin appearance of the ACL resembling a "ribbonlike" ligament. The average width was 12.2 mm and the average thickness was only 3.5 mm. Our findings reconfirmed reports of Smigielski et al. [32] (see Chap. 4).

We found the ACL midsubstance fibers to insert in a narrow C-shaped way from along the medial tibial spine toward the anterior aspect of the anterior root of the lateral meniscus around a central and posterolateral area. The latter was the place of the bony insertion of the anterior root of the lateral meniscus. It was covered by fat and overpassed by the flat ACL anteriorly.

As described for the femoral ACL insertion [19], the tibial insertion could macroscopically be divided into a "direct" and "indirect" part. The "direct" insertion was the 3.3 mm narrow but 13.7 mm long C-shaped attachment of the midsubstance fibers, and the "indirect" part was the anterior and broader attachment of the "fanlike" extension fibers, which extended from the midsubstance fibers and broadly spread underneath the transverse ligament toward the anterior rim of the tibial plateau. Both parts together formed a "duckfoot-like" bony footprint of the ACL, which was found by several authors in earlier dissection studies [4].

The reason for these different findings may lie in the different way of dissecting the tibial ACL insertion. The first step of our dissections was to carefully remove the synovial layer of the root of the lateral meniscus and to follow its shiny fibers down to its bony insertion in the central aspect of the area intercondylaris anterior. Then the overlaying fat was removed and the C-shaped direct insertion of the midsubstance ACL fibers was uncovered. The flat midsubstance ACL was also cleaned very carefully from the surrounding synovial and fat tissue down to its direct and indirect insertion. The cutting of the ACL was performed in knee extension after freezing the ACL with ice spray, which prevents the ACL fibers from losing its flat anatomical appearance [32].

The macroscopic anatomical separation of the ACL into bundles remains very difficult and controversial. From our dissections the distal flat part of the ACL midsubstance consisted of several small fiber bundles. However – and similar to the dissections by Śmigielski [32] – the collagen fibers could not clearly be separated into bundles. Several authors described the ACL midsubstance as a collection of individual fascicles that fan out over a broad flattened area with no histological evidence for two separate bundles [4, 8, 9, 20, 26, 34]. In contrast others differentiated between two [1, 5, 6, 10–13, 15, 16, 21, 24, 31, 35] or even three separate ACL bundles [2, 25, 27]. According to Amis and Dawkins [2], it was "sometimes difficult to separate the ACL into three discrete bundles" but "that the ACL wrinkles into the appearance of three bundles as the knee flexes." However, "in older specimens, the separate bundles were often obvious" [2]. We agree that the appearance of macroscopic "bundles" may be depending on the age of the specimen. It may also be artificially created by the twisted, flat, ribbonlike structure of the ACL from the femoral to tibial as well as the different alignment of the bony insertions during flexion [13]. Schutte et al. reported that the characteristic "twist" of the ACL begins approximately 5 mm distal to the femoral insertion [30]. When dissecting cadaveric knees, preparation is usually done in flexion increasing the amount of twisting of the ACL and the impression of bundles.

As for the femur the flat tibial ligament with its flat and long "direct" C-shaped insertion would support a flat footprint reconstruction. Sasaki et al. [29] concluded from their femoral dissections that whereas the indirect insertion plays a role as a dynamic anchorage of soft tissue to bone allowing certain shear movements, the strength of anchoring is weaker than the direct insertion. Mochizuki et al. [23] concluded that it is very difficult to reconstruct the fanlike indirect extension fibers by a bone tunnel; however, the midsubstance fibers of the ACL can be reconstructed. From our dissections we conclude that it would be ideal to reconstruct the "functional" direct insertion of the ACL (see Chap. 29). We also recommend to avoid a central or posterolateral tibial bone tunnel placement, as it is non-anatomical, may compromise biomechanics, and may damage the anterior root of the lateral meniscus. The most efficient technique for ACL reconstruction has to be proven in prospectively designed clinical long-term studies.

A weak point of this study is that all dissections were only performed by the first author. However, dissections were controlled by the whole team of investigators. Magnifying lenses were used for all dissections. Morphometric measurements were performed using calipers and on digital photography. Recent (pending) anatomical studies support the results of our macroscopic dissections.

Memory

The tibial midsubstance of the ACL was found to be a flat and ribbon-shaped ligament with a "C"-shaped "direct" tibial insertion. This "direct" "C"-shaped insertion runs from along the medial tibial spine to the anterior aspect of the anterior root of the lateral meniscus. No ACL fibers inserted in the center of the "C" nor posterolateral, which was the place of the bony attachment of the anterior root of the lateral meniscus. No PL bundle was found but posteromedial (PM) fibers. Together with its broader "indirect" ACL insertion, the "direct" insertion formed a "duckfoot-like" tibial footprint.

These new findings may change the approach to tibial ACL footprint SB and DB reconstruction and graft choice.

References

1. Adachi N, Ochi M, Uchio Y et al (2004) Reconstruction of the anterior cruciate ligament. Single- versus double-bundle multistranded hamstring tendons. J Bone Joint Surg Br 86(4):515–520
2. Amis AA, Dawkins GP (1991) Functional anatomy of the anterior cruciate ligament. Fibre bundle actions related to ligament replacements and injuries. J Bone Joint Surg Br 73(2):260–267
3. Anderson AF, Dome DC, Gautam S et al (2001) Correlation of anthropometric measurements, strength, anterior cruciate ligament size, and intercondylar notch characteristics to sex differences in anterior cruciate ligament tear rates. Am J Sports Med 29(1):58–66
4. Arnoczky SP (1983) Anatomy of the anterior cruciate ligament. Clin Orthop Relat Res 172:19–25
5. Baer GS, Ferretti M, Fu FH (2008) Anatomy of the ACL. In: Fu FH, Cohen S (eds) Current concepts in ACL reconstruction. SLACK, Thorofare, pp 21–32
6. Buoncristiani AM, Tjoumakaris FP, Starman JS et al (2006) Anatomic double-bundle anterior cruciate ligament reconstruction. Arthroscopy 22(9):1000–1006
7. Colombet P, Robinson J, Christel P et al (2006) Morphology of anterior cruciate ligament attachments for anatomic reconstruction: a cadaveric dissection and radiographic study. Arthroscopy 22(9):984–992
8. Dargel J, Pohl P, Tzikaras P et al (2006) Morphometric side-to-side differences in human cruciate ligament insertions. Surg Radiol Anat 28(4):398–402
9. Duthon VB, Barea C, Abrassart S et al (2006) Anatomy of the anterior cruciate ligament. Knee Surg Sports Traumatol Arthrosc 14(3):204–213
10. Edwards A, Bull AM, Amis AA (2007) The attachments of the anteromedial and posterolateral fibre bundles of the anterior cruciate ligament: Part 1: tibial attachment. Knee Surg Sports Traumatol Arthrosc 15(12):1414–1421
11. Ferretti M, Levicoff EA, Macpherson TA et al (2007) The fetal anterior cruciate ligament: an anatomic and histologic study. Arthroscopy 23(3):278–283
12. Fu FH, Karlsson J (2010) A long journey to be anatomic. Knee Surg Sports Traumatol Arthrosc 18(9): 1151–1153
13. Girgis FG, Marshall JL, Monajem A (1975) The cruciate ligaments of the knee joint. Anatomical, functional and experimental analysis. Clin Orthop Relat Res 106:216–231
14. Gray H, Gross CM (1973) Anatomy of the human body. Lea & Febiger, Philadelphia
15. Hamada M, Shino K, Horibe S et al (2001) Single- versus bi-socket anterior cruciate ligament reconstruction using autogenous multiple-stranded hamstring tendons with endoButton femoral fixation: a prospective study. Arthroscopy 17(8):801–807
16. Harner CD, Baek GH, Vogrin TM et al (1999) Quantitative analysis of human cruciate ligament insertions. Arthroscopy 15(7):741–749
17. Hashemi J, Mansouri H, Chandrashekar N et al (2011) Age, sex, body anthropometry, and ACL size predict the structural properties of the human anterior cruciate ligament. J Orthop Res 29(7):993–1001
18. Iriuchishima T, Yorifuji H, Aizawa S et al (2014) Evaluation of ACL mid-substance cross-sectional area for reconstructed autograft selection. Knee Surg Sports Traumatol Arthrosc 22:207–213
19. Iwahashi T, Shino K, Nakata K et al (2010) Direct anterior cruciate ligament insertion to the femur assessed by histology and 3-dimensional volume-rendered computed tomography. Arthroscopy 26(9 Suppl):S13–S20
20. Jacobsen K (1977) Osteoarthrosis following insufficiency of the cruciate ligaments in man. A clinical study. Acta Orthop Scand 48(5):520–526
21. Luites JW, Wymenga AB, Blankevoort L et al (2007) Description of the attachment geometry of the anteromedial and posterolateral bundles of the ACL from arthroscopic perspective for anatomical tunnel

placement. Knee Surg Sports Traumatol Arthrosc 15(12):1422–1431

22. Mochizuki T, Muneta T, Nagase T et al (2006) Cadaveric knee observation study for describing anatomic femoral tunnel placement for two-bundle anterior cruciate ligament reconstruction. Arthroscopy 22(4):356–361

23. Mochizuki T, Fujishiro H, Nimura A et al (2014) Anatomic and histologic analysis of the mid-substance and fan-like extension fibers of the anterior cruciate ligament during knee motion, with special reference to the femoral attachment. Knee Surg Sports Traumatol Arthrosc 22(2):336–344

24. Muneta T, Sekiya I, Yagishita K et al (1999) Two-bundle reconstruction of the anterior cruciate ligament using semitendinosus tendon with endobuttons: operative technique and preliminary results. Arthroscopy 15(6):618–624

25. Norwood LA, Cross MJ (1979) Anterior cruciate ligament: functional anatomy of its bundles in rotatory instabilities. Am J Sports Med 7(1):23–26

26. Odensten M, Gillquist J (1985) Functional anatomy of the anterior cruciate ligament and a rationale for reconstruction. J Bone Joint Surg Am 67(2):257–262

27. Otsubo H, Shino K, Suzuki D et al (2012) The arrangement and the attachment areas of three ACL bundles. Knee Surg Sports Traumatol Arthrosc 20(1):127–134

28. Outerbridge RE (2001) The etiology of chondromalacia patellae. 1961. Clin Orthop Relat Res 389:5–8

29. Sasaki N, Ishibashi Y, Tsuda E et al (2012) The femoral insertion of the anterior cruciate ligament: discrepancy between macroscopic and histological observations. Arthroscopy 28(8):1135–1146

30. Schutte MJ, Dabezies EJ, Zimny ML et al (1987) Neural anatomy of the human anterior cruciate ligament. J Bone Joint Surg Am 69(2):243–247

31. Siebold R, Ellert T, Metz S et al (2008) Tibial insertions of the anteromedial and posterolateral bundles of the anterior cruciate ligament: morphometry, arthroscopic landmarks, and orientation model for bone tunnel placement. Arthroscopy 24(2):154–161

32. Śmigielski R (2012) The ribbon concept of the anterior cruciate ligament. Presentation at ACL Study Group meeting. Jackson Hole, Wyoming

33. Starman JS, Vanbeek C, Armfield DR et al (2007) Assessment of normal ACL double bundle anatomy in standard viewing planes by magnetic resonance imaging. Knee Surg Sports Traumatol Arthrosc 15(5):493–499

34. Welsh RP (1980) Knee joint structure and function. Clin Orthop Relat Res 147:7–14

35. Yasuda K, Kondo E, Ichiyama H et al (2004) Anatomic reconstruction of the anteromedial and posterolateral bundles of the anterior cruciate ligament using hamstring tendon grafts. Arthroscopy 20(10):1015–1025

Variations of the Tibial Insertion of the Anterior Cruciate Ligament: An Anatomical Study

4

Robert Śmigielski, Urszula Zdanowicz, Michał Drwięga, Bogdan Ciszek, Christian Fink, and Rainer Siebold

Contents

R. Śmigielski, MD (✉)
Head of Orthopaedic and Sports Traumatology
Department, Carolina Medical Center,
Pory 78, Warsaw 02-757, Poland
e-mail: robert.smigielski@carolina.pl

U. Zdanowicz • M. Drwięga
Orthopaedic and Sports Traumatology
Department, Carolina Medical Center,
Pory 78, Warsaw 02-757, Poland

B. Ciszek
Department of Descriptive and Clinical Anatomy,
Medical University of Warsaw,
Chalbinskiego 5, Warsaw 02-004, Poland

C. Fink
OSM Research Foundation, Sportsclinic Austria,
Olympiastr.39, Innsbruck 6020, Austria

R. Siebold
Institute for Anatomy and Cell Biology,
Ruprecht-Karls University Heidelberg,
Im Neuenheimer Feld 307, Heidelberg 69120,
Germany

HKF: Center for Specialised Hip-Knee-Foot Surgery,
ATOS Hospital Heidelberg,
Bismarckstr. 9-15, Heidelberg 69115, Germany

An anatomical cadaveric study was performed in 111 knees to evaluate the macroscopic appearance of the tibial midsubstance of the ACL and its tibial insertion. The ACL was flat like a ribbon with a tibial insertion along the medial tibial spine to the anterior aspect of the anterior horn of the lateral meniscus. Three variations of the tibial insertion were found. The bony insertion of the anterior horn of the lateral meniscus is in the center of the tibial ACL insertion. Fibers of the anterior and posterior horn of the lateral meniscus blend with the tibial ACL insertion [1].

4.1 Materials and Methods

One-hundred and eleven fresh frozen cadaveric knees from 81 people were used in this anatomical study: 45 male (of which 17 with both knees) and 36 female (of which 13 with both knees) from the MedCure tissue bank in Portland, Oregon, USA. Knees with severe osteoarthritic changes (Grade IV according to the Outerbridge classification) were excluded from the study. The demographic data of the study subjects are displayed in Table. 4.1 (see Chap. 1).

All dissections were performed by the first author. After exposing the anterior aspect of the knee joint, the synovial tissue and Hoffa fat pad were carefully dissected and separated from the articular soft tissue structures (menisci and transverse ligament). The key point in the dissections

R. Siebold et al. (eds.), *Anterior Cruciate Ligament Reconstruction*,
DOI 10.1007/978-3-642-45349-6_4, © ESSKA 2014

Table 4.1 Detailed demographic data of the study subjects

Sex	Side	Age	Height	BMI	Weight	Races
66 females 45 males	49 right 62 left	Mean 67 year (32–74 year)	Mean 1.70 m (1.50–1.96 m)	Mean 22.6 (12.1–34.7)	Mean 64.3 kg (36–116 kg)	104 Caucasians 6 African Americans 1 Indian American

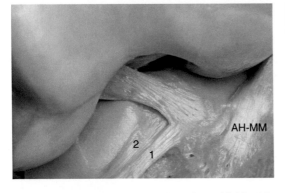

Fig. 4.1 Anterior fibers of lateral meniscus (*1*) blend in ACL, and posterior fibers of anterior horn of lateral meniscus (*2*) insert posterior to tibial ACL insertion in area intercondylaris anterior. *AH-MM* insertion of anterior horn of medial meniscus

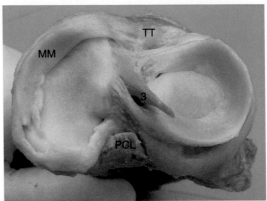

Fig 4.2 "Ribbonlike" midsubstance of ACL (*3*) and neighborhood to anterior horn (AH) and posterior horn (PH) of lateral meniscus. The ACL forms a ring structure with the lateral meniscus. *TT* tub. tibiae, *MM* medial meniscus, *PCL* posterior cruciate ligament

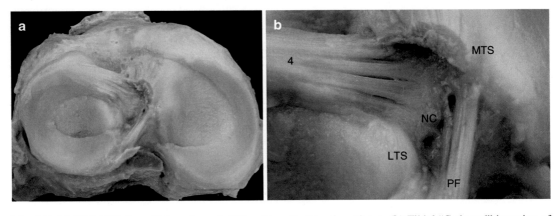

Fig. 4.3 (**a**) Tibial "C-shaped" insertion of ACL with neighborhood to lateral meniscus. The most anterior and most posterior fibers of the lateral meniscus blend with the ACL. The ACL forms a "ring structure" with the lateral meniscus. (**b**) Tibial "C-shaped" insertion of ACL. (*4*) *PF* posterior fibers of lateral meniscus, *NC* nutrition channels, *MTS* medial tibial spine, *LTS* lateral tibial spine

was the very careful and accurate removal of the synovial tissue surrounding the collagen fibers of the ACL. After achieving good visualization of the knee joint and ACL – anthropometric measurements were taken with VIS vernier calipers (VIS, Poland). Digital photographs were performed by a professional photographer using a Canon EOS 1 with a 24–70 mm lens for documentation.

4.2   Results

In all 111 dissected knees, the ACL was in the shape of a "ribbon" from midsubstance to its tibial insertion (Figs. 4.1 and 4.2). The tibial insertion was a continuation of that flat ribbon appearance in the shape of a crescent. The fibers of the ACL tibial footprint surrounded the attachment of the anterior horn of the lateral meniscus (Figs. 4.1 and 4.3a–b).

Three main types of the shape of the tibial insertion site were observed: C type (67 % of knees) (Fig. 4.4a–b), J type (24 %) (Fig. 4.4c), and Cc type (9 %) (Fig. 4.4d–h).

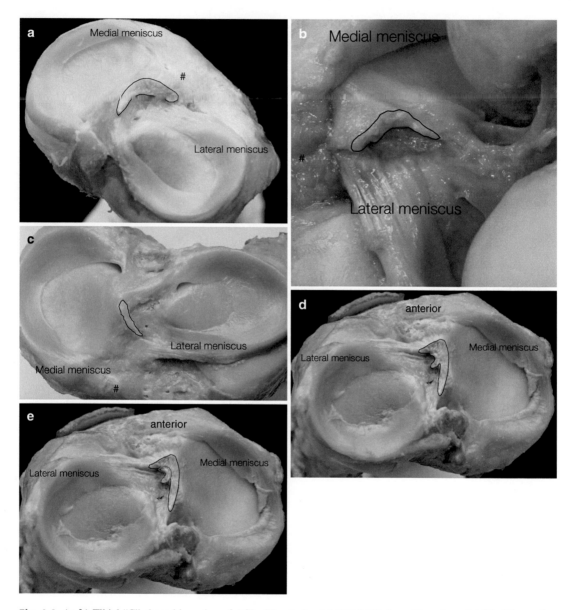

Fig. 4.4 (**a, b**) Tibial "C"-shaped insertion of ACL. (#) anterior. (**c**) Tibial "J"-shaped insertion of ACL. (#) anterior. (**d–h**) Tibial "Cc"-shaped insertion of ACL

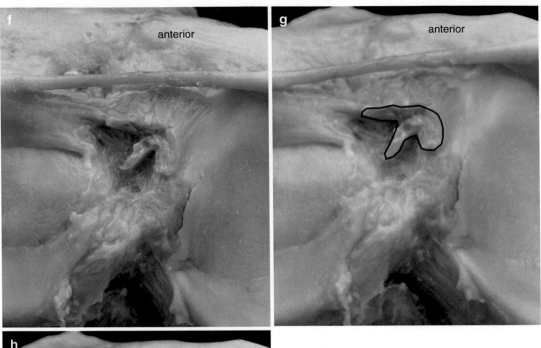

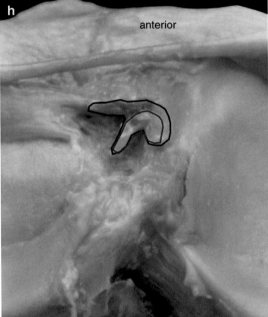

Fig. 4.4 (continued)

Reference

1. Śmigielski R (2012) The ribbon concept of the anterior cruciate ligament. ACL Study Group Meeting, Jackson Hole

Arthroscopic Appearance of the "C" –Shaped Insertion of the Anterior Cruciate Ligament

Rainer Siebold and Robert Śmigielski

Arthroscopic orientation of the tibial ACL insertion is essential for anatomical bone tunnel placement. The best individual landmark for orientation is the ACL stump itself. Other important landmarks are the anterior horn of the lateral meniscus, the transverse (intermeniscal) ligament, the medial and lateral tibial spine, and the posterior horn of the lateral meniscus. These landmarks are especially important in revision surgery when ACL remnants are lacking.

In acute ACL ruptures, the "C"-shaped tibial insertion of the ACL was carefully dissected with a small shaver. Arthroscopic pictures were taken to demonstrate the tibial ACL anatomy with associated landmarks (Figs. 5.1, 5.2, 5.3, and 5.4).

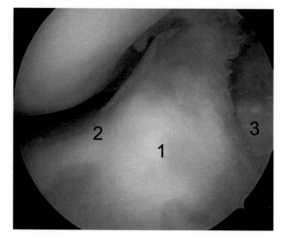

Fig. 5.1 Arthroscopic aspect of ACL in the left knee joint (*1*). Excellent landmarks are the medial tibial spine (*2*) and the anterior horn of the lateral meniscus (*3*). The anterior fibers of the ACL insertion cross the bony insertion of the lateral meniscus

R. Siebold (✉)
Institute for Anatomy and Cell Biology, Ruprecht-Karls University Heidelberg,
Im Neuenheimer Feld 307, Heidelberg, 69120, Germany

HKF: Center for Spezialised Hip-Knee-Foot Surgery, ATOS Hospital Heidelberg,
Bismarckstr. 9-15, Heidelberg, 69115, Germany
e-mail: rainer.siebold@atos.de

R. Śmigielski
Orthopaedic and Sports Traumatology Department,
Carolina Medical Center,
Pory 78, Warsaw, 02-757, Poland

R. Siebold et al. (eds.), *Anterior Cruciate Ligament Reconstruction*,
DOI 10.1007/978-3-642-45349-6_5, © ESSKA 2014

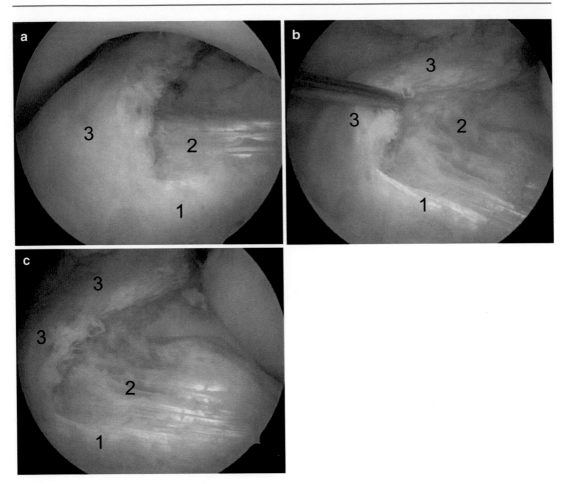

Fig. 5.2 (**a–c**) Anterior fibers (*1*) of the anterior horn of the lateral meniscus (*2*) blend into the anterior ACL insertion (*3*). The majority of the fibers of the lateral meniscus insert in the center of the tibial "C-shaped" ACL insertion in the area intercondylaris anterior in left knee joint

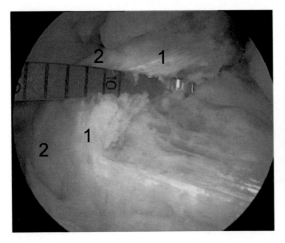

Fig. 5.3 Measurement of anteroposterior dimension of tibial ACL insertion (*1*) aligned along the medial tibial spine (*2*) in left knee joint

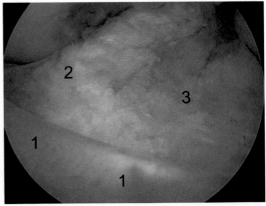

Fig. 5.4 Relationship between transverse ligament (*1*) and tibial "C"-shaped ACL insertion (*2*) as well as lateral meniscus (*3*) in left knee joint

Memory

The anterior and posterior borders of the anterior horn of the lateral meniscus are excellent landmarks for the anteroposterior length of the tibial ACL insertion. The tibial "C"-shaped ACL insertion is aligned along the medial tibial spine from the tuberculum intercondylare mediale and is curved toward the anterior border of the lateral meniscus. The anteriorly inserting ACL fibers cross over the bony insertion of the anterior root of the lateral meniscus. An anatomical "C"-shaped ACL reconstruction using hamstrings is described in Chap. 29.

Part II

Biomechanics

Biomechanics of the Knee with Intact Anterior Cruciate Ligament

6

Milos Dordevic and Michael T. Hirschmann

Contents

6.1   Introduction

The knee joint is a complex joint consisting of the medial tibiofemoral, the lateral tibiofemoral, the patellofemoral and the proximal tibiofibular joint. A number of ligaments provide passive stability in all directions to the knee joint. In our daily activities, the knee carries a large portion of our body weight, allowing a wide range of motion for flexion–extension and internal–external rotation. The cruciate ligaments have been known for almost 2,000 years and were first named by Claudius Galen of Pergamon [1].

Biomechanics, as a branch of mechanics investigating mechanical behaviour of biological materials, aims to provide a deeper understanding of the function and mechanical relationship of different anatomical structures such as the anterior cruciate ligament (ACL). Till today, a tremendous amount of biomechanical studies have been investigating the function of the ligaments of the knee. In particular, these have been given a better insight into the complex function and structure of the normal ACL, as well as reconstructed ACL [2].

With this chapter, we present an extensive review of the current knowledge of biomechanical research dealing with function of the anterior cruciate ligament. Other scientific fields have also been briefly reviewed in order to aid a comprehensive understanding of both intact and ruptured ACL. It was our purpose to present the biomechanical knowledge about the ACL in a simple and concise manner and illustrate the findings using self-explaining images.

6.2   Biomechanics of the Knee with Intact ACL

Ligaments consist of a multitude of collagenous small bundles which are impossible to count. Aiming for more simplicity most of the researchers investigating the ACL distinguish two or three bigger bundles (anteromedial, posterolateral, intermediate). One of the most important reasons for this simplification was an easier understanding of the biomechanical

M. Dordevic • M.T. Hirschmann, MD (✉)
Department of Orthopaedics and Traumatology,
Kantonsspital Baselland-Bruderholz,
Bruderholz CH-4101, Switzerland
e-mail: michael.hirschmann@unibas.ch

R. Siebold et al. (eds.), *Anterior Cruciate Ligament Reconstruction*,
DOI 10.1007/978-3-642-45349-6_6, © ESSKA 2014

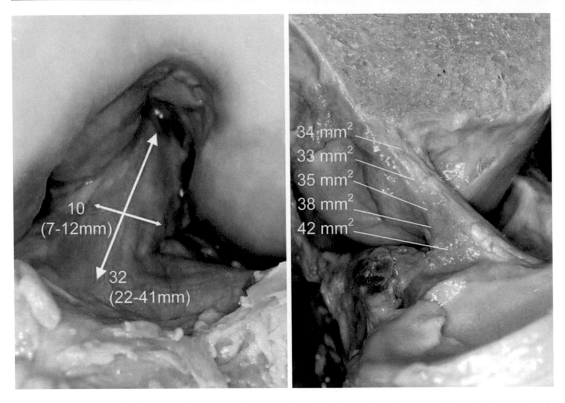

Fig. 6.1 Left knee ACL. Frontal view shows the measurements of ACL length and width (*left picture*). Cross-sectional area of the whole ACL is greatest at the tibial insertion site and smallest near the midsubstance (*right picture*) (Reprinted with permission from Duthon et al. [4])

function of the ACL. Most of the authors propose the concept of a double bundle structure of ACL, dividing the ACL in two main bundles, anteromedial (AM) bundle and posterolateral (PL) bundle, named based on the locations of their tibial insertions [1, 3–10]. These two bundles are considered to change their lengths and tension throughout the whole arc of flexion. A fact, which at least partially explains different ACL injury patterns such as partial or complete ACL tears.

To better understand the biomechanical aspects with regard to the ACL, here we briefly review the anatomy of the ACL. Although anatomical studies have shown large variance in the size of the bundles of the ACL, the average length of the AM bundle is considered to be between 28 and 38 mm; this is longer than the PL bundle, which is on average 17.8 mm long (Fig. 6.1). Both bundles have similar diameters, with a total width of 7–17 mm (average 11 mm) [6, 11, 12].

At the femoral and tibial insertion sites, the AM bundle is thicker than the PL bundle [13].

The cross-sectional shape of the ACL is considered to be "irregular" rather than circular, elliptical, or any other simple geometric form. This shape varies with the angle of flexion. The cross-sectional area increases from the femur to the tibia, being the smallest usually at midsubstance (Fig. 6.1). The femoral origin site of the ACL may be best described as semilunar, with a length and a width of 13–25 mm and 6–13 mm, respectively [7, 14, 15]. Approximated insertion sites of both AM bundle and PL bundle are shown in Fig. 6.2. Coming from the lateral femoral condyle, the ACL fibres fan out onto the tibial attachment [4]. The tibial insertion site is approximately 3.5 times larger than the diameter at its midsubstance and 120 % that of the femoral origin. It has been hypothesized that the tibial attachment is stronger than the femoral attachment [4, 6, 9, 11, 12, 16, 17].

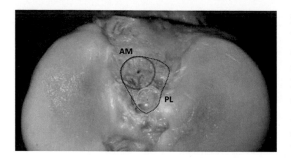

Fig. 6.2 Tibial insertion sites of AM and PL bundles (Reprinted with permission from Tsukada et al. [18])

multi-bundle structure of more than 1,000 fibres, which are individually recruited during the whole arc of motion. Some authors have reported difficulties to divide the ACL into the AM bundle and PL bundle. This fact clearly shows the problem of oversimplification. For a better understanding and technical feasibility in surgery, the orthopaedic fraternity came up with a double- or triple-bundle concept, which should be more precisely called a multi-bundle concept with regard to its biomechanical characteristics.

6.2.1 Properties of the ACL

To review the structural properties of the ACL, basic engineering terminology must be introduced here. When the ACL is subjected to tensile loading, the resulting load–elongation curve represents the structural properties of the ACL (Fig. 6.3a). The shape of this curve reflects the mechanical properties of the ACL and its bone insertion site. The most important structural properties are the linear stiffness, ultimate load, ultimate deformation, and energy absorbed at failure (area beneath the curve). The mechanical properties of the ACL can be derived from the stress–strain curve (Fig. 6.3b). Stress is defined as force per unit area (unit is MPa). Strain is defined as a ratio of the length change versus the original length (in percentage of the original length). These values can be calculated from the information in the load–elongation curve.

The resultant load–elongation curve (Fig. 6.3a) is divided into four distinct regions according to the structural properties of the ACL. The initial non-linear region (toe region) reflects the function of the collagen fibre architecture, which is able to compensate for low axial forces. This is also known as "creeping effect" of the ACL.

The toe region is followed by a quasi-linear region where collagen fibres reversibly deform. After load application, the ACL returns to its original length and no permanent plastic changes have occurred. The slope of the linear region allows for reproducible determination of ligament stiffness (N/mm) and corresponds to the

The tibial insertion begins approximately 10–14 mm posterior to the anterior border of the tibia and extends to the medial and lateral tibial spine, anterior to the spine itself. It most frequently has a triangular or ovular shape. The width ranges from 10 to 13 mm and the length 9 to 19 mm. However, these are depending on the size of the knee joint. The average insertion site of the AM bundle covers 56 % and that of the PL bundle 44 % of the entire insertion area [9].

In full extension, there is a significant difference in length between the bundles, with the AM bundle being longer than the PL bundle [4, 12]. It should be also noted that the orientation of the AM and PL bundles changes as the knee flexes. As the knee flexes, the AM bundle moves posteriorly behind the PL bundle and begins to spiral around it. Clearly, the lengths of the two bundles change with varying degrees of knee flexion, meaning that they are not isometric. The AM bundle lengthens and tightens in flexion, while the PL bundle shortens and becomes slack in flexion. In extension, the AM bundle is slack and the PL bundle tight. Thus, the AM bundle represents the main restraint against anterior translation of the tibia [1, 4, 14]. The AM and PL bundles are horizontally aligned when the knee is flexed beyond 90° [15, 19]. A physiological impingement between the AM bundle and the anterior intercondylar notch has been regularly noted. During ACL reconstruction, it is not replicated to avoid an unphysiological impingement [1, 11, 20].

However, Friederich reported in his professorial thesis that the ACL is organized in a

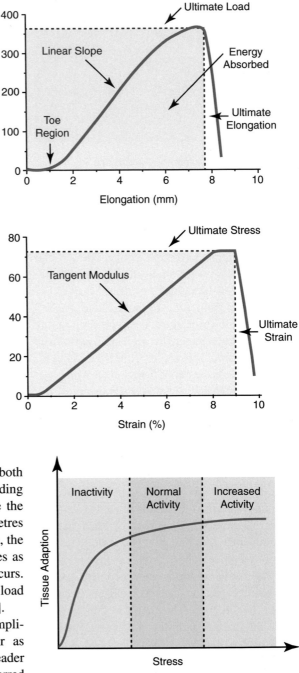

Fig. 6.3 (a) Structural properties of femur–ACL–tibia complex (FATC), showing the variables of load–elongation curve.
(b) Mechanical properties of ACL substance are calculated from its structural properties and morphological characteristics (Modified from Takeda et al. [21])

loads acting on the ACL. In the intact knee, both the toe and the linear region of the ACL loading curve represent the clinical situation where the tibia translates anteriorly for several millimetres during knee motion. With additional loading, the slope of the load–elongation curve decreases as plastic deformation of the collagen fibres occurs. Finally, the curve reaches the ultimate load (Fig. 6.3a) leading to failure of the ACL [19].

The viscoelasticity of the ACL can be simplified as quasi-linear viscoelastic behaviour as shown by Kwan et al. in 1993 [22]. The reader interested in the mathematical analysis is referred to it and similar ones explaining the viscoelasticity of ligaments in detail.

Figure 6.4 shows an approximation of the effect of immobilization on the properties of ligament. With normal activity and even strenuous exercise (to the right), the variation in properties is not very large. However, if prolonged inactivity

Fig. 6.4 Homeostatic response of ligaments to exercise and immobilization, showing a marked decrease in properties after a long-term inactivity and only a minor increase after prolonged exercise

takes place, after a period of time the properties begin to deteriorate at a fast rate.

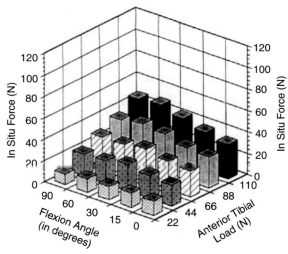
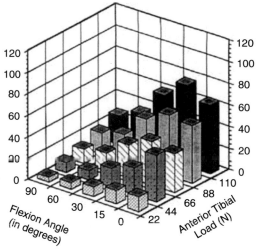

Fig. 6.5 Variation of the in situ force in the two ACL bundles. Tension in AM bundle increases as the knee flexes (*left picture*), while the PM bundle is more tensed in angles near full extension (*right picture*) (Reprinted with permission from Sakane et al. [29])

6.2.2   Function of ACL

The ACL is the primary restraint against anterior translation of the tibia in relation to the femur. This has been discovered by sectioning the ACL, as a result of which a significant increase in anteroposterior knee laxity occurred, being largest at full extension [11, 12, 19, 21, 23–26].

Contribution of the ACL to 100 N 1° of freedom (df) anterior drawer test is about 82–90 % of the total anterior restraint between 0° and 90° of knee flexion. However, when allowing unconstrained 5° of freedom knee motion, ACL restraint falls to 74–83 %, indicating that other soft-tissue structures aid to the ACL in restraining anterior tibial translation [21].

Ligament isometry has been defined as nearly equal length and tension of a ligament throughout a full range of motion. In the native ACL, there is no true isometry due to the different kinematic properties of its individual fibres and bundles and its complex geometry [1, 2, 12, 21].

Sakane et al. have shown that the in situ force in the ACL at 30° flexion is approximately equal to the magnitude of anterior-directed force applied to the tibia. Similar pattern can be observed if the knee is flexed 15° [26]. However, when the knee flexion angle is increased to more than 30°, the ACL in situ force gradually decreases (the curve becomes less steep) [27, 28]. The highest in situ forces were measured at about 15° flexion [29]. Hosseini et al. showed that even under full weight-bearing conditions, the ACL tension is highest between 15° and 30° [30].

During passive flexion and extension, the AM portion of the ACL lengthens with knee flexion, while the PL portion of the ACL shortens [1, 6, 12, 21]. The PL bundle is dominant at 20° of knee flexion [23, 31, 32].

Figure 6.5 represents the functional loading of each of the two ACL bundles over the 90° knee range of motion when various anterior tibial loads are applied. Sakane et al. highlighted that the in situ force of the PL bundle is similar to that of the ACL as a whole for all knee flexion angles. In contrast, the force distribution of the AM bundle is different, having the highest values at higher flexion angles [29].

Near extension and under anterior tibial loading, the PL bundle carries a higher load than the AM bundle. The AM bundle carries a higher load in flexion angles larger than 30° [2, 29, 33–35]. This load sharing between the two ACL bundles has led to the development of a concept named "reciprocal function of AM and PL bundles". However, this concept is only partially accepted

Fig. 6.6 The in situ forces in the AM bundle and PL bundle in response to a 134 N anterior tibial load. The PL bundle carried significantly lower in situ force than the AM bundle at all flexion angles. The AM bundle in situ force has not increased with knee flexion (Reprinted with permission from Wu et al. [37])

Fig. 6.7 Relative elongation of the anteromedial bundle (*AMB*) and posterolateral bundle (*PLB*) in response to full body weight at various knee flexion angles (Reprinted with permission from Hosseini et al. [30])

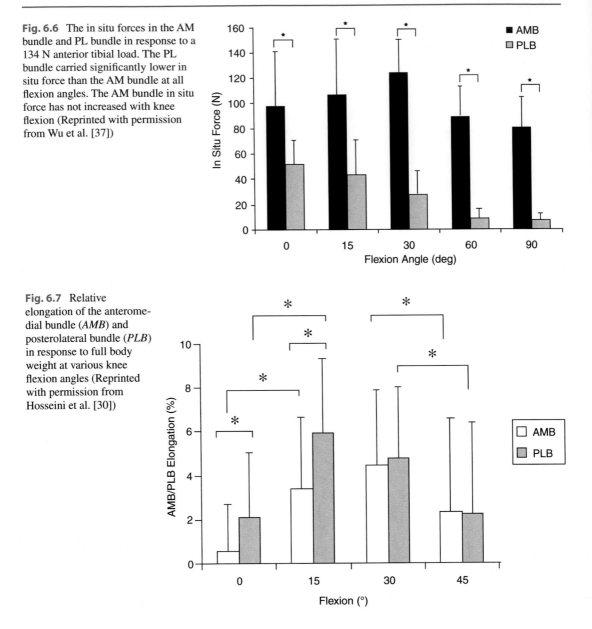

as some authors have reported a decrease in AM bundle length and strain with increased knee flexion angles which contradicts the concept of reciprocal function of the two bundles (Fig. 6.6) [25, 32, 36, 37].

During 150 N anterior tibial shear load, significant differences between the strains developed in the AM bundle of the ACL at 30° and 90° knee flexion were observed. Anterior shear testing at 30° produced more strain than testing at 90° flexion [25, 27, 32]. As a similar pattern

of behaviour was observed for the strain in the PL bundle, it has been suggested that the two bundles are rather complementary (Fig. 6.7) [30, 36].

Fleming et al. further investigated the effect of weight bearing and external loading on ACL strain [38]. In non-weight-bearing condition, the anterior shear loads as well as internal torques led to higher strains in the ACL, while external torques as well as varus–valgus moments did not.

Fig. 6.8 In situ force in the ACL and its AM and PL bundles in response to simultaneous internal tibial torque of 5 Nm and valgus torque of 10 Nm (Reprinted with permission from Gabriel et al. [34])

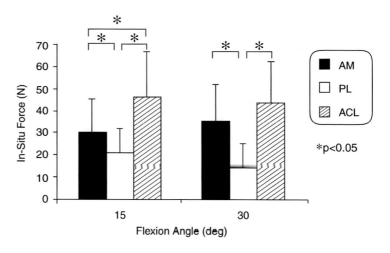

In weight-bearing condition, the ACL was also strained by external torques and varus–valgus. moments.

Keeping these differences in mind, there is no consensus on the exact pattern of force distribution in the different ACL bundles when the knee is in various degrees of flexion. Most authors agree that the PL shows highest strains at knee angles near extension (up to 30° flexion). However, it remains unclear when the AM bundle becomes strained and what the portion of the overall ACL strain it represents.

The secondary role of the ACL is to resist internal tibial rotation, which is most pronounced in knee extension [11, 21, 39–41]. The ACL lets the tibia internally rotate during anterior tibial translation [19]. This is a result of the oblique orientation of the femoral and tibial ACL attachment site, which runs from the posterolateral femoral condyle to the anteromedial tibia. In unconstrained knee compression experiments, peak forces of 5kN were observed at flexion angles of 30°, 60°, 90°, and 120°. Interestingly, during this experiment, the tibia rotated internally until the ACL ruptured. Then, the tibia started to rotate externally [38, 42, 43]. The mean peak torque value at internal torsion test was 33 Nm with tibia internally rotated by 58° and in 20° of valgus [43].

As far as the ACL bundles are concerned, the AM bundle is oriented more vertically in the intercondylar notch in the coronal plane, and it is thought to have little ability to restrain tibial internal–external rotation as it is located close to the vertical axis of rotation. In contrast, the PL bundle has a more horizontal orientation and is more distant to the axis of tibial internal–external rotation. Hence, it is able to restrain tibial rotation more than the AM bundle [23].

It is unclear if the ACL acts as a secondary restraint to varus–valgus rotation. If such a function of the ACL exists, it is considered to be very small. However, it has been reported that the ACL acts as a secondary restraint to simultaneous varus–valgus angulation and external [38] or internal tibial rotation [34] (Fig. 6.8).

It has also been found that when the knee was under combined rotatory loads of valgus and internal tibial torques, the AM and PL bundles almost evenly shared the load at 15° of knee flexion. In summary, it is common knowledge that the smaller PL bundle does play a significant role in controlling rotatory stability due to its more lateral femoral attachment site [2].

In a landmark paper, Taylor et al. used a combination of MRI, biplanar fluoroscopy, and marker-based motion capture techniques to assess the in vivo strain within the ACL during a single gait cycle [44]. The relative strain in the ACL was highest at mid-stance with the knee near full extension. The second highest values were found near the end of the swing phase prior to the heel strike.

Table 6.1 Effect of specimen age and orientation on structural properties of femur–ACL–tibia complex (mean ± standard error of the mean)

Age group	Specimen orientation	Stiffness (N/mm)	Ultimate load (N)	Energy absorbed (Nm)
Younger (22–35 years)	Anatomical	242 ± 28	2,160 ± 157	11.6 ± 1.7
	Tibial	218 ± 27	1,602 ± 167	8.2 ± 2.0
Middle aged (40–50 years)	Anatomical	220 ± 24	1,503 ± 83	6.1 ± 0.5
	Tibial	192 ± 17	1,160 ± 104	4.3 ± 0.5
Older (60–97 years)	Anatomical	180 ± 25	658 ± 129	1.8 ± 0.5
	Tibial	124 ± 16	495 ± 85	1.4 ± 0.3

Modified from Woo et al. [28]

6.2.3 Ultimate Load to Failure of ACL

Profound knowledge about the ultimate strength and load to failure is important for both designing prevention programmes for ACL injury and decision making for ACL reconstructive surgery. There is a considerable body of literature, mainly cadaveric studies, published regarding testing of the ultimate load to failure of the ACL. Striving for as realistic testing conditions as possible, various knee flexion angles, different directions of force application, as well as different strain rates have been investigated.

Typical types of failure are ligamentous midsubstance tear, cleavage at one of the zones of ligament–bone insertion, and an avulsion fracture. An avulsion most commonly occurs at the cancellous bone directly beneath the more dense cortical bone at the ACL insertion site [45].

Woo et al. [28] investigated the load to failure of ACLs in cadaveric knees from three age groups, younger (22–35 years), middle aged (40–50 years), and older (60–97 years). The experiment was performed at knee flexion angles of 30°. One knee of each donor pair was randomly assigned to be tested in line with the anatomical orientation (along the axis of the ACL) and tibial orientation (along the tibial axis), respectively (Table 6.1). In the 22–35-year-old group, the stiffness, ultimate load, and energy absorbed at failure were 242 ± 28 N/mm, 2.160 ± 157 N, and 11.6 ± 1.7 Nm, respectively, for the anatomical orientation. The corresponding values for tibial orientation were significantly lower (218 ± 27 N/mm, 1.602 ± 167 N, and 8.3 ± 2.0 Nm). This effect of specimen orientation on ultimate failure load was also found in the other two age groups.

It could be speculated if the increased ACL fibre recruitment while testing in anatomical orientation leads to higher ultimate load to failure.

The values given in the table can be used as a measure of the structural properties of ACL.

Noyes et al. [46] highlighted that ACLs from younger humans failed at an ultimate load to failure, which is on average 2.4 times higher than in older humans. The knees were tested in 45° of flexion at velocity of 1 ligament length per second. In this study, mechanical properties were also reported. The mean elastic modulus of the ACL from younger adult humans was 1.7-fold than that of older humans. The maximum stress and strain to failure in the ACL from younger humans were 2.8 and 3.3 times the respective values of the older group.

In addition, there was a significant difference in failure mode and site of failure in these ACLs. The ACLs from younger humans failed predominantly as midsubstance tear, whereas older humans also showed bony avulsions [46, 47]. The latter do not represent failure of the ligament per se. When older (40–60 years) ACLs failed midsubstance, they did not show lower ultimate load to failure than younger ones.

Furthermore, it has been found in ACL experiments on rhesus monkeys that elongation of the ACL is similar at the slow and fast rate of deformation. However, the ACL failed at fast rate at a higher load and at increased strain, and absorbs more energy, prior to failure. At slow deformation rate, the tibial bony insertion area was the weakest link, whereas at fast deformation rate, which more closely approximates physiological loading conditions, an increased frequency of ligamentous failure was observed [45].

References

1. Petersen W, Zantop T (2007) Anatomy of the anterior cruciate ligament with regard to its two bundles. Clin Orthop Relat Res 454:35–47
2. Woo SL et al (2006) Biomechanics and anterior cruciate ligament reconstruction. J Orthop Surg Res 1:2
3. Cimino F, Volk BS, Setter D (2010) Anterior cruciate ligament injury: diagnosis, management, and prevention. Am Fam Physician 82(8):917–922
4. Duthon VB et al (2006) Anatomy of the anterior cruciate ligament. Knee Surg Sports Traumatol Arthrosc 14(3):204–213
5. Ferretti M et al (2007) The fetal anterior cruciate ligament: an anatomic and histologic study. Arthroscopy 23(3):278–283
6. Giuliani JR, Kilcoyne KG, Rue JP (2009) Anterior cruciate ligament anatomy: a review of the anteromedial and posterolateral bundles. J Knee Surg 22(2):148–154
7. Steckel H et al (2007) Anatomy of the anterior cruciate ligament double bundle structure: a macroscopic evaluation. Scand J Med Sci Sports 17(4):387–392
8. Tena-Arregui J et al (2003) Arthroscopic study of the knee joint in fetuses. Arthroscopy 19(8):862–868
9. Siebold R et al (2008) Tibial insertions of the anteromedial and posterolateral bundles of the anterior cruciate ligament: morphometry, arthroscopic landmarks, and orientation model for bone tunnel placement. Arthroscopy 24(2):154–161
10. Siebold R, Fu FH (2008) Assessment and augmentation of symptomatic anteromedial or posterolateral bundle tears of the anterior cruciate ligament. Arthroscopy 24(11):1289–1298
11. Bicer EK et al (2010) Current knowledge in the anatomy of the human anterior cruciate ligament. Knee Surg Sports Traumatol Arthrosc 18(8):1075–1084
12. Zantop T et al (2006) Anterior cruciate ligament anatomy and function relating to anatomical reconstruction. Knee Surg Sports Traumatol Arthrosc 14(10):982–992
13. Katouda M et al (2011) Relationship between thickness of the anteromedial bundle and thickness of the posterolateral bundle in the normal ACL. Knee Surg Sports Traumatol Arthrosc 19(8):1293–1298
14. Giron F et al (2006) Femoral attachment of the anterior cruciate ligament. Knee Surg Sports Traumatol Arthrosc 14(3):250–256
15. Steckel H et al (2009) Arthroscopic evaluation of the ACL double bundle structure. Knee Surg Sports Traumatol Arthrosc 17(7):782–785
16. Dargel J et al (2006) Morphometric side-to-side differences in human cruciate ligament insertions. Surg Radiol Anat 28(4):398–402
17. Zantop T, Petersen W, Fu FH (2005) Anatomy of the anterior cruciate ligament. Oper Tech Orthop 15(1):20–28
18. Tsukada H et al (2008) Anatomical analysis of the anterior cruciate ligament femoral and tibial footprints. J Orthop Sci 13(2):122–129
19. Dargel J et al (2007) Biomechanics of the anterior cruciate ligament and implications for surgical reconstruction. Strategies Trauma Limb Reconstr 2(1):1–12
20. Tallay A, Lim MH, Bartlett J (2008) Anatomical study of the human anterior cruciate ligament stump's tibial insertion footprint. Knee Surg Sports Traumatol Arthrosc 16(8):741–746
21. Takeda Y et al (1994) Biomechanical function of the human anterior cruciate ligament. Arthroscopy 10(2):140–147
22. Kwan MK, Lin TH, Woo SL (1993) On the viscoelastic properties of the anteromedial bundle of the anterior cruciate ligament. J Biomech 26(4–5):447–452
23. Amis AA (2012) The functions of the fibre bundles of the anterior cruciate ligament in anterior drawer, rotational laxity and the pivot shift. Knee Surg Sports Traumatol Arthrosc 20(4):613–620
24. Christel PS et al (2012) The contribution of each anterior cruciate ligament bundle to the Lachman test: a cadaver investigation. J Bone Joint Surg Br 94(1):68–74
25. Fleming BC et al (1993) An in vivo comparison of anterior tibial translation and strain in the anteromedial band of the anterior cruciate ligament. J Biomech 26(1):51–58
26. Sakane M et al (1999) Relative contribution of the ACL, MCL, and bony contact to the anterior stability of the knee. Knee Surg Sports Traumatol Arthrosc 7(2):93–97
27. Livesay GA et al (1995) Determination of the in situ forces and force distribution within the human anterior cruciate ligament. Ann Biomed Eng 23(4):467–474
28. Woo SL et al (1991) Tensile properties of the human femur-anterior cruciate ligament-tibia complex. The effects of specimen age and orientation. Am J Sports Med 19(3):217–225
29. Sakane M et al (1997) In situ forces in the anterior cruciate ligament and its bundles in response to anterior tibial loads. J Orthop Res 15(2):285–293
30. Hosseini A, Gill TJ, Li G (2009) In vivo anterior cruciate ligament elongation in response to axial tibial loads. J Orthop Sci 14(3):298–306
31. Amis AA, Dawkins GP (1991) Functional anatomy of the anterior cruciate ligament. Fibre bundle actions related to ligament replacements and injuries. J Bone Joint Surg Br 73(2):260–267
32. Beynnon B et al (1992) The measurement of anterior cruciate ligament strain in vivo. Int Orthop 16(1):1–12
33. Akgun I et al (2009) Evaluation of the functional effects of anterior cruciate ligament bundles: a cadaveric experiment. J Knee Surg 22(4):317–324
34. Gabriel MT et al (2004) Distribution of in situ forces in the anterior cruciate ligament in response to rotatory loads. J Orthop Res 22(1):85–89
35. Markolf KL et al (2008) Contributions of the posterolateral bundle of the anterior cruciate ligament to anterior-posterior knee laxity and ligament forces. Arthroscopy 24(7):805–809
36. Jordan SS et al (2007) The in vivo kinematics of the anteromedial and posterolateral bundles of the anterior cruciate ligament during weightbearing knee flexion. Am J Sports Med 35(4):547–554

37. Wu JL et al (2010) In situ forces in the anteromedial and posterolateral bundles of the anterior cruciate ligament under simulated functional loading conditions. Am J Sports Med 38(3):558–563

38. Fleming BC et al (2001) The effect of weightbearing and external loading on anterior cruciate ligament strain. J Biomech 34(2):163–170

39. Andersen HN, Dyhre-Poulsen P (1997) The anterior cruciate ligament does play a role in controlling axial rotation in the knee. Knee Surg Sports Traumatol Arthrosc 5(3):145–149

40. Monaco E et al (2010) Navigated knee kinematics after tear of the ACL and its secondary restraints: preliminary results. Orthopedics 33(10 Suppl):87–93

41. Oh YK et al (2012) What strains the anterior cruciate ligament during a pivot landing? Am J Sports Med 40(3):574–583

42. Meyer EG, Haut RC (2005) Excessive compression of the human tibio-femoral joint causes ACL rupture. J Biomech 38(11):2311–2316

43. Meyer EG, Haut RC (2008) Anterior cruciate ligament injury induced by internal tibial torsion or tibio-femoral compression. J Biomech 41(16):3377–3383

44. Taylor KA et al (2013) In vivo measurement of ACL length and relative strain during walking. J Biomech 46(3):478–483

45. Noyes FR, DeLucas JL, Torvik PJ (1974) Biomechanics of anterior cruciate ligament failure: an analysis of strain-rate sensitivity and mechanisms of failure in primates. J Bone Joint Surg Am 56(2):236–253

46. Noyes FR, Grood ES (1976) The strength of the anterior cruciate ligament in humans and Rhesus monkeys. J Bone Joint Surg Am 58(8):1074–1082

47. Jones RS et al (1995) Mechanical properties of the human anterior cruciate ligament. Clin Biomech (Bristol, Avon) 10(7):339–344

Injury Mechanisms of ACL Tear

7

Milos Dordevic and Michael T. Hirschmann

Contents

More than 200,000 new ACL injuries occur in the United States each year, from either direct or indirect forces on the knee, making it overall one of the most common knee injuries worldwide [1, 2]. More than three quarters of ACL injuries have been reported to occur in noncontact situations (no direct contact to the knee when knee is injured), mostly while performing sports. In team sports 50–80 % of ACL injuries occur in noncontact situations [3–6]. Noncontact injury means that there is no contact of the knee with any object in the moment of injury [1, 3, 7]. Typically, an ACL injury occurs when the foot strikes the ground with the knee close to full extension while landing manoeuvres, sudden deceleration or lateral cutting manoeuvres [8]. The likely loading conditions for a noncontact injury are an anterior tibial shear force, knee abduction and tibial internal rotation moments. In a cadaveric study Levine et al. did not find a relationship between ACL disruption pattern (partial versus complete ACL tear, femoral insertion versus midsubstance versus tibial inser-

tion) and different loading situations in simulated landings from a jump [9] (Fig. 7.1).

Hewitt et al. identified four sites of biomechanical deficits influencing ACL injury pattern and named it as ligament dominance, quadriceps dominance, leg dominance and trunk dominance [10]. Their aim is to implement specific prevention programmes for each type of neuromuscular disbalance.

It has been highlighted that the primary function of the ACL is to prevent anterior translation of the tibia, accounting for about 80 % of all resistance to anterior tibial translation [11, 12]. Quadriceps muscles have the ability to pull the tibia anteriorly, causing thereby increased tension in the ACL [13]. When simulating an aggressive quadriceps load (e.g. 4,500 N for 1 s) on cadaveric knees at 20° of flexion, the tibia displaces anteriorly by on average 19.5 mm. It also rotates the tibia internally by approximately 5.5°. Hence, aggressive quadriceps loading might be a key player in a noncontact ACL injury [1]. Generally, the ACL is loaded from full extension to 80° of flexion during maximum, isolated contraction of the quadriceps muscle. In contrast, isolated contractions of the hamstrings and gastrocnemius muscles protect the ACL for almost the entire range of knee flexion until full extension (<10°) [14, 15]. Considering that the ACL load increases with knee extension, it can be at least partly explained why noncontact ACL injuries occur primarily during deceleration of the lower extremity, with the quadriceps maximally contracted and the knee at or near full extension [3, 11].

M. Dordevic • M.T. Hirschmann, MD (✉)
Department of Orthopaedics and Traumatology,
Kantonsspital Baselland-Bruderholz,
Bruderholz CH-4101, Switzerland
e-mail: michael.hirschmann@unibas.ch

R. Siebold et al. (eds.), *Anterior Cruciate Ligament Reconstruction*,
DOI 10.1007/978-3-642-45349-6_7, © ESSKA 2014

In the sense of the aforementioned findings, a landing position, which is prone for ACL injury, can be identified (Fig. 7.2). In combination with a 2–18-fold body weight, landing on the rear foot could easily lead to an ACL tear. For instance, if a person's body weight is 800 N and during land-ing the impact force is 10 G, then 8,000 N of vertical ground reaction force can cause the quadriceps tangential component of force to pull the tibia with more than 2,160 N (reported as average ACL rupture load) and thereby cause the injury. In a safer position, with the femur and the tibia more vertically oriented during landing on a forefoot, this is not likely to occur.

Clearly ACL injury is more likely to occur even in knee flexion angles greater than those near full extension when there is a disbalance of ham-string to quadriceps strength. However, in reality there is no standardized loading condition. It is mostly a combined anterior tibial loading and rotational torque. Due to the additional internal tibial torque, the loading of the ACL at full exten-sion and hyperextension is dramatically increased. An additional varus moment increases the force in extension and hyperextension, whereas an addi-tional valgus moment increases the force at flexed positions. An additional external tibial rotation moment decreases ACL loading in higher knee flexion angles [16, 17]. The combination of val-gus and internal rotation moments that occur in vivo during landing can cause ACL strains high enough to cause ACL injury [18]. Other mecha-nisms that have been reported to lead to ACL injury include lateral trunk displacement with

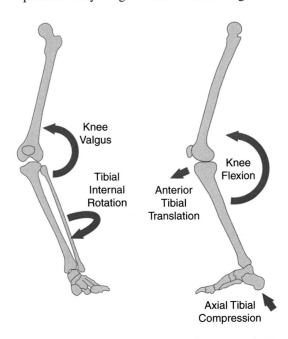

Fig. 7.1 Multidirectional loading which leads to ACL injury

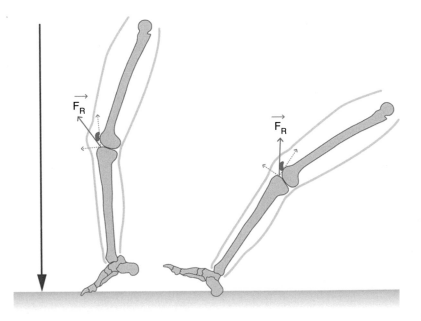

Fig. 7.2 Safe (*left*) and dangerous (*right*) landing manoeuvre

Table 7.1 Sports participation of male and female athletes in Japan who have suffered from ACL injury

Males			Females		
Sports	n	Rate (%)	Sports	n	Rate (%)
Soccer	154	18.3	Basketball	333	37.8
Ski	118	14.1	Ski	134	15.2
Basketball	113	13.5	Handball	106	12.0
Rugby	109	13.0	Volleyball	81	9.2
Handball	57	6.8	Track and field	27	3.1
Baseball	50	6.0	Judo	26	3.0
Judo	47	5.6	Gymnastics	21	2.4
Amer. football	30	3.6	Badminton	20	2.3
Volleyball	17	2.0	Softball	19	2.2
Sumo	16	1.9	Tennis	14	1.6

Modified Kobayashi et al. [22]

increased knee abduction moments and tibial rotation as well as uncoordinated contraction of the quadriceps muscle as in landing or twisting while off balance [5, 19, 20].

7.1 Partial Tears

Generally partial tears occur due to almost the same injury mechanisms as those resulting in complete ACL tears. The most important differences lie in the direction and magnitude of the injury force, affecting thereby only a portion of the ACL rather than the whole. Partial AM bundle tears are thought to be caused by a high velocity trauma to the knee. The direction of the force is predominantly in the anterior direction. In contrast, partial PL bundle tears are more commonly due to a low velocity and less energetic pivoting injury with a predominantly rotational component. A partial tear of one of those ACL bundles was observed in up to 25 % of cases [21].

7.2 Specific Sport Activities

Compared with running, there is a significant increase in ACL load during sidestepping, pivoting and cutting manoeuvres. This is the result of a large increase in varus/valgus and internal/external rotation movements, which have been considered to be the reason for ACL injuries [2]. Kobayashi et al. investigated the type of sports 1,718 Japanese athletes participated in when getting injured (Table 7.1).

Most commonly ACL injuries occur while playing football, skiing or doing gymnastics [2]. In particular, football players put great demands on their knees. Sudden change of direction, hard cutting as well as pivoting put the player's knees at great risk for an ACL injury [23].

Typical noncontact injury mechanisms in football are the following: change of direction, cutting manoeuvres combined with deceleration, landing from a jump with the knee at full extension, pivoting with knee near full extension and a planted foot [24]. Knee hyperextension and hyperflexion are additional injury mechanisms [6, 24].

In alpine skiing 50 % of knee injuries are ACL tears. A number of different noncontact injuries occur. One mechanism is that the knee gets hyperextended and internally rotated during a forward fall. Typically this happens when the tip of the skis cross or the outer edge of the ski gets caught in the snow [25]. Another mechanism is when the ski gets caught with the inner edge in the snow. Then a flexion-valgus-external rotation force acts on the knee. The third mechanism is the so-called phantom foot phenomenon [16]. Here, the ACL injury occurs while high-speed downhill skiing during backward fall in the landing phase following a jump [26]. Ruedl et al. emphasized that since the introduction of carving skiing, the forward twisting fall caused by catching an edge was the most common ACL injury mechanism [27].

The rare ACL injuries in snowboarders are considered to be quadriceps induced due to maximum eccentric quadriceps contraction [28]. Typically ACL injuries occur during a flat landing from a jump on a flexed knee with significant compression.

Typical injury situations in handball and basketball are a "plant-and-cut" faking movement (to change direction and pass by an opponent) or landing on one leg after a jump shot.

Professional dancers sustain ACL injuries when landing from a jump with the hip and foot turned outwards leading to a valgus stress on the knee joint [29]. ACL injuries in badminton are related to (a) single-leg landing after overhead striking and (b) plant-and-cut while sidestepping or backward stepping [30]. Wilson et al. reported an unusual mechanism of ACL injury in figure skating. It occurred during the execution of a Biellmann spin in the overhead non-weight-bearing knee [31].

References

1. DeMorat G et al (2004) Aggressive quadriceps loading can induce noncontact anterior cruciate ligament injury. Am J Sports Med 32(2):477–483
2. Siegel L, Vandenakker-Albanese C, Siegel D (2012) Anterior cruciate ligament injuries: anatomy, physiology, biomechanics, and management. Clin J Sport Med 22(4):349–355
3. Cimino F, Volk BS, Setter D (2010) Anterior cruciate ligament injury: diagnosis, management, and prevention. Am Fam Physician 82(8):917–922
4. Ali N, Rouhi G (2010) Barriers to predicting the mechanisms and risk factors of non-contact anterior cruciate ligament injury. Open Biomed Eng J 4:178–89
5. Georgoulis AD et al (2010) ACL injury and reconstruction: clinical related in vivo biomechanics. Orthop Traumatol Surg Res 96(8 Suppl):S119–S128
6. Rochcongar P et al (2009) Ruptures of the anterior cruciate ligament in soccer. Int J Sports Med 30(5):372–378
7. Boden BP et al (2010) Noncontact anterior cruciate ligament injuries: mechanisms and risk factors. J Am Acad Orthop Surg 18(9):520–527
8. Hughes G, Watkins J (2006) A risk-factor model for anterior cruciate ligament injury. Sports Med 36(5):411–428
9. Levine JW et al (2013) Clinically relevant injury patterns after an anterior cruciate ligament injury provide insight into injury mechanisms. Am J Sports Med 41(2):385–395
10. Hewett TE et al (2010) Understanding and preventing acl injuries: current biomechanical and epidemiologic considerations – update 2010. N Am J Sports Phys Ther 5(4):234–251
11. Dargel J et al (2007) Biomechanics of the anterior cruciate ligament and implications for surgical reconstruction. Strategies Trauma Limb Reconstr 2(1):1–12
12. Karmani S, Ember T (2003) The anterior cruciate ligament—1. Curr Orthop 17(5):369–377
13. Takeda Y et al (1994) Biomechanical function of the human anterior cruciate ligament. Arthroscopy 10(2):140–147
14. Imran A, O'Connor JJ (1998) Control of knee stability after ACL injury or repair: interaction between hamstrings contraction and tibial translation. Clin Biomech (Bristol, Avon) 13(3):153–162
15. Shelburne KB, Pandy MG (1997) A musculoskeletal model of the knee for evaluating ligament forces during isometric contractions. J Biomech 30(2):163–176
16. Krosshaug T et al (2007) Biomechanical analysis of anterior cruciate ligament injury mechanisms: three-dimensional motion reconstruction from video sequences. Scand J Med Sci Sports 17(5):508–519
17. Markolf KL et al (1995) Combined knee loading states that generate high anterior cruciate ligament forces. J Orthop Res 13(6):930–935
18. Shin CS, Chaudhari AM, Andriacchi TP (2011) Valgus plus internal rotation moments increase anterior cruciate ligament strain more than either alone. Med Sci Sports Exerc 43(8):1484–1491
19. Jones RS et al (1995) Mechanical properties of the human anterior cruciate ligament. Clin Biomech (Bristol, Avon) 10(7):339–344
20. Pappas E et al (2012) Lessons learned from the last 20 years of ACL-related in vivo-biomechanics research of the knee joint. Knee Surg Sports Traumatol Arthrosc 21(4):755–766
21. Siebold R, Fu FH (2008) Assessment and augmentation of symptomatic anteromedial or posterolateral bundle tears of the anterior cruciate ligament. Arthroscopy 24(11):1289–1298
22. Kobayashi H et al (2010) Mechanisms of the anterior cruciate ligament injury in sports activities: a twenty-year clinical research of 1,700 athletes. J Sports Sci Med 9(4):6
23. Delfico AJ, Garrett WE Jr (1998) Mechanisms of injury of the anterior cruciate ligament in soccer players. Clin Sports Med 17(4):779–785, vii
24. Alentorn-Geli E et al (2009) Prevention of non-contact anterior cruciate ligament injuries in soccer players. Part 1: mechanisms of injury and underlying risk factors. Knee Surg Sports Traumatol Arthrosc 17(7):705–729
25. Ruedl G et al (2011) ACL injury mechanisms and related factors in male and female carving skiers: a retrospective study. Int J Sports Med 32(10):801–806
26. Gerritsen KG, Nachbauer W, van den Bogert AJ (1996) Computer simulation of landing movement in downhill skiing: anterior cruciate ligament injuries. J Biomech 29(7):845–854
27. Ruedl G et al (2009) Distribution of injury mechanisms and related factors in ACL-injured female carving skiers. Knee Surg Sports Traumatol Arthrosc 17(11):1393–1398

28. Davies H et al (2009) Anterior cruciate ligament injuries in snowboarders: a quadriceps-induced injury. Knee Surg Sports Traumatol Arthrosc 17(9): 1048–1051

29. Meuffels DE, Verhaar JA (2008) Anterior cruciate ligament injury in professional dancers. Acta Orthop 79(4):515–518

30. Kimura Y et al (2010) Mechanisms for anterior cruciate ligament injuries in badminton. Br J Sports Med 44(15):1124–1127

31. Wilson EK, Lahurd AP, Wilckens JH (2012) An unusual mechanism for injury of the anterior cruciate ligament in figure skating. Clin J Sport Med 22(2): 160–162

Biomechanics of the Knee After Complete and Partial ACL Tear

8

Milos Dordevic and Michael T. Hirschmann

Contents

Disruption of the ACL inevitably results in alterations of knee kinematics as a transfer of loads can be effective only if the joint is mechanically stable [1].

Complete ACL tears involving the entire ACL can be differentiated from partial ACL tears, which only involve the AM or PL bundle [2]. Partial ACL tear frequency ranges from 5 to 28 % of isolated ACL tears. Compared to healthy subjects, the ACL-deficient subjects usually exhibit decreased gait variability. The decreased gait variability indicates that a patient with ACL tear is more "careful" in the way he or she walks in order to eliminate any extra movements, exhibiting thereby increased rigidity in movement patterns [3]. Gait analysis performed by Waite et al. found that an ACL-deficient knee is in greater extension during the stance phase of running activities than ACL-intact knees. This finding is in agreement with Roberts et al. pointing out that there is no quadriceps avoidance gait in ACL-deficient knees.

M. Dordevic • M.T. Hirschmann, MD (✉)
Department of Orthopaedics and Traumatology,
Kantonsspital Baselland-Bruderholz,
Bruderholz CH-4101, Switzerland
e-mail: michael.hirschmann@unibas.ch

8.1 Complete ACL Tears

The biomechanical function of ACL remnants in anterior-posterior and rotational stability in patients with a complete ACL injury was investigated using intraoperative navigation-based arthrometry [4]. Arthrometry was performed intraoperatively before and after resection of the ACL remnants. They found that at 30° knee flexion, ACL remnants contributed to anterior-posterior stability till 1 year after ACL injury, but not to rotational stability.

In patients with a complete ACL tear, an anterior tibial loading (134 N) leads to an increase in MCL strain by 120–177 % at 30°–90° of knee flexion. There is also an increase in strain in the posterolateral structures of the knee by 123 % at full knee extension and 413 % at 15° of knee flexion [5].

Biomechanical studies have shown that ACL-deficient knees remain in higher flexion angles during most of the stance phase compared to the normal knees (Fig. 8.1) [6, 7].

The ACL-deficient knees also show significant differences in anterior tibial translation during the late stance phase of the gait cycle (Fig. 8.2). A significantly increased external rotation of the tibia has also been associated with ACL-deficient knees [8, 9].

Restraining tibial anterior displacement relative to the femur may be the most important function of the ACL. A loss of the ACL eliminates such restraint, and the posterior pulling generated by the hamstrings and other tissues cannot fully compensate for this. This observation is

R. Siebold et al. (eds.), *Anterior Cruciate Ligament Reconstruction*,
DOI 10.1007/978-3-642-45349-6_8, © ESSKA 2014

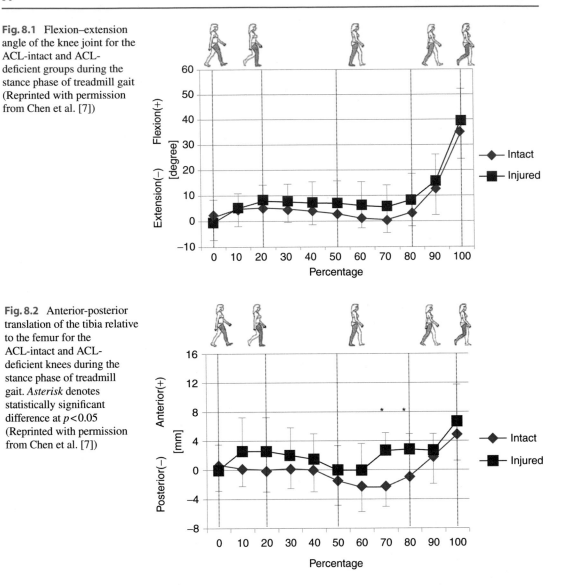

Fig. 8.1 Flexion–extension angle of the knee joint for the ACL-intact and ACL-deficient groups during the stance phase of treadmill gait (Reprinted with permission from Chen et al. [7])

Fig. 8.2 Anterior-posterior translation of the tibia relative to the femur for the ACL-intact and ACL-deficient knees during the stance phase of treadmill gait. *Asterisk* denotes statistically significant difference at $p < 0.05$ (Reprinted with permission from Chen et al. [7])

supported by a greater hamstring EMG activity in the injured knee compared to the hamstring activity of the healthy knee [6, 7, 9–11]. Anterior tibial translation was found to be greater for ACL-deficient knee during squatting over the entire flexion arc as compared to healthy knee. Also greater anterior tibial translation in ACL-deficient knees was found during pivoting tasks [12].

Results of leg press experiments indicated a significantly larger anterior tibial translation for the ACL-deficient knee than the normal knee at 30° knee flexion, but not at 45° [13]. This reflects the fact that at 45° the quadriceps muscles are not able to pull on the tibia as strongly as at 30° and the hamstrings are then able to compensate the anterior-directed quadriceps force.

While in the ACL-intact knees the step-up (closed chain exercise) causes more anterior tibial translation than the active extension (open chain), in the ACL-deficient knee it is similar during both activities. Kozanek et al. further reported that during step-up exercise, patients with ACL-deficient knees showed increases in anterior tibial translation, medial tibial translation and external tibial rotation [14]. However, the difference here was only significant in the terminal stance phase.

In gait analysis the ACL-deficient knee is significantly more flexed than the ACL-intact one when ascending stairs. Greater knee flexion occurs also before foot strike during stair descent, thereby constantly avoiding positions of the knee near full extension [15].

Shefelbine et al. analysed the meniscal and tibiofemoral kinematics in normal and ACL-deficient patients under axial loading conditions using MRI [16]. MR images were obtained at full extension and partial flexion (45°) with a 125 N compressive load applied to the foot. The authors showed that an ACL injury lead to a significant change in tibiofemoral kinematics, but no change in meniscal kinematics.

8.2 Partial ACL Tears

Approximately 40–50 % of patients with a partial ACL tear evolve into a complete tear.

Patients with a symptomatic AM bundle tear often suffer from an anterior instability similar to that of a complete ACL tear. These patients usually have a positive anterior drawer test at 90° of knee flexion and a KT-1000 side-to-side difference >3 mm. The anterior translation in the Lachman test at 30° is rather small and the pivot-shift test is negative or only slightly positive [17]. In contrast, patients with a symptomatic PL bundle tear complain about rotational instability rather than anterior instability. Non-pivoting activities are typically not limited in a patient with PL bundle tear. They often show a positive pivot-shift test (1+), while the anterior drawer test and the Lachman test might be 0 to 1+. The KT-1000 usually shows a small side-to-side difference of 1–3 mm [17].

References

1. Dargel J et al (2007) Biomechanics of the anterior cruciate ligament and implications for surgical reconstruction. Strategies Trauma Limb Reconstr 2(1):1–12
2. Georgoulis AD et al (2010) ACL injury and reconstruction: clinical related in vivo biomechanics. Orthop Traumatol Surg Res 96(8 Suppl):S119–S128
3. Pappas E et al (2013) Lessons learned from the last 20 years of ACL-related in vivo-biomechanics research of the knee joint. Knee Surg Sports Traumatol Arthrosc 21(4):755–766
4. Nakamae A et al (2010) Biomechanical function of anterior cruciate ligament remnants: how long do they contribute to knee stability after injury in patients with complete tears? Arthroscopy 26(12):1577–1585
5. Kanamori A et al (2000) In-situ force in the medial and lateral structures of intact and ACL-deficient knees. J Orthop Sci 5(6):567–571
6. Beard DJ et al (1996) Gait and electromyographic analysis of anterior cruciate ligament deficient subjects. Gait Posture 4(2):83–88
7. Chen CH et al (2012) Anteroposterior stability of the knee during the stance phase of gait after anterior cruciate ligament deficiency. Gait Posture 35(3):467–471
8. Fuentes A et al (2011) Gait adaptation in chronic anterior cruciate ligament-deficient patients: pivot-shift avoidance gait. Clin Biomech (Bristol, Avon) 26(2):181–187
9. Zhang LQ et al (2003) Six degrees-of-freedom kinematics of ACL deficient knees during locomotion-compensatory mechanism. Gait Posture 17(1):34–42
10. Andriacchi TP, Dyrby CO (2005) Interactions between kinematics and loading during walking for the normal and ACL deficient knee. J Biomech 38(2):293–298
11. Liu W, Maitland ME (2000) The effect of hamstring muscle compensation for anterior laxity in the ACL-deficient knee during gait. J Biomech 33(7):871–879
12. Yamaguchi S et al (2009) In vivo kinematics of anterior cruciate ligament deficient knees during pivot and squat activities. Clin Biomech (Bristol, Avon) 24(1):71–76
13. Esfandiarpour F et al (2013) Comparison of kinematics of ACL-deficient and healthy knees during passive flexion and isometric leg press. Knee 20(6):505–510
14. Kozanek M et al (2011) Kinematic evaluation of the step-up exercise in anterior cruciate ligament deficiency. Clin Biomech (Bristol, Avon) 26(9):950–954
15. Gao B, Cordova ML, Zheng NN (2012) Three-dimensional joint kinematics of ACL-deficient and ACL-reconstructed knees during stair ascent and descent. Hum Mov Sci 31(1):222–235
16. Shefelbine SJ et al (2006) MRI analysis of in vivo meniscal and tibiofemoral kinematics in ACL-deficient and normal knees. J Orthop Res 24(6):1208–1217
17. Siebold R, Fu FH (2008) Assessment and augmentation of symptomatic anteromedial or posterolateral bundle tears of the anterior cruciate ligament. Arthroscopy 24(11):1289–1298

Part III

ACL Augmentation

Mark Bergin, Marcus Hofbauer, Bruno Ohashi, and Volker Musahl

Contents

M. Bergin, MD • B. Ohashi, MD
Department of Orthopaedic Surgery,
University Pittsburgh Medical Center,
Pittsburgh, PA, USA

M. Hofbauer, MD
Department of Orthopaedic Surgery, University
Pittsburgh Medical Center,
Pittsburgh, PA, USA

Department of Trauma Surgery,
Medical University of Vienna, Wien, Austria

V. Musahl, MD (✉)
Department of Orthopaedic Surgery, University
Pittsburgh Medical Center,
Pittsburgh, PA, USA

UPMC Center for Sports Medicine,
3200 S Water St., Pittsburgh, PA, USA
e-mail: musahlv@upmc.edu

The aim of this chapter is to briefly describe the anatomy of the ACL, including the anatomy and biomechanics of the AM and PL bundles; to provide an overview of the history and physical examination of a patient when evaluating for a potential ACL injury, and specifically detecting a partial rupture; and to discuss imaging methods and correlate them with intraoperative findings and examination to determine the best modalities to help diagnose a partial ACL rupture.

9.1 Introduction

Complete anterior cruciate ligament (ACL) rupture is a common injury; however, partial ruptures (rupture of either the anteromedial (AM) or posterolateral (PL) bundle in isolation) have been reported to occur in between 5 and 28 % of all ACL-injured knees [9, 14]. A partial rupture is likely secondary to the fact that the two bundles of the ACL have a synergistic yet distinctly different biomechanical function at different knee flexion angles.

The increase in understanding of the individual roles that the AM and PL bundles play in stabilizing the knee has led to a better appreciation of the persistent instability that patients with a rupture of just one of these bundles may experience. The continuous advancement of imaging techniques, particularly magnetic resonance imaging (MRI), has also enhanced our ability to diagnose these partial tears. Unstable

R. Siebold et al. (eds.), *Anterior Cruciate Ligament Reconstruction*,
DOI 10.1007/978-3-642-45349-6_9, © ESSKA 2014

partial ruptures of the ACL can potentially result in altered knee kinematics, meniscal damage, and subsequent early degenerative changes of the articular cartilage, eventually resulting in posttraumatic osteoarthritis (OA) [12]. Due to these potential negative outcomes, single bundle-augmentation surgery, as opposed to traditional ACL reconstruction, has recently been recognized for its ability to restore proprioceptive and biomechanical function to the knee [1, 17, 25].

There are many definitions of partial ACL rupture. For the purpose of this chapter, partial ACL rupture will be defined as an isolated rupture of either the AM or PL bundle of the ACL. The diagnosis is made with the aid of history, physical exam, and imaging but needs to be confirmed at the time of arthroscopy with intraoperative findings. Surgeons must also differentiate between the "functional" and "non-functional" ACL. A "functional ACL" that has sustained a partial rupture will likely result in clinical symptoms and may have a detectable increase in anterior translation relative to the uninjured knee; however, the pivot shift examination will be normal. A "non-functional ACL" that has sustained a partial rupture will have the above findings and a positive pivot shift examination [3, 4]. The surgeon must have a high index of suspicion for these injuries and, furthermore, must perform a thorough examination under anaesthesia followed by arthroscopic examination, including visualization, probing, and intraoperative performance of clinical tests for rotation and translation.

9.2   Anatomy and Biomechanics

The ACL consists of two functional bundles, the AM and PL bundles, based on their attachment sites on the proximal tibia. On the femur the bundles attach on the medial aspect of the lateral femoral condyle, just posterior to the lateral intercondylar ridge [24]. The AM bundle is located proximal to the PL bundle, and the bifurcate ridge separates the two bundles [2]. The two bundles have a crossing appearance when the knee is flexed and are parallel when the knee is fully extended [2, 27].

The AM bundle is the primary restraint against anterior translation and is tight in flexion. The PL bundle is taut in full extension and primarily limits tibial internal rotation [18]. These biomechanical concepts are important to consider when obtaining the patients' history and performing the physical examination.

9.3   Patient Evaluation

An accurate diagnosis of ACL injury begins with a comprehensive history including details of the specific injury mechanism and a thorough physical exam. The diagnosis of a partial ACL rupture still remains a challenge and can be aided by radiographs and MRI and ultimately by intraoperative findings. The challenge for the orthopaedic surgeon is to use all these available tools and put together a specific treatment plan individualized to each patient [11].

9.3.1   History

A detailed history should be obtained from the patient. Important questions include the following: When did the injury occur? What activity the patient was participating in when the injury occurred? Has the patient ever had any previous injury to the knee in question? These questions will help determine a baseline for the patient and the acuity of the injury. Although patients with a partial ACL rupture may present in a similar manner to those with a complete rupture, this is not always the case. Frequently, patients with only a partial ACL injury will be able to return to sports or activity, and will not complain of gross instability, but will complain of recurrent knee pain and swelling [19]. This is contrary to patients with a complete ACL rupture who may acutely hear a "pop" and experience an immediate, large amount of swelling in the knee. They will likely not be able to return to competition and may have a grossly unstable knee.

It is also important to determine the mechanism of injury. Was it a contact or noncontact injury? The majority of ACL injuries are caused by noncontact mechanisms. A more detailed knowledge of the injury mechanism may even help to determine which bundle has ruptured. The AM bundle is frequently torn with high-energy trauma, while the PL bundle may be torn with a more subtle, rotational mechanism [17]. One must always be concerned about a fracture when the mechanism is suspicious.

Further questioning must determine whether or not the knee is painful, where the pain is located, and whether the patient is able to ambulate. The clinician must also be alert for concomitant injuries such as other ligamentous injuries; meniscal tears, which frequently present with mechanical symptoms of catching and locking; or damage to the articular cartilage.

9.3.2 Physical Examination

A detailed physical examination will help to distinguish between partial and complete ACL ruptures. A description of the complete knee examination is beyond the scope of this chapter; however, careful attention must be paid to several key aspects of the examination. First, it must be determined whether or not an effusion or haemarthrosis is present. The presence of an effusion is highly suggestive of intra-articular knee pathology.

Next, with regard to the Lachman examination, a careful comparison to the contralateral knee must be made. In the event of an isolated AM or PL bundle rupture, it is likely that the Lachman test will be increased relative to the other knee (0 to 1+) but may still have an endpoint, and the difference may be difficult to detect [19]. One study found that a significant difference in translation was not detected until at least 75 % of the ACL was transected (this included the entire PL bundle and half of the AM bundle). In this same study, only 2 of 18 exams led to the correct diagnosis of a partially transected ACL [7].

The anterior drawer test is another important test when evaluating the integrity of the ACL; however, it can be an unreliable measure of anterior knee laxity due to the inability to eliminate interference from secondary knee stabilizers [10]. The examiner must keep in mind that the anterior drawer test might be more affected in cases of isolated AM bundle rupture and the Lachman test greater in cases of isolated PL bundle rupture [17].

The next important examination to consider is the pivot shift examination. The pivot shift exam, when performed under anaesthesia, can frequently yield more information than the Lachman exam and is considered indicative of clinically significant, or "functional", instability. It is likely in the scenario of a partial ACL rupture that the pivot shift exam will be negative to slightly positive (0 to 1+) due to the remaining intact bundle [23]. Some clinicians advocate that any difference in pivot shift from side to side should be treated as a complete ACL injury [3].

In the future, quantitative pivot shift examination will help to increase sensitivity and specificity of the pivot shift test and perhaps allow us to differentiate between isolated AM and PL bundle ruptures. In an effort to quantify these small differences, Zaffagnini et al. have used non-invasive inertial sensors to measure the acceleration of the tibia during the reduction phase of the pivot shift test [26]. Nishizawa et al. used electromagnetic tracking to show that small side-to-side differences in acceleration (3.0 vs. 1.2 mm/s^2) can indicate partial ACL injury [13]. Using simple image analysis, enhanced by an iPad$^©$ application, Hoshino et al. showed that differences between pivot shift test grades can be both detected and quantified [8].

There are several other instruments that can be useful in quantifying anterior translation in the ACL-injured knee. The KT-1000 (MEDmetric, San Diego, CA) side-to-side difference has been found to frequently be less than 3 mm in a knee with a partial ACL rupture [19]. Radiological examination, by applying anterior stress to the leg with the Telos$^©$ device, has been shown to have a high correlation in detecting and differentiating between a complete and a partial ACL tear. Panisset et al. recently found that they could reliably predict a complete ACL rupture versus a partial ACL rupture based on physical exam findings confirmed with Telos© stress radiography. They did not find the same predictive benefit when using the Rolimeter© device. All results were confirmed with intraoperative findings [16].

9.3.3 Imaging

Based on clinical suspicion, ACL injuries can be confirmed with MRI, which is considered by many as the "gold standard" for diagnosis of an ACL rupture and allows for determination of concomitant intra-articular pathology. Radiographs are frequently obtained to rule out fracture and to determine the amount of pre-existing joint space narrowing in these patients. There are several other studies, which may also be beneficial when evaluating for partial ACL rupture.

9.3.4 Magnetic Resonance Imaging (MRI)

Although the ACL can be visualized with T1- or T2-weighted images on "standard" views in the coronal axial and sagittal planes, special MRI sequences, such as views in the oblique coronal and oblique sagittal planes, were developed and allow for a clear and predictable recognition of partial ACL ruptures [19, 21] (Figs. 9.1 and 9.2). In our institution, we use these oblique views routinely when performing MRI examination with concern for ACL injury. It is simple to do and adds an additional 5 min to the patient's MRI examination. Additionally, these views also allow for excellent visualization of the anterior and posterior roots of the menisci [21].

Starman et al. assessed the reliability of detecting partial ACL ruptures and found that the AM bundle could be identified on most standard views; however, the PL bundle was frequently unable to be visualized. They concluded that the standard coronal and sagittal views were inadequate to reliably detect a tear in the individual bundles [20]. Steckel et al. evaluated the ability to detect partial ACL rupture using oblique

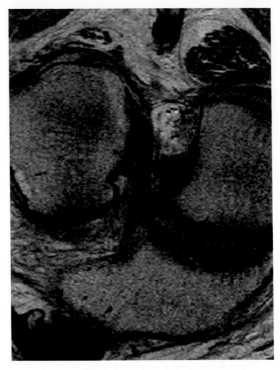

Fig. 9.1 Oblique coronal MRI showing an intact AM bundle

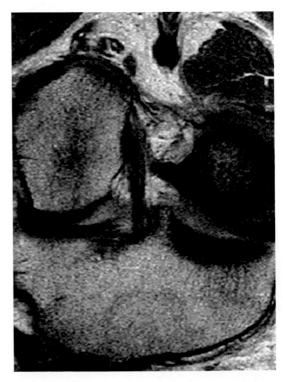

Fig. 9.2 Oblique coronal MRI showing an intact PL bundle

coronal and oblique sagittal MRI cuts as described above. They determined that the AM bundle was easier to visualize on a consistent basis, and that the oblique coronal view was the best view to look at both the AM and PL bundles. They were able to correctly diagnose 90 % of isolated AM bundle ruptures on both oblique views, 80 % of isolated PL bundle ruptures in the oblique coronal plane, and 67 % when using the oblique sagittal plane alone. They concluded that partial ACL tears could predictably be recognized using these oblique views and 3 T technology [22].

Several other types of MRI may be beneficial in detecting a partial ACL rupture as well. Okazaki et al. found that by placing patients in an open MRI with the knee in a position replicating that of the Slocum's Anterolateral Rotatory Instability test (ALRI test), they could predict the grade of the pivot shift test based on the anterior translation of the lateral compartment [15]. Haughom et al. also showed that they were able to detect small changes in tibial rotation in ACL-deficient knees using kinematic MRI. Sequential MRI images were obtained as internal and external rotational forces were applied to the knee [6].

9.3.5 Three-Dimensional Computed Tomography (3D CT) Scan

The recent addition of 3D CT has been of added benefit when determining the exact location of the ACL insertion, particularly on the femoral side. Not only can the intercondylar ridge be seen, but the bifurcate ridge separating the AM and PL bundles can be reliably located as well. Forsythe et al. recently adopted the quadrant system and measured eight cadaver knees after drilling AM and PL tunnels in the tibia and femur. These tunnel positions were then quantified based on their quadrant system. Thus, a preoperative 3D CT gives even more information when determining where to place either the AM or PL bundle when performing ACL augmentation for a partial ACL rupture [5].

9.4 Correlation with Intraoperative Findings and Examination

Case 1: Isolated PL Bundle Tear, AM Bundle Intact

A 23-year-old male who was involved in motorcycle accident. Examination revealed a 2A Lachman (5 mm vs. 2 mm), 1+ pivot shift, 1+ anterior drawer, and 5 mm opening to varus stress at 30° of knee flexion (Figs. 9.3, 9.4, 9.5, 9.6, 9.7, and 9.8).

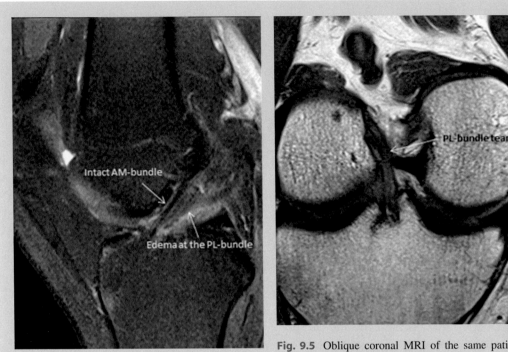

Fig. 9.5 Oblique coronal MRI of the same patient showing a PL bundle oedema and tear

Fig. 9.3 Oblique sagittal MRI of this patient shows an intact AM bundle, with PL bundle tear and oedema

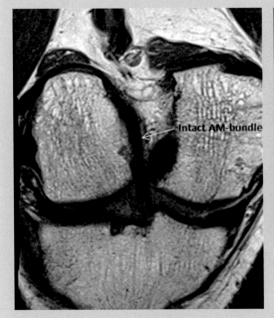

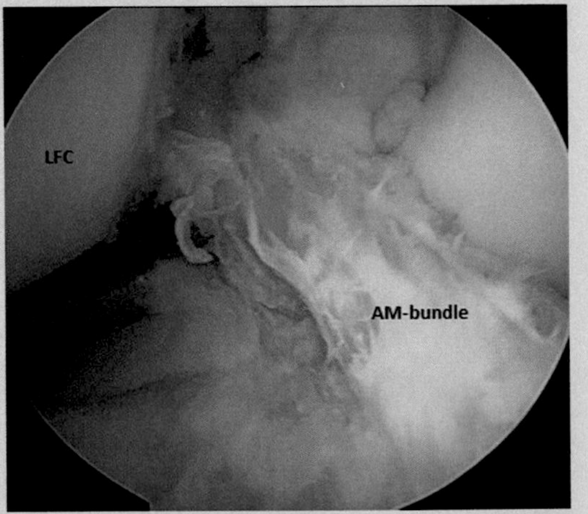

Fig. 9.6 This same 23-year-old male underwent arthroscopic evaluation and the image shows the intact AM bundle. *LFC* lateral femoral condyle

Fig. 9.4 Oblique coronal MRI of the same patient showing an intact AM bundle

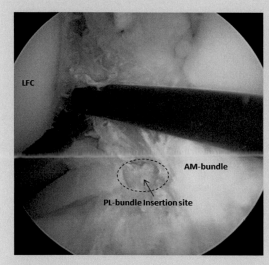

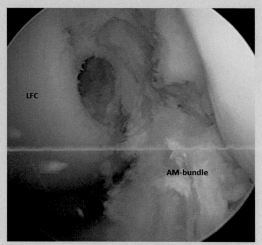

Fig. 9.7 The same patient with a probe on the intact AM bundle and a tear of the PL bundle from the femoral insertion site. *LFC* lateral femoral condyle

Fig. 9.8 View of the notch in the same patient showing an intact AM bundle and the newly drilled tunnel for PL reconstruction. *LFC* lateral femoral condyle

Case 2: Isolated PL Bundle Tear, AM Bundle Intact

A 15-year-old male who sustained a twisting injury to his knee while playing soccer. Examination revealed a 1B Lachman, 1+ anterior drawer, negative posterior drawer, and 1+ pivot shift exam (Figs 9.9, 9.10, 9.11, 9.12, 9.13, and 9.14).

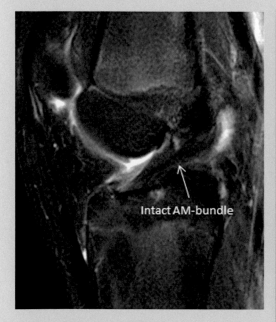

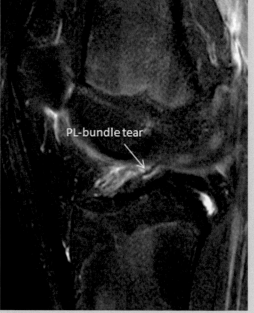

Fig. 9.9 Oblique sagittal MRI on this patient showing an intact AM bundle

Fig. 9.10 Oblique sagittal MRI of the same patient showing a PL bundle tear

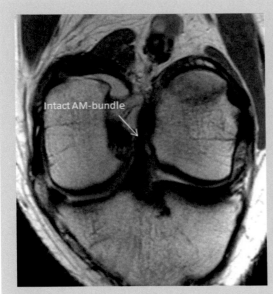

Fig. 9.11 Oblique coronal MRI on this 15-year-old male showing the AM bundle intact

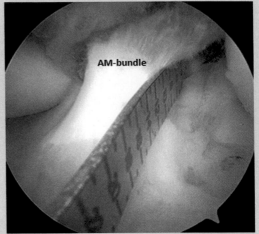

Fig. 9.13 This patient also underwent arthroscopic evaluation and the image shows an intact AM bundle

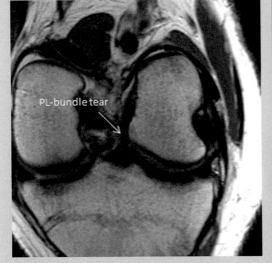

Fig. 9.12 Oblique coronal MRI of the same patient showing a PL bundle tear

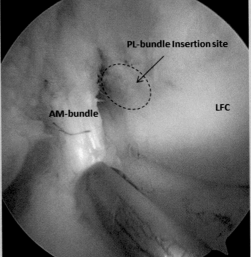

Fig. 9.14 The same patient with an arthroscopic image showing intact AM bundle and tear of PL bundle from femoral insertion in the upper right of the photo. *LFC* lateral femoral condyle

Case 3: AM Bundle Rupture, PL Bundle Intact
A 37-year-old female who fell while playing volleyball. Examination showed a 1B Lachman exam and 1+ pivot shift exam with 1+ anterior drawer (Figs. 9.15, 9.16, 9.17, 9.18, and 9.19).

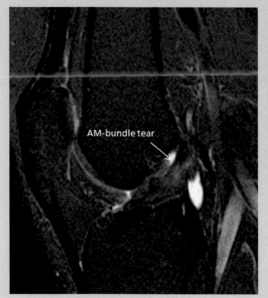

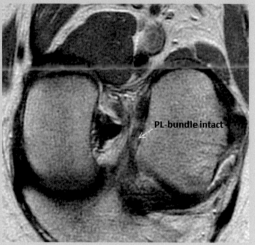

Fig. 9.17 Oblique coronal MRI from same MRI shows the PL bundle intact

Fig. 9.15 Oblique sagittal MRI of this patient showing an AM bundle tear

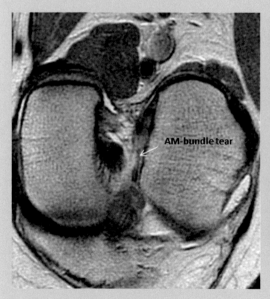

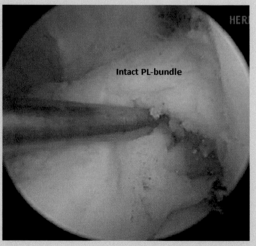

Fig. 9.18 Image during diagnostic arthroscopy of this patient shows intact PL bundle with probe

Fig. 9.16 Oblique coronal MRI of the same patient showing an AM bundle tear

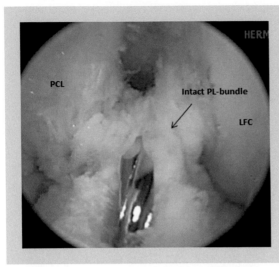

Fig. 9.19 Arthroscopic image from the same patient showing PL bundle intact with AM bundle rupture. Guide pin within the AM bundle insertion site on the tibia. *LFC* lateral femoral condyle, *PCL* posterior cruciate ligament

Memory

The diagnosis of partial ACL rupture is challenging and relies on many different tools at the physician's disposal. A thorough history must be obtained, as the presenting symptoms will quite possibly be different than the "classic" ACL rupture presentation. Next, a detailed examination must be performed including the Lachman examination and the pivot shift test. MRI can be an invaluable asset when diagnosing a partial ACL rupture as well, with oblique coronal and oblique sagittal views being the most reliable. Suspicion for a partial ACL rupture based on all of the above findings must be confirmed intraoperatively at the time of arthroscopy. Ultimately, partial ACL reconstruction aims at improving patient outcomes.

References

1. Adachi N, Ochi M, Uchio Y, Sumen Y (2000) Anterior cruciate ligament augmentation under arthroscopy. A minimum 2-year follow-up in 40 patients. Arch Orthop Trauma Surg 120(3–4):128–133
2. Amis AA, Beynnon B, Blankevoort L, Chambat P, Christel P, Durselen L, Friederich N, Grood E, Hertel P, Jakob R, Müller W, O'Brien M, O'Connor J (1994) Proceedings of the ESSKA scientific workshop on reconstruction of the anterior and posterior cruciate ligaments. Knee Surg Sports Traumatol Arthrosc 2(3):124–132
3. Bach BR Jr, Warren RF, Flynn WM, Kroll M, Wickiewiecz TL (1990) Arthrometric evaluation of knees that have a torn anterior cruciate ligament. J Bone Joint Surg Am 72(9):1299–1306
4. DeFranco MJ, Bach BR Jr (2009) A comprehensive review of partial anterior cruciate ligament tears. J Bone Joint Surg Am 91(1):198–208
5. Forsythe B, Kopf S, Wong AK, Martins CA, Anderst W, Tashman S, Fu FH (2010) The location of femoral and tibial tunnels in anatomic double-bundle anterior cruciate ligament reconstruction analyzed by three-dimensional computed tomography models. J Bone Joint Surg Am 92(6):1418–1426
6. Haughom BD, Souza R, Schairer WW, Li X, Ma CB (2012) Evaluating rotational kinematics of the knee in ACL-ruptured and healthy patients using 3.0 Tesla magnetic resonance imaging. Knee Surg Sports Traumatol Arthrosc 20(4):663–670
7. Hole RL, Lintner DM, Kamaric E, Moseley JB (1996) Increased tibial translation after partial sectioning of the anterior cruciate ligament. The posterolateral bundle. Am J Sports Med 24(4):556–560
8. Hoshino Y, Araujo P, Irrgang JJ, Fu FH, Musahl V (2012) An image analysis method to quantify the lateral pivot shift test. Knee Surg Sports Traumatol Arthrosc 20(4):703–707
9. Jacquot L, Selmi TAS, Servien E, Neyret P (2003) Lésions ligamentaires récentes du genou. Encyclopédie medico-chirurgicale appareil locomoteur 14(080):20
10. Lubowitz JH, Bernardini B, Reid JB 3rd (2008) Current concepts review: comprehensive physical examination for instability of the knee. Am J Sports Med 36(3):577–594
11. Musahl V, Kopf S, Rabuck S, Becker R, van der Merwe W, Zaffagnini S, Fu FH, Karlsson J (2012) Rotatory knee laxity tests and the pivot shift as tools

for ACL treatment algorithm. Knee Surg Sports Traumatol Arthrosc 20(4):793–800

12. Nakamae A, Ochi M, Deie M, Adachi N, Kanaya A, Nishimori M, Nakasa T (2010) Biomechanical function of anterior cruciate ligament remnants: how long do they contribute to knee stability after injury in patients with complete tears? Arthroscopy 26(12): 1577–1585

13. Nishizawa Y, Kuroda R, Matsushita T, Kubo S, Nagamune K, Kurosaka M (2012) Preoperative and postoperative biomechanical analysis of the knee with partial anterior cruciate ligament disruption: quantitative evaluation using an electromagnetic measurement system. Abstract only. ESSKA Congress, Geneva, 2–5 May 2012

14. Noyes FR, Bassett RW, Grood ES (1980) Arthroscopy in acute traumatic hemarthrosis of the knee. Incidence of anterior cruciate tears and other injuries. J Bone Joint Surg Am 62:687–695, 757

15. Okazaki K, Tashiro Y, Izawa T, Matsuda S, Iwamoto Y (2012) Rotatory laxity evaluation of the knee using modified Slocum's test in open magnetic resonance imaging. Knee Surg Sports Traumatol Arthrosc 20(4):679–685

16. Panisset JC, Ntagiopoulos PG, Saggin PR, Dejour D (2012) A comparison of Telos stress radiography versus Rolimeter in the diagnosis of different patterns of anterior cruciate ligament tears. Orthop Traumatol Surg Res 98(7):751–758

17. Petersen W, Zantop T (2006) Partial rupture of the anterior cruciate ligament. Arthroscopy 22(11):1143–1145

18. Sakane M, Fox RJ, Woo SL, Livesay GA, Li G, Fu FH (1997) In situ forces in the anterior cruciate ligament and its bundles in response to anterior tibial loads. J Orthop Res 15(2):285–293

19. Siebold R, Fu FH (2008) Assessment and augmentation of symptomatic anteromedial or posterolateral bundle tears of the anterior cruciate ligament. Arthroscopy 24(11):1289–1298

20. Starman JS, Vanbeek C, Armfield DR, Sahasrabudhe A, Baker CL 3rd, Irrgang JJ, Fu FH (2007) Assessment

of normal ACL double bundle anatomy in standard viewing planes by magnetic resonance imaging. Knee Surg Sports Traumatol Arthrosc 15(5): 493–499

21. Steckel H, Vadala G, Davis D, Fu FH (2006) 2D and 3D 3-tesla magnetic resonance imaging of the double bundle structure in anterior cruciate ligament anatomy. Knee Surg Sports Traumatol Arthrosc 14(11): 1151–1158

22. Steckel H, Vadala G, Davis D, Musahl V, Fu FH (2007) 3-T MR imaging of partial ACL tears: a cadaver study. Knee Surg Sports Traumatol Arthrosc 15(9):1066–1071

23. van Eck CF, Schreiber VM, Liu TT, Fu FH (2010) The anatomic approach to primary, revision and augmentation anterior cruciate ligament reconstruction. Knee Surg Sports Traumatol Arthrosc 18(9): 1154–1163

24. Wang JH, Kim JG, Ahn JH, Lim HC, Hoshino Y, Fu FH (2012) Is femoral tunnel length correlated with the intercondylar notch and femoral condyle geometry after double-bundle anterior cruciate ligament reconstruction using the transportal technique? An in vivo computed tomography analysis. Arthroscopy 28(8): 1094–1103

25. Yagi M, Kuroda R, Nagamune K, Yoshiya S, Kurosaka M (2007) Double-bundle ACL reconstruction can improve rotational stability. Clin Orthop Relat Res 454:100–107

26. Zaffagnini S, Lopomo N, Signorelli C, Marcheggiani Muccioli GM, Bonanzinga T, Grassi A, Visani A, Marcacci M (2013) Innovative technology for knee laxity evaluation: clinical applicability and reliability of inertial sensors for quantitative analysis of the pivot-shift test. Clin Sports Med 32(1):61–70

27. Zantop T, Herbort M, Raschke MJ, Fu FH, Petersen W (2007) The role of the anteromedial and posterolateral bundles of the anterior cruciate ligament in anterior tibial translation and internal rotation. Am J Sports Med 35(2):223–227

Arthroscopic Assessment of Partial ACL Tears

10

Rainer Siebold

Contents

The anterior cruciate ligament (ACL) is a continuum of fibers, which is organized in multiple small fascicles. Based on anatomical and biomechanical findings, it was divided into two main bundles – the anteromedial (AM) and posterolateral (PL) bundles [5–11, 13–17, 20, 24]. Histological investigations showed that AM and PL are separated by a fine septum [11]. Recently there is increasing anatomical evidence that the ACL is flat and that the tibial ACL insertion is in the shape of a "C" with fibers inserting anteromedial (AM) and posteromedial (PM named accordigly by the authors, see Chap. 1) along the medial tibial spine. This new finding is of importance especially for tibial PM bone tunnel placement.

10.1   Arthroscopic Assessment of a Partial ACL Tear or Elongation

The anterior cruciate ligament (ACL) consists of a continuum of fibers separated by fine septums. Therefore, it is very unlikely to find a true "isolated" bundle tear. Most often a partial tear of the ACL is a combined injury of the anterior and posterior fibers. An overview of different injury patterns of AM and PL was reported by Zantop et al. [23]. In most cases the bundles (Fig. 10.1a–c) (Fig. 10.2) were torn from their femoral insertion site. The second bundle was still intact or partially torn. Partial intraligamentous or tibial insertion site tears are less frequent. The diagnosis of a partial ACL tear is difficult and should always be a combination of patient history, clinical examination, MRI, and arthroscopy.

R. Siebold, MD
Institute for Anatomy and Cell Biology,
Ruprecht-Karls University Heidelberg,
Im Neuenheimer Feld 307, Heidelberg 69120,
Germany

HKF: Center for Specialised Hip-Knee-Foot Surgery,
ATOS Hospital Heidelberg,
Bismarckstr. 9-15, Heidelberg 69115, Germany
e-mail: rainer.siebold@atos.de

R. Siebold et al. (eds.), *Anterior Cruciate Ligament Reconstruction*,
DOI 10.1007/978-3-642-45349-6_10, © ESSKA 2014

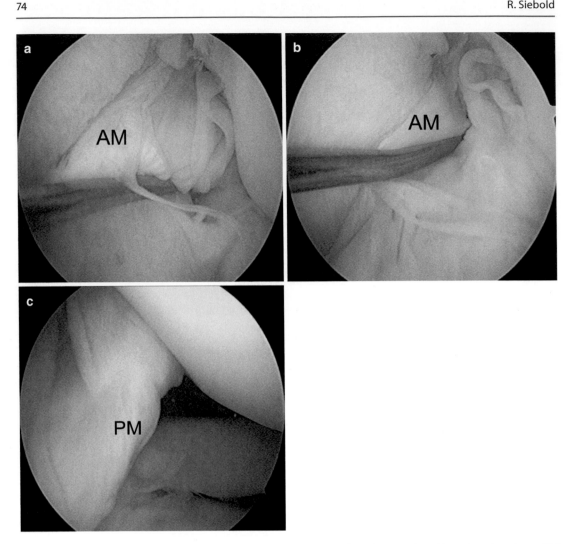

Fig. 10.1 (**a–c**) Left knee: (**a, b**) proximal rupture of AM fibers with fatty degeneration; (**c**) same patient, intact PM fibers

10.1.1 Examination of Bundles

The surgical procedure has to start with patient examination under anesthesia. Two tests are essential: the Lachman test and the pivot shift test, which are much more pertinent under anesthesia [4]. The pivot shift test is usually negative or glide, which is one of the characteristic of ACL partial tear [18].

The arthroscopic examination of the anterior and posterior ACL fibers is performed in various knee flexion angles with a probe to consider the different tensioning patterns of the different parts of the ACL. The *AM fibers* have relatively con-stant levels of in situ forces during knee flexion [1–3, 12, 19, 21, 22] and might best be probed arthroscopically in 90° of knee flexion. The ante-rior drawer test under arthroscopic visualization might help to establish the diagnosis. The Lachman test and pivot shift test are difficult to be performed during arthroscopic visualization.

In contrast, the *PM fibers* may have high in situ forces between 0° and 30° of flexion as found previously for PL fibers [1–3, 12, 19, 21, 22]. The intercondylar notch cannot be examined arthroscopically close to extension. These fibers might be best probed with the knee in a "figure of four." In this position the PM fibers are stretched,

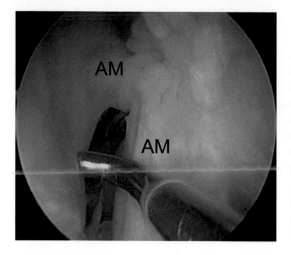

Fig. 10.2 Right knee: view from medial portal. PM fibers rupture, probe showing PM insertion site; AM bundle with proximal partial tear but good stability

and the femoral PM footprint is rotated and exposed in the shallow aspect of the lateral femoral intercondylar wall.

10.1.2 Femoral Partial Tear

Especially on the femoral insertion site, a thorough arthroscopic probing is necessary to assess the injury pattern (Fig. 10.1a, b). The diagnosis is easy when the injury is acute or the torn fibers are retracted exposing the lateral femoral intercondylar wall (Fig. 10.2). In case of a chronic injury with scar tissue, the tear might only be observed with thorough probing of the fibers at the femoral insertion site. A femoral AM or PM fiber tear is best probed in flexion. The "figure of four" position might give some additional information on the condition of the PM fibers.

10.1.3 Intraligamentous Partial Tears

An acute intraligamentous tear of fibers is less frequent but usually exposed and easy to be diagnosed. Chronic tears with scar tissue are difficult to be diagnosed and need thorough probing of the insufficient part of the ACL.

10.1.4 Tibial Partial Tear

A tear of the AM fibers from its tibial insertion site is easy to be seen arthroscopically as it is in the anterior aspect of the tibial ACL insertion. In contrast a rupture of the PM fibers from the posteromedial aspect of the ACL insertion site close to the medial tibial spine is difficult to be observed as it is hidden behind the AM fibers. Both injury patterns are rather rare.

> **Memory**
> According to their distinct insertions sites, the ACL fibers contribute individually to the overall stability of the knee [1–3, 12, 19, 21, 22]. The diagnosis of a partial ACL tear is difficult and should always be a combination of patient history, clinical examination, MRI, and arthroscopy. A detailed experience of the arthroscopic ACL anatomy with its tensioning pattern is very helpful to establish the right diagnosis of a partial ACL tear.

References

1. Amis AA, Dawkins GP (1991) Functional anatomy of the anterior cruciate ligament. Fibre bundle actions related to ligament replacements and injuries. J Bone Joint Surg Br 73(2):260–267
2. Amis AA, Zavras TD (1995) Isometricity and graft placement during anterior cruciate ligament reconstruction. Knee 2(1):5–17
3. Bach JM, Hull ML (1998) Strain inhomogeneity in the anterior cruciate ligament under application of external and muscular loads. J Biomech Eng 120(4):497–503
4. Bach BR Jr, Warren RF, Wickiewicz TL (1988) The pivot shift phenomenon: results and description of a modified clinical test for anterior cruciate ligament insufficiency. Am J Sports Med 16(6):571–576
5. Chhabra A, Starman JS, Ferretti M et al (2006) Anatomic, radiographic, biomechanical, and kinematic evaluation of the anterior cruciate ligament and its two functional bundles. J Bone Joint Surg Am 88(Suppl 4):2–10
6. Colombet P, Robinson J, Christel P et al (2006) Morphology of anterior cruciate ligament attachments for anatomic reconstruction: a cadaveric dissection and radiographic study. Arthroscopy 22(9):984–992
7. Dodds JA, Arnoczky SP (1994) Anatomy of the anterior cruciate ligament a blueprint for repair and reconstruction. Arthroscopy 10(2):132–139

8. Duthon VB, Barea C, Abrassart S et al (2006) Anatomy of the anterior cruciate ligament. Knee Surg Sports Traumatol Arthrosc 14(3):204–213

9. Edwards A, Bull AM, Amis AA (2007) The attachments of the anteromedial and posterolateral fibre bundles of the anterior cruciate ligament: Part 1: tibial attachment. Knee Surg Sports Traumatol Arthrosc 15(12):1414–1421

10. Edwards A, Bull AM, Amis AA (2008) The attachments of the anteromedial and posterolateral fibre bundles of the anterior cruciate ligament. Part 2: femoral attachment. Knee Surg Sports Traumatol Arthrosc 16(1):29–36

11. Ferretti M, Levicoff EA, Macpherson TA et al (2007) The fetal anterior cruciate ligament: an anatomic and histologic study. Arthroscopy 23(3):278–283

12. Gabriel MT, Wong EK, Woo SL et al (2004) Distribution of in situ forces in the anterior cruciate ligament in response to rotatory loads. J Orthop Res 22(1):85–89

13. Girgis FG, Marshall JL, Monajem A (1975) The cruciate ligaments of the knee joint. Anatomical, functional and experimental analysis. Clin Orthop Relat Res (106):216–231

14. Giron F, Cuomo P, Aglietti P et al (2006) Femoral attachment of the anterior cruciate ligament. Knee Surg Sports Traumatol Arthrosc 14(3):250–256

15. Harner CD, Baek GH, Vogrin TM et al (1999) Quantitative analysis of human cruciate ligament insertions. Arthroscopy 15(7):741–749

16. Mochizuki T, Muneta T, Nagase T et al (2006) Cadaveric knee observation study for describing anatomic femoral tunnel placement for two-bundle anterior cruciate ligament reconstruction. Arthroscopy 22(4):356–361

17. Odensten M, Gillquist J (1985) Functional anatomy of the anterior cruciate ligament and a rationale for reconstruction. J Bone Joint Surg Am 67(2):257–262

18. Panisset JC, Duraffour H, Vasconcelos W et al (2008) Clinical, radiological and arthroscopic analysis of the ACL tear. A prospective study of 418 cases. Rev Chir Orthop Reparatrice Appar Mot 94(8 Suppl):362–368

19. Sakane M, Fox RJ, Woo SL et al (1997) In situ forces in the anterior cruciate ligament and its bundles in response to anterior tibial loads. J Orthop Res 15(2):285–293

20. Siebold R, Ellert T, Metz S et al (2008) Tibial insertions of the anteromedial and posterolateral bundles of the anterior cruciate ligament: morphometry, arthroscopic landmarks, and orientation model for bone tunnel placement. Arthroscopy 24(2):154–161

21. Woo SL, Debski RE, Withrow JD et al (1999) Biomechanics of knee ligaments. Am J Sports Med 27(4):533–543

22. Yagi M, Wong EK, Kanamori A et al (2002) Biomechanical analysis of an anatomic anterior cruciate ligament reconstruction. Am J Sports Med 30(5):660–666

23. Zantop T, Brucker PU, Vidal A et al (2007) Intraarticular rupture pattern of the ACL. Clin Orthop Relat Res 454:48–53

24. Zantop T, Petersen W, Sekiya JK et al (2006) Anterior cruciate ligament anatomy and function relating to anatomical reconstruction. Knee Surg Sports Traumatol Arthrosc 14(10):982–992

Conservative versus Operative Treatment

11

Jürgen Höher and Christoph Offerhaus

Contents

J. Höher (✉)
Clinic for Sports Traumatology at Merheim Medical
Center, Cologne, University of Witten-Herdecke,
Ostmerheimer Str. 200, Cologne 51109, Germany
e-mail: jhoeher@t-online.de

C. Offerhaus
St. Vinzenz Hospital Cologne, Clinic for Trauma,
Orthopaedics, Hand- and Reconstructive Surgery,
University of Cologne, Merheimer Str. 221-223,
Cologne 50733, Germany

11.1   Introduction

An anterior cruciate ligament (ACL) tear is a common injury and arises most frequently in athletes from a noncontact pivoting injury, typically by a change of direction or deceleration manoeuvre. The annual incidence in the United States is about 200,000 with at least 100,000 receiving arthroscopic reconstruction [2]. The frequency of a partial tear of the ACL ranges from 10 to 35 % which is reported to be symptomatic in 5–10 % of the cases [3, 24].

Recently, a well-designed clinical review reported that conservative treatment could be a valid treatment option for avoiding systematic surgical reconstruction in partial ACL tears [7]. However, 38 % of partial lesions may evolve into complete tears requiring reconstruction of the ACL at a later point in time. Early ACL augmentation with preserving remnants of the torn ACL was shown to have biomechanical, vascular and proprioceptive advantages for the patient [22, 24].

In the following chapter, we aim to give the surgeon the scientific background of conservative and operative treatment of ACL rupture and provide an algorithm that may help to decide whether a patient should receive nonoperative treatment, ACL augmentation or standard ACL reconstruction.

R. Siebold et al. (eds.), *Anterior Cruciate Ligament Reconstruction*,
DOI 10.1007/978-3-642-45349-6_11, © ESSKA 2014

11.2 Literature

As the ACL secures the tibia against anterior forces, the loss of its function leads to anterolateral instability that may be noticed by the patient as a "giving way". As the posterolateral (PL) bundle is tight in extension and the anteromedial (AM) bundle is tight in flexion, the particular fibres have a varying contribution to stability and the potential for partial ruptures at different knee positions. Whereas the AM bundle is the primary restraint against anterior tibial translation in flexion, the PL bundle stabilizes the knee near full extension, specifically against rotatory moments. Thus, an isolated rupture of the AM bundle has a larger effect on the anterior drawer sign than on the Lachman test, whereas the effect of an isolated rupture of the PL bundle is vice versa. A tear of the PL bundle leads to rotational instability which may be documented by a positive pivot shift test. Vice versa a pivot shift usually remains negative in cases of an isolated AM bundle tear [26].

The often cited "knee cascade" describes the osteoarthritic changes in a chronic instable knee. Several studies showed a growing incidence of meniscal lesions in the untreated ACL-deficient knee [6, 15, 25]. The loss of meniscal function as well as high shearing and compressive force in pivoting moments may lead to secondary chondral injury [15]. Therefore, surgical reconstruction after ACL injury is commonly recommended to prevent secondary meniscal damage and decrease the risk of degenerative osteoarthritis in high-demand athletes. However, conservative treatment is a valid option in patients with low impact sports participation and at a higher age.

At present, there is no evidence that ACL reconstruction can prevent osteoarthritis in the long run [7, 12]. Several long-term follow-up studies showed an increasing frequency of abnormal radiographs in 24 % up to 86 % of the cases with untreated ACL rupture [4, 21, 25]. The incidence of abnormal radiographs after ACL reconstruction varied between 10 % and 71 % of the patients at a minimum follow-up of 5 years [9, 16, 19]. The great variation of the incidence of osteoarthritis between these studies may be

explained by differences in study population with respect to age, activity level, accompanying injuries as well as by discrepancies with respect to radiographic techniques and osteoarthritis classification. In some studies, early reconstructed patients had an even higher degree of osteoarthritis on radiographs than conservatively treated patients, but Tegner scores were significantly lower in these non-reconstructed patients [10]. Another bias of these studies may be that patients choosing ACL reconstruction rather than nonoperative treatment have a higher pre-injury activity level. Whereas the rates of degenerative changes increase over time in both the operative and nonoperative groups, Fink et al. indicated a higher level of sports participation in patients after ACL reconstruction [9]. Nevertheless, operative treatment is not the prerequisite for sports participation, nor does it guarantee the ability to return to high-level sports. Besides biomechanical behaviour of the knee, the psychological profile of the patient was shown to be an important factor influencing return to previous sports level [14].

In contrast, partial meniscectomy is well accepted as a risk factor for developing osteoarthritis. Even in knees with an intact ACL, degenerative changes are 3–7 times more frequent than in the contralateral uninjured knee 20 years after partial meniscectomy [23]. After ACL rupture it was demonstrated that no matter if the treatment was surgical or conservative, patients who sustained a meniscus injury associated with the ACL rupture had a higher rate of radiographically documented osteoarthritic changes [29]. It is well demonstrated that the risk of further meniscal damage after an ACL rupture was significantly higher with conservative treatment [8]. Even though some authors mention that the reduction of further meniscus lesion not necessarily would be due to the surgical reconstruction rather than to a decrease of high pivoting activities or a more aggressive (surgical) management of small meniscal tears when the ACL was reconstructed early [7, 12].

In 2010 Frobell et al. published a randomized controlled trial (RCT) on treatment of acute ACL tears including 121 young active adults comparing early ACL reconstruction plus structural rehabilitation and early rehabilitation with the option of delayed reconstruction [12]. Of 59 patients assigned to rehabilitation plus optional delayed ACL reconstruction, 23 underwent delayed ACL surgery while the other 36 patients underwent rehabilitation alone. That means with the use of the delayed reconstruction strategy, ACL reconstruction could be avoided in 61 % of the cases, and there were no differences between the patient reported outcomes of the two groups at 2 years follow-up. However, objective knee-stability tests showed better results in the early-surgery group as well as a lower frequency of meniscal resections.

There are various attempts to distinguish between "high-risk" patients who should be treated with early-surgery and "low-risk" patients who should be treated nonsurgically. The well-known surgical risk factor (SURF) algorithm of Daniel et al. assessed patients according to their activity level and side-to-side laxity values [6]. Following this algorithm, patients with high activity levels and/or great side-to-side laxity differences should be treated surgically. Another study identified a positive pivot shift test in an awake patient 3 months after ACL rupture as the strongest predictor for the need of ACL reconstruction [20]. However, some authors were able to demonstrate that knee laxity measurements were not able to differentiate between "potential copers" and "noncopers". They estimated that clinical tests that capture neuromuscular adaptations such as the hop test may be more useful in decision-making whether a patient should be treated by surgery or not than only knee laxity measurements and pre-injury activity level as used by the SURF algorithm [17, 18].

Compared to complete ACL ruptures, there are fewer studies investigating the outcome of partial ruptures of the ACL. In a meta-analysis Pujol et al. concluded that the conservatively treated partial ACL tears ensure good functional results, although a long-time follow-up is missing [27]. The mean rates of delayed ACL reconstruction (8 %) and secondary meniscectomy (7 %) were low. However, just 30–50 % of the conservatively treated patients returned to their pre-injury sports level [1, 27]. Noyes et al. reported a

progression to complete ACL deficiency in 38 % of the cases in a 7-year follow-up [24]. Predicting factors for the evolution into a complete ACL deficiency were a subtle increase in initial anterior translation, the occurrence of subsequent reinjury with giving way and the initial amount of ligament tearing. Thus, tears involving one-half and three-fourths of the ligament progressed frequently (50 and 86 %), whereas one-fourth tears rarely progressed. If surgery is needed in case of a partial ACL rupture, augmentation has several advantages to a standard ACL reconstruction. Keeping ACL remnants intact preserves its blood supply and may maintain proprioceptive innervation providing a support for the healing process [3, 5, 22]. In the early postoperative period, the augmentation may be protected by the intact bundle guaranteeing mechanical strength allowing faster rehabilitation and an earlier return to sports. Finally, the intact bundles may optimize the accuracy of bone tunnel placement by increased arthroscopic orientation.

> **Memory**
> There is no evidence that ACL reconstruction reduces the incidence of osteoarthritis. The risk of further lesions remains high, no matter if surgical or conservative treatment is selected. Although studies present inconsistent results, return to sports tends to be higher in operated patients, whereas the risk of further meniscal damage seems to be lower. As conservative treatment is still a valid alternative and maybe an underestimated option after ACL lesion, patients should accurately be evaluated clinically to identify "potential copers" that could be treated by structured rehabilitation with the option of later ACL reconstruction if needed. With respect to partial ACL tears, the results of conservative treatment are good over medium terms, especially if patients limit their sports activities. With symptomatic partial tears or in athletes practising pivoting sports, ligament reconstruction may be

required. If so, ACL augmentation preserving the intact bundle shows vascular, proprioceptive and biomechanical advantages. Surgical indications are thus very much the same in partial as in complete tears.

11.3 Clinical Approach to Patients with ACL Injuries

When a patient comes into the office with a suspicion of having sustained an acute ACL injury, a structured work up is necessary to evaluate the patient and find the appropriate treatment. First of all the patient should be asked for the history of the accident. From this the mechanism of injury may be concluded. After asking for previous injuries and the kind of treatment yet received, a thorough clinical examination has to follow (Fig. 11.1).

Besides general parameters such as range of motion, existence of joint effusion and joint line tenderness, the two crucial tests for the ACL are the Lachman test and the pivot shift test [11]. The Lachman test has two features: the extent of the translation of the tibia relative to the femur compared to the contralateral side and the quality of the endpoint indicating if remnant fibres of the ACL get taught at the end of the motion limit (Fig. 11.2). In addition an instrumented Lachman test should be performed in order to semiobjectively quantify the Lachman test and as it is helpful in evaluating the extent of the injury. While originally a KT-1000 was introduced for instrumented testing, meanwhile a Rolimeter device has been established in our clinic as it has been proven to deliver similar test results [13] and has strong advantages such as its availability/versatility (presence in each examination room) and its low cost. However, it is important for the reliability of the device to have a constant platform available to underlie the patient's thigh in order to have a consistent flexion angle of the knee at each time (Fig. 11.3). Additionally an MRI is usually available and the ACL injury may further be classified.

According to the patient's history, the clinical examination and the MRI findings, the ACL injury may then be classified into no tear, partial tear (AM or PL) or complete tear. For complete tears it has to be considered if patients have an isolated ACL tear or if an additional lesion is present that may require surgery such as a meniscus, cartilage or other ligament injury.

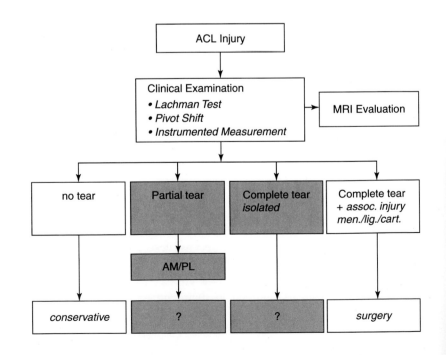

Fig. 11.1 Diagnostic algorithm for acute ACL injuries

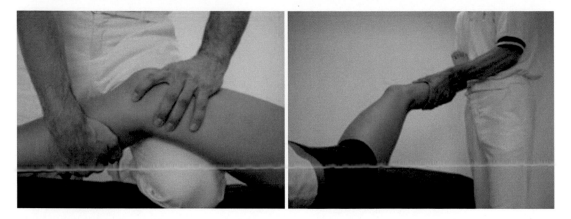

Fig. 11.2 Modified Lachman test (*left*), pivot shift test (*right*) -> crucial steps for clinical evaluation of an ACL injury

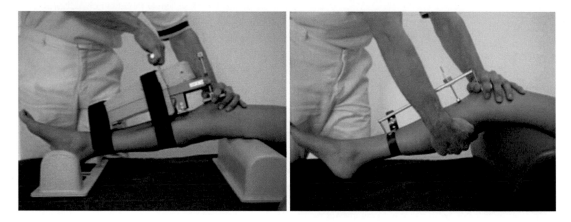

Fig. 11.3 Instrumented laxity measurement (*left*, KT-1000; *right*, Rolimeter®) -> crucial step for clinical evaluation of ACL injury

When the injury to the ACL has been evaluated in the described way as detailed as possible, it is crucial in finding the appropriate treatment for the patient to have a face-to-face interview with him (Fig. 11.4). In the course of the interview, it is important to talk about the sports activity of the patient, his/her profession, the expectation into the treatment and if a return to play in the old sports is desired or if a modification of the sports activities could be accepted by him/her (Table 11.1). With respect to sports activities, the patient may be classified according to the Tegner activity scale (scale 0–10) [28] or the IKDC definition of high- and low-level sports (level 1–4) (Fig. 11.5). At the end of the interview, the doctor should be able to come to an individual conclusion about the ideal treatment for the specific person and he should explain this

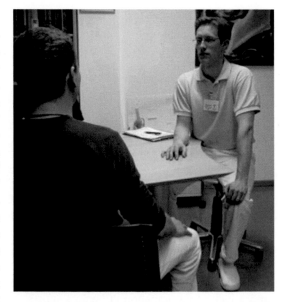

Fig. 11.4 Face-to-face patient interview -> crucial step to develop an individual treatment plan after ACL injury

Table 11.1 Variables being analyzed during patient interview

| Sports participation (kind and level) |
| Expectation of treatment (desire for return to play?) |
| Motivation for rehabilitation |
| Profession |
| Social environment |

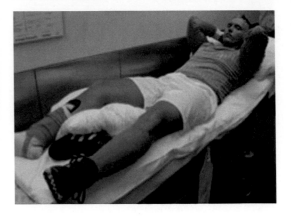

Fig. 11.6 Typical high-demand athlete 19-year-old male, football player 3rd league, Lachman + no firm end point -> no option for conservative treatment of ACL tear

Fig. 11.5 Treatment algorithm for ACL injuries (partial tear/complete isolated tear)

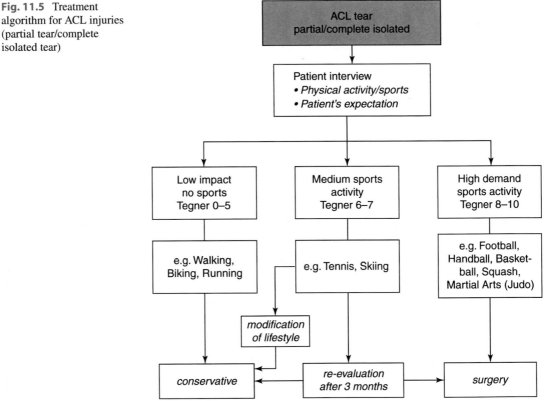

to the patient (Figs. 11.6 and 11.7). If a partial tear or an isolated complete tear of the ACL is present, a conservative treatment may be initiated. This will include physical therapy and, in some patient groups, a modification of lifestyle and a lack of participation in contact sports. In

Figs. 11.6 and 11.7, two typical patient examples are revealed with an indication for either operative or conservative treatment of an ACL tear.

If a conservative treatment has been initiated, a reevaluation of the patient is strongly recommended. We prefer a reevaluation at 3 and 6

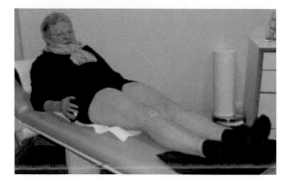

Fig. 11.7 Typical low-demand patient, 59-year-old female, ACL tear during hiking in the Himalaya, Lachman + firm end point, pivot shift test negative, expectation for sports participation hiking (Tegner 4, walk on uneven grounds) -> good option for conservative treatment of ACL tear

months, and 1 year after the injury. In case that giving-way episodes are reported by the patient or clinical examination reveals increased laxity or a positive pivot shift, delayed ACL reconstruction has to be considered.

> **Memory**
> Both conservative and operative treatment may be performed in patients with a partial or complete isolated tear of the ACL. After a thorough clinical work up, a face-to-face interview with the patient is crucial to find out about the sports activities and the expectations on the treatment. If a conservative treatment is initiated, a clinical reevaluation of the patient should be performed to verify if compensation of the injury can really be achieved.

References

1. Bak K, Scavenius M, Hansen S et al (1997) Isolated partial rupture of the anterior cruciate ligament. Long-term follow-up of 56 cases. Knee Surg Sports Traumatol Arthrosc 5:66–71
2. Beynnon BD, Johnson RJ, Abate JA et al (2005) Treatment of anterior cruciate ligament injuries, part I. Am J Sports Med 33:1579–1602
3. Borbon CA, Mouzopoulos G, Siebold R (2012) Why perform an ACL augmentation? Knee Surg Sports Traumatol Arthrosc 20:245–251
4. Casteleyn PP, Handelberg F (1996) Non-operative management of anterior cruciate ligament injuries in the general population. J Bone Joint Surg Br 78:446–451
5. Colombet P, Dejour D, Panisset JC et al (2010) Current concept of partial anterior cruciate ligament ruptures. Orthop Traumatol Surg Res 96:S109–S118
6. Daniel DM, Stone ML, Dobson BE et al (1994) Fate of the ACL-injured patient. A prospective outcome study. Am J Sports Med 22:632–644
7. Delince P, Ghafil D (2012) Anterior cruciate ligament tears: conservative or surgical treatment? Knee Surg Sports Traumatol Arthrosc 20:48–61
8. Dunn WR, Lyman S, Lincoln AE et al (2004) The effect of anterior cruciate ligament reconstruction on the risk of knee reinjury. Am J Sports Med 32:1906–1914
9. Fink C, Hoser C, Hackl W et al (2001) Long-term outcome of operative or nonoperative treatment of anterior cruciate ligament rupture–is sports activity a determining variable? Int J Sports Med 22:304–309
10. Fithian DC, Paxton EW, Stone ML et al (2005) Prospective trial of a treatment algorithm for the management of the anterior cruciate ligament-injured knee. Am J Sports Med 33:335–346
11. Frank CB, Jackson DW (1997) The science of reconstruction of the anterior cruciate ligament. J Bone Joint Surg Am 79:1556–1576
12. Frobell RB, Roos EM, Roos HP et al (2010) A randomized trial of treatment for acute anterior cruciate ligament tears. N Engl J Med 363:331–342
13. Ganko A, Engebretsen L, Ozer H (2000) The rolimeter: a new arthrometer compared with the KT-1000. Knee Surg Sports Traumatol Arthrosc 8:36–39
14. Gobbi A, Francisco R (2006) Factors affecting return to sports after anterior cruciate ligament reconstruction with patellar tendon and hamstring graft: a prospective clinical investigation. Knee Surg Sports Traumatol Arthrosc 14:1021–1028
15. Hawkins RJ, Misamore GW, Merritt TR (1986) Followup of the acute nonoperated isolated anterior cruciate ligament tear. Am J Sports Med 14:205–210
16. Hertel P, Behrend H, Cierpinski T et al (2005) ACL reconstruction using bone-patellar tendon-bone press-fit fixation: 10-year clinical results. Knee Surg Sports Traumatol Arthrosc 13:248–255
17. Hurd WJ, Axe MJ, Snyder-Mackler L (2008) A 10-year prospective trial of a patient management algorithm and screening examination for highly active individuals with anterior cruciate ligament injury: part 1, outcomes. Am J Sports Med 36:40–47
18. Hurd WJ, Axe MJ, Snyder-Mackler L (2008) A 10-year prospective trial of a patient management algorithm and screening examination for highly active individuals with anterior cruciate ligament injury: part 2, determinants of dynamic knee stability. Am J Sports Med 36:48–56
19. Kessler MA, Behrend H, Henz S et al (2008) Function, osteoarthritis and activity after ACL-rupture: 11 years follow-up results of conservative versus reconstructive treatment. Knee Surg Sports Traumatol Arthrosc 16:442–448

20. Kostogiannis I, Ageberg E, Neuman P et al (2008) Clinically assessed knee joint laxity as a predictor for reconstruction after an anterior cruciate ligament injury: a prospective study of 100 patients treated with activity modification and rehabilitation. Am J Sports Med 36:1528–1533

21. Meunier A, Odensten M, Good L (2007) Long-term results after primary repair or non-surgical treatment of anterior cruciate ligament rupture: a randomized study with a 15-year follow-up. Scand J Med Sci Sports 17:230–237

22. Mifune Y, Ota S, Takayama K et al (2013) Therapeutic advantage in selective ligament augmentation for partial tears of the anterior cruciate ligament: results in an animal model. Am J Sports Med 41: 365–373

23. Neyret P, Donell ST, Dejour H (1993) Results of partial meniscectomy related to the state of the anterior cruciate ligament. Review at 20 to 35 years. J Bone Joint Surg Br 75:36–40

24. Noyes FR, Mooar LA, Moorman CT 3rd et al (1989) Partial tears of the anterior cruciate ligament. Progression to complete ligament deficiency. J Bone Joint Surg Br 71:825–833

25. Noyes FR, Mooar PA, Matthews DS et al (1983) The symptomatic anterior cruciate-deficient knee. Part I: the long-term functional disability in athletically active individuals. J Bone Joint Surg Am 65: 154–162

26. Petersen W, Zantop T (2006) Partial rupture of the anterior cruciate ligament. Arthroscopy 22: 1143–1145

27. Pujol N, Colombet P, Cucurulo T et al (2012) Natural history of partial anterior cruciate ligament tears: a systematic literature review. Orthop Traumatol Surg Res 98:S160–S164

28. Tegner Y, Lysholm J (1985) Rating systems in the evaluation of knee ligament injuries. Clin Orthop Relat Res 198:43–49

29. Von Porat A, Roos EM, Roos H (2004) High prevalence of osteoarthritis 14 years after an anterior cruciate ligament tear in male soccer players: a study of radiographic and patient relevant outcomes. Ann Rheum Dis 63:269–273

Reasons for ACL Augmentation

12

Philippe Colombet and Rainer Siebold

Content

P. Colombet, MD (✉)
Clinique Du Sport, Bordeaux-Merignac,
2 rue Negrevergne, Mérignac 33700, France
e-mail: philippe.colombet5@wanadoo.fr

R. Siebold, MD
Institute for Anatomy and Cell Biology,
Ruprecht-Karls University Heidelberg,
Im Neuenheimer Feld 307,
Heidelberg 69120, Germany

HKF: Center for Specialised Hip-Knee-Foot Surgery,
ATOS Hospital Heidelberg,
Bismarckstr. 9-15, Heidelberg 69115, Germany

12.1 Biomechanical Stability

First, ACL remnants, bridging from the tibia to the femur, may add biomechanical strength in the immediate postoperative period to the reconstruction, while the graft strength depends primarily on the fixation device. In this period, the augmentation may be protected by the intact remnants and bundle and may allow accelerated rehabilitation and an earlier return to sports.

Different types of ACL remnants were reported by Crain et al. [10]. In the majority of its cases, femoral attachment is the posterior cruciate ligament (PCL), but in some cases, the ACL remnant bridges the femur and tibia, although its diameter is attenuated and its femoral attachment positions are slightly different from the normal anatomical origin. To some extent, this type of ACL remnant helps to prevent anterior knee laxity. In contrast, the ACL remnant attached to the PCL does not contribute to stabilization of the ACL-deficient knee. The authors examined the anterior laxity before and after ACL remnant debridement using a KT-1000 knee arthrometer in 48 patients and found that ACL remnants scarred to the roof of the notch (8 %) or to the lateral wall of the notch or the medial aspect of the lateral femoral condyle (12 % or 20 % of their series) contributed to the prevention of tibial anterior laxity. They concluded that ACL remnants may act like a biomechanical restraint against anterior translation.

The importance of the ACL remnants was reconfirmed by a modeling study of partial ACL injury with simulated KT-2000 tests by Liu et al.

R. Siebold et al. (eds.), *Anterior Cruciate Ligament Reconstruction,*
DOI 10.1007/978-3-642-45349-6_12, © ESSKA 2014

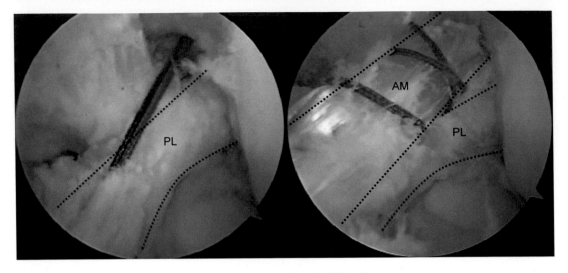

Fig. 12.1 ACL augmentation: PL bundle intact, reconstruction of AM bundle

in 2002 [15]. A computer model in sagittal plane was designed to simulate different levels of AM and PL bundle tears. Results showed that the degree of anterior instability was related to the amount of partial ACL disruption, and remnants may add to postoperative mechanical stability of the injured knee.

The importance of the ACL remnants, with conservative treatment, was also shown by Bak et al. [2]. They evaluated the natural history of partial ACL tears 5 years after the initial injury. Of 34 knees, 73 % had a negative Lachman test and 27 % a +1 or +2 positive Lachman test. Instrumental laxity testing in 24 knees showed 2 mm or less difference in laxity, compared with the uninjured knee. The largest side-to-side difference was 4.5 mm. However, only 62 % had a good or excellent knee function, and a significant decline in activity was seen. They concluded that ACL remnant may have an important role in the immediate rehabilitation period by providing additional mechanical strength while the graft is in the healing process.

12.2 Vascularization

A second important advantage of saving fibers may be that the residual portion of the ACL may maintain its blood supply, providing a support for the healing process in the graft. In an animal study by Bray et al. [6], standardized partial injuries were surgically induced to the anterior cruciate ligament in rabbits, and 4 months after the injury, the ACL was dissected and compared to a control group. The results showed direct injury induced significant increase in blood flow and vascular volume.

The vascularization of the human native ACL was investigated by Dodds et al. [12]. They described a vascularized synovial envelope around the intact ACL and periligamentous vessels penetrating the ligament transversely and anastomosing with a longitudinal network of endoligamentous vessels. Spared parts of the native ACL tissue may enhance the vascularization of the ACL augmentation. The authors also stated that the extremities of ACL have a greater vascular density, and the proximal part has greater vascularity compared to the distal part.

The time interval for maturity and remodeling, following arthroscopically assisted ACL reconstruction, was described by Falconiero et al. [13]. Superficial and deep biopsy specimens at different intervals from 3 to 120 months after ACL reconstruction were examined under light microscopy in 48 patients. The authors concluded that revascularization and ligamentization occur over a 12-month period following autogenous ACL reconstruction, with peak maturity evident after 1 year. By the 12-month period, the graft maturity resembles that of a normal ACL. Additionally, two of the four parameters observed, vascularity and fiber pattern, show statistically significant evidence that maturity may occur at an earlier time ranging from 6 to 12 months.

12.3 Proprioception

Saving ACL fibers may also maintain some proprioceptive innervation of the ACL. The joint position sense may be increased which may allow a faster and safer return to sports.

Schultz et al. described mechanoreceptors that resemble Golgi tendon organs beneath the synovial membrane of the ACL [16]. They published the first detailed description of mechanoreceptors in human ACL and suggested that they may have proprioceptive function. Schutte et al. reported that human ACL is extensively innervated and that neural elements comprise approximately about 1 % of the area of the ligament [17]. Proprioception of the knee has been measured in various ways, such as the joint position sense test by Co et al. [7] and Corrigan et al. [9], threshold to detection of passive motion by Barrack et al. [3], and latency of reflex hamstring contraction by Beard et al. [4]. It has been reported that in an ACL-deficient knee, proprioceptive function is less than that found in a normal knee.

An important study was performed by Adachi et al. [1]. They showed that the proprioceptive function of the ACL is correlated to the number of mechanoreceptors in the ACL. The authors measured the correlation between the number of mechanoreceptors and the accuracy of joint position sense in 29 knees. Interestingly, they also found mechanoreceptors in patients having a long interval between the ACL injury and the surgery and concluded that surgeons should consider preserving ACL remnants during ACL reconstruction.

These findings were reconfirmed by Georgoulis et al. [14]. They investigated the presence of neural mechanoreceptors in the remnants of the ruptured ACL as a possible source of reinnervation of the ACL autologous graft. The remainder of the torn ACL was selected for histological investigation from 17 patients during ACL reconstruction 3 months to 3.5 years after injury. They noted free neural ends in all patients.

In patients with an ACL remnant adapted to the PCL, mechanoreceptors exist even 3 years after injury. The authors also stated that if the theory accepts that restoration of proprioception is the result of reinnervation of the ACL, leaving the ACL remnants as a source may be a potential benefit to the patient.

Ochi et al. explained the restoration of knee function not only in terms of the reconstruction of the ACL as a mechanical restraint but also as a result of a sensory reinnervation of the reconstructed ACL [5]. They found somatosensory evoked potentials in about 50 % of the investigated ACL remnants as confirmation that the original sensory neurons are preserved to some extent in the ACL remnants. The occurrence of this in patients means that the ACL remnant may be an important source of neuralization for the graft. Denti et al. [11] and Barrack et al. [3] reconfirmed these findings for bone–patellar tendon bone grafts which were reinnervated 3–6 months postoperatively in animals.

12.4 Arthroscopic Orientation

Finally, intact fibers may also allow optimized accuracy of bone tunnel placement at the insertion sites. The bundle may serve as a guide for orientation and point of reference for the proper placement of the graft as described by Siebold et al. [19] and others.

> **Memory**
> Sparing intact ACL remnants during ACL augmentation or selective bundle reconstruction (Fig. 12.1) may have biomechanical, vascular and proprioceptive advantages [8, 18].

References

1. Adachi N, Ochi M, Uchio Y et al (2002) Mechanoreceptors in the anterior cruciate ligament contribute to the joint position sense. Acta Orthop Scand 73(3):330–334
2. Bak K, Scavenius M, Hansen S et al (1997) Isolated partial rupture of the anterior cruciate ligament. Long-term

follow-up of 56 cases. Knee Surg Sports Traumatol Arthrosc 5(2):66–71

3. Barrack RL, Buckley SL, Bruckner JD et al (1990) Partial versus complete acute anterior cruciate ligament tears. The results of nonoperative treatment. J Bone Joint Surg Br 72(4):622–624

4. Beard DJ, Kyberd PJ, Fergusson CM et al (1993) Proprioception after rupture of the anterior cruciate ligament. An objective indication of the need for surgery? J Bone Joint Surg Br 75(2):311–315

5. Boisgard S, Levai JP, Geiger B et al (1999) Study of the variations in length of the anterior cruciate ligament during flexion of the knee: use of a 3D model reconstructed from MRI sections. Surg Radiol Anat 21(5):313–317

6. Bray RC, Leonard CA, Salo PT (2002) Vascular physiology and long-term healing of partial ligament tears. J Orthop Res 20(5):984–989

7. Co FH, Skinner HB, Cannon WD (1993) Effect of reconstruction of the anterior cruciate ligament on proprioception of the knee and the heel strike transient. J Orthop Res 11(5):696–704

8. Colombet P, Dejour D, Panisset JC et al (2010) Current concept of partial anterior cruciate ligament ruptures. Orthop Traumatol Surg Res 96(8 Suppl): S109–S118

9. Corrigan JP, Cashman WF, Brady MP (1992) Proprioception in the cruciate deficient knee. J Bone Joint Surg Br 74(2):247–250

10. Crain EH, Fithian DC, Paxton EW et al (2005) Variation in anterior cruciate ligament scar pattern: does the scar pattern affect anterior laxity in anterior cruciate ligament-deficient knees? Arthroscopy 21(1): 19–24

11. Denti M, Monteleone M, Berardi A et al (1994) Anterior cruciate ligament mechanoreceptors. Histologic studies on lesions and reconstruction. Clin Orthop Relat Res (308):29–32

12. Dodds JA, Arnoczky SP (1994) Anatomy of the anterior cruciate ligament: a blueprint for repair and reconstruction. Arthroscopy 10(2):132–139

13. Falconiero RP, DiStefano VJ, Cook TM (1998) Revascularization and ligamentization of autogenous anterior cruciate ligament grafts in humans. Arthroscopy 14(2):197–205

14. Georgoulis AD, Pappa L, Moebius U et al (2001) The presence of proprioceptive mechanoreceptors in the remnants of the ruptured ACL as a possible source of re-innervation of the ACL autograft. Knee Surg Sports Traumatol Arthrosc 9(6):364–368

15. Liu W, Maitland ME, Bell GD (2002) A modeling study of partial ACL injury: simulated KT-2000 arthrometer tests. J Biomech Eng 124(3):294–301

16. Schultz RA, Miller DC, Kerr CS et al (1984) Mechanoreceptors in human cruciate ligaments. A histological study. J Bone Joint Surg Am 66(7): 1072–1076

17. Schutte MJ, Dabezies EJ, Zimny ML et al (1987) Neural anatomy of the human anterior cruciate ligament. J Bone Joint Surg Am 69(2):243–247

18. Siebold R (2008) One-bundle anterior cruciate ligament augmentation using the anatomic reconstruction concept. Oper Tech Sports Med 16(3):148–156

19. Siebold R, Fu FH (2008) Assessment and augmentation of symptomatic anteromedial or posterolateral bundle tears of the anterior cruciate ligament. Arthroscopy 24(11):1289–1298

Surgical Technique

13

Bertrand Sonnery-Cottet, Philippe Colombet,
Rainer Siebold, Pooler Archbold, Pierre Chambat,
Jacopo Conteduca, and Mathieu Thaunat

Contents

B. Sonnery-Cottet, MD (✉) • P. Chambat, MD
J. Conteduca, MD • M. Thaunat, MD
Centre Orthopédique Santy,
24 Avenue Paul Santy, Lyon 69008, France
e-mail: sonnerycottet@aol.com

P. Colombet, MD (✉)
Clinique Du Sport, Bordeaux-Merignac,
2 rue Negrevergne, Mérignac, 33700, France
e-mail: philippe.colombet5@wanadoo.fr

R. Siebold, MD
Institute for Anatomy and Cell Biology,
Ruprecht-Karls University Heidelberg,
Im Neuenheimer Feld 307, Heidelberg
69120, Germany

HKF: Center for Spezialised Hip-Knee-Foot Surgery,
ATOS Hospital Heidelberg,
Bismarckstr. 9-15, Heidelberg 69115, Germany

P. Archbold, MD
Musgrave Park Hospital,
Stockmans Lane, Belfast BT9 7JB, UK

13.1   Tibial Bone Tunnel Drilling

Bertrand Sonnery-Cottet, Jacopo Conteduca,
Mathieu Thaunat, Pooler Archbold, and Pierre
Chambat

13.1.1 Introduction

A number of studies have defined the ideal location for tibial tunnel placement. In addition a beneficial role of ACL remnant preservation has been proposed [1–11]. Based on these findings, it could be beneficial to develop a more biological technique for ACL reconstruction that preserves the cellular and neurovascular capacity of the ACL remnant [12, 13]. The technique described below has been developed in an attempt to achieve this.

13.1.2 Anatomy

Precise knowledge of the tibial attachment area of the anterior cruciate ligament (ACL) and its orientation in relation to the roof of the intercondylar fossa are prerequisites for successful intra-articular ACL reconstruction (Fig. 13.1). A number of studies have described the tibial footprint of the ACL insertion [14–20]. This attachment site is broad based. The distal insertion is located at the anterior intercondylar area of the tibia. In the sagittal plane, the anterior most part of the attachment is beneath the transverse ligament [21].

R. Siebold et al. (eds.), *Anterior Cruciate Ligament Reconstruction,*
DOI 10.1007/978-3-642-45349-6_13, © ESSKA 2014

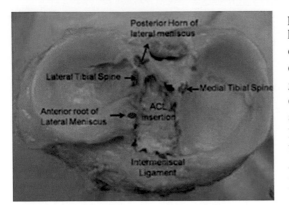

Fig. 13.1 Gross anatomy of the ACL tibial attachment and its relationship with anatomic landmarks (Reprinted with permission from the *Knee Surgery Sports Traumatology Journal*, Inc. [23])

Medially, the attachment is bound by the articular cartilage border of the medial tibial plateau; laterally, it is located near the articular cartilage border of the lateral tibial plateau with the most posterior part of the ACL attaching to the posterior third of the anterior intercondylar area on the upward slope of the intercondylar eminence.

Various anatomic landmarks have been described to aid correct guide pin and tunnel placement. These include the posterior border of the anterior horn of the medial or lateral meniscus, the medial tibial eminence, the ACL stump, the anterior border of the PCL, the roof of the notch and the "over-the-back" position located at the change of slope of the tibial plateau that occurs just anterior to the PCL. Jackson and Gasser proposed referencing four anatomic landmarks when placing the tibial tunnel, the posterior border of the anterior horn of the lateral meniscus, the medial tibial eminence, the PCL and the ACL stump [22]. Another important anatomic reference point described is the transverse ligament [23–25], which is arthroscopically identifiable at the anterior edge of the ACL tibial footprint.

13.1.3 Surgical Technique

13.1.3.1 Arthroscopic Portals
The correct placement of the arthroscopic portals is crucial for a successful and uncomplicated

procedure. The anterolateral portal is sited at the highest possible position just off the lateral edge of the patellar tendon and just off the inferior border of the patella. This position allows the surgeon to avoid the infrapatellar fat pad (IPFP) and ensures an excellent wide view of the intra-articular structures, in particular the intercondylar notch. The anteromedial portal is sited just below the inferior border of the patella and about 4 mm medially to the medial border of the patellar tendon [26]. Once inside the articulation, the first structure found and resected is the ligamentum mucosum. This is performed with a 90° flexed knee orienting the scope toward the anterior aspect of the notch. When the ligamentum mucosum is released, the IPFP is pushed anteriorly by the pressure of the intra-articular liquid (Fig. 13.2).

The IPFP may also impede adequate visualisation when positioning the tibial guide. When placing the tibial guide aiming hook on the ACL footprint, the arthroscope can enter the IPFP and vision can be reduced. To avoid this problem, the knee is held in 40° flexion. This helps to move the IPFP anteriorly with the patellar tendon, taking it away from the arthroscopic view (Fig. 13.3).

13.1.3.2 Tibial Tunnel Placement and Drilling
With the knee at 30° of flexion, the tibial ACL remnant is inspected. If fixed to the PCL or a non-anatomic site on the femoral condyle, it is carefully mobilised preserving its entire synovial cover and tibial attachment. The tibial guide is introduced through the anteromedial portal and positioned so that the guide wire either splits (Fig. 13.4a) or stays within the centre of the ACL tibial stump (Fig. 13.4b). If the location of the guide wire is satisfactory, the tunnel is drilled with increasing drill-bit diameters, stopping as soon as the bone of the tibial plateau is breached. The drill remains strictly within the ACL remnant to conserve residual tissue. A shaver is passed through the tibial tunnel, into the remnant to emerge at its upper end, so that the remnant is hollowed out for passage of the graft. The interior of the synovial sleeve is debrided to avoid

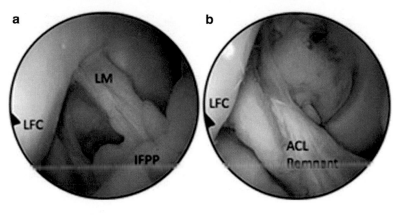

Fig. 13.2 Arthroscopic view of the knee. The ligamentum mucosum (*LM*) extends from the infrapatellar fat pad (*IFPP*) to the apex of the intercondylar notch impeding vision (**a**). The notch vision is considerably improved after ligamentum mucosum resection without additional notch debridement (**b**). *LFC* lateral femoral condyle

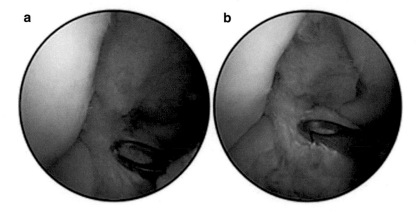

Fig. 13.3 Arthroscopic view of tibial guide placement. (**a**) Knee in 90° of flexion. (**b**) Holding the knee in 40° of flexion moves the IPFP anteriorly allowing an excellent vision of the ACL footprint without further shaving (Reprinted with permission from the *Orthopaedic Traumatology Surgery Research Journal*, Inc. [26])

overpacking of the intercondylar notch with the consequence of anterior tissue impingement and extension deficit (Fig. 13.4b).

Tricks and Pearls
- Use a guide with a ring-shaped target to easily visualise the emergence of the guide pin inside the ACL stump.
- During drilling whilst enlarging the tunnel, ensure that the entire tip of the drill has passed through the intra-articular cortex. Using a low rpm, the ACL remnant should "shake" when the drill gently turns inside it.

- During drilling reposition the guide pin manually through the tunnel and push it through the entire length of the ACL remnant before enlarging the tunnel by increasing drill-bit diameter.

Avoid Pitfalls
- Use a slower motor speed when enlarging the tibial tunnel with increasing drill-bit diameter. This avoids abruptly exiting with the drill into the joint and subsequent intra-articular damage.

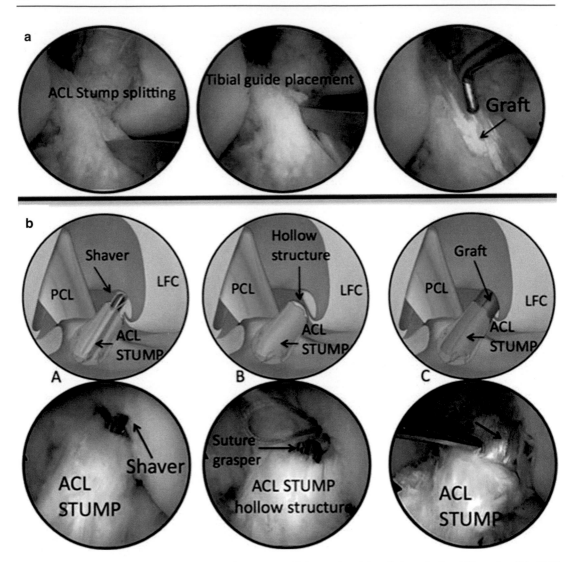

Fig. 13.4 ACL tibial stump preservation: ACL stump splitting option (**a**) and through the ACL socket (**b**) (*PCL* Posterior Cruciate ligament, *LFC* Lateral Femoral Condyle)

13.1.3.3 Partial Tear

Partial ACL tears are very common and account for 10–28 % of all ACL lesions. By placing the knee in the figure-of-four position, the ACL is observed from its femoral to its tibial insertion [27]. The augmentation of isolated AM or PL bundle tears is performed in a similar way to a "traditional" single-bundle technique whilst sparing intact ACL tissue. Remnants of the AM or PL bundle are useful landmarks for orientation of the tibial tunnel, and care should be taken to preserve these intact ACL fibres. If the AMB is to be restored, the tibial tunnel is placed within the anatomic footprint of this bundle; in PLB recon-

> **Tricks and Pearls**
> - Adapt the size of the graft; avoid use of a large graft (>8 mm) in presence of a large AM or PL remnant bundle.

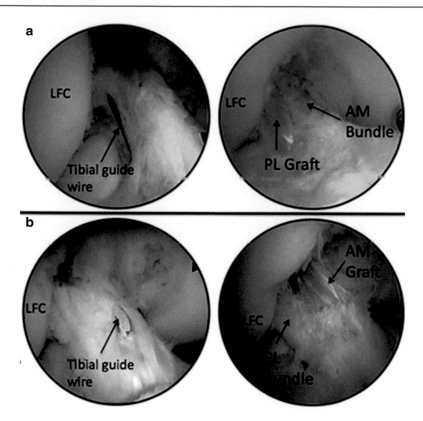

Fig. 13.5 Tibial tunnel for partial ACL tear augmentation. PL bundle reconstruction with guide wire placement in the posterolateral aspect of the ACL footprint (**a**) and AM bundle reconstruction with the guide wire in the anteromedial aspect of the ACL footprint (**b**)

struction, the tibial tunnel exits just posterolateral to the insertion of the AMB (Fig. 13.5).

13.1.3.4 Memory

The optimal location for the tibial tunnel remains a subject of considerable debate. However, the technique described in this chapter fulfils many of the criteria required to achieve this. By using the residual remnant of the ACL, it attempts to reproduce normal anatomy and can be easily applied for single-bundle, double-bundle and partial reconstructions. In addition it is proposed that by preserving the remnant of the ACL, it improves proprioception, graft vascularisation and integration.

13.2 Anteromedial and Posteromedial Bundle Reconstruction

Philippe Colombet and Rainer Siebold

This surgery is quite similar to a standard procedure for ACL reconstruction with some differences in the graft choice, notch cleaning, tunnel positions and drilling. Saving ACL fibres in the notch decrease the arthroscopic vision of bony landmarks and could lead to surgical errors, especially in tunnel positioning.

The patient setting is classic with a leg holder or not, depending on surgeon's habit. As it is a technically demanding surgery, the non-experienced surgeon has to stay in his own marks. Portals stay the same, an anterolateral arthroscopic portal is done close to the patellar tendon and an anteromedial instrumental portal 15 mm medial to the patellar tendon. Some authors propose to add a third low anteromedial portal to make the posteromedial (PM) bundle reconstruction easier [10] (see also Chapter 1.3).

An ACL augmentation requires a perfect vision of the notch, so start with the knee close to extension (20°–30° of flexion). This position provides a good view with the largest space of the anterior part of the notch and tibial ACL insertion. Carefully remove interfering parts of the fat pad with a shaver to have a good visualisation of the tibial ACL insertion and residual parts of the anteromedial (AM) bundle retracted under the intermeniscal ligament. Be aware to not remove too much fat pad as the Hoffa fat pad tends to scar causing postoperative trouble.

The next step is to assess the remaining ACL fibres. On the tibial side, it is quite easy because the vision is perfect and usually the ACL rupture occurs on the proximal femoral part of the ACL. There are two possible situations: (1) either one bundle is torn and the remaining bundle is intact or stretched, in anatomical situation on the lateral wall of the intercondylar notch or (2) both bundles are torn and the ACL remaining fibres are healed somewhere to the intercondylar notch (to

the posterior cruciate ligament (PCL) or to the femoral condyle). It is difficult to give a ruling on the exact lesion; a perfect knowledge of the anatomical ACL footprint is required [14].

Do not hesitate to shift the portals and to use the anteromedial portal for the arthroscope to improve the vision on the lateral side of the intercondylar notch. The shaver is helpful to better individualise the bundles and to clarify the type of lesion. Take care to use the shaver in a continuous function and high speed of rotation; in these conditions you will not be too aggressive on residual fibres, and the suction must be activated by small touch. Alternatively use a nonmotorised instrument which is much more harmless to use if you are not an expert.

The next question is to assess the mechanical properties of the bundles. The first test is to use the probe to pull on the remnants. Are they strong enough? How is the mechanical quality? Is it justified to take the risk of bad tunnel placement just to save these fibre remnants? A very good trick is to place the knee in the figure-of-four position [28] (Fig. 13.6). In this situation the PM bundle is tighten and can be better tested with the probe.

Two other points have to be considered: (1) the blood supply of each bundle, which might help graft healing [1, 29] and (2) the width of the intercondylar notch. Measurements can be done with an arthroscopic ruler [30] to match the graft size to the size of the insertion site and to the

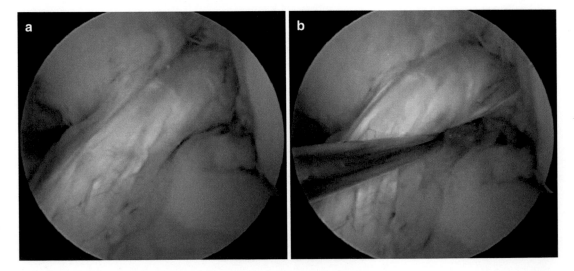

Fig. 13.6 (a, b) Probing of proximal PM-bundle in "figure-of-four" position

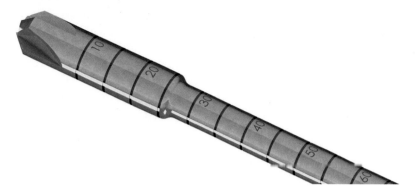

Fig. 13.7 Compaction drill for femoral bone tunnel drilling in "inside-out" technique. The drill is a safe instrument to protect remnants

remnants. Intercondylar notch impingement, especially with the roof, may lead to a postoperative extension deficit [27].

13.2.1 Graft Selection

It can be systematic according to the surgeon's experience. However, such a procedure is easier when using a none-bone block graft. Hamstring graft is widely used for such reconstruction [2, 8, 10, 11]. If you use a bone-tendon-bone graft, it could be difficult to manage the graft passage in the notch and its insertion in the second tunnel whatever the way of graft from the femur to the tibia or the opposite. The size of the graft is another issue. Pay attention with a too big diameter graft which can lead to a notch impingement. The space left in the notch by the intact bundle makes 7–8 mm graft to be the ideal size [4, 27]. The use of quadrupled semitendinosus (ST) graft should be a limitation for this technique. Three strands ST is the perfect graft setting for this use (Fig. 13.7).

13.2.2 AM Bundle Reconstruction

AM bundle reconstruction represents the large majority of cases [27, 31, 32]. The debridement must be done carefully to avoid any damage to the PM bundle. On the tibial side, the risk is to damage the remnant when the drill comes inside the notch, so decrease the drill speed when you

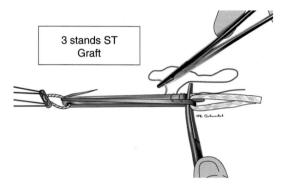

3 stands ST Graft

Fig. 13.8 Preparation of 3-fold hamstring graft

feel the cortical bone of the tibial plateau. It could be safer to use a router to drill the tibial tunnel; it is less aggressive than a classic drill (Fig. 13.8).

Siebold and Fu [10] recommend to set the tibial drill guide to 60° and the tunnel will start 1.5 cm medial to the anterior tibial tuberosity. The landmark is quite easy to find; it is represented by the anteromedial part of the native ACL footprint. It is recommended to save 3–4 mm of native ACL to help healing and to seal the internal aperture of the tibial tunnel by avoiding penetration of joint fluid inside the tunnel. The femoral tunnel is much more difficult to perform because the femoral AM footprint is located behind the PM, so the bony landmarks are not easy to find. The reference is the posterior part of the lateral condyle. A good trick is to place the shaver in a triangle represented by the notch, the PCL and the PM bundle, to go through, and to use the shaver as a bur in continuous rotation and high speed. Go in contact with the condyle and clean a small socket. This small socket will help you to stabilise the K-wire in a good place when the knee is placed in full flexion.

> **Tips and Tricks**
> Especially in ACL augmentation with restricted arthroscopic view, it is important to control the intended tunnel position on the femoral side. Therefore, we recommend to place a microfracture awl at the intended femoral tunnel position. Perform a lateral fluoroscopy to reconfirm anatomical positioning *before* definitive bone tunnel drilling (see Chap. 18).

When using an inside-out technique, insert a femoral K-wire into the marked femoral position in 90°. Increase knee flexion to 130° and advance the K-wire through the lateral femoral condyle. Overdrill the femoral K-wire carefully without damaging the remnants to the final graft diameter.

When using an outside-in technique, a specific aimer is required. Use a retrodrill to make the definitive socket. Think about protection of the PM bundle with a cannula when drilling the definitive socket from inside out and prefer a router, headed reamer or impactor to preserve PL fibres.

13.2.3 PM Bundle Reconstruction

Posteromedial (PM, see Chap. 1) bundle reconstruction is exactly the opposite, easier on the femur and more difficult on the tibial side because the tibial PM insertion is situated behind the AM bundle. The outside aperture of the tibial tunnel must be placed 3.5 cm medial to the tibial tuberosity [10]. Inside the joint the landmarks are medially in between the AM bundle insertion and the PCL close to the medial tibial spine (see Chap. 1).

On the femur, the tunnel must be placed close to the cartilage and just under and in front of the AM bundle when the knee is flexed to 90°. We recommend to mark this place with a chondropic to keep this situation when the knee will be fully

flexed. Siebold [10] proposed to set up the position an average of 5 mm posterior to the shallow articular cartilage of the lateral femoral condyle. Perform a lateral fluoroscopy to reconfirm anatomical positioning *before* definitive bone tunnel drilling (see Chap. 18). For easy drilling of the femoral bone tunnel, use an accessory anteromedial portal, just above the anterior horn of the medial meniscus. Be careful with the articular cartilage of the medial condyle which can be damaged by an aggressive drill and prefer a router or a headed reamer. You can also use an outside-in guide to be sure to prevent any condyle damage on the femoral side.

13.2.4 Graft Fixation

Many authors [2, 8, 10, 33] use a suspensory fixation such as Endobutton® system (Smith and Nephew, Andover, USA) for the femoral graft fixation and an absorbable interference screw on the tibial side. But the fixation is not specific and it is related to the technique used. The PM bundle has to be fixed at 20° of flexion, whilst there is no consensus for the AM bundle fixation angle. However, a fixation around 20° of flexion can be advised, too, from our clinical experience. Before fixation, conditioning of both the graft is recommended by bringing the knee through a range of motion for at least 20 times. After graft fixation finish the surgery by an arthroscopic control to exclude soft tissue impingement with the intercondylar notch.

> **Memory**
> A perfect arthroscopic assessment of the remnants is fundamental to know which ACL fibres are torn. Test the mechanical properties of the remaining fibres. An appropriated selection of portal is needed and a medial accessory portal can be used. Perfect adapted instruments are required to preserve fibres. The size of the notch can be an issue so the graft size needs to be matched to the empty space. Perform a lateral fluoroscopy to reconfirm anatomical positioning *before* definitive bone tunnel drilling.

References

1. Adachi N, Ochi M, Uchio Y, Iwasa J, Ryoke K, Kuriwaka M (2002) Mechanoreceptors in the anterior cruciate ligament contribute to the joint position sense. Acta Orthop Scand 73:330–334
2. Adachi N, Ochi M, Uchio Y, Sumen Y (2000) Anterior cruciate ligament augmentation under arthroscopy. A minimum 2-year follow-up in 40 patients. Arch Orthop Trauma Surg 120:128–133
3. Arnoczky SP, Tarvin GB, Marshall JL (1982) Anterior cruciate ligament replacement using patellar tendon. An evaluation of graft revascularization in the dog. J Bone Joint Surg Am 64:217–224
4. Buda R, Ferruzzi A, Vannini F, Zambelli L, Di Caprio F (2006) Augmentation technique with semitendinosus and gracilis tendons in chronic partial lesions of the ACL: clinical and arthrometric analysis. Knee Surg Sports Traumatol Arthrosc 14:1101–1107
5. Crain EH, Fithian DC, Paxton EW, Luetzow WF (2005) Variation in anterior cruciate ligament scar pattern: does the scar pattern affect anterior laxity in anterior cruciate ligament–deficient knees? Arthroscopy 21:19–24
6. Lee BI, Min KD, Choi HS, Kwon SW, Chun DI, Yun ES, Lee DW, Jin SY, Yoo JH (2009) Immunohistochemical study of mechanoreceptors in the tibial remnant of the ruptured anterior cruciate ligament in human knees. Knee Surg Sports Traumatol Arthrosc 17:1095–1101
7. Murray MM, Martin SD, Martin TL, Spector M (2000) Histological changes in the human anterior cruciate ligament after rupture. J Bone Joint Surg Am 82:1387–1397
8. Ochi M, Adachi N, Uchio Y, Deie M, Kumahashi N, Ishikawa M, Sera S (2009) A minimum 2-year follow-up after selective anteromedial or posterolateral bundle anterior cruciate ligament reconstruction. Arthroscopy 25:117–122
9. Ochi M, Iwasa J, Uchio Y, Adachi N, Sumen Y (1999) The regeneration of sensory neurones in the reconstruction of the anterior cruciate ligament. J Bone Joint Surg Br 81:902–906
10. Siebold R, Fu F (2008) Assessment and augmentation of symptomatic anteromedial or posterolateral bundle tears of the anterior cruciate ligament. Arthroscopy 24:1289–1298
11. Sonnery-Cottet B, Lavoie F, Scussiato RG, Kidder JF, Ogassawara R, Chambat P (2010) Selective anteromedial bundle reconstruction in partial ACL tears: a series of 36 patients with mean 24 months follow-up. Knee Surg Sports Traumatol Arthrosc 18:47–51
12. Gohil S, Annear PO, Breidahl W (2007) Anterior cruciate ligament reconstruction using autologous double hamstrings: a comparison of standard versus minimal debridement techniques using MRI to assess revascularisation. A randomised prospective study with a 1-year follow-up. J Bone Joint Surg Br 89: 1165–1171
13. Lee BI, Kwon SW, Kim JB, Choi HS, Min KD (2008) Comparison of clinical results according to amount of preserved remnant in arthroscopic anterior cruciate ligament reconstruction using quadrupled hamstring graft. Arthroscopy 24:560–568
14. Colombet P, Robinson J, Christel P, Franceschi JP, Djian P, Bellier G, Sbihi A (2006) Morphology of anterior cruciate ligament attachments for anatomic reconstruction: a cadaveric dissection and radiographic study. Arthroscopy 22:984–992
15. Cuomo P, Edwards A, Giron F, Bull AM, Amis AA, Aglietti P (2006) Validation of the 65 degrees Howell guide for anterior cruciate ligament reconstruction. Arthroscopy 22:70–75
16. Dargel J, Pohl P, Tzikaras P, Koebke J (2006) Morphometric side to-side differences in human cruciate ligament insertions. Surg Radiol Anat 28:398–402
17. Heming JF, Rand J, Steiner ME (2007) Anatomical limitations of transtibial drilling in anterior cruciate ligament reconstruction. Am J Sports Med 35:1708–1715
18. Kasten P, Szczodry M, Irrgang J, Kropf E, Costello J, Fu FH (2010) What is the role of intra-operative fluoroscopic measurements to determine tibial tunnel placement in anatomical anterior cruciate ligament reconstruction? Knee Surg Sports Traumatol Arthrosc 18:1169–1175
19. Purnell ML, Larson AI, Clancy W (2008) Anterior cruciate ligament insertions on the tibia and femur and their relationships to critical bony landmarks using high-resolution volume-rendering computed tomography. Am J Sports Med 36:2083–2090
20. Tállay A, Lim MH, Bartlett J (2008) Anatomical study of the human anterior cruciate ligament stump's tibial insertion footprint. Knee Surg Sports Traumatol Arthrosc 16:741–746
21. Arnoczky SP (1983) Anatomy of the anterior cruciate ligament. Clin Orthop Relat Res 172:19–25
22. Jackson DW, Gasser SI (1998) Tibial tunnel placement in ACL reconstruction. Arthroscopy 10: 124–131
23. Ferretti M, Doca D, Ingham SM, Cohen M, Fu FH (2012) Bony and soft tissue landmarks of the ACL tibial insertion site: an anatomical study. Knee Surg Sports Traumatol Arthrosc 20:62–68
24. Kongcharoensombat W, Ochi M, Abouheif M, Adachi N, Ohkawa S, Kamei G, Okuhara A, Shibuya H, Niimoto T, Nakasa T, Nakamae A, Deie M (2011) The transverse ligament as a landmark for tibial sagittal insertions of the anterior cruciate ligament: a cadaveric study. Arthroscopy 27:1395–1399
25. Nelson EW, LaPrade RF (2000) The anterior intermeniscal ligament of the knee. An anatomic study. Am J Sports Med 28:74–76
26. Sonnery-Cottet B, Archbold P, Zayni R, Thaunat M, Bortolletto J, Fayard JM, Chambat P (2011) High lateral portal for sparing the infrapatellar fat-pad during ACL reconstruction. Orthop Traumatol Surg Res 97: 870–873

27. Sonnery-Cottet B, Barth J, Graveleau N, Fournier Y, Hager JP, Chambat P (2009) Arthroscopic identification of isolated tear of the posterolateral bundle of the anterior cruciate ligament. Arthroscopy 25:728–732

28. Sonnery-Cottet B, Chambat P (2007) Arthroscopic identification of the anterior cruciate ligament posterolateral bundle: the figure-of-four position. Arthroscopy 23(10):1128.e1121–1123

29. Georgoulis AD, Pappa L, Moebius U et al (2001) The presence of proprioceptive mechanoreceptors in the remnants of the ruptured ACL as a possible source of re-innervation of the ACL autograft. Knee Surg Sports Traumatol Arthrosc 9(6):364–368

30. Siebold R (2011) The concept of complete footprint restoration with guidelines for single- and double-bundle ACL reconstruction. Knee Surg Sports Traumatol Arthrosc 19(5):699–706

31. Ochi M, Adachi N, Deie M et al (2006) Anterior cruciate ligament augmentation procedure with a 1-incision technique: anteromedial bundle or posterolateral bundle reconstruction. Arthroscopy 22(4):463. e461–465

32. Panisset JC, Duraffour H, Vasconcelos W et al (2008) Clinical, radiological and arthroscopic analysis of the ACL tear. A prospective study of 418 cases. Rev Chir Orthop Reparatrice Appar Mot 94(8 Suppl):362–368

33. Colombet P, Dejour D, Panisset JC et al (2010) Current concept of partial anterior cruciate ligament ruptures. Orthop Traumatol Surg Res 96(8 Suppl): S109–S118

Literature Results

14

Bertrand Sonnery-Cottet, Jacopo Conteduca, Pooler Archbold, and Mathieu Thaunat

Contents

B. Sonnery-Cottet, MD (✉) • J. Conteduca, MD
M. Thaunat, MD
Department of Sport Medecine,
Centre Orthopédique Santy,
24 Avenue Paul Santy, Lyon 69008, France
e-mail: sonnerycottet@aol.com

P. Archbold, MD
Department of Orthopaedic, Musgrave Park Hospital,
Stockmans Lane, Belfast BT9 7JB, Northern Ireland

14.1   Introduction

Although partial injuries of the ACL have been recognised for nearly 50 years, the optimal treatment for these injuries continues to be a subject of considerable debate. A question remains whether it is advantageous to preserve the ACL remnant and augment it with a graft or to debride it and proceed with a standard ACL reconstruction unhindered by the remnant within the notch.

Increasing scientific evidence suggests that augmentation of the intact remnant is beneficial in terms of vascularity, proprioception and kinematics. With this knowledge a number of surgeons have pioneered techniques to augment the intact bundle of the ACL in partial tears or to biologically enhance standard reconstructions by preserving the ACL remnant in complete tears. The objective of this chapter was to determine the clinical outcome of augmentation of the ACL.

14.1.1   Search and Study Selection

A literature search was performed using 'ACL reconstruction and remnant', 'partial bundle ACL reconstruction' and 'ACL augmentation'. Pubmed (http://www.ncbi.nlm.nih.gov/pubmed/), Cochrane database (http://www.cochrane.org/) and medline databases were searched on 29 December 2012 to search English language publications. At the first electronic search, 816 articles were identified. Full-text versions were obtained

R. Siebold et al. (eds.), *Anterior Cruciate Ligament Reconstruction*,
DOI 10.1007/978-3-642-45349-6_14,© ESSKA 2014

to include or exclude the study. The reference lists of the selected articles were reviewed by hand to identify articles not identified at the electronic search. All journals were considered and all relevant articles were retrieved. Studies focusing on clinical status of patients who had undergone ACL augmentation procedure with preservation of the remnant were selected. Finally, 13 publications relevant to the topic were included and evaluated (Table 14.1).

A total of 672 patients who had undergone ACL surgery with an augmentation technique were involved. Of the 13 studies analysed, only three included a control group without augmentation [1, 5, 13], the others reported the postoperative results of a single technique. The size of the studies was generally small, with only two studies reporting more than 60 patients [12, 13].

The PL bundle reconstruction is less investigated within the literature. Out of the 672 patients, only 106 cases described an isolated PL bundle reconstruction (16 %), and no studies showed the results of this isolated augmentation technique (Fig. 14.1).

14.2 Clinical Outcome

All the selected studies presented the clinical outcome of ACL surgery, measured by subjective and objective tests. The most used clinical outcome measures were the IKDC Score (9 studies), the pivot shift test (7 studies), the Lysholm Score (6 studies), the Lachman test (4 studies) and the Tegner Score (3 studies). The KT-1000 and KT-2000, Telos and Rolimeter were used to assess anteroposterior laxity.

Significant improvement of objective and subjective scores following augmentation was reported in all studies [1–13]. Of the three studies including a standard ACL reconstruction group [1, 5, 13], a significant difference was reported for instrumented side-to-side laxity in one study [1] with a lower side-to-side laxity in the augmentation group. No other significant differences were reported regarding clinical outcome in these comparative studies. We have found only one

multicenter study [12] involving 168 partial reconstructions of the AM bundle with preservation of the PL bundle. This confirms that irrespective of the graft or technique used, selective ACL reconstruction of the AM bundle restores knee stability and function.

Interestingly, in one study [6], satisfactory results were achieved suturing the partially disrupted fibres of the ACL and promoting their healing with bone marrow stimulation. However, this is the only study investigating this treatment option, and although the outcomes seem promising, there is not enough data to fully evaluate this technique.

14.3 MRI Evaluation

Postoperative MRI evaluation is reported in five studies [1–3, 6, 8]. Large discrepancies in MRI protocol and time points of evaluation exist among these different studies. Minimal tunnel widening and correlation between clinical findings and MRI appearance is reported in one study [3].

A correlation between graft coverage at the index procedure and graft incorporation at MRI follow-up is reported in another study as well as an increased incidence of a cyclops-like mass lesion without clinical significance [2]. A specific preoperative MRI protocol has been evaluated as a useful tool to diagnose ACL partial tear [12].

14.4 Second-Look Arthroscopy

Three studies reported evaluation of the augment by second-look arthroscopy [1, 2, 9] accounting for a total of 64 patients. Fair synovial coverage was reported in 58 knees and poor synovial coverage in six knees. In two studies and a total of 52 knees [2, 9], assessment of graft tension and continuity was performed at second-look arthroscopy. Thirty-six grafts were evaluated as taut, 10 slightly or mildly lax and 2 lax. The grafts were intact in 49 cases; partial graft tears were observed in 3 cases.

Table 14.1 Clinical studies

Study	Technique	Patients	Evaluation	Main results	Complications
Adachi et al. [1]	Augmentation. Femur: over the top. Standard ACLR. ST, STG graft +5 allogeneic fascia lata	Augmentation = Group 40 Standard ACLR = Group 40	Final FU >2 years Clinical evaluation + MRI ($n = 38$), J.P.S, second look at 1.5 years ($n = 12$)	*Augmentation > control group for KT 2000 and J.P.S $p < 0.05$* No significant difference in other objective and subjective evaluation Second look: good synovial coverage MRI: graft not distinguishable from remnan	No complication reported
Ahn et al [2]	Preservation and femoral tensioning of remnant. STG graft	53 patients	Final FU >2 years. Clinical evaluation + MRI at 6 months ($n = 48$), second look at 1 year ($n = 33$)	Subjective score significantly improved $p < 0.001$ KT 2000 preop 5.6 ± 2.7; postop 1.8 ± 2 $p < 0.001$ MRI: graft incorporation fair (27) poor (21), cyclops-like mass lesion (12) Second look: graft taut (27), mild laxity (6), partial tear (3) *Graft incorporation correlated with graft coverage at reconstruction* *Graft coverage at reconstruction correlated with time from injury to surgery*	Cyclops-like mass lesion without symptoms One graft rupture at 3 months
Buda et al. [3]	Augmentation of partial tear. Femur: over the top. STG graft	28 patients. 12 AMB tear, 16 PLB tear	Final FU = 27 ± 9.2 months. MRI study and clinical evaluation	Objective IKDC 25 A, 1 B, 2 C Subjective IKDC, 25 excellent 3 fair. MRI: tibial tunnel 6 slight enlargement, 22 decreased Graft continuity in 25 patients (grade 1 Yamato). Graft integration (Howell) 20 grade 1, 5 grade 2, 2 grade 3, 1 grade 4 *Excellent clinical results correlated with decrease in tunnel size and normal graft appearance at MRI*	One graft failure at MRI

(continued)

Table 14.1 (continued)

Study	Technique	Patients	Evaluation	Main results	Complications
Buda et al. [4]	Augmentation of partial tear. Femur: over the top. STG graft	47 patients (12 AM lesion and 35PL lesion)	Final FU 5 years. Clinical evaluation	IKDC last FU: 31 A, 14B, 2C. Tegner pre-injury 6.8, last FU 6.1 KT 2000: 41 <3 mm; 6 between 3 and 5 mm *No difference for AMB and PLB groups* *No graft rupture at 5 years*	No complication reported
Demirag et al. [5]	Augmentation group (PL bundle recons.) and standard ACLR. STG graft	Prospective randomised study. 40 patients, 20 in each group	Final FU 24.3 months. Clinical evaluation. Arthrofibrosis incidence. Tunnel widening	No differences in clinical outcome, arthrofibrosis incidence and femoral tunnel widening *Less tibial tunnel widening in the augmentation group (p=0.001)*	1 cyclops syndrome in the augmentation group
Gobbi et al. [6]	Primary repair with bone marrow stimulation of acute partial tears	26 athletes with arthroscopically confirmed partial tear	Final FU 25.3 months. Clinical evaluation. MRI at 6 months and final FU. Second look (n=4)	Final FU: IKDC 23 A, 2 B, 1 D. Rolimeter side-to-side diff improved from 3.7 to 1.3 mm at final FU. Pre-injury Tegner similar to Tegner at last FU. MRI at last FU: 9 normal, 6 normal insertion and local oedema 7 hyperintensity, 3 chronic rupture and 1 ACL lesion. Second look (n=6) good healing and stable to traction. *Effective in selected patients*	No complication reported
Jung et al. [7]	Augmentation + remnant tensioning (group 1)/ augmentation alone (Group 2), STG graft	33 in remnant tensioning group and 43 in augmentation alone	Final FU >24 months. Clinical evaluation	*Significant improvement of clinical scores* *No difference between the two groups* KT 1000 side-to-side difference at final FU 1.8 mm	Arthrofibrosis in 3 patients (2 in tensioning group, 1 in remnant preservation alone)
Ochi et al. [8]	Augmentation of partial tear, ST graft	45 patients, 37 AM bundle recons and 8 PL bundle recons	Final FU minimum 2 years. Clinical evaluation, J.P.S, MRI	43 patients with negative pivot shift, 2 glide. KT 1000 side-to-side difference, improved from 3.4 to 0.5 mm at last FU *Joint position sense significantly improved* MRI, 20 cases resembled one bundle, 9 cases 2 bundles	No complication reported

Ohsawa et al. [9]	Augmentation of partial tear. ST graft	19 patients, 5 AM recons. 14 PL recons	Final FU 40.9 months. Clinical evaluation. Second look at 12.4 months	At last FU: IKDC, objective: 10 A and 9 B. Pivot shift, equal in 17, glide in 2. *Second look, 13 graft taut, 4 slightly lax, 2 lax. 2 partial tear. No cyclops*	No complication reported
Serrano-Fernandez et al. [10]	Augmentation of partial tear. Femur: over the top. ST graft	24 patients, 20 AM recons. 4 PL recons.	Median final FU 6.2 years (minimum 2 years). Clinical evaluation	IKDC Final FU: 16 A, 8 B, 1 C, 1 D. No residual pivot shift. *KT*000 side-to-side diff: no diff for 11. 1 mm diff for 10 and 2 mm for 3 patients*	No complication reported
Sonnery-Cottet et al. [11]	Augmentation of ACL AM bundle tear. Out/in femoral tunnel. ST, STG graft	36 patients	Final FU 24 months. Clinical evaluation	IKDC at Final FU (n=33): 24 A, 8 B, 1 C. *Rolimeter side-to-side laxity improved from 4.8 to 0.8 mm*	2 cyclops syndromes (large graft) one traumatic graft rupture
Sonnery-Cottet et al. [12]	Augmentation of ACL AM bundle tear. Multicentric study. ST and STG (n=108), PT (n=55) and QT graft (n=5)	168 patients	Final FU 26 months. Clinical evaluation	IKDC at Final FU: 114 A, 40B, 6 C, 8 D. Objective, subjective IKDC and Lysholm significantly improved. Side-to-side instrumented laxity improved from 5.5 to 1.1 mm. *13% of patients with postop residual pain, correlated with postop flexum, correlated with type of graft (large PT graft)*	13 % residual pain. 9 cyclops syndromes. 3 % graft failure
Yoon et al. [13]	Augmentation of ACL partial tear. STG graft and standard ACLR	82 standards ACLR, 40 AM augmentation and 42 PL augmentation	Final FU 24.3 months. Clinical evaluation. Validity of preop MRI diagnosis	*No significant diff. Between the three groups for postop ROM, pivot shift, anterior draw test, Lachman test, instrumented side-to-side laxity and objective IKDC. 3 T MRI useful for partial tear diagnosis. AM tear associated with higher MCL tear incidence*	Limited ROM, 1 in the standard recons group, 1 in the AM recons group

ST semitendinosus, *STG* semitendinosus gracilis, *PT* patella tendon, *QT* quadriceps tendon, *JPS* joint sense position

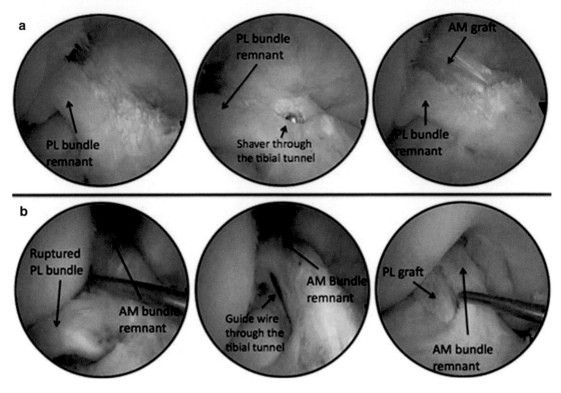

Fig. 14.1 Isolated AM reconstruction (**a**) and PL reconstruction (**b**)

14.5 Joint Position Sense

In an effort to assess postoperative knee proprioceptive function, joint position sense was reported in two studies [1, 8]. Significant improvement of joint position sense was reported after ACL augmentation procedure [8]. In a comparative study [8], the joint sense position was significantly better in the augmentation group than in the standard reconstruction group.

14.6 Complications

Cyclops syndromes associated with extension deficit were reported in augmentation procedure in three studies [5, 11, 12]. A total of nine cyclops syndromes have been reported in the largest series of ACL augmentation [12]. In this study, the cyclops lesion was significantly associated with a large patellar tendon graft, and several authors recommend to limit the graft size in order to avoid excess tissue in the intercondylar notch [4, 11, 12].

In a series of 76 patients comparing remnant preservation alone against a remnant tensioning technique, Jung et al. reported three cases of postoperative arthrofibrosis [7].

Graft ruptures are reported in three studies [2, 11, 12]. Two traumatic graft ruptures occurred in the earlier postoperative period (<4 months) [2, 11]. A 3 % rate of graft rupture is reported in the largest series of ACL augmentation [12].

> **Memory**
> The clinical outcome of studies investigating ACL augmentation in patients with preserved AM or PL bundle is encouraging. Nevertheless, there is a lack of comparative studies, which would allow a more vigorous evaluation of this technically demanding procedure compared to standard ACL reconstruction. Moreover, it is difficult to report on the benefits of leaving the ACL remnant using only clinical scores.

A standardised and validated evaluation tool to assess graft incorporation and proprioception function would be beneficial.

References

1. Adachi N, Ochi M, Uchio Y, Sumen Y (2000) Anterior cruciate ligament augmentation under arthroscopy. A minimum 2-year follow-up in 40 patients. Arch Orthop Trauma Surg 120:128–33
2. Ahn JH, Wang JH, Lee YS, Kim JG, Kang JH, Koh KH (2011) Anterior cruciate ligament reconstruction using remnant preservation and a femoral tensioning technique: clinical and magnetic resonance imaging results. Arthroscopy 27:1079–89
3. Buda R, Di Caprio F, Giuriati L, Luciani D, Busacca M, Giannini S (2008) Partial ACL tears augmented with distally inserted hamstring tendons and over-the-top fixation: an MRI evaluation. Knee 15:111–6
4. Buda R, Ferruzzi A, Vannini F, Zambelli L, Di Caprio F (2006) Augmentation technique with semitendinosus and gracilis tendons in chronic partial lesions of the ACL: clinical and arthrometric analysis. Knee Surg Sports Traumatol Arthrosc 14:1101–7
5. Demirağ B, Ermutlu C, Aydemir F, Durak K (2012) A comparison of clinical outcome of augmentation and standard reconstruction techniques for partial anterior cruciate ligament tears. Eklem Hastalik Cerrahisi 23:140–4
6. Gobbi A, Bathan L, Boldrini L (2009) Primary repair combined with bone marrow stimulation in acute anterior cruciate ligament lesions results in a group of athletes. Am J Sports Med 37:571–8
7. Jung YB, Jung HJ, Siti HT, Lee YS, Lee HJ, Lee SH, Cheon HY (2011) Comparison of anterior cruciate ligament reconstruction with preservation only versus remnant tensioning technique. Arthroscopy 27:1252–8
8. Ochi M, Adachi N, Uchio Y, Deie M, Kumahashi N, Ishikawa M, Sera S (2009) A minimum 2-year follow-up after selective anteromedial or posterolateral bundle anterior cruciate ligament reconstruction. Arthroscopy 25:117–22
9. Ohsawa T, Kimura M, Kobayashi Y, Hagiwara K, Yorifuji H, Takagishi K (2012) Arthroscopic evaluation of preserved ligament remnant after selective anteromedial or posterolateral bundle anterior cruciate ligament reconstruction. Arthroscopy 28:807–17
10. Serrano-Fernandez JM, Espejo-Baena A, Martin Castilla B, De La Torre-Solis F, Mariscal-Lara J, Merino-Ruiz ML (2010) Augmentation technique for partial ACL ruptures using semitendinosus tendon in the over-the-top position. Knee Surg Sports Traumatol Arthrosc 18:1214–8
11. Sonnery-Cottet B, Lavoie F, Ogassawara R, Scussiato RG, Kidder JF, Chambat P (2010) Selective anteromedial bundle reconstruction in partial ACL tears: a series of 36 patients with mean 24 months follow-up. Knee Surg Sports Traumatol Arthrosc 18:47–51
12. Sonnery-Cottet B, Panisset JC, Colombet P, Cucurulo T, Graveleau N, Hulet C, Potel JF, Servien E, Trojani C, Djian P, Pujol N, French Arthroscopy Society (SFA) (2012) Partial ACL reconstruction with preservation of the posterolateral bundle. Orthop Traumatol Surg Res 98:S165–70
13. Yoon KH, Bae DK, Cho SM, Park SY, Lee JH (2009) Standard anterior cruciate ligament reconstruction versus isolated single-bundle augmentation with hamstring autograft. Arthroscopy 25:1265–74

Part IV

Single Bundle ACL Reconstruction

Diagnostics

15

Rainer Siebold, Volker Musahl, Yuichi Hoshino,
Christopher D. Murawski, and Georgios Karidakis

Contents

R. Siebold, MD (✉) • G. Karidakis, MD
Institute for Anatomy and Cell Biology, Ruprecht-Karls
University Heidelberg, Im Neuenheimer Feld 307,
Bismarckstr, 9-15, Heidelberg 69115, Germany

HKF: Center for Specialised Hip- Knee- Foot
Surgery, ATOS Hospital Heidelberg,
Bismarckstr, 9-15, Heidelberg
69115, Germany
e-mail: rainer.siebold@atos.de

V. Musahl (✉) • C.D. Murawski
Department of Orthopaedic Surgery,
University Pittsburgh Medical Center,
Pittsburgh, PA, USA
e-mail: musahlv@upmc.edu

Y. Hoshino
Department of Orthopaedic Surgery, University
Pittsburgh Medical Center, Pittsburgh, PA, USA

Department of Orthopaedic Surgery, Kobe University,
Kobe Kaisei Hospital, Kobe, Japan

15.1 Clinical Symptoms and Findings with ACL Rupture

Rainer Siebold and Georgios Karidakis

15.1.1 Introduction

A rupture of the ACL is the most common ligament injury in the knee. Increased participation
in sports and other recreational activities expose
more individuals to the risk of ACL rupture.
Despite the improvement that occurred in recent
years in imaging techniques, clinical evaluation
including a careful history and physical examination is the first step for establishing a precise
diagnosis after an ACL injury.

15.1.2 History

Clinical evaluation of the knee should begin with
a complete history of the symptoms and a full
description of the mechanism of injury. In general

R. Siebold et al. (eds.), *Anterior Cruciate Ligament Reconstruction*,
DOI 10.1007/978-3-642-45349-6_15, © ESSKA 2014

50–80 % of ACL injuries occur in non-contact situations [1–3]; thus, a patient may describe a pivoting injury pattern on a fixed foot an abrupt deceleration or hyperextension [2].

Symptoms depend on the timing of assessment after trauma: in *acute* cases, the patient may present with a limp or even inability to load on the affected knee. The knee might be slightly flexed because of a painful effusion (maximum joint volume capacity) or might be flexed because of collateral ligament injuries. The patient may also complain of an inability to fully extend and/or flex the knee, painful movements, sensation of strain in the joint, and sometimes locking in a fixed angle. In *chronic* ACL insufficiency, the patient is usually able to walk but may complain of various degrees of instability from regularly to only in certain situations, such as descending stairs or pivoting sports. He/she may report pain and joint effusion periodically, especially after athletic activities. History also comprises questions about past injuries to the affected and the contralateral limb.

15.1.3 Physical Examination

The physical examination should include both the injured and contralateral limbs and begins with an observation and inspection: the patient may limp or may be unable to walk without support (crutches). Clinical effusion may be apparent visually, especially in acute cases where the patients usually develop a hemarthrosis, while a significant muscle atrophy could be present in chronic cases. Active range of motion, if feasible, should be recorded along with any limitations to full extension or flexion so that active range of motion can be further evaluated with palpation and passive range of motion of the knee. The next step is palpation, where the examiner should record any pain produced by pressing the bony landmarks around the knee and the joint line with the meniscus.

15.1.4 Special Tests

Abnormal anterior tibial translation is the basis for clinical diagnosis of an ACL-deficient knee. It is clinically assessed with the Lachman and anterior drawer tests or instrumentally with, e.g., the KT-1000 or KT-2000 knee arthrometer (MEDmetric, San Diego, CA) or the Rolimeter (Aircast Europa, Neubeuern, Germany) [4]. The ACL is the primary restraint to anterior translation of the tibia on the femur, and the ligament's greatest contribution occurs at 30° of flexion [5]. In an in vivo study [6], Beynnon et al. found that the ACL undergoes greater strain in response to an anterior force at 30° than at 90°. When the ACL is sectioned, maximum anterior translation occurs at 30°. After sectioning of the medial collateral ligament (MCL), anterior translation increases only in 90°, suggesting that the Lachman test at 30° carries diagnostic specificity for ACL deficiency [7]. Consequently, the Lachman test is the clinical examination of choice for detection of an ACL insufficiency, while the anterior drawer test (performed at 90°) places less strain on the ACL. Unfortunately, in the acutely injured knee, both tests (especially the anterior drawer test) may be of less value as a result of hemarthrosis and patient's pain and resistance. De Haven [8] showed that after acute ACL rupture, the Lachman test was positive in 80 % of patients examined without anesthesia but in almost 100 % of patients examined under anesthesia. Concerning the anterior drawer test, it was positive in only 10 % of patients without anesthesia and in 50 % of patients under anesthesia. Both tests had higher diagnostic value in chronic ACL insufficiency [8].

15.1.4.1 The Lachman-Noulis Test
The Lachman-Noulis test, as Pässler and Michel reported [9], was originally described by Georgios K. Noulis (1849–1919) in his doctoral thesis "Entorse du genou" at the University of Paris in 1875. This test, widely known as "Lachman test" described by Joseph Torg, MD [10], was named for his mentor John Lachman, MD, chairman and professor of orthopedic surgery at Temple University, Philadelphia. Although originally the author recommended holding the knee between full extension and 15° of flexion, now it is common to place the knee in 30° of flexion. The tibia must rest in neutral rotation, because in internal

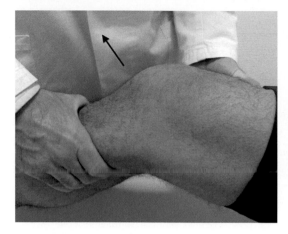

Fig. 15.1 The Lachman-Noulis test

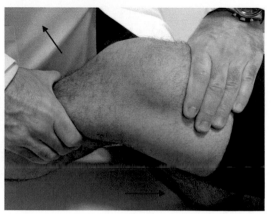

Fig. 15.2 The Lachman-Noulis test with leg support

or external rotation, secondary stabilizers will be activated, thereby confounding assessment of the ACL. Another point to mention is that the tibia must not be subluxated posteriorly as in posterior cruciate ligament (PCL)-deficient knee to avoid a false-positive test. The Lachman test has high sensitivity and specificity (about 95 %) [11], while false-negative results may be found in concomitant bucket-handle meniscal tears with anterior tibial translation [10], although other data indicate that additional injuries do not alter the test sensitivity [12].

The test is performed with the patient supine and the knee positioned in 30° of flexion. The examiner stabilizes the anterolateral distal femur with one hand and applies pressure on the posterior aspect of proximal tibia with the other, in an attempt to produce anterior displacement. A visible anterior translation of the tibia on the femur with "soft" endpoint represents a positive test result [10]. The results of the test can be described qualitatively and quantitatively, in comparison to the contralateral knee: An anterior translation of 1–5 mm is defined as grade I laxity, 6–10 mm as grade II laxity, and >10 mm as grade III. The quality of the endpoint is graded as firm, soft, or absent [13]. The Lachman test is illustrated in Fig. 15.1. A variation to the above proposed technique, especially when a disproportion between patient's leg and examiner's hands exists, is illustrated in Fig. 15.2. In this, the examiner's knee is placed flexed under the patient's femur so as his/her knee is flexed to 30° and stabilized by one hand, while the other attempts to produce anterior dislocation.

15.1.4.2 The Anterior Drawer Test

The anterior drawer test, as mentioned before, has many limitations, mainly because of the need to be performed in 90° of flexion, where the ACL is not the primary restraint for anterior translation. Also, the posterior meniscal horns and the bony contour may interfere with the test. Additional limitation may be the inability to flex to 90° in an acutely injured or swollen knee. Although the test accuracy is higher in patients with chronic injury, the sensitivity in an alert patient varies and is reported to be from 22 to 95 %, whereas in anesthetized patients improves and is from 50 to 90 % [11, 12, 14].

The patient lies supine and the knee is flexed to 90° with the tibia in neutral rotation. The examiner must ensure that the tibia is not subluxated posteriorly before performing the test to avoid misdiagnosis in a PCL-deficient knee and encourage the patient to fully relax the hamstring muscles so as to minimize their resistance to anterior translation. The test is performed with the examiner grasping the proximal tibia with both hands, placing both thumbs on the anterior joint line. The test is positive with increased anterior translation and a soft endpoint compared to the contralateral knee and graded similar to the Lachman test (Fig. 15.3).

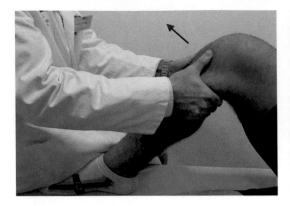

Fig. 15.3 The anterior drawer test

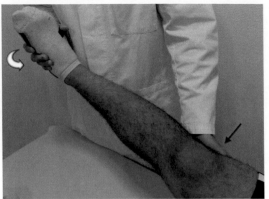

Fig. 15.4 The pivot shift test, starting position

15.1.4.3 The Pivot Shift Test

The *pivot shift* is both a clinical phenomenon that results in a sensation of giving way of the knee and a physical sign that can be elicited on examination. The phenomenon is characterized as an anterior subluxation of the lateral tibial plateau in relation to the femoral condyle when the knee approaches extension with reduction produced with knee flexion. Several studies have been performed to determine the diagnostic sensitivity and specificity of the pivot shift test in the diagnosis of ACL injuries. The sensitivity of the pivot shift test in ACL injuries varies from 84 to 98.4 %, with a specificity of >98 % when the test is performed with the patient under anesthesia, while in the alert patient, values as low as 35 % have been described [11, 12, 15].

The patient lies supine attempting to relax the leg muscles as much as possible. With one hand, the examiner holds the leg in full extension from the foot applying internal rotation to the tibia and with the other hand on the lateral aspect of the knee applies valgus stress while flexing it. In an ACL-deficient knee, the lateral tibial plateau will be initially subluxated (in less than 30° of flexion) and will reduce while flexion continues. This is palpable and sometimes also audible (Figs. 15.4 and 15.5). The pivot shift test is graded estimating the relocation event: grade 0 is considered normal, without reduction, grade I represents a smooth glide with slight shift, grade II is assumed when the tibia is reduced with moderate shift, and grade III when the reduction is abrupt with large shift.

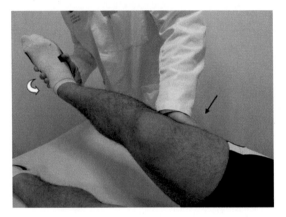

Fig. 15.5 The pivot shift test, ending position

15.1.4.4 Instrumented Manual Measurement Systems

The clinical tests described above are the most widely, single-plane tests used to evaluate an ACL rupture. Although the examiner should grade them quantitatively and qualitatively, this is not always feasible or precise and the result varies greatly between surgeons because of the inherent variability in the magnitude, direction, and rate of force application. The need of higher accuracy led to the development of various arthrometers and measurement systems. The first device of this type was the KT-1000 Knee Ligament Arthrometer (MEDmetric, San Diego, CA), developed by Dale Daniel and Larry Malcolm [16]. The newer version is named KT-2000. Many other systems followed, e.g., the Rolimeter (Aircast Europa, Neubeuern, Germany) [4], the CA-4000 Electrogoniometer (OSI, Hayward, CA) [17], the Genucom Knee Analysis System (FARO Medical

Technologies, Montreal, Ontario Canada) [18], the Kneelax3 (Monitored Rehab Systems, Haarlem, the Netherlands) [19], and the Stryker Knee Laxity Tester (Stryker, Kalamazoo, MI) [20].

KT-1000 and KT-2000 Arthrometer

These devices are widely used to quantify anterior tibial translation. They provide an objective measure of anterior laxity and have been shown to be both accurate and reliable [21]. Patient relaxation, correct positioning, and application of an anterior directed force are required, as with Lachman and anterior drawer tests [16].

The patient is positioned supine with the thigh support in a position to flex his/her knees to 30°. Then, patient's heels are placed on footrest to ensure neutral rotation. The device is placed on the knee to be tested (usually first the contralateral normal knee), with the arrows of the arthrometer pointing directly at the joint line and the measurement pads secured against the tibial tubercle and patella using the straps provided. The next step is to secure the device, placing the thumb of the hand not to be used for the application of anterior force on the patellar pad and the remaining fingers on the patient's lateral thigh aspect. The zero calibration point should be established next by applying alternating anterior and posterior forces to the handle of the device. After the reference point has been established, anterior translation measurements are recorded as three different forces are applied through the arthrometer handle. First, an anterior force of 67 N is applied, indicated by an initial audible tone. Second, a force of 89 N is applied, indicated by a different audible tone. Finally, a manual maximum force is applied to the posterior aspect of the proximal tibia, as in the Lachman test. A result that correlates with an ACL insufficiency is a maximum side-to-side difference of >3 mm, a maximum manual translation of >10 mm, or a difference in translation between the first two tests (67 and 89 N) of >2 mm [22]. The KT-1000 use is displayed in Figs. 15.6, 15.7, and 15.8.

Rolimeter

Rolimeter is another arthrometer developed for objective measurement of anterior laxity and

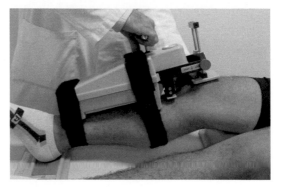

Fig. 15.6 The KT-2000, starting position

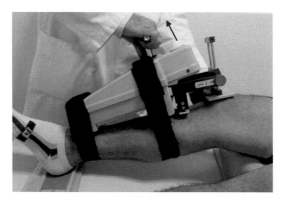

Fig. 15.7 The KT-2000, ending position

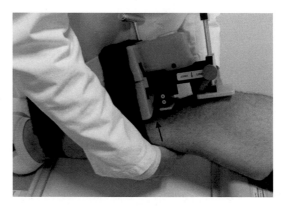

Fig. 15.8 The KT-2000, manual shifting

is found to have similar accuracy and reliability as KT-1000/2000 [4, 23]. It was also found to have inter- and intraobserver reliability [24], with the advantages of being less expensive, sterilizable, and simple in use. The patient is positioned supine with a thigh support so as the knee is flexed to 30°. Rolimeter is positioned with its patella pad on mid patella and secured with the

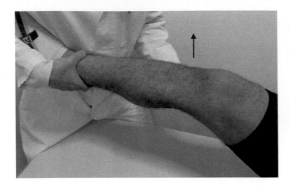

Fig. 15.9 The flexion-rotation drawer test, starting position

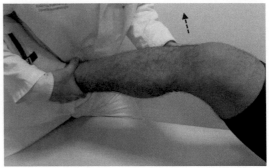

Fig. 15.10 The flexion-rotation drawer test, ending position

tibia strap. Then the stylus is slid so as to rest against the center of the tibial tuberosity and secured, and the white indicator is slid against the adjustment knob for calibration. Stabilizing the patella pad with one hand, the examiner tries to produce anterior translation with the other. The extent of translation can be read on the stylus.

15.1.4.5 Other Clinical Tests

Except for the Lachman, anterior drawer, and pivot shift tests, other clinical tests have been described to evaluate an ACL-deficient knee based on rotational instability in addition to anterior.

The *flexion-rotation drawer test* is built on the Lachman test and notes tibial motion and femoral rotation from 15° to 30° of flexion [25]. It is performed with the leg stabilized between examiner's armpit and hands that apply anterior force to the tibia starting at 15° of flexion. This leads to anterior subluxation, while further knee flexion leads to a reduction of the tibia beneath the femur with a noticeable "clunk" and internal rotation of the femur. This test is illustrated in Figs. 15.9 and 15.10.

The following tests are based on anterolateral motion of the tibia against the femur and are difficult to perform on an acutely injured knee.

The *jerk test* begins with the knee in flexion. The examiner holds the leg with one hand on the foot applying internal rotation and the other on the lateral aspect of the knee with the thumb applying a forward force to the fibular head and the other fingers valgus stress. This combination subluxes

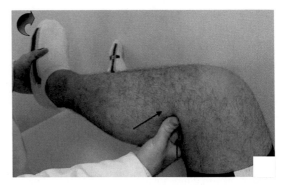

Fig. 15.11 The jerk test, starting position

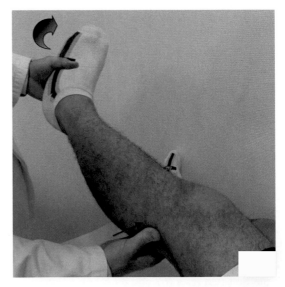

Fig. 15.12 The jerk test, ending position

the lateral tibial condyle anteriorly. As the knee is brought into extension, the tibia reduces with a palpable clunk (Figs. 15.11 and 15.12).

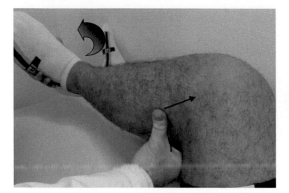

Fig. 15.13 The Losee test, starting position

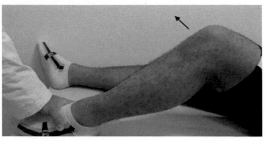

Fig. 15.15 The quadriceps active test

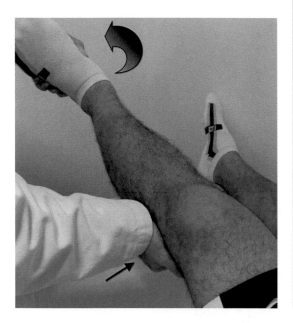

Fig. 15.14 The Losee test, ending position

The *Losee test* [26] is similar to the jerk test. The examiner holds the leg the same way (in flexion and applying valgus stress), but with the tibia initially held in external rotation. Subsequently, as the knee is gradually extended, the tibia is rotated internally and the clunk is again felt as reduction occurs (Figs. 15.13 and 15.14).

The *quadriceps active test for the ACL* [27] is performed with the knee held at 30° of flexion. The patient is asked to contract the quadriceps muscle, and this action will pull first the tibia slightly forward before the lower part of the leg begins to extend (Fig. 15.15).

> **Memory**
> The clinical evaluation is essential in the diagnosis of ACL rupture. The diagnostic sequence should begin with a history followed by a thorough physical examination including clinical tests. Several limitations are present, especially in the acute setting, and the examiner should consider them. Even a thoroughly performed clinical examination cannot be always feasible or precise. The results may vary greatly between examiners because of the inherent variability in the magnitude, direction, and rate of force application. The need of higher accuracy led to the development of various practicable arthrometers and measurement systems. However, further instrumental developments are necessary to assess the amount of multidirectional laxity and instability including the pivot shift test of the injured knee.

15.2 Imaging of ACL Rupture and Bone Tunnels

Yuichi Hoshino, Christopher D. Murawski, and Volker Musahl

15.2.1 Introduction

Anterior cruciate ligament (ACL) reconstruction has traditionally been conducted by placing a single ACL graft into the knee joint to replicate the native ACL. Although double-bundle ACL reconstruction has gained popularity to mimic the two functional bundles of the native ACL [28], single-bundle (SB) ACL reconstruction is still the most common technique for the ACL reconstruction. However, conventional (i.e., transtibial) ACL reconstruction has been proven to lead to abnormal knee kinematics [29, 30] and long-term degenerative changes [31]. Non-anatomic placement of the ACL graft has been suggested to contribute to unsatisfactory clinical results [32, 33]. The inability of the anatomic placement by conventional SB techniques has been demonstrated by advanced imaging techniques [34, 35]. This imaging technology could also provide useful anatomic information to improve the anatomic ACL graft placement.

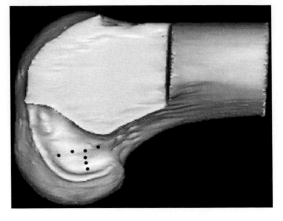

Fig. 15.16 Three-dimensional CT scan demonstrating native anatomical landmarks on the lateral wall of the intercondylar notch for the femoral insertion site of the ACL. The horizontal line (marked by *dots*) designates the lateral intercondylar ridge, whereas the vertical line signifies the lateral bifurcate ridge

15.2.2 Imaging of ACL Rupture

15.2.2.1 Radiography

In general, ACL rupture cannot be visualized by simple radiography. However, some secondary bony lesions due to ACL injury can be demonstrated on a radiograph.

A lateral tibial avulsion fracture, known as a Segond fracture [36], can be observed in around 9 % of ACL-injured patients [37]. The typical location of the Segond fracture is the mid-third of the lateral meniscotibial attachment, whereby traction force of the lateral capsular ligament is considered to produce this avulsion fracture [38].

Lateral femoral condyle and posterior aspect of the lateral tibial plateau is supposed to collide with each other while bucking the knee at the time of the ACL injury. This bony contusion can be often seen on the MRI [39], but radiographically visible bony depression on the femoral condyle, i.e., more than 1.5 mm, is relatively rare [40, 41].

The ACL is commonly torn at the ligament portion, but, especially in the pediatric population, tibial avulsion fracture at the ACL attachment site happens [42].

15.2.2.2 Computed Tomography

Three-dimensional computed tomography (3D-CT) can provide clinically relevant anatomic references. Purnell et al. [43] demonstrated that the lateral intercondylar ridge, also known as "resident's ridge" [44, 45], was clearly shown by 3D-CT images and can be defined as the anterior edge of the native ACL insertion site [43]. Moreover, Feretti et al. [46] described the bifurcate ridge on the lower third of the lateral wall which separates the AM and PL bundles [46], which can also be recognized via 3D-CT images [47] (Fig. 15.16). Although these small bony ridges are not always visible arthroscopically [48], they serve as landmarks from which useful information for identifying the original ACL insertion site and for performing ACL reconstruction in an anatomic fashion can be obtained [44, 47, 49, 50].

15.2.2.3 MRI

The ability of magnetic resonance imaging (MRI) to display soft tissues and the recent advancement of its resolution have boosted anatomic research for the ACL insertion site using MRI. MRI can identify the intact ACL, and only minimal side-to-side differences exist [51, 52] (Fig. 15.17). Therefore, identification of the individual ACL footprint in the contralateral knee using MRI may provide a truly anatomic reference for ACL graft placement in each patient. However, it has yet to be defined how to replicate the location indicated by the MRI during an arthroscopic procedure. Further research and technological development is warranted to utilize this anatomic information derived from the MRI as intra-operative references for the anatomic placement of the ACL graft.

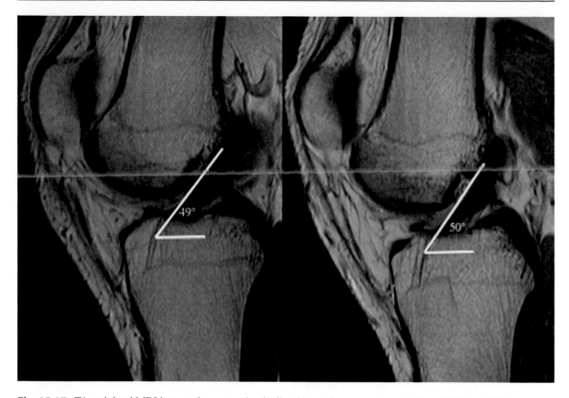

Fig. 15.17 T1-weighted MRI images demonstrating inclination angle measurements of intact bilateral ACLs

15.2.3 Postoperative Assessment of the ACL Graft Placement

15.2.3.1 Radiography

Simple radiography has long been used for determining the ACL tunnel placement. Traditional radiographic references for the femoral tunnel position in ACL reconstruction were the "clock-face" reference [53] and quadrant method [54], which were independently developed as fixed and universal scaling methods to describe the anatomical location of the ACL insertion site and graft placement. The "clock-face" reference has been utilized for referring the coronal position of the ACL insertion site and graft placement [55, 56]. This reference system can also be adopted for arthroscopic images [53]. However, the "clock-face" reference has been frequently criticized, and its reliability is now questioned [57–59]. On the other hand, the quadrant method, originally described by Bernard et al. [54], is still widely used for the location of the femoral ACL tunnel on the lateral X-ray of the distal femur [60–62]. This reference system can be utilized in a computer navigation system, which can accurately guide the operator to a fixed location [63] (Fig. 15.18). However, the anatomic location of the ACL in each individual patient varies on this reference system [60–62]. The indicated graft position is normally the averaged location by the navigation system and is thus not always anatomically correct for each individual patient. The clinical applicability of this system is also questioned, as the coordinate system is largely based on the Blumensaat's line. This reference line is not always clearly recognizable [64] and is subject to anatomic variation [65]. Also, intraoperative imaging of the distal femur affords the use of expensive fluoroscopy equipment and technical ability to achieve a true lateral view.

For the tibial ACL location, there are two reference methods for the anteroposterior position of the ACL; one was reported by Amis and Jacob [53] and the other by Staubli and Rauschning [66]. The difference between the two methods is the reference line. Amis and Jacob line is determined by the tibial plateau, while Staubli and

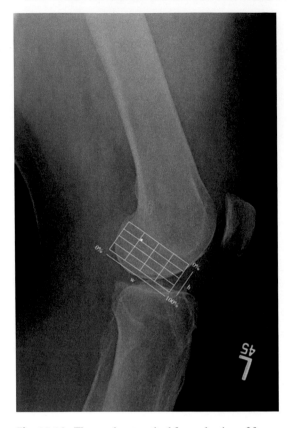

Fig. 15.18 The quadrant method for evaluation of femoral tunnel placement for the ACL based on Blumensaat's line on a lateral radiograph. The tunnel location is located at 23 % height of the quadrant (*h*) and 28 % width of the quadrant (*w*)

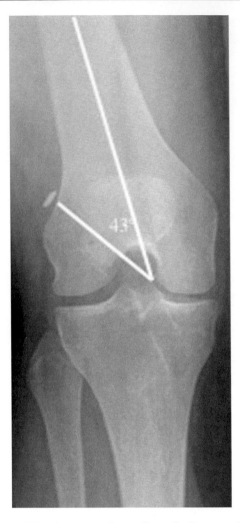

Fig. 15.19 Anteroposterior radiograph demonstrating the femoral tunnel angle relative to the long axis of the femur after single-bundle ACL reconstruction. A femoral tunnel angle greater than 32° is suggestive of anatomic tunnel placement [59]

Rauschning line is drawn based on the tibial axis. Both reference techniques can be used when the lateral view of the tibia is obtained. There is few established reference method for the mediolateral position of the ACL insertion which can be used intraoperatively. However, for the research purpose, the percentage or distance from the edge of the tibial plateau is often used for determining the ACL attachment location [67].

Imaging technology is often used for postoperative evaluation of ACL graft placement. Radiographic assessment of the ACL graft orientation using a plain anteroposterior (AP) radiograph can distinguish non-anatomic placement of the ACL tunnel relative to the long axis of the femur [68] (Fig. 15.19). This technique cannot provide any surgical reference for the ACL graft placement, but nevertheless serves as a reliable postoperative assessment of anatomic placement.

This assessment revealed that the ACL tunnel drilling via the transtibial technique frequently positions the tunnel outside of an anatomic position [68].

15.2.3.2 Computed Tomography

The advantage of CT imaging is the ability to reconstruct it three-dimensionally and to arrange the rotation of the three-dimensional image in a standardized orientation, providing consistent mapping of the ACL tunnel location [69] (Fig. 15.20). This technique can be used for accurate and repeatable analysis of the ACL graft tun-

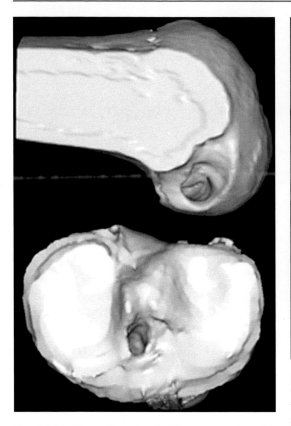

Fig. 15.20 Three-dimensional CT reconstruction of a single-bundle ACL reconstruction demonstrating anatomic placement of both the femoral (*top*) and tibial (*bottom*) tunnels

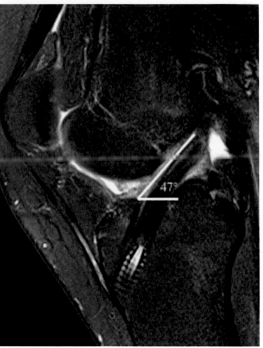

Fig. 15.21 Sagittal T2-weighted MRI image of a patient 7 months status post single-bundle ACL reconstruction using quadriceps tendon autograft. The inclination angle measurement is 47°

nel locations after reconstruction. The progress of CT imaging technique from a two- to three-dimensional modality has contributed significantly to the anatomic research of the ACL. Kopf et al. [35] demonstrated that, again, conventional transtibial drilling techniques failed to place the ACL graft into an anatomic position [35].

15.2.3.3 MRI
Similar to the CT imaging studies, recent studies using three-dimensional MRI assessment revealed that the ACL graft location after transtibial ACL reconstruction tends to miss the anatomic position [34, 70]. Inclination angle of the native ACL and/or the ACL graft can be simply measured on a sagittal cut of the MRI and can assess the anatomic adequacy of the ACL graft orientation [68] (Fig. 15.21). Although imaging assessment of ACL graft placement has made significant progress, it is mainly used for

postoperative assessment. To the best of our current knowledge, bony landmarks indicated by CT imaging studies can provide clinically available intraoperative references for anatomic graft placement. There still remains a problem of individual anatomic variation of the ACL footprint. Further research and development of MRI could facilitate individualized ACL reconstruction by using the contralateral intact ACL location determined by the MRI.

Memory
Imaging technology and its clinical application for the ACL reconstruction has evolved secondary to clinical demand for more anatomic ACL graft placement. The goal of anatomic ACL reconstruction is to be precise and to individualize the surgery. Therefore, universal radiographic references have lost popularity as a result of their two-dimensionality and the inability

to appraise anatomical variability. Three-dimensional CT can provide useful bony landmarks, which can be used as an anatomic reference for anatomic ACL placement during an arthroscopic procedure. Furthermore, MRI has an enormous potential to facilitate an individualized ACL reconstruction by using the contralateral intact knee as a template for true anatomic reference of the ACL footprint.

References

1. Arendt EA, Agel J, Dick R (1999) Anterior cruciate ligament injury patterns among collegiate men and women. J Athl Train 34(2):86–92
2. Boden BP, Dean GS, Feagin JA Jr et al (2000) Mechanisms of anterior cruciate ligament injury. Orthopedics 23(6):573–578
3. Cochrane JL, Lloyd DG, Buttfield A et al (2007) Characteristics of anterior cruciate ligament injuries in Australian football. J Sci Med Sport 10(2):96–104
4. Balasch H, Schiller M, Friebel H et al (1999) Evaluation of anterior knee joint instability with the Rolimeter. A test in comparison with manual assessment and measuring with the KT-1000 arthrometer. Knee Surg Sports Traumatol Arthrosc 7(4):204–208
5. Butler DL, Noyes FR, Grood ES (1980) Ligamentous restraints to anterior-posterior drawer in the human knee. A biomechanical study. J Bone Joint Surg Am 62(2):259–270
6. Beynnon B, Howe JG, Pope MH et al (1992) The measurement of anterior cruciate ligament strain in vivo. Int Orthop 16(1):1–12
7. Haimes JL, Wroble RR, Grood ES et al (1994) Role of the medial structures in the intact and anterior cruciate ligament-deficient knee. Limits of motion in the human knee. Am J Sports Med 22(3):402–409
8. DeHaven KE (1980) Diagnosis of acute knee injuries with hemarthrosis. Am J Sports Med 8(1):9–14
9. Paessler HH, Michel D (1992) How new is the Lachman test? Am J Sports Med 20(1):95–98
10. Torg JS, Conrad W, Kalen V (1976) Clinical diagnosis of anterior cruciate ligament instability in the athlete. Am J Sports Med 4(2):84–93
11. Katz JW, Fingeroth RJ (1986) The diagnostic accuracy of ruptures of the anterior cruciate ligament comparing the Lachman test, the anterior drawer sign, and the pivot shift test in acute and chronic knee injuries. Am J Sports Med 14(1):88–91
12. Donaldson WF 3rd, Warren RF, Wickiewicz T (1985) A comparison of acute anterior cruciate ligament examinations. Initial versus examination under anesthesia. Am J Sports Med 13(1):5–10
13. Lubowitz JH, Bernardini BJ, Reid JB 3rd (2008) Current concepts review: comprehensive physical examination for instability of the knee. Am J Sports Med 36(3):577–594
14. Jonsson T, Althoff B, Peterson L et al (1982) Clinical diagnosis of ruptures of the anterior cruciate ligament: a comparative study of the Lachman test and the anterior drawer sign. Am J Sports Med 10(2):100–102
15. Lucie RS, Wiedel JD, Messner DG (1984) The acute pivot shift: clinical correlation. Am J Sports Med 12(3):189–191
16. Daniel DM, Malcom LL, Losse G et al (1985) Instrumented measurement of anterior laxity of the knee. J Bone Joint Surg Am 67(5):720–726
17. Kvist J (2004) Sagittal plane translation during level walking in poor-functioning and well-functioning patients with anterior cruciate ligament deficiency. Am J Sports Med 32(5):1250–1255
18. Oliver JH, Coughlin LP (1987) Objective knee evaluation using the Genucom knee analysis system. Clinical implications. Am J Sports Med 15(6):571–578
19. Benvenuti JF, Vallotton JA, Meystre JL et al (1998) Objective assessment of the anterior tibial translation in Lachman test position. Comparison between three types of measurement. Knee Surg Sports Traumatol Arthrosc 6(4):215–219
20. Boniface RJ, Fu FH, Ilkhanipour K (1986) Objective anterior cruciate ligament testing. Orthopedics 9(3):391–393
21. Myrer JW, Schulthies SS, Fellingham GW (1996) Relative and absolute reliability of the KT-2000 arthrometer for uninjured knees. Testing at 67, 89, 134, and 178 N and manual maximum forces. Am J Sports Med 24(1):104–108
22. Bach BR Jr, Warren RF, Flynn WM et al (1990) Arthrometric evaluation of knees that have a torn anterior cruciate ligament. J Bone Joint Surg Am 72(9):1299–1306
23. Ganko A, Engebretsen L, Ozer H (2000) The rolimeter: a new arthrometer compared with the KT-1000. Knee Surg Sports Traumatol Arthrosc 8(1):36–39
24. Muellner T, Bugge W, Johansen S et al (2001) Inter- and intratester comparison of the Rolimeter knee tester: effect of tester's experience and the examination technique. Knee Surg Sports Traumatol Arthrosc 9(5):302–306
25. Nett MP, Pedersen HB, Roehrig GJ et al (2006) Clinical examination of the knee. Surgery of the knee. I. A. Scott. Elsevier Churchill Livingstone, New York, pp 47–61
26. Losee RE, Johnson TR, Southwick WO (1978) Anterior subluxation of the lateral tibial plateau. A diagnostic test and operative repair. J Bone Joint Surg Am 60(8):1015–1030
27. Daniel DM, Stone ML, Barnett P et al (1988) Use of the quadriceps active test to diagnose posterior cruciate-ligament disruption and measure posterior laxity of the knee. J Bone Joint Surg Am 70(3):386–391
28. Yasuda K, van Eck CF, Hoshino Y, Fu FH, Tashman S (2011) Anatomic single- and double-bundle anterior

cruciate ligament reconstruction, part 1: basic science. Am J Sports Med 39(8):1789–1799

29. Tashman S, Collon D, Anderson K, Kolowich P, Anderst W (2004) Abnormal rotational knee motion during running after anterior cruciate ligament reconstruction. Am J Sports Med 32(4):975–983

30. Ristanis S, Giakas G, Papageorgiou CD, Moraiti T, Stergiou N, Georgoulis AD (2003) The effects of anterior cruciate ligament reconstruction on tibial rotation during pivoting after descending stairs. Knee Surg Sports Traumatol Arthrosc 11(6): 360–365

31. Lohmander LS, Östenberg A, Englund M, Roos H (2004) High prevalence of knee osteoarthritis, pain, and functional limitations in female soccer players twelve years after anterior cruciate ligament injury. Arthritis Rheum 50(10):3145–3152

32. Marchant BG, Noyes FR, Barber-Westin SD, Fleckenstein C (2010) Prevalence of nonanatomical graft placement in a series of failed anterior cruciate ligament reconstructions. Am J Sports Med 38(10):1987–1996

33. Aglietti P, Buzzi R, Giron F, Simeone AJ, Zaccherotti G (1997) Arthroscopic-assisted anterior cruciate ligament reconstruction with the central third patellar tendon. A 5-8-year follow-up. Knee Surg Sports Traumatol Arthrosc 5(3):138–144

34. Abebe ES, Moorman CT 3rd, Dziedzic TS, Spritzer CE, Cothran RL, Taylor DC, Garrett WE Jr, DeFrate LE (2009) Femoral tunnel placement during anterior cruciate ligament reconstruction: an in vivo imaging analysis comparing transtibial and 2-incision tibial tunnel-independent techniques. Am J Sports Med 37(10):1904–1911

35. Kopf S, Forsythe B, Wong AK, Tashman S, Anderst W, Irrgang JJ, Fu FH (2010) Nonanatomic tunnel position in traditional transtibial single-bundle anterior cruciate ligament reconstruction evaluated by three-dimensional computed tomography. J Bone Joint Surg Am 92(6):1427–1431

36. Milch H (1936) Cortical avulsion fracture of the lateral tibial condyle. J Bone Joint Surg Am 18:159–164

37. Hess T, Rupp S, Hopf T, Gleitz M, Liebler J (1994) Lateral tibial avulsion fractures and disruptions to the anterior cruciate ligament. A clinical study of their incidence and correlation. Clin Orthop Relat Res 303:193–197

38. Goldman AB, Pavlov H, Rubenstein D (1988) The Segond fracture of the proximal tibia: a small avulsion that reflects major ligamentous damage. AJR Am J Roentgenol 151(6):1163–1167

39. Kaplan PA, Walker CW, Kilcoyne RF, Brown DE, Tusek D, Dussalt RG (1992) Occult fracture patterns of the knee associated with anterior cruciate ligament tears: assessment with MR imaging. Radiology 183:835–838

40. Warren RF, Kaplan N, Bach BR (1988) The lateral notch sign of anterior cruciate ligament insufficiency. Am J Knee Surg 1:119–124

41. Pao DG (2001) The lateral femoral notch sign. Radiology 219:800–801

42. Kendall NS, Hsu SY, Chan KM (1992) Fracture of the tibial spine in adults and children-a review of 31 cases. J Bone Joint Surg Br 74:848–852

43. Purnell ML, Larson AI, Clancy W (2008) Anterior cruciate ligament insertions on the tibia and femur and their relationships to critical bony landmarks using high-resolution volume-rendering computed tomography. Am J Sports Med 36(11):2083–2090

44. Shino K, Suzuki T, Iwahashi T, Mae T, Nakamura N, Nakata K, Nakagawa S (2010) The resident's ridge as an arthroscopic landmark for anatomical femoral tunnel drilling in ACL reconstruction. Knee Surg Sports Traumatol Arthrosc 18(9):1164–1168

45. Hutchinson MR, Ash SA (2003) Resident's ridge: assessing the cortical thickness of the lateral wall and roof of the intercondylar notch. Arthroscopy 19(9):931–935

46. Ferretti M, Ekdahl M, Shen W, Fu FH (2007) Osseous landmarks of the femoral attachment of the anterior cruciate ligament: an anatomic study. Arthroscopy 23(11):1218–1225

47. Fu FH, Jordan SS (2007) The lateral intercondylar ridge–a key to anatomic anterior cruciate ligament reconstruction. J Bone Joint Surg Am 89(10):2103–2104

48. van Eck CF, Morse KR, Lesniak BP, Kropf EJ, Tranovich MJ, van Dijk CN, Fu FH (2010) Does the lateral intercondylar ridge disappear in ACL deficient patients? Knee Surg Sports Traumatol Arthrosc 18(9):1184–1188

49. Ziegler CG, Pietrini SD, Westerhaus BD, Anderson CJ, Wijdicks CA, Johansen S, Engebretsen L, LaPrade RF (2011) Arthroscopically pertinent landmarks for tunnel positioning in single-bundle and double-bundle anterior cruciate ligament reconstructions. Am J Sports Med 39(4):743–752

50. Iwahashi T, Shino K, Nakata K, Otsubo H, Suzuki T, Amano H, Nakamura N (2010) Direct anterior cruciate ligament insertion to the femur assessed by histology and 3-dimensional volume-rendered computed tomography. Arthroscopy 26(9 Suppl):S13–S20

51. Scanlan SF, Lai J, Donahue JP, Andriacchi TP (2012) Variations in the three-dimensional location and orientation of the ACL in healthy subjects relative to patients after transtibial ACL reconstruction. J Orthop Res 30(6):910–918

52. Jamison ST, Flanigan DC, Nagaraja HN, Chaudhari AM (2010) Side-to-side differences in anterior cruciate ligament volume in healthy control subjects. J Biomech 43(3):576–578

53. Amis AA, Jakob RP (1998) Anterior cruciate ligament graft positioning, tensioning and twisting. Knee Surg Sports Traumatol Arthrosc 6(Suppl 1): S2–S12

54. Bernard M, Hertel P, Hornung H, Cierpinski T (1997) Femoral insertion of the ACL. Radiographic quadrant method. Am J Knee Surg 10(1):14–21; discussion 21-22

55. Loh JC, Fukuda Y, Tsuda E, Steadman RJ, Fu FH, Woo SL (2003) Knee stability and graft function following anterior cruciate ligament reconstruction:

comparison between 11 o'clock and 10 o'clock femoral tunnel placement. Arthroscopy 19(3):297–304

56. Rue JP, Ghodadra N, Bach BR Jr (2008) Femoral tunnel placement in single-bundle anterior cruciate ligament reconstruction: a cadaveric study relating transtibial lateralized femoral tunnel position to the anteromedial and posterolateral bundle femoral origins of the anterior cruciate ligament. Am J Sports Med 36(1):73–79

57. Fu FH (2008) The clock-face reference: simple but nonanatomic. Arthroscopy 24(12):1433; author reply 1434

58. Colvin AC, Shen W, Musahl V, Fu FH (2009) Avoiding pitfalls in anatomic ACL reconstruction. Knee Surg Sports Traumatol Arthrosc 17(8):956–963

59. Azzam MG, Lenarz CJ, Farrow LD, Israel HA, Kieffer DA, Kaar SG (2011) Inter- and intraobserver reliability of the clock face representation as used to describe the femoral intercondylar notch. Knee Surg Sports Traumatol Arthrosc 19(8):1265–1270

60. Colombet P, Robinson J, Christel P, Franceschi JP, Djian P, Bellier G, Sbihi A (2006) Morphology of anterior cruciate ligament attachments for anatomic reconstruction: a cadaveric dissection and radiographic study. Arthroscopy 22(9):984–992

61. Takahashi M, Doi M, Abe M, Suzuki D, Nagano A (2006) Anatomical study of the femoral and tibial insertions of the anteromedial and posterolateral bundles of human anterior cruciate ligament. Am J Sports Med 34(5):787–792

62. Zantop T, Wellmann M, Fu FH, Petersen W (2008) Tunnel positioning of anteromedial and posterolateral bundles in anatomic anterior cruciate ligament reconstruction: anatomic and radiographic findings. Am J Sports Med 36(1):65–72

63. Kawakami Y, Hiranaka T, Matsumoto T, Hida Y, Fukui T, Uemoto H, Doita M, Tsuji M, Kurosaka M, Kuroda R (2012) The accuracy of bone tunnel position using fluoroscopic-based navigation system in anterior cruciate ligament reconstruction. Knee Surg Sports Traumatol Arthrosc 20(8):1503–1510

64. Farrow LD, Chen MR, Cooperman DR, Goodfellow DB, Robbin MS (2008) Radiographic classification of the femoral intercondylar notch posterolateral rim. Arthroscopy 24(10):1109–1114

65. Berg GE, Ta'ala SC, Kontanis EJ, Leney SS (2007) Measuring the intercondylar shelf angle using radiographs: intra- and inter-observer error tests of reliability. J Forensic Sci 52(5):1020–1024

66. Staubli HU, Rauschning W (1994) Tibial attachment area of the anterior cruciate ligament in the extended knee position. Anatomy and cryosections in vitro complemented by magnetic resonance arthrography in vivo. Knee Surg Sports Traumatol Arthrosc 2:138–146

67. Doi M, Takahashi M, Abe M, Suzuki D, Nagano A (2009) Lateral radiographic study of the tibial sagittal insertions of the anteromedial and posterolateral bundles of human anterior cruciate ligament. Knee Surg Sports Traumatol Arthrosc 17(4):347–351

68. Illingworth KD, Hensler D, Working ZM, Macalena JA, Tashman S, Fu FH (2011) A simple evaluation of anterior cruciate ligament femoral tunnel position: the inclination angle and femoral tunnel angle. Am J Sports Med 39(12):2611–2618

69. Forsythe B, Kopf S, Wong AK, Martins CA, Anderst W, Tashman S, Fu FH (2010) The location of femoral and tibial tunnels in anatomic double-bundle anterior cruciate ligament reconstruction analyzed by three-dimensional computed tomography models. J Bone Joint Surg Am 92(6):1418–1426

70. Bowers AL, Bedi A, Lipman JD, Potter HG, Rodeo SA, Pearle AD, Warren RF, Altchek DW (2011) Comparison of anterior cruciate ligament tunnel position and graft obliquity with transtibial and anteromedial portal femoral tunnel reaming techniques using high-resolution magnetic resonance imaging. Arthroscopy 27(11):1511–1522

Timing of ACL Surgery: Any Evidence?

16

Michael E. Hantes and Alexander Tsarouhas

Contents

Establishing the optimal timing for ACL reconstruction is particularly important for patients, treating surgeons, and health-care systems. When ACL reconstruction is performed within the first weeks after injury, knee effusion, ROM deficits, and rehabilitation protocols more strongly affect the clinical outcome than the actual timing of surgery. Accumulated evidence from the existing body of literature suggests a significant relationship between the duration of ACL deficiency and the subsequent incidence of secondary chondral and medial meniscal injuries. Although prospective comparisons are lacking, most authors suggest that to avoid the risk of additional damage, ACL reconstruction should preferably be performed within 6 months from injury. Skeletally immature patients are at a similar risk of developing secondary lesions and should be prioritized for ACL reconstruction with appropriate physeal-sparing techniques.

16.1 Introduction

The optimal timing for the reconstruction of the anterior cruciate ligament (ACL) currently remains controversial. There has been considerable debate in the literature regarding both the earliest time that the reconstruction can be performed with safety and the time that surgery can be delayed without increasing the risk of developing secondary knee lesions. In a national survey among UK orthopedic surgeons in the early

M.E. Hantes, MD (✉)
Department of Orthopaedic Surgery,
Faculty of Medicine, School of Health Sciences,
University of Thessaly, 41110 Mezourlo area,
Larissa, Greece
e-mail: hantesmi@otenet.gr

A. Tsarouhas, MD
Department of Orthopaedic Surgery,
Trikala General Hospital,
16 Omogenon Amerikis str, Kalambaka, Thessaly
42200, Greece

R. Siebold et al. (eds.), *Anterior Cruciate Ligament Reconstruction*,
DOI 10.1007/978-3-642-45349-6_16, © ESSKA 2014

2000s [6], 81 % advocated that surgery should ideally be performed between 1 and 6 months post-injury. However, it was acknowledged that only 35 % of ACL reconstructions are performed within this time frame in National Health Service (NHS) hospitals. Additional concerns have been raised in the pediatric and adolescent population where the risk of damaging open physes should be weighted against that of secondary meniscal and chondral injury. It is clear that establishing the optimal timing for ACL reconstruction is particularly important for both the treating surgeons and the patients. Apart from the need to prioritize the patients, cost and cost-benefit issues may well ensue in health-care systems with extended waiting lists and finite resources.

16.2 How Early to Perform ACL Reconstruction

In their landmark study, Shelbourne et al. [16] demonstrated that ACL reconstructions performed beyond 3 weeks post-injury were at significantly lower risk of developing arthrofibrosis compared with those performed within the first 3 weeks. Delaying surgical intervention was considered to allow knee range of motion (ROM) to be restored to preoperative levels and surrounding soft tissues to recover from the initial injury. In addition, it offers the patient the opportunity to determine if he/she can ultimately cope without reconstructing the ligament.

In contrast, advocates of immediate surgical intervention have suggested that restoring tibiofemoral stability minimizes the risk of further meniscal and chondral injury. Although specific cost-benefit studies are lacking, early surgery also aims to expedite the return to sporting and occupational activities, with considerable economic consequences. In addition, it is considered to prevent significant quadriceps muscle atrophy and reduced strength, which is now acknowledged as a chief determinant of clinical outcomes and re-rupture risk [5, 12]. In their prospective level one study, Bottoni et al. [1] found that

excellent clinical results can be achieved after ACL reconstructions performed soon after injury using autograft hamstrings. However, the authors did not advocate all reconstructions to be performed acutely. In a recent meta-analysis of 370 ACL reconstructions in total, Smith et al. [18] found no significant difference in postoperative functional knee scores, tibiofemoral laxity, knee stability tests, and range of motion between patients who underwent early (within a mean of 3 weeks post-injury) compared to delayed (a minimum 6 weeks post-injury) ACL reconstruction. However, the authors documented a substantial heterogeneity and methodological limitations in the studies examined.

Recent research has focused on other factors that affect the outcomes of ACL reconstruction when performed early after injury. Mayr et al. [11] retrospectively reviewed a large cohort of 156 ACL-reconstructed patients with postoperative arthrofibrosis. They found that knee irritation, effusion, and swelling following the acute injury significantly correlated with the development of arthrofibrosis. Similarly, Cosgarea et al. [3] suggested that arthrofibrosis was significantly more likely in patients with a preoperative motion deficit of 10° or greater compared to those without. Presumably, in a recent survey, 993 American Orthopaedic Society for Sports Medicine members responded that they regarded knee ROM and effusion as the most important factors in deciding the timing of ACL reconstruction [5]. The use of an accelerated rehabilitation program has also been considered to significantly affect the incidence of arthrofibrosis [1, 16]. It is possible that evolutions in rehabilitation strategies and ACL reconstruction techniques have limited the effect of early surgical timing on knee stiffness and arthrofibrosis and partially explain the diversity between study outcomes. A most recent meta-analysis of studies that employed a modern accelerated rehabilitation protocol found no significant difference in the risk of adverse outcomes between early and delayed ACL reconstruction using multiple cutoff points (1–20 weeks). The authors concluded that if a modern surgical technique and accelerated rehabilitation protocol are used, ACL reconstruction can safely be performed as early as the first week after injury [10].

16.3 How Long Can ACL Reconstruction Be Delayed

The association between ACL injury and meniscal and chondral pathology has long been established. Several studies have demonstrated a predominance of lateral meniscal tears in the acute setting and an increase in the incidence of medial tears as the time from injury elapses. The complexity of the tears increases in the chronic stage, and, consequently, tears are less amenable to repair as time elapses [2].

Clinical and imaging studies have shown that the incidence of medial meniscal injuries presents a clear temporal relationship after the ACL ruptures [14, 21]. It is not clear whether secondary injuries occur as a consequence of tibiofemoral laxity and translation combined with long-term changes in dynamic joint loading or they are caused by the initial injury and subsequently deteriorate. On the contrary, the incidence of lateral meniscal tears does not increase significantly with time [9, 19], which suggests that these lesions result from the index injury.

An increase in the number and grade of cartilage lesions with increasing time from injury is a consistent finding in many studies [9, 20]. The medial femoral condyle is the most commonly affected. It is possible that these lesions evolve from a low-grade defect of the articular cartilage caused by the initial episode of tibiofemoral subluxation and subsequently tend to deteriorate as a result of both recurrent instability and attritional wear due to coexisting meniscal tears. Cartilage lesions have been found to occur nearly twice as frequently when a meniscal tear is also present, and vice versa [7].

Although a consensus has been reached regarding the benefits of timely restoring knee stability to significantly diminish the incidence of secondary meniscal and chondral lesions, the optimal timing of ACL reconstruction has only recently been elucidated. Studies reviewing large retrospective cohorts and national registries have offered stronger comparisons using multiple cut-off points. In a single-surgeon series of 300 patients, Kennedy et al. [9] found a significantly higher chance of a medial meniscal tear when ACL reconstruction was performed 6 months after injury and of knee degenerative changes with surgery performed a year post-injury. In a large retrospective cohort from the Norwegian National Knee Ligament Registry, Granan et al. [7] found that the odds of a cartilage lesion in the adult knee increased by nearly 1 % for each month that elapsed from injury to surgery. In a most recent study, Sri-ram et al. [19] reviewed 5,086 patients undergoing ACL reconstruction and found that the chances of requiring medial meniscal surgery increased by a factor of two if surgery was delayed by 5 months and by 6 if surgery was performed more than 12 months after injury. Overall, the odds of chondral damage also increased significantly when more than 5 months had elapsed from injury. In contrast, the incidence of lateral meniscal tears did not increase significantly with time. The authors suggested that ideally ACL reconstruction should not be delayed more than 5 months from injury.

It should be acknowledged, however, that the data available on this issue derive exclusively from the analysis of retrospective case series. Prospective randomized comparisons are not currently available and are realistically difficult to perform. In addition, data from national registries or multicenter cohorts are subject to considerable interobserver variability. Estimations of cartilage and meniscal injury location, size, and depth may vary considerably among surgeons. Most importantly, although the benefits of early intervention in regard to meniscal and chondral pathology are well appreciated, most authors agree that the ability of reconstructive ACL surgery to limit cartilage degeneration in the long term compared with nonoperative treatment has not yet been proven beyond doubt.

Apart from time from injury, other factors have been implicated in the occurrence of secondary meniscal and chondral injuries in the ACL-deficient knee and potentially interact with surgical timing, such as patient gender, age, previous surgery, and activity level. Male gender has been associated with an increased frequency and severity of meniscal tears and articular cartilage lesions [15, 17]. However, the risk of meniscal injury has been found to increase at a higher rate over time among women [13]. Similarly, increasing patient age has been acknowledged as a significant predictor of medial meniscal and grade 3 and 4 cartilage lesions.

16.4 ACL Reconstruction in the Skeletally Immature Patient

Anterior cruciate ligament injuries in pediatric and adolescent patients have long been considered to be best treated conservatively until skeletal maturity was reached. Advantages of delaying surgery include better skeletal and psychological maturity, which increases surgical options for reconstruction, reduces the risk of growth arrest, and facilitates adherence to rehabilitation protocols. However, current evidence suggests that a long delay in ligament reconstruction may predispose the patient to further episodes of instability, subsequently increasing meniscal and chondral injuries. Among 370 pediatric patients that underwent ACL reconstruction, Dumont et al. [4] found a significantly higher rate of medial meniscal tears in those treated over 150 days after injury. In addition, chondral injuries were significantly associated with the presence of meniscal tear in the same knee compartment. Similarly, in a subgroup of 431 patients aged <17 years, Sriram et al. [19] found that the odds of medial meniscal pathology were doubled when surgery was delayed between 5 and 12 months and were quadrupled with a delay of more than 12 months. The authors advocated early reconstruction of the ligament in this age group to timely restore knee stability. With the advent of modern physeal-sparing techniques for ACL reconstruction, the objective of restoring tibio-femoral stability can theoretically be achieved without significantly compromising future physeal growth [8].

Memory
When ACL reconstruction is performed within the first weeks after injury, knee effusion, ROM deficits, and rehabilitation protocols more strongly affect the clinical outcomes than the actual timing of surgery. Accumulated evidence from the existing body of literature suggests a significant relationship between the duration of ACL deficiency and the incidence of secondary chondral and medial meniscal injuries. Although prospective comparisons are lacking, most authors suggest that to avoid the risk of additional damage, ACL reconstruction should preferably be performed within 6 months from injury. Skeletally immature patients are at a similar risk of developing secondary lesions and should be prioritized for ACL reconstruction with appropriate physeal-sparing techniques.

References

1. Bottoni CR, Liddell TR, Trainor TJ, Freccero DM, Lindell KK (2008) Postoperative range of motion following anterior cruciate ligament reconstruction using autograft hamstrings: a prospective, randomized clinical trial of early versus delayed reconstructions. Am J Sports Med 36(4):656–662
2. Chhadia AM, Inacio MC, Maletis GB, Csintalan RP, Davis BR, Funahashi TT (2011) Are meniscus and cartilage injuries related to time to anterior cruciate ligament reconstruction? Am J Sports Med 39(9): 1894–1899
3. Cosgarea AJ, Sebastianelli WJ, DeHaven KE (1995) Prevention of arthrofibrosis after anterior cruciate ligament reconstruction using the central third patellar tendon autograft. Am J Sports Med 23(1):87–92
4. Dumont GD, Hogue GD, Padalecki JR, Okoro N, Wilson PL (2012) Meniscal and chondral injuries associated with pediatric anterior cruciate ligament tears: relationship of treatment time and patient-specific factors. Am J Sports Med 40(9)
5. Duquin TR, Wind WM, Fineberg MS, Smolinski RJ, Buyea CM (2009) Current trends in anterior cruciate ligament reconstruction. J Knee Surg 22(1):7–12
6. Francis A, Thomas RD, McGregor A (2001) Anterior cruciate ligament rupture: reconstruction surgery and rehabilitation. A nation-wide survey of current practice. Knee 8(1):13–18

7. Granan LP, Bahr R, Lie SA, Engebretsen L (2009) Timing of anterior cruciate ligament reconstructive surgery and risk of cartilage lesions and meniscal tears: a cohort study based on the Norwegian National Knee Ligament Registry. Am J Sports Med 37(5):955–961

8. Hui C, Roe J, Ferguson D, Waller A, Salmon L, Pinczewski L (2012) Outcome of anatomic transphyseal anterior cruciate ligament reconstruction in Tanner stage 1 and 2 patients with open physes. Am J Sports Med 40(5):1093–1098

9. Kennedy J, Jackson MP, O'Kelly P, Moran R (2010) Timing of reconstruction of the anterior cruciate ligament in athletes and the incidence of secondary pathology within the knee. J Bone Joint Surg Br 92(3):362–366

10. Kwok CS, Harrison T, Servant C (2013) The optimal timing for anterior cruciate ligament reconstruction with respect to the risk of postoperative stiffness. Arthroscopy 29(3):556–565. doi:10.1016/j.arthro.2012.09.005, S0749-8063(12)01730-6 [pii]

11. Mayr HO, Weig TG, Plitz W (2004) Arthrofibrosis following ACL reconstruction and outcome. Arch Orthop Trauma Surg 124(8):518–522

12. Myer GD, Paterno MV, Ford KR, Hewett TE (2008) Neuromuscular training techniques to target deficits before return to sport after anterior cruciate ligament reconstruction. J Strength Cond Res 22(3):987–1014

13. O'Connor DP, Laughlin MS, Woods GW (2005) Factors related to additional knee injuries after anterior cruciate ligament injury. Arthroscopy 21(4):431–438

14. Papastergiou SG, Koukoulias NE, Mikalef P, Ziogas E, Voulgaropoulos H (2007) Meniscal tears in the ACL-deficient knee: correlation between meniscal tears and the timing of ACL reconstruction. Knee Surg Sports Traumatol Arthrosc 15(12)

15. Rotterud JH, Sivertsen EA, Forssblad M, Engebretsen L, Aroen A (2011) Effect of gender and sports on the risk of full-thickness articular cartilage lesions in anterior cruciate ligament-injured knees: a nationwide cohort study from Sweden and Norway of 15 783 patients. Am J Sports Med 39(7):1387–1394

16. Shelbourne KD, Wilckens JH, Mollabashy A, DeCarlo M (1991) Arthrofibrosis in acute anterior cruciate ligament reconstruction. The effect of timing of reconstruction and rehabilitation. Am J Sports Med 19(4):332–336

17. Slauterbeck JR, Kousa P, Clifton BC, Naud S, Tourville TW, Johnson RJ et al (2009) Geographic mapping of meniscus and cartilage lesions associated with anterior cruciate ligament injuries. J Bone Joint Surg Am 91(9):2094–2103

18. Smith TO, Davies L, Hing CB (2010) Early versus delayed surgery for anterior cruciate ligament reconstruction: a systematic review and meta-analysis. Knee Surg Sports Traumatol Arthrosc 18(3):304–311

19. Sri-Ram K, Salmon LJ, Pinczewski LA, Roe JP (2013) The incidence of secondary pathology after anterior cruciate ligament rupture in 5086 patients requiring ligament reconstruction. Bone Joint J 95-B(1):59–64

20. Tandogan RN, Taser O, Kayaalp A, Taskiran E, Pinar H, Alparslan B et al (2004) Analysis of meniscal and chondral lesions accompanying anterior cruciate ligament tears: relationship with age, time from injury, and level of sport. Knee Surg Sports Traumatol Arthrosc 12(4):262–270

21. Yoo JC, Ahn JH, Lee SH, Yoon YC (2009) Increasing incidence of medial meniscal tears in nonoperatively treated anterior cruciate ligament insufficiency patients documented by serial magnetic resonance imaging studies. Am J Sports Med 37(8):1478–1483

Graft Harvest and Preparation

17

Juan Carlos Monllau, Wolf Petersen, Christian Fink,
Sven U. Scheffler, Pablo Eduardo Gelber,
and Christian Hoser

Contents

J.C. Monllau, MD, PhD (✉)
Department of Orthopaedic Surgery, Hospital de Sant
Pau, Universitat Autònoma de Barcelona,
C/Sant Quintí 89, Barcelona 08041, Spain
e-mail: jmonllau@santpau.cat

W. Petersen (✉)
Department of Orthopaedic and Trauma Surgery,
Martin Luther Hospital, Berlin Grunewald,
Caspar Theyss Strasse 27-34,
Berlin D-14193, Germany
e-mail: w.petersen@mlk-berlin.de

C. Fink (✉) • C. Hoser
OSM Research Foundation, Sportsclinic Austria,
Olympiastr. 39, Innsbruck 6020, Austria
e-mail: christian.fink@sportsclinicaustria.com

S.U. Scheffler (✉)
Department of Orthopaedic Surgery and Traumatology,
COPV – Chirurgisch Orthopädischer PraxisVerbund,
Breitenbachplatz 8, 14195 Berlin, Germany
e-mail: sven.scheffler@gmx.com

P.E. Gelber, MD, PhD
Catalan Institute of Traumatology and Sports
Medicine (ICATME). Hospital Universitari Quirón
Dexeus, Universitat Autònoma de Barcelona (UAB),
Barcelona, Spain

17.1   Hamstrings

Juan Carlos Monllau and Pablo Eduardo Gelber

Among the various surgical procedures for correcting knee instability after ACL injury, the standard method of treatment is intra-articular ACL reconstruction with autogenous tissues. The bone-patellar tendon-bone autograft had been traditionally considered as the gold-standard surgical option. However, in an effort to minimize the donor-site morbidity associated to its harvest, semitendinosus tendon (ST) and gracilis tendon (GT) are increasingly used for ACL reconstruction. The doubled ST and GT grafts have greater mechanical strength than a bone-patellar tendon-bone complex [22], and the donor-site morbidity

R. Siebold et al. (eds.), *Anterior Cruciate Ligament Reconstruction*,
DOI 10.1007/978-3-642-45349-6_17, © ESSKA 2014

is reduced [26]. In fact, patients treated with hamstring tendon grafts are less likely to have patellofemoral pain and extension loss and more likely to a better recovery of quadriceps muscle strength [14, 29, 34]. Another advantage of the hamstring tendon graft technique is preservation of hamstring muscle strength. In spite of tendon harvest, most of the reported series have shown almost full recovery of knee flexor strength [34]. This could be due to the known postoperative regeneration of the previously harvested tendons in up to 75 % of the patients, although they usually do not restore their full cross-sectional area [3]. The downside of hamstring autograft is the limited quantity of tissue available. Thus, a way of providing a hamstring graft with the required diameter and thus mechanical strength is to triple the tendons.

Although reproducible, a requisite to successful hamstring graft harvest is a sound understanding of the insertional anatomy of the ST and GT to minimize tendon amputation. In addition and in meeting patient expectations, harvesting techniques for autogenous hamstrings are becoming increasingly minimally invasive. This blind hamstring harvest through a mini-incision carries an additional risk of nerve injury, from either direct transection during release of accessory insertions or blunt trauma during passage of the tendon stripper between layers I and II of the medial aspect of the knee [28]. There is also controversy regarding the most appropriate skin incision for semitendinosus-gracilis tendon harvest.

With all these in mind, the purpose of this chapter is to show step by step a way of easy, reproducible, and minimally invasive hamstring harvesting. Subsequent optimal preparation of double and triple hamstring graft is also detailed.

17.1.1 Hamstring Tendon Harvest

17.1.1.1 Skin Incision

First, it is mandatory to identify the exact proximal-distal location of the ST and GT. The easiest way is to palpate them medially to the tibial tuberosity (TT). However, in many cases, this

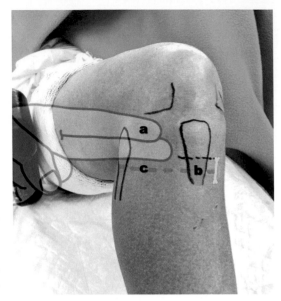

Fig. 17.1 The three recommended landmarks to identify the exact location of the semitendinosus tendon (ST) and gracilis tendon (GT) are (**a**) 2–3 finger widths distal to the joint line, (**b**) the lower half of the tibial tuberosity (TT), and (**c**) a line perpendicular to the fibular neck

is hardly possible due to either a thick subcutaneous tissue or a thin diameter of the tendons. Thus, three different landmarks can be used (Fig. 17.1):

- Two to three fingers widths distal to the joint line
- Within the lower half of the TT
- On a line perpendicular to the fibular neck

Regarding the medial-lateral location, controversy exists in the literature as the best way to perform the skin incision [35]. Most of the studies have recommended performing oblique incisions to minimize the risk of nerve injury. These studies have compared long (3–4 cm) vertical and oblique incisions and have concluded that the line of the longitudinal incision runs across the nerve branches which were distributed to the infrapatellar region and the anterior lower leg region. These branches originate from the saphenous nerve (IPSBN: infrapatellar branch of saphenous nerve) and medial femoral cutaneous nerve (SBSN: sartorial branch of sensory nerve) [20, 24]. While an oblique incision has less incidence of IPSBN transections, injury to SBSN is not

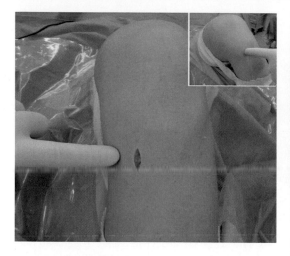

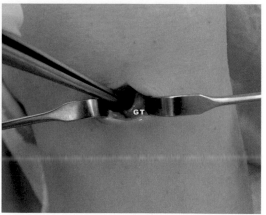

Fig. 17.2 The skin vertical incision is performed 2 cm medial to the tibial tuberosity as long as it allows the introduction of the index finger through it

Fig. 17.3 The GT is identified by sliding any solid instrument in a proximal to distal direction on the sartorial fascia and feeling a soft bump. This indicates the presence of the tendon underneath it

affected by the type of incision used [27]. In any case, and in agreement with our own observations, it has been concluded that daily living is nothing or only slightly affected by these sensory changes [21]. In addition, although it cannot be considered the main reason for the sensory disturbance [20], the possibility of nerve injury during harvesting of the ST and GT with a tendon stripper cannot be overlooked, and the use of the tendon stripper may in some cases be responsible for injury not only of the SBSN but also of the IPBSN at a more proximal level [28]. Regardless of the type of chosen incision, the complicated anatomic variations of the nerve branches in the infrapatellar region and the anterior lower leg region preclude their absolute avoidance in any surgical knee incision, and a completely safe zone cannot be found [20]. Based on the aforementioned considerations and in the belief of a more subtle cosmetic disturbance, once the desire landmark has been chosen, we currently recommend performing a vertical incision 2 cm medial to the TT with only the length that allows the introduction of the index finger through it (Fig. 17.2). Subsequently, after careful low-intensity electrocoagulation of the subcutaneous vessels, the virtual space between the crural fascia and the subcutaneous tissue is cleared off

with the help of the index finger. An assistant with two small retractors (e.g., two Senn-Müller) stands from the lateral side of the patient.

17.1.1.2 Identification of Tendons
Then, the GT, which inserts more proximally in relation to the ST, is identified by sliding any solid instrument in a proximal to distal direction and feeling a soft bump indicating that the GT is right below the sartorial or crural fascia (Fig. 17.3). Next, the membranous insertion of the sartorius muscle parallel with its fiber orientation is split (Fig. 17.4). One of the two retractors pulls up the sartorial fascia, and the GT and ST can be seen through this window. The GT and ST insert in a conjoined structure about 2.25 cm medial to the apex of the tibial tuberosity, and they become distinct structures at 1.8 cm proximal to their combined insertion site (i.e., about 4 cm medial to the TT) [23]. In case of any difficulty to properly identify both tendons as individual structures, it is easier to locate them just posterior to the superficial medial collateral ligament, where they can be easily palpated as round, separate, distinct structures. Only if the surgeon still finds difficulties to identify both tendons, we recommend to perform an inverted "L"-shaped incision placed medially from the proximal aspect of the sartorial fascia incision line to enhance tendon exposure (Fig. 17.5).

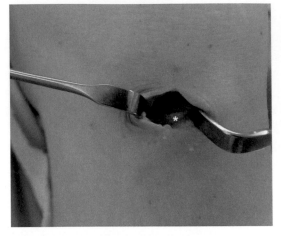

Fig. 17.4 The membranous insertion of the sartorius muscle is split parallel with its fiber orientation

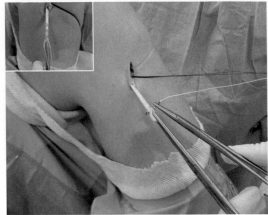

Fig. 17.6 Once GT and ST insertions are released from its tibial insertion, their ends are whip stitched for a distance of 30 mm with a high-resistance #2 suture

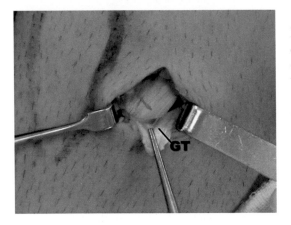

Fig. 17.5 In case of difficulty identifying the tendons through the short transversal split of the sartorius fascia, a complementary lateral vertical incision configuring an inverted "L"-shaped incision enhances tendon exposure

17.1.1.3 Harvest with a Closed Tendon Stripper

The tendon is first released from the pes anserine and is then stripped of the muscle belly: The GT is first identified, isolated, and pulled strongly with a small 90° curved dissector. It is then released from its tibial insertion. The free end is then whip stitched for a distance of 30 mm with a high-resistance #2 suture (Fig. 17.6), which has shown to withstand considerable maximum failure loads [25]. These sutures allow pulling from them in the next step; thus, commonly pulling with an aggressive

Kocher forceps is avoided, and the tendon is not damaged. While pulling from the sutures, the GT is freed from its few and tenuous fascial bands by sliding an opened Metzenbaum scissors. A closed-loop tendon stripper is then inserted over the tendon, and the tendon stripper is advanced. If the tendon stripper meets considerable resistance, then tendon adherences can be ruled out with the help of the index finger inserted through the incision before final advancement of the tendon stripper is done.

It is very important to keep the ST with you: Once the GT is harvested, due to the release of their adherences with the ST, the latter consequently displaces distally, which can make more difficult to harvest it. Thus, a simple way to keep it in "our hands" is to isolate it with a #1 Vicryl suture before GT extraction to pull it up later toward the surgical incision (Fig. 17.7).

Semitendinosus tendon harvest is performed in a similar way, but the tendon is usually more difficult to harvest. Up to five accessory bands or insertions must be released when dissecting the tendon to avoid its premature amputation by the tendon stripper. The most consistent of these insertions is described as diverging from the semitendinosus at a mean distance of 5.5 cm proximal to the conjoined insertion site (i.e., about 7 cm from the TT) joining the medial head of the gastrocnemius [31]. Another

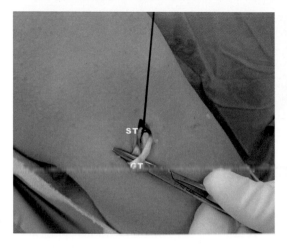

Fig. 17.7 Before the GT is released, the ST should be marked with a #1 suture. This will considerably help on later harvesting of the ST pulling it toward the surgical incision

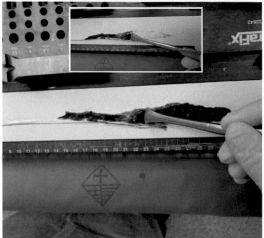

Fig. 17.9 A periosteotome allows blunt removal of the muscle fibers and fatty tissue from the harvested tendons with a low risk of tendon damage

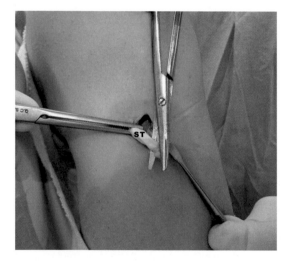

Fig. 17.8 Prevent proximal retraction of the ST during its release by grasping it with a Kocher forces about 4 cm medial to the insertion site

17.1.1.4 Harvest with an Open Tendon Stripper

The tendon is stripped of first from the muscle belly then released from the pes anserine. The tendons have to be located, and the accessory bands have to be released as described above. Then the open tendon stripper is introduced, and the gracilis and the semitendinosus tendons are stripped of the muscles.

> **Tricks and Pearls**
> - Find the hamstring tendons on a line perpendicular to the fibular neck.
> - Open the sartorial fascia 5 mm more proximal than the palpated proximal border of the GT to avoid its accidental injury.
> - It is easier to locate the hamstring tendons just posterior to the superficial medial collateral ligament.
> - Open the sartorial fascia with an inverted "L"-shaped incision placed medially to enhance tendon exposure if necessary.
> - Close the sartorial fascia once the hamstring tendons are harvested. You will forget it later!

important issue is to prevent proximal retraction of the ST when its insertion is released, as it is usually under much higher tension from the muscle belly than the GT is. This proximal pulling is counterbalanced by grasping the ST with a Kocher forceps about 4 cm medial to the insertion site during its releasing (Fig. 17.8). The harvested tendons are cleaned of adherent muscle fibers and surrounding soft tissue (Fig. 17.9).

Avoid Pitfalls

- Identify and release every accessory band of the hamstring tendons to avoid their premature amputation by the tendon stripper.
- Prevent proximal retraction of the distally released hamstring tendons by pulling them with a Kocher forceps.
- Avoid ST retraction from the incision once the GT is harvested by isolating the ST with a #1 Vicryl suture to pull it up later toward the surgical incision.

17.1.2 Graft Preparation

17.1.2.1 Quadruple Hamstring Graft

The ends of both tendons are whip stitched for a distance of 30 mm with a high-resistance #2 suture. Use two suture colors and stitch each tendon with the same suture color on both ends. This facilitates to identify the two limbs of each tendon at the end for pulling during tibial fixation. Now the GT and ST are doubled to form a quadruple hamstring graft. In case of an extracortical fixation with a button, the tendons are both doubled over the loop of the button, and in case of a femoral screw fixation, the tendons are both doubled over a strong pulling suture (Fig. 17.10). At

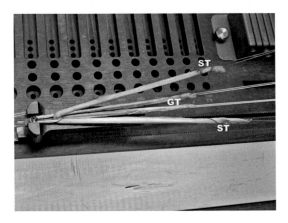

Fig. 17.10 Quadruple hamstring graft. Two suture colors are used to stitch each tendon with the same suture color on both ends. In this case, the GT and ST were doubled over the loop of an extracortical fixation to form a quadruple hamstring graft

the end of graft preparation, the diameter is measured on both ends with a sizing block with 0.5 mm diameter increments. In our hands, we only perform a quadruple hamstring graft when its diameter measures at least 9 mm.

17.1.2.2 Multifolded Hamstring Graft

It is also possible to triplicate the ST and/or the GT to achieve a larger-diameter graft, e.g., five-folded graft $(3x+2x)$ or a six-folded graft $(3x+3x)$. In the hands of the authors, the ST and the GT is triplicated in almost every procedure to achieve a strong six-folded graft.

A disadvantage when using hamstring autografts is the limited quantity of tissue available. Despite that hamstring tendon diameter can be reliably predicted with ultrasonography and magnetic resonance imaging [4], due to the small diameter that it is sometimes obtained, one potential way of providing one or two grafts with the required diameters and thus mechanical strength is to triple the hamstring grafts. It has been shown that the strength and stiffness of hamstring tendons increase with the number of strands included in the graft [11, 18], and that anterior tibial translation has an inverse relationship with graft diameter [9]. On the other hand, it has been recently questioned that there is a risk of failure to suitably incorporate the third limb into the fixation leading to a weakened graft, and that there is no mechanical difference in the overall properties between a doubled tendon and a tripled tendon graft at time zero [30]. In addition, the best method of incorporating the tripled strand into the construct of a suspensory fixation is unknown [19].

In the triplicating procedure, at least 21 cm of tendon is necessary to obtain 7 cm of usable graft. The procedure is illustrated and explained in Fig. 17.11a–c.

The second tendon may be added in the same way—either doubled or tripled—resulting in a five-folded or six-folded graft. The diameter of the graft is finally measured at both ends as the proximal end can be up to 1 mm thinner than the distal end, which would require different drilling sizes of the femoral and tibial tunnels.

The graft construct is kept in sterile gauze soaked in 5 mg/mL vancomycin solution.

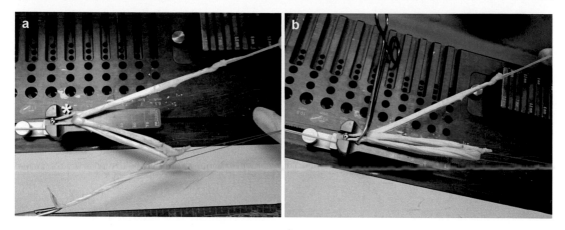

Fig. 17.11 (**a, b**) Triplicating method of the tendon. A 2 cm long end of the tendon is flipped over the loop of the extracortical fixation device. The tendon end is fixed to the long part by a whip stitch using a 2-0 high-resistance nonresorbable suture. The other end (thick end) of the tendon is passed again through the loop of the fixation device resulting in a triple-stranded graft. Distally the single free tendon end is whip stitched with a high-resistance nonab- sorbable No. 2 suture, and a nonresorbable suture tape is passed through the created tendon loop. The distal tendon loop and free tendon end are balanced to the same length over the loop of the device and pretensioned in this position. Then, finally the proximal 3 cm at the device loop is again whip stitched with the 2-0 nonresorbable suture resulting in a stable graft

The vancomycin solution is prepared by dissolving 500 mg of vancomycin powder in 100 mL of sterile saline solution, as has been previously reported (14). Prophylactic vancomycin presoaking of hamstring autografts statistically reduced the infection rate (14). Intravenous antibiotics have shown its difficulty to achieve antibiotic tissue levels above the minimum inhibitory concentration of *Staphylococcus* in the tendon because of the poor vascularity of tendons [13].

Pretensioning of Graft

Some studies have suggested that—as the ST has an elongation at plastic failure of 4–8 % and an elongation at rupture of 10 % [37]—repeated postoperative constraining mechanism of different activities could lead to secondary slackening of the hamstring graft. Among the solutions introduced to reduce that effect, intraoperative pretensioning has been adopted by many surgeons to balance all limbs of the construct to a similar tension and to tighten the interface between the tendons and the sutures.

However, pretensioning is controversial. Scanning electron microscopy (SEM) evaluation of pretensioned tendons has shown significant alterations of its collagen fibrillar ultrastructure through loss of cohesion, integrity, and parallelism of the collagen fibrils [10]. Thus, no conclusive scientific data exist regarding any advantage of pretensioning the tendons.

Pearls and Tricks
- Triple your hamstring tendons if the quadruple ST and GT construct has a diameter thinner than 9 mm. More collagen for your graft!
- Keep the graft in a sterile gauze soaked in 5 mg/mL vancomycin solution to reduce your infection rate [36].
- If you are running out of time, skip pretensioning of the graft! No conclusive scientific data supports this practice.

Memory
In an effort to minimize donor-site morbidity, semitendinosus tendon (ST) and gracilis tendon (GT) are increasingly used for ACL reconstruction. The doubled ST and GT graft has a greater mechanical strength

than a bone-patellar tendon-bone complex. Both tendons are harvested through a small incision at the pes anserine. Care should be taken to release all accessory bands before harvest to avoid its premature amputation by the tendon stripper. Most surgeons use a quadruple hamstring graft for ACL reconstruction. However, depending on the graft diameter, the tendons may be tripled to achieve a stronger tendon graft.

17.2 Bone-Patellar Tendon-Bone (BPTB)

Wolf Petersen

The purpose of this chapter is to discuss different aspects of patellar tendon harvest using a minimally invasive approach.

17.2.1 BPTB Harvest

The patellar tendon can be harvested by either a short longitudinal section medial to the patellar tendon or two horizontal sections. When a transtibial drilling technique is used, two horizontal sections are favorable since the tibial drill hole can be created in this way far medially. We prefer a short longitudi-

nal incision because the femoral tunnel is drilled via the anteromedial portal. The longitudinal incision reaches from the distal patella pole to the tibial tuberosity (Fig. 17.12a). The patellar tendon is exposed after transection of the paratenon. Depending on the width of the tendon, a graft of 8–10 mm width is excised with the scalpel (Fig. 17.12b). The middle, lateral, or medial third of the tendon can be harvested (Fig. 17.13). In our clinical practice, the medial one third is typically used.

Then the tibial bone block with a length between 15 and 20 mm is excised. For arthroscopic BPTB reconstruction with anteromedial portal drilling, we prefer a 15 mm bone block because the intra-articular handling of a shorter bone block is easier. First, the tendon tissue over the bone is incised with a scalpel. Then the cortical bone of the tibial tuberosity is cut with a small oscillating saw (Fig. 17.12c), a 2 mm hole is drilled in the distal one third of the bone block, and then the bone block is mobilized with a chisel (Fig. 17.12d).

If the tendon is long enough (75–80 mm with tibial bone block), the graft can be harvested without a patellar bone block. This might reduce donor-site morbidity. If the tendon is shorter, a patellar bone block has to be excised as well.

For harvesting the patellar bone block, the prepatellar bursa is opened to expose the tendon. Then the tendon tissue is cut in the form of the desired bone block. If a tibial press-fit technique

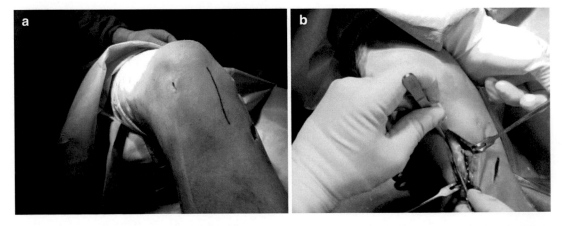

Fig. 17.12 (a) Longitudinal incision from the distal patella pole to the tibial tuberosity, (b) a graft of 8–10 mm width is excised with the scalpel, (c) the cortical bone of the tibial tuberosity is cut with a small oscillating saw, (d) the tibial bone block is mobilized with a chisel, and (e) after tendon harvesting, the paratenon is closed with a suture

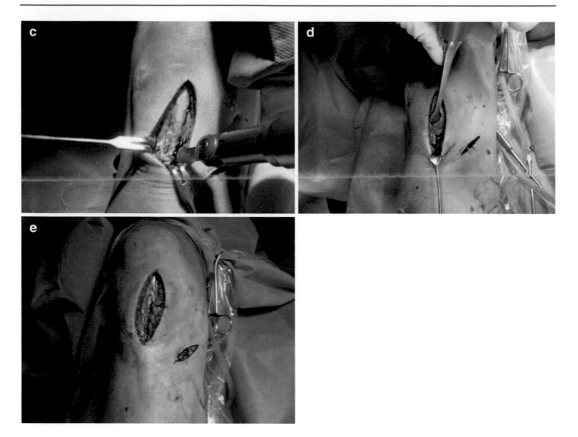

Fig. 17.12 (continued)

is chosen, the block should be a little wider than the graft (Fig. 17.14). Care should be taken to ensure that the harvest defect is flat in order to minimize harvest site morbidity.

The bone defects can be filled either with autologous bone material gained from the bone tunnels when a mill is used or by ceramic bone substitutes.

17.3   Quadriceps Tendon Harvest

Christian Fink and Christian Hoser

While many knee surgeons use the quadriceps tendon (QT) as a graft for anterior cruciate (ACL) revision surgery, it has never achieved universal acceptance for primary ACL reconstruction. The main reason in our opinion is that QT graft

harvest is technically more demanding and a scar on the thigh cosmetically less favorable, despite excellent clinical results in the literature [1, 2, 7, 8, 16, 17]. In the late 1990s, HU Stäubli from Switzerland published anatomical and biomechanical details of the QT and was the first advocate of its use as a primary ACL graft [32, 33]. For ACL revision surgery, QT has also documented an excellent clinical outcome [6].

The QT is a very versatile graft which can be harvested in different widths, thicknesses, and lengths and used with or without a bone block. It can be harvested in an open technique or using a new minimally invasive approach [5]. If a preoperative MRI is available, it is helpful to examine the QT and evaluate the thickness. Following a few guidelines, QT harvest is safe and associated with minimum donor-site morbidity [12].

Fig. 17.13 (**a**) Central BPTP graft, (**b**) medial BPTP graft, (**c**) conical patellar bone block, (**d**) flat patellar bone block, and (**e**) conical block of the tuberosity

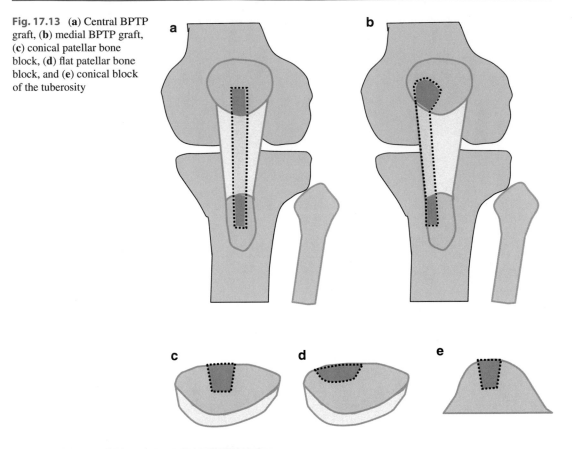

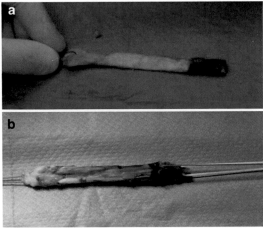

Fig. 17.14 (**a**) BPTB graft with two bone blocks. (**b**) BPTB graft with a tibial bone block

17.3.1 Open QT Harvest

1. A 5–6 cm longitudinal incision is made midline over the thigh starting 1 cm distal to the superior boarder of the patella (Fig. 17.15a).

2. The QT is carefully exposed. The prepatellar bursa is incised longitudinally and can be closed over a harvested bone block later.

3. The width (commonly 8–12 mm) is determined, and the QT incised parallel starting in the middle or slightly lateral to the middle at the patella. Care should be taken not to go too deep with the knife in order to prevent opening of the joint.

4. The thickness (commonly 5–8 mm) of the QT is determined about 1 cm proximal to the bony insertion. A suture is passed through (Fig. 17.16a). The suture loop is then pulled proximally, and the tendon strip carefully released along the suture with a knife (Fig. 17.16b). The graft is then cut proximally at the desired length (commonly 6 cm when using a bone block or 7–8 cm without a bone block) (Fig. 17.16c).

5. If the QT is used with a bone block, the tendon strip is elevated and then followed distally until its bony attachment. The dimensions of

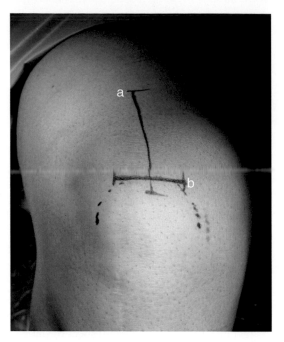

Fig. 17.15 Skin incisions for (*a*) open technique, (*b*) minimally invasive technique

the bone block (1.5 cm length and respective graft width) are outlined. The bone cuts are made with an oscillating saw, starting with the longitudinal cuts. The graft is then elevated, and the final cut determining the thickness of the bone block is made from proximal to distal. The bone block is then easily elevated with a chisel (Fig. 17.16d). These steps avoid extensive use of chisel and hammer in order to remove the block and reduce the risk of a patella fracture (Fig. 17.17).

Do not start your QT harvest with taking the bone block first. This is commonly associated with taking an unnecessary amount of bone and also an increased risk of opening the joint capsule.

6. The tendon defect is closed with a running suture. The stitches should be placed in the superficial aspect of the tendon to avoid shortening of the tendon ("fanlike closure") (Fig. 17.18a, b). If the joint capsule has been opened (which

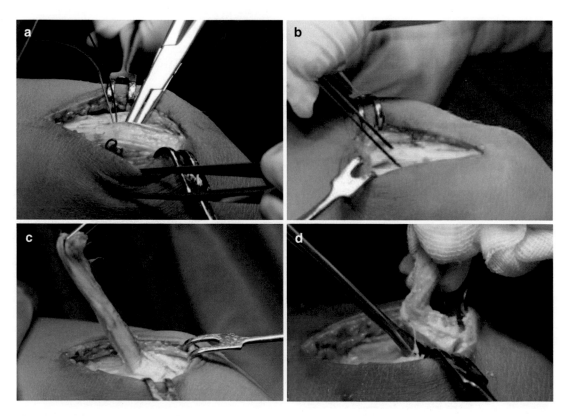

Fig. 17.16 Open QT harvest. (**a**) After incising the tendon longitudinally, the thickness is determined using a clamp with a suture loop. (**b**) The suture is moved proximally and the graft carefully released. (**c**) The graft is cut proximally and elevated. (**d**) After cutting the bone with an oscillating saw, the block is elevated from proximal with a chisel

happens only occasionally if you follow the steps described above), the defect should be carefully closed first. The prepatellar bursa is carefully closed over the bony defect.

17.3.2 Minimally Invasive QT Harvest

1. In 90° of knee flexion, a 2.5–3 cm transverse skin incision is placed over the superior boarder of the patella. The prepatellar bursa is incised longitudinally, and the quadriceps tendon is then carefully exposed (Fig. 17.19a).
2. A long Langenbeck retractor is then introduced, and the quadriceps tendon subcutaneously exposed proximal to the patella.

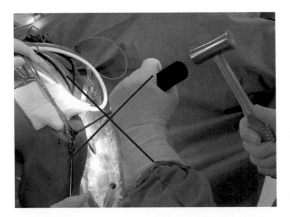

Fig. 17.17 Do not use the chisel extensively toward the patella (*red lines*). Due to the hard bone, there is a high risk of patella fracture

3. The double knife (KARL STORZ, Tuttlingen) in 8–12 mm width is then introduced starting over the middle or slightly lateral to the middle of the superior patella border and pushed up to a minimum of 6 cm (if used with bone block for ACL or 8 cm for PCL) (Fig. 17.19b).
4. The thickness of the graft (5 or 6 mm) is then determined using a second special knife (KARL STORZ, Tuttlingen). The knife is pushed proximal to the same mark (Fig. 17.19c).
5. Finally, the tendon strip is cut subcutaneously by a special tendon cutter (KARL STORZ, Tuttlingen) (Fig. 17.19d).
6. The bone block is then outlined (approx 1.5 cm long) and cut with an oscillating saw as described above for the open technique (Fig. 17.20a–c).
7. A long Langenbeck retractor is reintroduced, and tendon defect closed. The stitches should be placed in the superficial aspect of the tendon to avoid shortening of the tendon ("fan-like closure"). The prepatellar bursa is carefully closed over the bony defect.

> **Memory**
> Quadriceps tendon harvest is a safe and reliable procedure regardless if performed open or minimally invasive. However, the cosmetical outcome can be markedly improved (Fig. 17.21), and the surgical time reduced using a minimally invasive technique with special instrumentation.

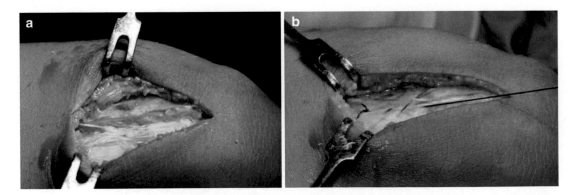

Fig. 17.18 The tendon defect (**a**) is then closed with running sutures superficially (**b**)

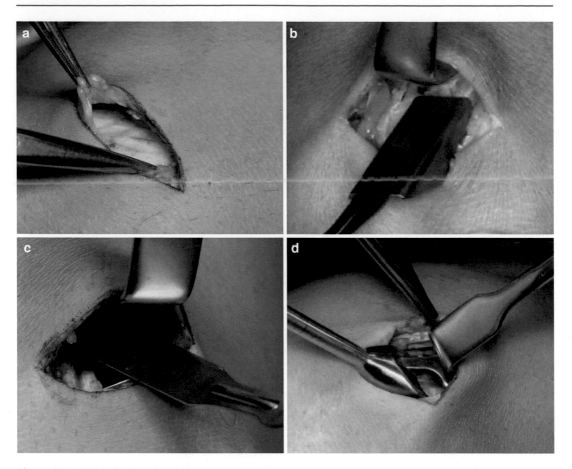

Fig. 17.19 Minimally invasive QT harvest. (**a**) After placing a 2.5–3 cm transverse skin incision, the quadriceps tendon is carefully exposed. (**b**) The double knife (KARL STORZ, Tuttlingen) is then introduced starting over the middle or slightly lateral to the middle of the superior patella border and pushed up. (**c**) Graft thickness is then determined using a second special knife (KARL STORZ, Tuttlingen). (**d**) The tendon strip is cut subcutaneously by a special tendon cutter (KARL STORZ, Tuttlingen)

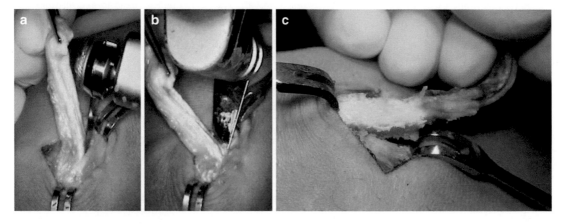

Fig. 17.20 The bone block is harvested using an oscillating saw. First, the longitudinal and transverse cuts are made (**a**). The last cut is determining the thickness of the bone block and is made from proximal to distal (**b**). Finally, the block is easily elevated (**c**)

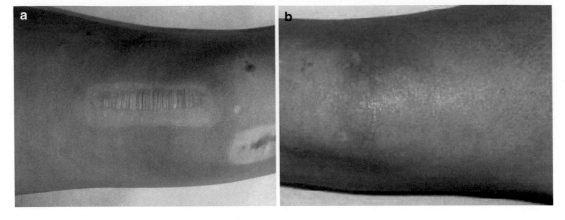

Fig. 17.21 Cosmetic appearance at 12 months post-op. (**a**) Open technique. (**b**) Minimally invasive technique

17.4 Anterior Half Peroneus Longus Tendon Graft

Sven U. Scheffler

Surgeons are often confronted with the problem of limited autologous graft sources in revision and ligamentous reconstructions of complex knee injuries.

This can become an even more imminent problem when allograft tissue is not available. The peroneus longus tendon is an alternative autograft to the commonly used patellar, quadriceps, and hamstring tendons. This graft can be harvested as a whole or as an anterior half split graft.

For the first time, Kerimoglu et al. mentioned the peroneus longus tendon as a source for reconstructive procedures of the knee joint in 2008, stating its use since 1997 [15]. Zhao et al. reported on a technique, using only the anterior half of the peroneus longus tendon (AHPLT) for reconstructive procedures of the ACL, PCL, and MPFL, thereby preserving the function of the peroneus longus muscle [38]. They found that the biomechanical properties of the AHPLT were comparable to the semitendinosus and gracilis tendons and that overall harvest site morbidity was minimal [38].

The author of this chapter regularly uses the AHPLT since 2010 for reconstructive procedures of the ACL, PCL, and MPFL. The details of the harvest procedure are outlined in the following chapter.

17.4.1 Anatomy Peroneus Longus Tendon

The peroneus longus muscle originates from the head and proximal two thirds of the lateral surface of the fibula, from the deep surface of the fascia, and from the intermuscular septa between it and the muscles on the front and back of the lower leg. The common fibular nerve runs through a small gap between its attachments to the head and to the body of the fibula to the front of the leg. The muscle continues in a long tendon, which runs behind the lateral malleolus, in a groove right on top of the fibularis brevis tendon; the groove is converted into a canal by the superior fibular retinaculum with the tendons contained in a common mucous sheath. The peroneus longus tendon continues distally below the trochlear process, and the tendon of the fibularis brevis, and under cover of the inferior fibular retinaculum. It crosses the lateral side of the cuboid, continuing across the sole of the foot obliquely and inserting into the lateral side of the base of the first metatarsal and the lateral side of the medial cuneiform bone. The peroneus longus muscle is responsible for plantar flexion of the talocrural joint and eversion of the subtalar joint.

17.4.2 Patient Positioning

The patient must lie in a prone position. The ankle must be moved from neutral position to

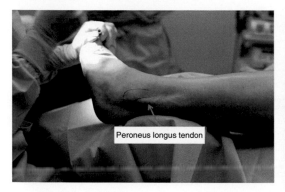

Fig. 17.22 Patient positioning

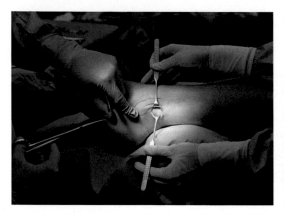

Fig. 17.23 Skin incision

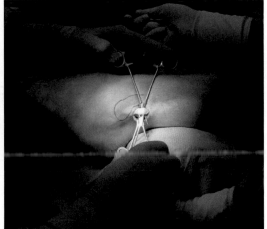

Fig. 17.24 Identification of peroneus longus tendon

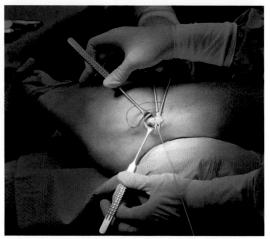

Fig. 17.25 Preparation of anterior half of peroneus longus tendon

plantar flexion and supination. In this position, the tendon can be easily identified about 2 cm proximal from the lateral malleolus (Fig. 17.22).

17.4.3   Skin Incision

A 3 cm long skin incision is done starting 2 cm proximal from the distal tip of the lateral malleolus extending in proximal fashion directly above the peroneus longus tendon (Fig. 17.23).

17.4.4   Preparation of Peroneus Longus Tendon

The peroneus longus tendon can be readily identified directly under the skin. It is wrapped in a mucous sheath (Fig. 17.24). The sheath is opened with a pair of scissors along its fibers. A small clamp is used to separate the peroneus longus from the underlying peroneus brevis tendon. A stab incision is performed in the middle of the peroneus longus tendon, extending the cut proximally for about 1 cm along its fiber orientation. A second small clamp is used to sling a suture loop around the anterior half of the peroneus longus tendon (AHPLT) (Fig. 17.25).

17.4.5   Distal Release of the AHPLT

The ankle is placed in plantar flexion and eversion, easing the access to the distal part of the

AHPLT. With the use of a scalpel, the AHPLT is released about 1 cm proximal from the distal tip of the lateral malleolus. This ensures the continuity of the superior fibular retinaculum, which is eminent to prevent subluxation of the peroneus longus tendon. After the distal release of AHPLT, its free end can be either augmented with holding sutures or grasped with a tendon clamp (Fig. 17.26).

The free end of the AHLPT is placed in an open or closed tendon harvester (Fig. 17.27). The harvester is moved proximally below the skin while applying manual tension to the free end of the AHPLT. Under gentle pressure, the tendon harvester is further moved proximally until release of the tendon can be felt. The free AHPLT graft can then be retrieved through its distal skin incision (Fig. 17.28).

17.4.6 Closure

The mucous sheath around the peroneus brevis and remaining half of the peroneus longus tendons is closed with resorbable 3-0 sutures (Fig. 17.29). This is followed by subcutaneous and skin sutures (Fig. 17.30).

17.4.7 Advantages

Main advantages of the AHPLT are that the graft can be easily identified, even in obese people. Due to its subcutaneous location, graft preparation and harvest can be achieved with ease. Only

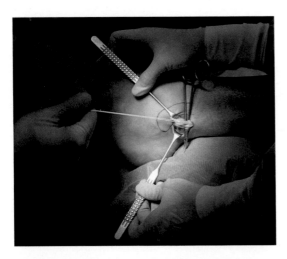

Fig. 17.26 Distal release and suture augmentation of AHPLT

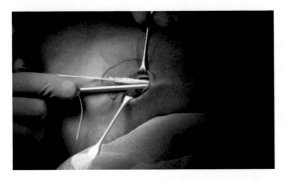

Fig. 17.27 AHLPT harvest

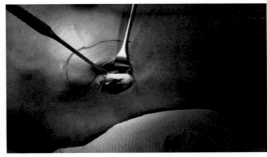

Fig. 17.29 Remaining intact posterior half of peroneus longus tendon

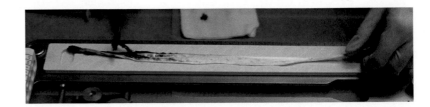

Fig. 17.28 Anterior half peroneus longus tendon

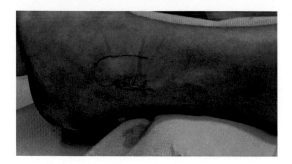

Fig. 17.30 Skin closure

a small incision of 2–3 cm is required with little compromise of patient cosmesis. No irritation of neuronal sensoric function exists as it is often observed following harvest of the patellar or hamstring tendons. Average distance between proximal tendon end and branching point of the deep peroneus nerve is 4.6–10.4 cm [38]. Tendon length of 24–28 cm can be obtained, which makes the graft suitable for MPFL, ACL, or PCL reconstruction. Function of the peroneus longus muscle is preserved through the posterior half, allowing immediate full weight bearing as tolerated.

17.4.8   Disadvantages/ Complications

Hematoma is commonly seen following tendon harvest. Temporal dysesthesia can be observed at the skin incision, which usually subsides around 1–3 weeks post surgery. Care has to be taken to avoid release of the complete tendon, sacrificing peroneus tendon function. Also, it must be avoided to injure the superior fibular retinaculum. Injury would result into sub- or even dislocation of the remaining posterior half of the peroneus longus tendon.

> **Memory**
> The harvest of the anterior half of Peroneus Longus tendon is a valuable option in case of graft shortness.

References

1. Chen CH, Chuang TY, Wang KC et al (2006) Arthroscopic anterior cruciate ligament reconstruction with quadriceps tendon autograft: clinical outcome in 4–7 years. Knee Surg Sports Traumatol Arthrosc 14:1077–1085
2. Eriksson E (2007) Patellar tendon or quadriceps tendon grafts for ACL reconstruction. Knee Surg Sports Traumatol Arthrosc 15:1283
3. Eriksson K, Hamberg P, Jansson E et al (2001) Semitendinosus muscle in anterior cruciate ligament surgery: morphology and function. Arthroscopy 17:808–817
4. Erquicia J, Gelber PE, Doreste JL et al (2013) How to improve the prediction of quadruple semitendinosus and gracilis autograft sizes with magnetic resonance imaging and ultrasonography. Am J Sports Med 41:1857–1863
5. Fink C, Hoser C (2013) Einzelbündeltechnik: Quadrizepssehne in Portaltechnik. Arthroskopie 26: 35–41
6. Garofalo R, Djahangiri A, Siegrist O (2006) Revision anterior cruciate ligament reconstruction with quadriceps tendon-patellar bone autograft. Arthroscopy 22:205–214
7. Geib TM, Shelton WR, Phelps RA et al (2009) Anterior cruciate ligament reconstruction using quadriceps tendon autograft: intermediate-term outcome. Arthroscopy 25:1408–1414
8. Gorschewsky O, Klakow A, Putz A et al (2007) Clinical comparison of the autologous quadriceps tendon (BQT) and the autologous patella tendon (BPTB) for the reconstruction of the anterior cruciate ligament. Knee Surg Sports Traumatol Arthrosc 15:1284–1292
9. Grood ES, Walz-Hasselfeld KA, Holden JP et al (1992) The correlation between anterior-posterior translation and cross-sectional area of anterior cruciate ligament reconstructions. J Orthop Res 10:878–885
10. Guillard C, Lintz F, Odri GA et al (2012) Effects of graft pretensioning in anterior cruciate ligament reconstruction. Knee Surg Sports Traumatol Arthrosc 20:2208–2213
11. Hamner DL, Brown CH Jr, Steiner ME et al (1999) Hamstring tendon grafts for reconstruction of the anterior cruciate ligament: biomechanical evaluation of the use of multiple strands and tensioning techniques. J Bone Joint Surg Am 81:549–557
12. Hoeher J, Balke M, Albers M et al (2012) Anterior cruciate ligament (ACL) reconstruction using a quadriceps tendon autograft and press-fit fixation has equivalent results compared to a standard technique using semitendinosus graft: a prospective matched-pair analysis after 1 year. Knee Surg Sports Traumatol Arthrosc 20:147
13. Judd D, Bottoni C, Kim D et al (2006) Infections following arthroscopic anterior cruciate ligament reconstruction. Arthroscopy 22:375–384

14. Kartus J, Movin T, Karlsson J (2001) Donor-site morbidity and anterior knee problems after anterior cruciate ligament reconstruction using autografts. Arthroscopy 17:971–980

15. Kerimoğlu S, Aynaci O, Saraçoğlu M, Aydin H, Turhan AU (2008) Anterior cruciate ligament reconstruction with the peroneus longus tendon. Acta Orthop Traumatol Turc 42:38–43

16. Kim SJ, Kumar P, Oh KS (2009) Anterior cruciate ligament reconstruction: autogenous quadriceps tendon-bone compared with bone-patellar tendon-bone grafts at 2-year follow-up. Arthroscopy 25:137–144

17. Lee S, Seong SC, Jo H et al (2004) Outcome of anterior cruciate ligament reconstruction using quadriceps tendon autograft. Arthroscopy 20:795–802

18. Ma CB, Keifa E, Dunn W et al (2010) Can preoperative measures predict quadruple hamstring graft diameter? Knee 17:81–83

19. Maeda E, Asanuma H, Noguchi H et al (2009) Effects of stress shielding and subsequent restressing on mechanical properties of regenerated and residual tissues in rabbit patellar tendon after resection of its central one-third. J Biomech 42:1592–1597

20. Mochizuki T, Akita K, Muneta T et al (2003) Anatomical bases for minimizing sensory disturbance after arthroscopically-assisted anterior cruciate ligament reconstruction using medial hamstring tendons. Surg Radiol Anat 25:192–199

21. Mochizuki T, Muneta T, Yagishita K et al (2004) Skin sensory change after arthroscopically-assisted anterior cruciate ligament reconstruction using medial hamstring tendons with a vertical incision. Knee Surg Sports Traumatol Arthrosc 2:198–202

22. Noyes FR, Butler DL, Grood ES et al (1984) Biomechanical analysis of human ligament grafts used in knee-ligament repairs and reconstructions. J Bone Joint Surg 66:344–352

23. Pagnani MJ, Warner JJP, O'Brien SJ et al (1993) Anatomic considerations in harvesting the semitendinosus and gracilis tendons and a technique of harvest. Am J Sports Med 21:565–571

24. Papastergiou SG, Voulgaropoulos H, Mikalef P et al (2006) Injuries to the infrapatellar branch(es) of the saphenous nerve in anterior cruciate ligament reconstruction with four-strand hamstring tendon autograft: vertical versus horizontal incision for harvest. Knee Surg Sports Traumatol Arthrosc 14:789–793

25. Petri M, Ettinger M, Drtzidis A et al (2012) Comparison of three suture techniques and three suture materials on gap formation and failure load in ruptured tendons: a human cadaveric study. Arch Orthop Trauma Surg 132:649–654

26. Rosenberg TD, Deffner KT (1997) ACL reconstruction: semitendinosus tendon is the graft of choice. Orthopedics 20:396–398

27. Sabat D, Kumar V (2012) Nerve injury during hamstring graft harvest: a prospective comparative study of three different incisions. Knee Surg Sports Traumatol Arthrosc. doi:10.1007/s00167-012-2243-8

28. Sanders B, Rolf R, McClelland W et al (2007) Prevalence of saphenous nerve injury after autogenous hamstring harvest: an anatomical and clinical study of sartorial branch injury. Arthroscopy 23:956–963

29. Shaieb MD, Kan DM, Chang SK et al (2002) A prospective randomized comparison of patellar tendon versus semitendinosus and gracilis tendon autografts for anterior cruciate ligament reconstruction. Am J Sports Med 30:214–220

30. Snow M, Cheung W, Mahmud J (2012) Mechanical assessment of two different methods of tripling hamstring tendons when using suspensory fixation. Knee Surg Sports Traumatol Arthrosc 20:262–267

31. Solman CG Jr, Pagnani MJ (2003) Hamstring tendon harvesting. Reviewing anatomic relationships and avoiding pitfalls. Orthop Clin North Am 34:1–8

32. Stäubli H, Bollmann C, Kreutz R et al (1999) Quantification of intact quadriceps tendon, quadriceps tendon insertion, and suprapatellar fat pad: MR arthrography, anatomy, and cryosections in the sagittal plane. Am J Roentgenol 173:691–698

33. Stäubli H, Schatzmann L, Brunner P et al (1999) Mechanical tensile properties of the quadriceps tendon and patellar ligament in young adults. Am J Sports Med 27:27–34

34. Tashiro T, Kurosawa H, Kawakami A et al (2003) Influence of medial hamstring tendon harvest on knee flexor strength after anterior cruciate ligament reconstruction. Am J Sports Med 31:522–529

35. Tillet E, Madsen R, Rogers R et al (2004) Localization of the semitendinosus-gracilis tendon bifurcation point relative to the tibial tuberosity: an aid to hamstring tendon harvest. Arthroscopy 20:51–54

36. Vertullo CJ, Quick M, Jones A et al (2012) A surgical technique using presoaked vancomycin hamstring graft to decrease the risk of infection after anterior cruciate ligament reconstruction. Arthroscopy 28:337–342

37. Wang JH (2006) Mechanobiology of tendon. J Biomech 39:1563–1582

38. Zhao J, Huangfu X (2012) The biomechanical and clinical application of using the anterior half of the peroneus longus tendon as an autograft source. Am J Sports Med 40:662–671

Tibial Bone Tunnel Placement (Arthroscopically and with Fluoroscopy)

18

Christophe Hulet, Goulven Rochcongar, and Valentin Chapus

Contents

C. Hulet, MD (✉) • G. Rochcongar • V. Chapus
Orthopedic Department, Caen University Hospital,
Comete INSERM U1075 – UCBN EA 3917,
Avenue de la Côte de Nacre,
Caen 14033, France
e-mail: hulet-c@chu-caen.fr

18.1   Introduction

The choice of the tibial tunnel position has a significant effect on the outcome of ACL reconstruction. This issue is really relevant, and the most common surgical error is thought to be poor tunnel position, which leads to poor rotational stability or increased graft stress and early failure with nonanatomic reconstruction [1]. Graft placement in single-bundle ACL reconstruction is essential for knee mechanic and transplant survival, but to know if the tibial bone tunnel is in an optimal position, it is primordial to define what is an "ideal tibial tunnel." Karlson defines four major principles to perform anatomic reconstruction: restore the native insertion site anatomy, restore the two functional bundles and they may be restored as one single graft "anatomic single-bundle reconstruction," address the tension behavior of the native ACL, and, at least, individualize the surgical procedure for each patient.

Biomechanically, Kato [2] compared three different tunnel positions (AM–AM, PL–PL, PL–high AM) for single-bundle ACL reconstruction to the reference position MID–MID. He found that the AM–AM graft yielded a high in situ force in response to the external loads at all flexion angles. Also, the AM–AM gave better rotational stability, and the MID–MID reconstruction did not have any major weakness. For anatomic single-bundle ACL reconstruction, both tunnels are drilled in the middle of the AM and the PL footprints (MID–MID reconstruction). Achieving optimal tunnel placement position

Fig. 18.1 Bony landmarks of the ACL tibial footprint (Courtesy R. Seil)

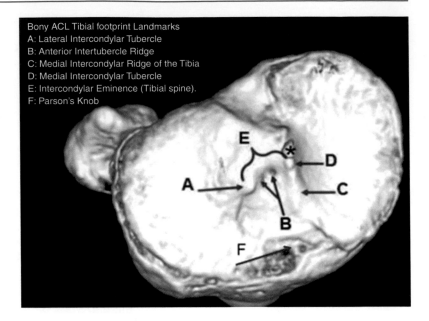

Bony ACL Tibial footprint Landmarks
A: Lateral Intercondylar Tubercle
B: Anterior Intertubercle Ridge
C: Medial Intercondylar Ridge of the Tibia
D: Medial Intercondylar Tubercle
E: Intercondylar Eminence (Tibial spine).
F: Parson's Knob

increases the likelihood of clinical success. Focus is now changing toward anatomic reconstruction with greater emphasis on tunnel position in the native ACL footprint [1, 3].

18.2 Tibial Bone Tunnel placement

Basic knowledge of the dimensions and the natural position of the ACL insertion sites and knowledge of anatomic landmarks during surgery are essential [3]. Anatomic dissections of the human knee have provided accurate description of the anatomy of the tibial attachment of the ACL [4]. The ACL tibial insertion is located between the medial and the lateral tibial spines and other bony landmarks [5]. The tibial plateau also had distinct bony margins for the ACL footprint that could be identified from an axial, sagittal, and a simulated arthroscopic view. These boundaries were quite consistently seen: the lateral intercondylar tubercle, the tibial ACL ridge, the medial intercondylar ridge of the tibia, the medial intercondylar tubercle, and the intercondylar eminence (medial tibial spine). Sometimes there is also a bony prominence anterior to the tibial footprint which is the confluent insertion of the anterior horn of medial meniscus and the medial fibers of the anterior cruciate ligament (ACL). The prominence has been called "Parsons' knob" by anato-

mists and the "tuberculum intercondylare tertium" by radiologists [6] (Fig. 18.1).

The insertion site is a broad oval area or duck footprint (triangular region) [7]. For Ferretti [8], the length of the ACL tibial insertion was 18.1 ± 2.8 mm, and the width was 10.7 ± 1.9 mm. The ACL tibial insertion had 206.2 ± 10.3 mm^2 of cross-sectional area with eight knees. In a large study of 50 cadaveric knees, Siebold [9] found an average width of 10 ± 2 mm (7–15 mm^2) and the average length was 14 ± 2 mm and the average tibial insertion area of the ACL of all cadavers was 114 ± 36 mm^2 (67–259 mm^2) (Fig. 18.2).

It is important to better characterize the anatomic centrum of the tibial footprint with radiographic evaluation with X-rays and 3D CT and also arthroscopic landmarks for routine use in ACL reconstruction [10].

Several studies evaluated radiographically the position of the AM and PM bundle and the variability of the tibial insertions [11–14].

With reference to the Amis and Jakob line, in seven cadaver knees, Colombet [11] found that the center of AM was at 36 % and the center of the PL bundle was at 52 %. The values were respectively 30 and 44 % for Zantop [13] with 20 cadaveric knees. Iriuchishima [14] did measurement in both the AP and medial-to-lateral directions with 20 cadaveric knees. In the AP direction, the center of the AM tunnel was at

Fig. 18.2 Morphometry of the AM and PL bundle insertions of the ACL tibial footprint from Siebold [7]

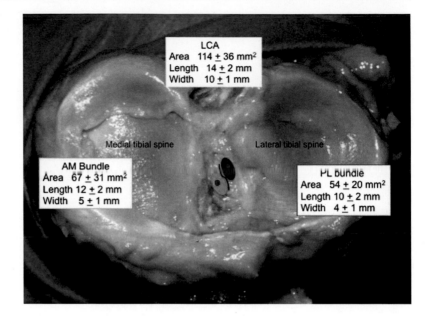

LCA
Area   114 ± 36 mm²
Length 14 ± 2 mm
Width   10 ± 1 mm

Medial tibial spine   Lateral tibial spine

AM Bundle
Area   67 ± 31 mm²
Length 12 ± 2 mm
Width   5 ± 1 mm

PL bundle
Area   54 ± 20 mm²
Length 10 ± 2 mm
Width   4 ± 1 mm

31 ± 3 %, and the PL tunnel was at 50 ± 3 %. On the mediolateral direction, the center point of the AM tunnel was located at 49 ± 4 % from the medial border at the tibia, and the PL was at 47 ± 3 %.

In vivo with fluoroscopic measurements on 67 patients, Kasten [12] found the AM bundle to be at 35 ± 4 % (23–42 %) of the AP distance on the Amis and Jakob line. The center of the PL bundle was 48 ± 4 % (39–58 %). For the single bundle, the center of the tibial footprint was 42 ± 6.7 % (35–56 %) and 41 % ± 4.4 % (37–52 %) of the AP distance relatively to the medial joint line and the Amis and Jakob line, respectively.

More recently with the use of 3D CT scan, three publications [15–17] evaluated the position of the tibial tunnel in both AP and medial-to-lateral plateau directions.

	AP	Med–lat
Lertwanich [15] (3D CT n=52)	38.7 ± 11.1 % (12.4–66.1)	49.1 ± 3.2 % (39.2–55.8)
Ahn [16] (3 D CT n=69)	35.7 %	51.45 %
Forsythe [17] (3D CT n=8)	AM: 25 ± 2.8 % PL: 46.4 ± 3.7 %	AM: 50.5 ± 4.2 % PL: 52.4 + 2.5 %
Pietrini [18] X-rays, n=12	AM: 36 ± 3.8 % PL: 51 ± 4 %	AM: 44.2 ± 3.4 % PL: 50.1 ± 2.1 %

In the study performed by Pietrini [18], the anterior and posterior edges of the AM and PL bundle were measured. Therefore, the center of the tibial footprint was at 44.1 % on the lateral view.

Arthroscopic assessment is very important during surgery, but there is some disagreement regarding optimal tunnel placement due to the heterogeneity of landmarks used to identify the center of the tibial ACL footprint [10]. For Ferretti [8], the ACL center was 9.1 ± 1.5 posterior to the intermeniscal ligament and 5.7 ± 1.1 anterior to a projected line from the apex of the medial tibial eminence. This tibial eminence also demonstrated a constant relationship with the ACL tibial insertion center. Morgan [19], in an anatomic MRI study, found that the ACL sagittal central insertion point was on the inter condylar notch 7 mm sagittally anterior to the anterior margin of the PCL with the knee flexed at 90°. On the other hand, Hutchinson [20] found that the centrum of the ACL is 10.4 ± 2.4 mm anterior to the anterior margin of the PCL and posterior border of the ACL tibial footprint is 6.7 ± 1.2 mm anterior to PCL. Ziegler [21] evaluated also the position of the ACL center on the tibia. The ACL attachment center was 7.5 mm medial to the anterior horn of the lateral meniscus, 13.0 mm anterior to the retro-eminence ridge, and 15.7 mm anterior to the PCL. In summary for Hwang [10], the centrum of the ACL tibial footprint is located between 7 and 15 mm anterior to the PCL and

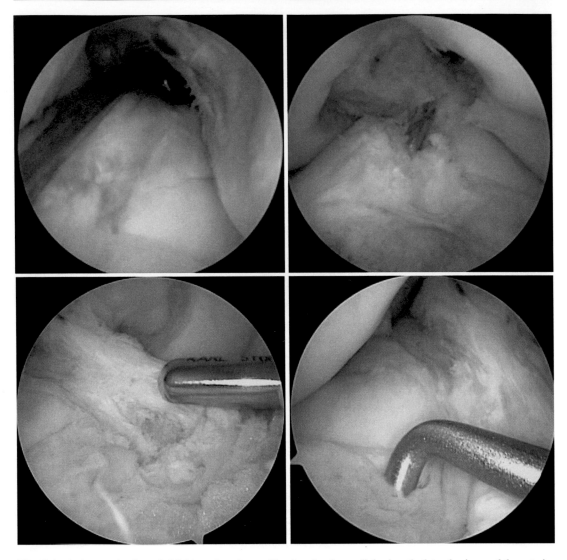

Fig. 18.3 Arthroscopic view of tibial insertion sites and landmarks: the medial spine, the lateral spine, and the anterior horn of the lateral meniscus and the PCL (left knee)

approximately two fifths of the interspinous distance from the medial to the lateral intercondylar eminence.

Before the start of the reconstruction, complete evaluation of the knee using arthroscopy is mandatory for treatment of cartilage defects and also meniscus preservation if required [3, 7]. During the procedure, arthroscopic technique is performed with at least three portals. Standard or high lateral portal for the arthroscope [22] to better visualize the ACL footprint. The medial portal and the accessory medial portal were used to analyze the whole lateral wall of the intercondylar

notch. Also, the medial portal is very relevant to analyze the tibial ACL insertion site [7].

Once the femoral starting point is marked with the awl, the anatomic tibial tunnel placement is accomplished with arthroscopic landmarks and fluoroscopy [6, 10] (Fig. 18.3).

In fact, the purpose of a well-made tibial tunnel in a single-bundle reconstruction is to match the initial ACL tibial insertion to preserve proprioceptors and create better isometric.

The posterior aspect of the soft tissue at the ACL footprint on the tibial surface is used as a landmark for tibial tunnel creation. Also, great care should be

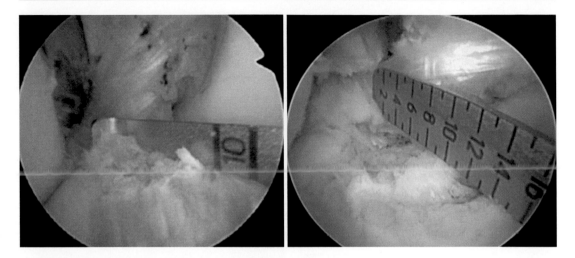

Fig. 18.4 Measurement of the tibial ACL footprint during arthroscopy

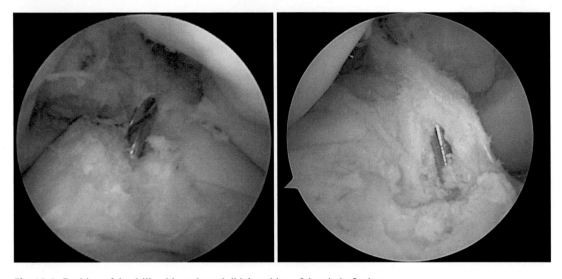

Fig. 18.5 Position of the drill guide and good tibial position of the pin in flexion

done to the posterior aspect of the anterior horn of the lateral meniscus and to the intermeniscal ligament. In addition, the length and width of the native ACL insertion sites are measured using a ruler to be used as a reference when drilling the tunnel with an appropriate diameter (Fig. 18.4).

We preserved as much as possible part of the remnants of the native ACL.

Borbon [23] justified that preserving the ACL remnants in surgical ACL reconstruction with four main effects: preservation of the intact remnants that played an important role in mechanical strength in the early postoperative period; reservation of the blood supply, which may aid in the healing process of the graft; maintenance of proprioceptive innervation with evident benefits for the subjective outcome and return to sports; and, at least, optimization of the accuracy of the procedure by improving the arthroscopic orientation and bone tunnel placement at the insertion site. During arthroscopy, the remnants of the ACL tibial footprint should be identified and used as a guide for the tibial tunnel placement.

The drill guide is placed through the medial portal and positioned with the use of several landmarks including anterior border of the PCL, posterior border of the anterior horn of the LM, and the interspinous area of the tibial plateau (Fig. 18.5).

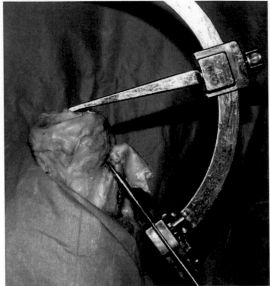

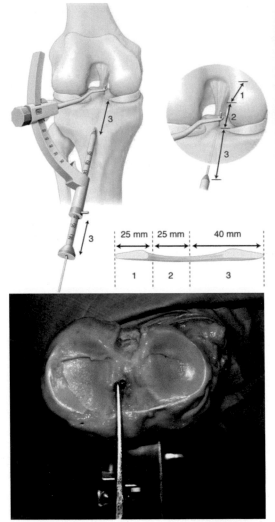

Fig. 18.6 Position of the tibial guide: extra-articular aspect of the drill guide in the sagittal and the transverse obliquity (from 10° to 20° of the transverse plane)

Morgan [21] said it is 7 mm anterior to the anterior border of the PCL with the knee flexed at 120°. For Staübli [24], the center of the intra-articular tibial hole is placed at 44.3 % of the anteroposterior length of the tibia. For Jackson [25], the intra-articular tissue of the tibial tunnel is open between the posterior extension of the anterior horn of lateral meniscus, the medial tibial spine, and the anterior insertion of the PCL. Therefore, the aspect of the tibial tunnel will be able to drape the PCL [25]. Kongcharoensombat [26] shows that the transverse ligament coincides with the anterior edge of the ACL tibial footprint in the sagittal plane. The transverse ligament is an easily identifiable anatomic structure and

is very close to the anterior edge of the attachments of the tibial ACL footprint.

On the tibial cortex, the starting point for the guide pine had some relevance. The entry point and the intra-articular exit do not only define the tibial tunnel: the orientation and the length are also a crucial part of the surgery [7, 27, 28] (Fig. 18.6).

Surgical technique [7] usually advocated the use of an intra- and extra-articular drill guide for the placement of the pine guide before the drilling of the tibial tunnel; usually this drill guide is adjusted to have an orientation between 55° and 65° regarding the horizontal. Once the pine guide is placed, the orientation of the future tunnel is defined; in spite of that, the tunnel is not drilled

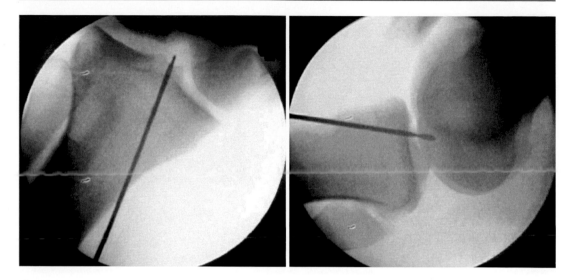

Fig. 18.7 Fluoroscopic evaluation with AP and lateral view before the tunnel drilling

yet. For Morgan [21], a well-made tibial tunnel takes its origin "1 cm above the superior (sartorial) border of the pes anserinus insertion and coronally 1.5 cm posteromedial from the medial margin of the tibial tubercle along the superior surface of the pes anserinus" or 4.5 cm under the articular edge.

To avoid tunnel enlargement risk and anterior misplacement, the length and the angle of the tunnel have to be considered. Length should be verified during pin guide placement; ideal tunnel length is 4–5 cm. If the tunnel is shorter than 4 cm, it can lead to two problems: firstly, a low-angle tunnel and oblong outlet cause tunnel enlargement. Secondly, short tunnel can mean anterior placement resulting intercondylar roof impingement, graft loosening, and loss of flexion. For Hulet, the tunnel is well oriented when it has a medial position with a 25° of obliquity in the frontal plan regarding the vertical and an anteroposterior obliquity between 40° and 60° regarding the horizontal. During patient review, Howell [29, 30] showed that patient with anteroposterior obliquity superior at 65° experiences instability and loss of flexion.

Orientation of the tibial tunnel will also define the section of the intra-articular aperture; in fact, the size of the outlet is greater in one direction than the tunnel diameter. Kopf [27] showed the influence of tibial drill guide angle on the drill bit diameter on the bone tunnel aperture area. The use of a 9 mm drill but at 45° drill guide created at 90 mm² bone tunnel aperture

area. Decreasing the drill guide angle from 65° to 30° increased the area of aperture of 81 %. The more horizontal the tunnel, the more the size of the outlet will increase. When outlet is far bigger than the tunnel, the inflection point of the graft is located within the tunnel itself, and the graft cannot stay in full contact with the tunnel walls. This mobility in the outlet can lead to the radiographic phenomenon of tunnel enlargement and at least graft loosening.

Also if you modified the transverse position of the drill guide, you increased the misplaced area of the tunnel aperture relatively to the theoretical area of the tibial footprint. At 15° from the transverse drill angle plane, the misplaced area is 5.5 % versus 15.3 % at 45° from the transverse drill angle plane. If the tunnel is too horizontal, the intra-articular outlet will show an ellipsoid section, and the contact between the graft and the tunnel will be inconstant; at least you will experience tunnel enlargement and graft loosening.

The pin position could be evaluated on lateral on AP fluoroscopic imaging [24, 31, 32] (Fig. 18.7).

On the lateral view, the pin should on the tibial plateau at the junction of the anterior and middle third of the tibial plateau. In extension, the tunnel should be posterior to extension of the Blumensaat line, and the anterior side of the tunnel must follow the extension of the anterior slope of the tibial spine. In flexion, it should be in line with the radiographic shadow indicating the roof of the notch with the Blumensaat line. Also,

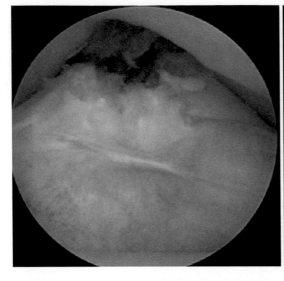
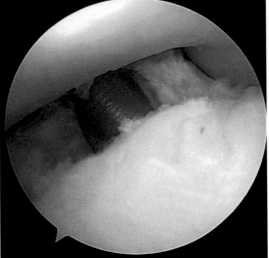

Fig. 18.8 Impingement checked before tibial tunnel drilling by putting the knee in full extension. Also the pin should not be in conflict with neither the medial nor the lateral condyle, and the anterior horn of the lateral meniscus is a reliable landmark

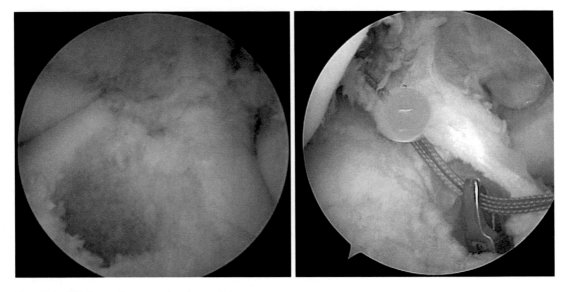

Fig. 18.9 Tibial tunnel aperture location and shape

this fluoroscopic evaluation could be done with the pin guide in place before the tunnel drilling, and the extended line of the pin has to be posterior and parallel of the Blumensaat line in lateral X-ray of the extended knee.

On the AP view, the pin should emerge into the joint on the down slope of the medial tibial spine.

When the guide pin is placed, the knee is brought in extension to check for knee impingement of the pin with the intercondylar notch [30, 33] (Fig. 18.8).

It is also interesting to evaluate the position of the pin relatively to the intermeniscal ligament and the anterior horn of the lateral meniscus. If the location is not acceptable, the pin can be moved with a 3–5 mm offset guide to get the correct position. Then, the tunnel is drilled to the appropriate size with a cannulated reamer (Fig. 18.9).

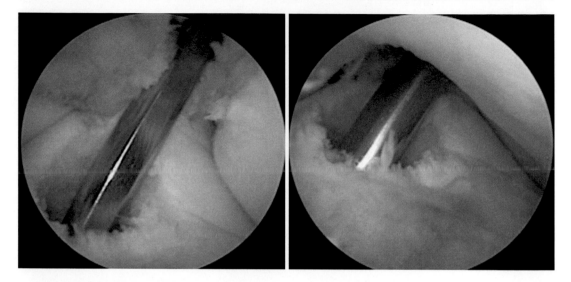

Fig. 18.10 Cannulated reamer in place to check for impingement in mid-flexion and then in full extension

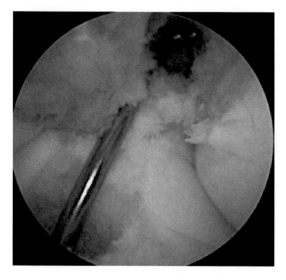

Fig. 18.11 After having realized the tibial tunnel, you can check that you are able to get the femoral footprint you would like to get

As a trip, a curette could be placed over the intra-articular end of the pin into the joint to prevent inadvertent pin migration during overdrilling. Care should be taken during this time to protect the PCL, the lateral wall of the notch, and the lateral femoral condyle.

It is also possible to use a cannulated trephine for drilling the tibial tunnel to get a bone plug for filling the bone gap in the patella or the tibia in case of BTB graft. This bone plug could be useful also for the tibial fixation in case of hamstring graft.

Tibial tunnel is then created with a cannulated reamer at the same size or 1 mm smaller than the graft size. The final dilator is left in place, and once again, the knee is brought in extension to check for knee impingement of the cannulated dilator with the notch. If there is any impingement, an appropriate technique with a notchplasty should be performed (Fig. 18.10).

The intra-articular edge of the tunnel could be cleaned by the shaver or a rasp, to be smooth. With the probe, impingement in both flexion and extension should be controlled. Probe could be used as a tool to get the target point for the femoral tunnel aperture (Fig. 18.11).

After the procedure, the optimal position of tunnel placement to achieve anatomic reconstruction should be controlled by X-ray evaluation by reliable technique as Aglietti recommended [32].

In the literature, there was a lot of interest about the quality for femoral tunnel location, but the tibial tunnel is also very relevant to allow good knee kinematics and therefore for the success of your procedure. This is available whatever the graft you decided to use (Fig. 18.12).

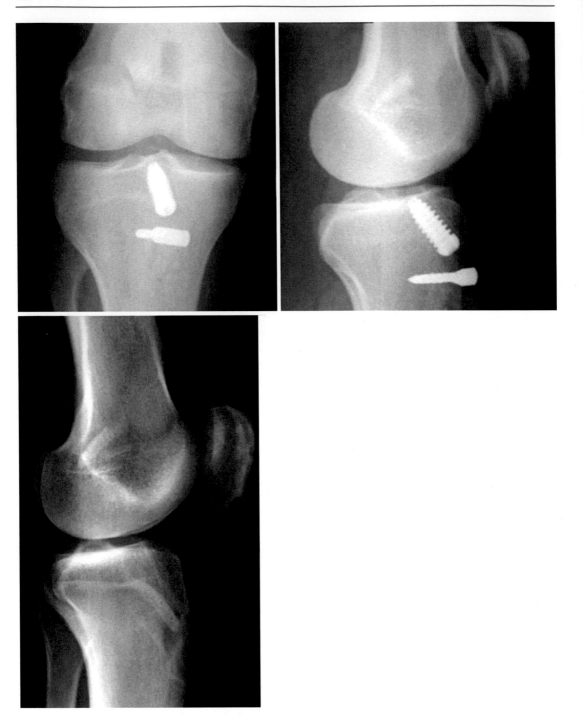

Fig. 18.12 Postoperative X-rays with AP and lateral view to control the anatomic position of both tunnels

References

1. Yasuda K, van Eck CF, Hoshino Y, Fu FH, Tashman S (2011) Anatomic single-and double-bundle anterior cruciate ligament reconstruction. Part 1: Basic science. Am J Sports Med 39:1789–1799
2. Kato Y, Maeyama A, Lertwanich P, Wang JH, Ingham SJ, Kramer S, Martins CQ, Smolinski P, Fu FH (2013) Biomechanical comparison of different graft positions for single-bundle anterior cruciate ligament reconstruction. Knee Surg Sports Traumatol Arthrosc 21:816 823
3. Karlsson J, Irrgang JJ, van Eck CF, Samuelsson K, Mejia HA, Fu FH (2011) Anatomic single- and double-bundle anterior cruciate ligament reconstruction. Part 2: Clinical application of surgical technique. Am J Sports Med 39:2016 2026
4. Purnell ML, Larson AI, Clancy W (2008) Anterior cruciate ligament insertions on the tibia and femur and their relationships to critical bony landmarks using high-resolution volume-rendering computed tomography. Am J Sports Med 36:2083–2090
5. Berg EE (1993) Parsons' knob (tuberculum intercondylare tertium). A guide to tibial anterior cruciate ligament insertion. Clin Orthop Relat Res 292:229–231
6. Kopf S, Musahl V, Tashman S, Szczodry M, Shen W, Fu FH (2009) A systematic review of the femoral origin and tibial insertion morphology of the ACL. Knee Surg Sports Traumatol Arthrosc 17:213–219
7. Hulet C, Lebel B, Colombet P, Pineau V, Locker B (2011) Traitement chirurgical des lésions du ligament Croisé antérieur. EMC (Elsevier Masson SAS, Paris), Techniques chirurgicales- Orthopedie traumatologie, pp 44–780
8. Ferretti M, Doca D, Ingham SM, Cohen M, Fu FH (2012) Bony and soft tissue landmarks of the ACL tibial insertion site: an anatomical study. Knee Surg Sports Traumatol Arthrosc 20:62–68
9. Siebold SR, Ellert T, Metz S, Metz J (2008) Tibial insertions of the anteromedial and posterolateral bundles of the anterior cruciate ligament: morphometry, arthroscopic landmarks, and orientation model for bone tunnel placement. Arthroscopy 24:154–161
10. Hwang MD, Piefer JW, Lubowitz JH (2012) Anterior cruciate ligament tibial footprint anatomy: systematic review of the 21st century literature. Arthroscopy 28:728–734
11. Colombet P, Robinson J, Christel P, Franceschi JP, Djian P, Bellier G, Sbihi A (2006) Morphology of anterior cruciate ligament attachments for anatomic reconstruction: a cadaveric dissection and radiographic study. Arthroscopy 22:984–992
12. Katsen P, Szczodry M, Irrgang J, Kropf E, Costello J, Fu FH (2010) What is the role of intra operative fluoroscopic measurements to determine tibial tunnel, placement in anatomical anterior cruciate ligament reconstruction? Knee Surg Sports Traumatol Arthrosc 18:1169–1175
13. Zantop T, Wellmann M, Fu FH, Peterson W (2008) Tunnel positioning of anteromedial and posterolateral bundles in anatomic anterior cruciate ligament reconstruction: anatomic and radiographic findings. Am J Sports Med 36:65–72
14. Iriuchishima T, Ingham SJ, Tajima G et al (2010) Evaluation of the tunnel placement in the anatomical double-bundle ACL reconstruction: a cadaver study. Knee Surg Sports Traumatol Arthrosc 18:1226–1231
15. Lertwanich P, Martins CA, Asai S, Ingham SJ, Smolinski P, Fu FH (2011) Anterior cruciate ligament tunnel position measurement reliability on 3-dimensional reconstructed computed tomography. Arthroscopy 27:391–398
16. Ahn JH, Jeong HJ, Ko CS, Ko TS, Kim JH (2013) Three-dimensional reconstruction computed tomography evaluation of tunnel location during single bundle anterior cruciate ligament reconstruction: a comparison of transtibial and 2-incision tibial tunnel-independent techniques. Clin Orthop Surg 5:26–35
17. Forsythe B, Kopf S, Wong AK, Martins CAQ, Anderst W, Tashman S, Fu FH (2010) The location of femoral and tibial tunnels in anatomic double-bundle anterior cruciate ligament reconstruction analyzed by three-dimensional computed tomography models. J Bone Joint Surg Am 92:1418–1426
18. Pietrini SD, Ziegler CG, Anderson CJ, Wijdicks CA, Westerhaus BD, Johansen S, Engebretsen L, LaPrade RF (2011) Radiographic landmarks for tunnel positioning in double-bundle ACL reconstructions. Knee Surg Sports Traumatol Arthrosc 19:792–800
19. Morgan CD, Kalman VR, Grawl DM (1995) Definitive landmarks for reproducible tibial tunnel placement in anterior cruciate ligament reconstruction. Arthroscopy 11:275–288
20. Hutchinson MR, Bae TS (2001) Reproducibility of anatomic tibial landmarks for anterior cruciate ligament reconstructions. Am J Sports Med 29:777–780
21. Ziegler CG, Pietrini SD, Westerhaus BD, Anderson CJ, Wijdicks CA, Johansen S, Engebretsen L, LaPrade RF (2011) Arthroscopically pertinent landmarks for tunnel positioning in single-bundle and double-bundle anterior cruciate ligament reconstructions. Am J Sports Med 39:743–752
22. Sonnery-Cottet B, Archbold P, Zayni R, Thaunat M, Bortolletto J, Fayard JM, Chambat P (2011) High lateral portal for sparing the infrapatellar fat-pad during ACL reconstruction. Orthop Traumatol Surg Res 97:870–873
23. Borbon CA, Mouzopoulos G, Siebold R (2012) Why perform an ACL augmentation? Knee Surg Sports Traumatol Arthrosc 20:245–251
24. Stäubli HU, Rauschning W (1994) Tibial attachment area of the anterior cruciate ligament in the extended knee position. Knee Surg Sports Traumatol Arthrosc 2:138–146
25. Jackson DW, Gasser SI (1994) Tibial tunnel placement in ACL reconstruction. Arthroscopy 10:124–131

26. Kongcharoensombat W, Ochi M, Abouheif M, Adachi N, Ohkawa S, Kamei G, Okuhara A, Shibuya H, Niimoto T, Nakasa T, Nakamae A, Deie M (2011) The transverse ligament as a landmark for tibial sagittal insertions of the anterior cruciate ligament: a cadaveric study. Arthroscopy 27:1395–1399

27. McConkey MO, Amendola A, Ramme AJ, Dunn WR, Flanigan DC, Britton CL, MOON Knee Group, Wolf BR (2012) Arthroscopic agreement among surgeons on anterior cruciate ligament tunnel placement. Am J Sports Med 40:2737–2746

28. Kopf S, Martin DE, Tashman S, Fu FH (2010) Effect of tibial drill angles on bone tunnel aperture during anterior cruciate ligament reconstruction. J Bone Joint Surg Am 92:871–881

29. Howell SM, Gittins ME, Gottlieb JE, Traina SM, Zoellner TM (2001) The relationship between the angle of the tibial tunnel in the coronal plane and loss of flexion and anterior laxity after anterior cruciate ligament reconstruction. Am J Sports Med 29:567–574

30. Howell SM, Taylor MA (1993) Failure of reconstruction of the anterior cruciate ligament due to impingement by the intercondylar roof. J Bone Joint Surg Am 5:1044–1055

31. Sullivan JP, Matava MJ, Flanigan DC, Gao Y, Britton CL, Amendola A, MOON Group, Wolf BR (2012) Reliability of tunnel measurements and the quadrant method using fluoroscopic radiographs after anterior cruciate ligament reconstruction. Am J Sports Med 40:2236–2241

32. Aglietti P, Zaccherotti G, Menchetti PPM, De Biase P (1995) A comparison of clinical and radiological parameters with two arthroscopic techniques for anterior cruciate ligament reconstruction. Knee Surg Sports Traumatol Arthrosc 3:2–8

33. Scheffel PT, Henninger HB, Burks RT (2013) Relationship of the intercondylar roof and the tibial footprint of the ACL: implications for ACL reconstruction. Am J Sports Med 41:396–401

Femoral Bone Tunnel Placement (Arthroscopically and with Fluoroscopy)

19

Tim Spalding, Curtis Robb, and Charles H. Brown Jr.

Contents

T. Spalding (✉) • C. Robb
Department of Orthopaedics,
University Hospital Coventry, Coventry, UK
e-mail: info@timspalding.com

C.H. Brown Jr.
International Knee and Joint Centre, Abu Dhabi,
United Arab Emirates

19.1 Introduction

Anatomic placement of the femoral tunnel is critical to the success and clinical outcome of anterior cruciate ligament (ACL) reconstruction [1–11]. Anatomic single-bundle ACL reconstruction is defined as a single-bundle ACL reconstruction in which the femoral and tibial bone tunnels are positioned at the center of the native ACL femoral and tibial attachment sites [1, 3, 12, 13]. Nonanatomic ACL tunnel placement is the most common technical error leading to recurrent instability and a failed ACL reconstruction [2, 4–11]. Proper placement of the ACL femoral tunnel is especially important because the length and tension of the ACL replacement graft is most influenced by the position of the ACL femoral tunnel [14–18]. Malposition of the ACL femoral tunnel can cause excessive tightening or loosening of the ACL graft, which may result in a loss of motion and or patholaxity of the knee [2, 4–11, 15–18]. Proper placement of the femoral tunnel during ACL reconstruction is therefore a critical part of the surgical procedure. A working knowledge of the anatomy of the ACL femoral attachment site is important to ensure anatomic placement of the ACL femoral tunnel. The anatomy of the ACL has been discussed in greater detail elsewhere in this book. To summarize, the ACL femoral attachment site is oval in appearance and is located along the lower third of the inner wall of the lateral femoral condyle [13, 14, 19–26]. The ACL femoral attachment site is defined by two bony ridges,

R. Siebold et al. (eds.), *Anterior Cruciate Ligament Reconstruction*,
DOI 10.1007/978-3-642-45349-6_19, © ESSKA 2014

the lateral intercondylar and the lateral bifurcate ridges [13, 20, 22–24, 26, 27] (Fig. 19.1). The lateral intercondylar ridge is an important anatomic landmark since the native ACL always attaches inferior (arthroscopic description) or posterior (anatomic description) to the lateral intercondylar ridge [3, 20, 22–24, 26–28] (Fig. 19.1). The lateral intercondylar ridge can be identified arthroscopically in 88 % of subacute and chronic ACL-deficient knees and therefore is a consistent anatomic landmark to assist the knee surgeon with placement of the ACL femoral tunnel [29]. The lateral bifurcate ridge which can be identified arthroscopically in 48 % of subacute and chronic knees runs perpendicular to the lateral intercondylar ridge and divides the ACL femoral attachment site into the attachment site areas for the posterolateral (PL) and anteromedial (AM) bundles [3, 12, 13, 20, 22, 24, 26] (Fig. 19.1). The center of the ACL femoral attachment site is 1.7 mm deep or proximal to the bifurcate ridge and 7.3–8.5 mm superior or anterior to the inferior or posterior articular cartilage margin of the lateral femoral condyle [21, 26]. For anatomic single-bundle ACL reconstruction, the center of

the ACL femoral attachment site is chosen as the position for the ACL femoral tunnel [1, 3, 5, 12, 13, 30–32]. Biomechanical and clinical studies have demonstrated that ACL reconstruction using a replacement graft placed at the center of the ACL femoral and tibial attachment sites is more effective at controlling anterior tibial translation and the combined motions of anterior tibial translation and internal tibial rotation (simulated pivot shift test) and restores knee kinematics more closely to that of the normal knee compared to "isometric" ACL femoral tunnel placement, other anatomic ACL tunnel placements, or techniques that have traditionally restored predominantly the AM bundle fibers [1, 6, 30–38].

19.2 Outline of the Surgical Technique

To obtain a clear view of the ACL femoral attachment site and to place the ACL femoral tunnel in the center of the ACL femoral attachment site, an orderly sequence of steps is recommended. This chapter details the following technical aspects of

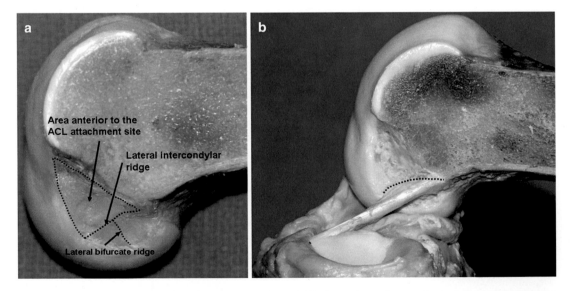

Fig. 19.1 Right knee, human cadaveric specimen. The medial femoral condyle has been removed. (**a**) The ACL femoral attachment site is located on the lower third of inner wall of the lateral femoral condyle. The

ACL femoral attachment site is defined by the lateral intercondylar and lateral bifurcate ridges. (**b**) The native ACL is seen to attach inferior to the lateral intercondylar ridge

each component of the surgical technique for anatomic single-bundle ACL femoral tunnel placement:

1. Patient positioning
2. Portal placement
3. Preparation of the intercondylar notch
4. Identification of the center of the ACL femoral attachment site
5. Use of intraoperative fluoroscopy
6. Drilling the ACL femoral tunnel
7. Assessment of the ACL femoral tunnel

19.3   Patient Positioning

When drilling the ACL femoral tunnel through an anteromedial (AM) or accessory anteromedial (AAM) portal, it is important to have the ability to achieve full, unrestricted knee flexion during the procedure. Hyperflexion of the knee is necessary to avoid having the femoral guide pin exit the lateral soft tissues too posteriorly. The peroneal nerve and posterior neurovascular structures are at risk for injury when the femoral guide pin exits the lateral soft tissues in a too posterior position. The requirement to achieve at least 120° of knee flexion while drilling the ACL femoral tunnel may present problems when a circumferential leg holder is used and the foot of the operating room table flexed down. Keeping the

operating room table flat and using a thigh post and one or two foot posts allow full unrestricted knee flexion and facilitate drilling the ACL femoral tunnel. The patient is positioned supine with the feet close to the end of the operating table. Time out is called and the correct operative side, site, and procedure confirmed. A foam heel protector is placed on the nonoperative leg. The operative knee is shaved and a padded tourniquet placed high on the operative leg. A padded thigh post is clamped to the side rail of the operating table on the operative side at the level of the tourniquet. A padded lateral hip positioner is clamped to the side rail of the operating table opposite the thigh post on the side of the nonoperative leg. The padded lateral hip positioner stabilizes the patient's pelvis on the operating table and prevents the patient's pelvis from sliding on the operating table during the application of valgus stress to open the medial compartment. Two padded foot posts are clamped to the operating table. The distal foot post is positioned to support the operative leg at 90° of flexion during graft harvest and during preparation of the intercondylar notch. The more proximal foot post is adjusted to position the knee at a minimum of 120° of flexion. The two foot posts allow the leg to be positioned during the surgery without requiring an assistant to hold the leg (Fig. 19.2). The ability to hold the leg in maximal flexion during drilling of

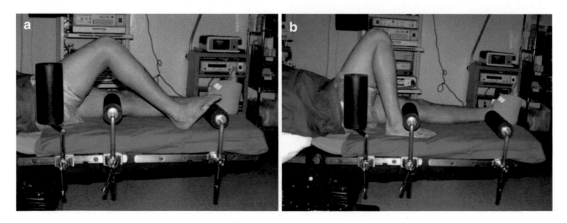

Fig. 19.2 (**a**) Distal foot post is adjusted to position the knee at 90° of knee flexion during graft harvest and preparation of the intercondylar notch. (**b**) Proximal foot rest is adjusted to maintain the knee in hyperflexion during drilling of the ACL femoral tunnel

the ACL femoral tunnel through an AM or AAM portal is essential to avoid a "blowout" of the posterior wall of the ACL femoral tunnel, to achieve an acceptable femoral tunnel length, to prevent bending of the femoral guide pin, and to protect the peroneal nerve.

19.4 Portal Placement

Proper placement of the arthroscopic portals is critical to the success of the procedure. Anatomic ACL femoral tunnel placement is facilitated by using three arthroscopic portals and drilling the femoral tunnel through an accessory anteromedial portal [3, 12, 39–41] (Fig. 19.3):

- The anterolateral (AL) portal—used as the primary viewing portal when performing diagnostic arthroscopy and meniscal surgery

- The anteromedial (AM) portal—used as the primary viewing portal for identification of the ACL femoral attachment site
- The accessory anteromedial portal (AAM)—used as a working portal to insert instrumentation into the notch and for drilling the ACL femoral tunnel

The use of three portals offers the following advantages:

1. The additional medial portal allows the ACL femoral attachment site to be viewed through the AM portal while working instrumentation is inserted into the notch through the AAM portal. As will be discussed later, viewing through the AM portal is the preferred method to visualize the ACL femoral attachment site.
2. Drilling the ACL femoral tunnel through an AAM portal increases the obliquity of the ACL femoral tunnel relative to lateral wall of the notch, resulting in a longer femoral tunnel length and a more elliptical ACL femoral tunnel aperture compared to drilling the femoral tunnel through the AM portal [41, 42].

19.4.1 Establish the Anterolateral Portal

A high AL portal is created at the level of the inferior pole of the patella, as close as possible to the lateral border of the patellar tendon using a #11 knife blade. A high AL portal places the arthroscope above the widest part of the fat pad, which minimizes interference of the visual field in the intercondylar notch when the knee is positioned in hyperflexion. A high AL portal also provides a better, "look down" view of the ACL tibial attachment site.

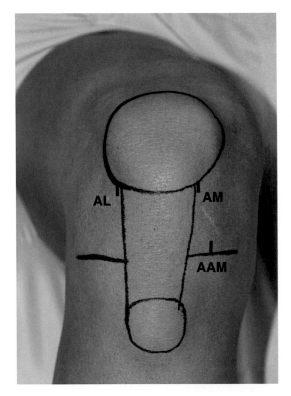

Fig. 19.3 Three arthroscopic portals and their relationship to the inferior pole of the patella, medial and lateral borders of the patellar tendon, and the medial and lateral joint lines (*marked*). *AL* high anterolateral portal, *AM* high anteromedial portal, *AAM* low accessory anteromedial portal

19.4.2 Establish the Anteromedial Portal

Creating the AM portal at the correct height above the medial joint line is extremely important. Placing the AM portal too close to the medial joint line will lead to instrument crowding when the AM and AAM portals are used simultaneously during the preparation of the intercondylar notch and during drilling of the ACL femoral tunnel. A 30° arthroscope is introduced into the knee joint through the AL portal and a diagnostic arthroscopy is performed. The knee is flexed to between 70° and 90° and the AM portal created under direct visualization using an 18-gauge spinal needle. The spinal needle is introduced into the knee joint as close as possible to the medial border of the patellar tendon and directed toward the roof of the intercondylar notch. The height of the spinal needle above the medial joint line is adjusted as needed to ensure that it comes to lie parallel to the roof of the intercondylar notch. Typically, the spinal needle is located at the height of the interior pole of the patella or slightly higher. Placing the spinal needle at this level ensures adequate spatial separation between the AM and the AAM portal which is created later and also results in the AM portal being positioned above the fat pad. The spinal needle position is too low if it enters the knee joint below the level of the roof of the intercondylar notch or passes through the fat pad. Placing the AM portal too low above the medial joint line will result in the arthroscope passing through the fat pad and the fat pad being dragged into the visual field by the sheath of the arthroscope. Placing the AM portal too low above the medial joint line will also result in instrument crowding when the AM and AAM portals are used simultaneously to view the ACL femoral attachment site and during drilling of the ACL femoral tunnel. A motored shaver is inserted into the knee joint through the AM portal, and the ligamentum mucosum resected. This step will release the fat pad and expose the intercondylar notch. Any necessary meniscal or chondral surgery can be carried out at this point.

19.4.3 Establish the Accessory Anteromedial Portal

Proper placement of the AAM portal is also critical to the success of the procedure as it is the *most* important factor affecting the length of the ACL femoral tunnel. The medial-lateral placement of the AAM portal determines both the length of the ACL femoral tunnel and the shape of the aperture of the femoral tunnel. Positioning the AAM portal more medially results in a more perpendicular orientation of the drill bit with respect to the lateral wall of the notch and produces a shorter ACL femoral tunnel and a more circular-shaped tunnel aperture [41, 42] (Fig. 19.4). However, placing the AAM portal too medially can result in damage to the medial femoral condyle when drilling the ACL femoral tunnel through the AAM portal.

Moving the AAM portal more laterally, toward the medial border of the patellar ligament, orients the drill bit more obliquely with respect to the lateral wall of the notch and produces a longer ACL femoral tunnel length and a more elliptically shaped tunnel aperture [41, 42] (Fig. 19.5).

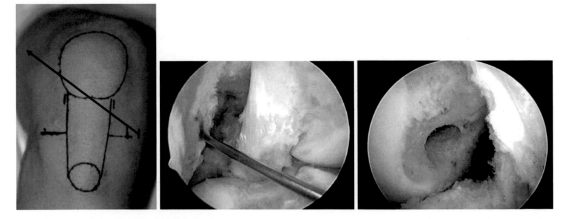

Fig. 19.4 Medial placement of the AAM portal results in a more perpendicular orientation of the spinal needle relative to the lateral wall of the notch. This orientation will produce a more circularly shaped aperture of the ACL femoral tunnel and a shorter femoral tunnel length

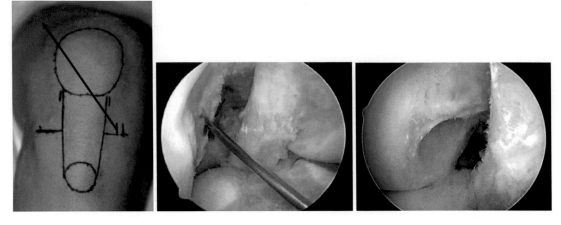

Fig. 19.5 A more lateral placement of the AAM portal results in a more oblique orientation of the spinal needle relative to the lateral wall of the notch. This orientation will result in a more elliptically shaped aperture of the ACL femoral tunnel and a longer femoral tunnel length

Based on the ACL graft type and femoral fixation method, the position of the AAM portal is adjusted to achieve the desired ACL femoral tunnel length. For example, if a bone-patellar tendon-bone ACL graft with interference screw fixation of the femoral bone block is used, the required length of the femoral tunnel is in the range of 20–25 mm, which will allow a 20-mm bone block to be fully inserted into the femoral socket. In this situation, the AAM portal can be positioned more medially. When performing hamstring ACL reconstructions using a cortical suspensory femoral fixation technique, it is desirable to achieve a femoral tunnel length of around 40 mm, with the minimum tunnel length being around 35 mm. These femoral tunnel lengths allow for 20–25 mm of the hamstring tendon graft to be inserted into the ACL femoral socket when a 15-mm polyester loop is selected for the cortical suspensory implant.

An 18-gauge spinal needle is used to locate the optimal position for the AAM portal. The AAM portal should be located as low as possible above the medial joint line while avoiding the anterior horn of the medial meniscus. The 30° arthroscope is rotated medially to determine if the spinal needle is positioned too close to the medial femoral condyle and the position adjusted accordingly. The AAM portal is created using a #11 knife blade, with the cutting edge of the blade oriented away from the anterior horn of the medial meniscus. The AAM portal is dilated by inserting the tips of the Metzenbaum scissors or a small clamp into the knee joint through the AAM portal incision and spreading the tips of the instrument in-line with the direction of the portal. This step will ease future instrument passage through the AAM portal.

19.5 Intercondylar Notch Preparation

The intercondylar notch is viewed through the AL portal and remnants of the torn ACL are resected using a basket punch and motorized shaver blade inserted into the knee joint through the AM portal. Some of the native ACL tissue is preserved at the femoral and tibial attachment sites to aid with later placement of the ACL femoral and tibial tunnels. To enhance biological healing and proprioception and to provide additional biomechanical support to the ACL replacement graft, an attempt should be made to preserve large ACL remnants with intact fiber connections from the femur to the tibia. The vertical fibers of lateral border of the posterior cruciate ligament (PCL) in the center of the notch should be identified and visualized by resecting some of the fat tissue surrounding the PCL with a motorized shaver blade. The distance from the lateral border of the PCL to the lateral wall of the intercondylar notch can be measured with an ACL ruler to ensure there is adequate space for

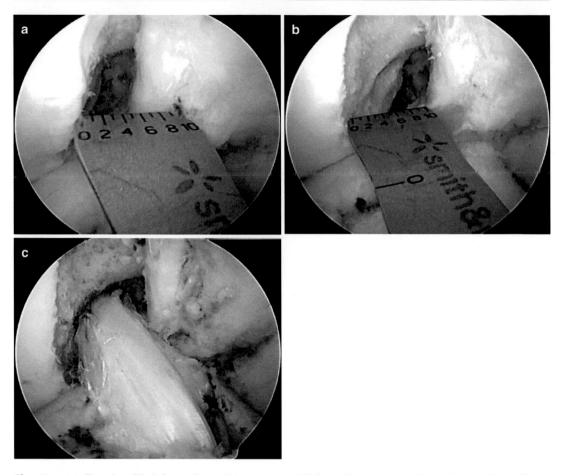

Fig. 19.6 (**a**) Chronic ACL-deficient knee with narrow notch width. The distance between the lateral border of the ACL and lateral wall of the notch measures 5 mm in this case. (**b**) A wallplasty was performed *after* drilling the ACL femoral tunnel. Note that the space between the deep part of the lateral wall of the notch at the site of the ACL femoral tunnel and the lateral border of the PCL was not changed. The distance between the lateral border of the PCL and the lateral wall of the notch was widened to 10 mm to accommodate an 8.5-mm, 5-stranded hamstring tendon graft. (**c**) 5-stranded, 8.5-mm hamstring tendon ACL graft. There is no lateral wall or PCL impingement

the ACL replacement graft (Fig. 19.6). In the case of large ACL grafts or small notch widths, a limited wallplasty may be required. However, the wallplasty should be performed after the ACL femoral tunnel is drilled to avoid removing remnants of the native ACL and the underlying bony landmarks which are valuable aids to help with placement of the ACL femoral tunnel. If a wallplasty is required, it is important to remove bone only at the shallow area of the notch and avoid removing bone in the area of the ACL femoral bone tunnel. Removing bone around the ACL femoral tunnel may lateralize the position of the tunnel, changing the axis of rotation of the ACL replacement graft.

The view of the intercondylar notch and the ACL femoral attachment site changes significantly depending on the arthroscopic portal utilized [3, 12, 39, 40]. Viewing the ACL femoral attachment site through the AM portal provides an orthogonal view of the lateral wall of the notch, allowing accurate assessment of the ACL femoral tunnel position in both the shallow-deep and high-low directions (Fig. 19.7). As a result, the AM portal is the preferred portal for viewing the anatomic ACL femoral attachment site. Viewing the ACL femoral attachment site through the AM portal also eliminates the need to perform a routine notchplasty for visualization purposes. Avoid using a curette, motorized shaver

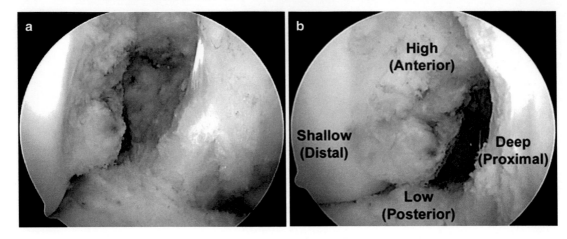

Fig. 19.7 (**a**) Right knee at 90°. View through the AL portal. This view provides a tangential view of the ACL femoral attachment site. (**b**) AM portal view at 90° of flexion. The native ACL femoral footprint is seen along the lower third of the lateral wall of the notch. In the arthroscopic terminology, directions along the lateral wall of the inter-condylar notch are referred to as high or superior, low or inferior, and shallow and deep. The directions using the corresponding anatomic description (shown in parenthesis) which references the knee in the extended position are anterior, posterior, distal, and proximal [3, 14]

blade, or burr to initially perform a notchplasty or to completely remove all of the soft tissue remnants from the lateral wall of the notch as this destroys the remaining native ACL tissue and underlying bony landmarks.

The arthroscope is switched to the AM portal and the knee positioned at 90° of flexion to identify the ACL femoral attachment site. Identification of the ACL femoral attachment can be facilitated by maintaining 90° of flexion and placing the knee in the figure-four position. This position will open the lateral compartment and elevate the femur off the tibia and the lateral meniscus providing a superior view of the inferior articular cartilage border which is an anatomic landmark for the lower border of the native ACL attachment site. Placing the knee in the figure-four position also protects the posterior horn of the lateral meniscus during drilling of the ACL femoral tunnel (Fig. 19.8).

19.6 Identification of the Center of the ACL Femoral Attachment Site

Although the clockface reference method has often been used to specify the location of the ACL femoral tunnel, the clockface reference method has several shortcomings: it ignores the depth of the intercondylar notch; there is no agreed-upon reference position for the 3 and 9 o'clock locations; it relies on no known anatomic landmarks; and it cannot be used when viewing the ACL femoral attachment site through the AM portal [3, 12]. Due to the above limitations, the clockface reference is not an accurate method to specify or locate ACL femoral tunnel position. ACL femoral tunnel position is more accurately located and specified using the following methods:

19.6.1 Native ACL Footprint

In most situations, there are remnants of the native ACL present to aid with anatomic ACL femoral tunnel placement (Fig. 19.9).

To use the native ACL footprint method, view the lateral wall of the notch with the 30° arthroscope positioned in the AM portal. Insert a 90° thermal probe through the AAM portal and mark the borders of the ACL femoral attachment site. Next, insert an angled microfracture awl through the AAM portal and mark the center of the ACL femoral attachment site. This "eyeball" technique is fairly accurate for estimating high-low positions. However, due to the visual distortion

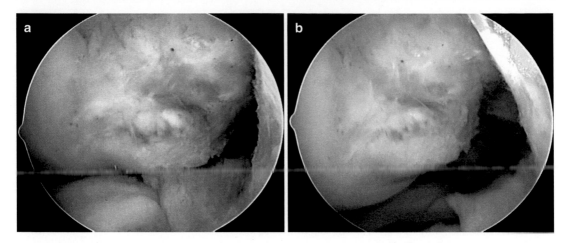

Fig. 19.8 Right knee. (**a**) View of the ACL femoral attachment site through the AM portal with the knee at 90° of flexion. Remnants of the native ACL are seen lying inferior to the lateral intercondylar ridge. (**b**) View of the ACL femoral attachment site through the AM portal with the knee at 90° in the figure-four position. The lateral compartment is opened and the femur elevated from the lateral meniscus. This position provides a better view of the inferior and deep aspects of the ACL femoral attachment site

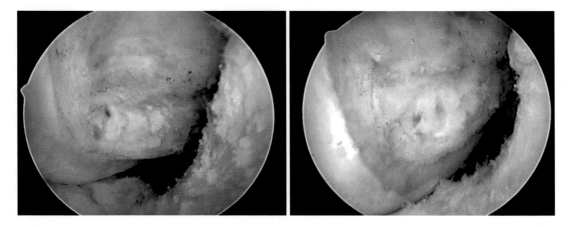

Fig. 19.9 AM portal view at 90° of flexion. The native ACL femoral footprint is clearly seen

associated with the use of a 30° arthroscope, using visual cues to locate the center of the ACL femoral attachment site tends to position the tip of the microfracture awl more shallow than the true center of the ACL femoral attachment site. The true center of the ACL attachment site can be more accurately located using an ACL ruler inserted through the AL portal oriented along the long axis of the ACL attachment site. To achieve the correct axis of measurement, the knee is flexed to 110–120° which orients the long axis of the ACL femoral attachment site parallel to the tibial plateau. The length of the ACL femoral footprint is measured from the deep (proximal) border to the shallow (distal) border along its long axis and the midpoint located and marked by inserting an angled microfracture awl through the AAM portal (Fig. 19.10).

19.6.2 Lateral Intercondylar and Bifurcate Ridges

When there are no remnants of the native ACL present, the underlying bony morphology of the ACL femoral attachment site can provide useful anatomic landmarks to assist with anatomic ACL femoral tunnel placement. The lateral

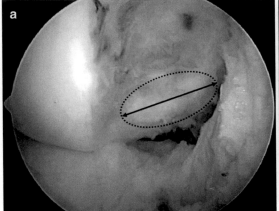

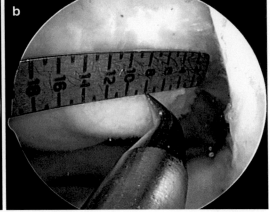

Fig. 19.10 (**a**) AM portal view at 90° of flexion. The margin of the native ACL footprint is outlined by the *dotted ellipse*. The knee is flexed to 110° and the length of the ACL femoral attachment site is measured along its long axis (*black line*). (**b**) The ACL ruler is inserted through the AL portal and an angled microfracture awl inserted through the AAM portal. In this case, the ACL femoral attachment site length measures 14 mm, so the center of the ACL femoral tunnel is placed at the 7-mm mark

intercondylar ridge, when present, is an important anatomic landmark to aid the knee surgeon with anatomic ACL femoral tunnel placement since the native ACL *always* attaches inferior to this ridge [3, 20, 22–24, 26–28]. The lateral intercondylar ridge, therefore, marks the upper limit of the superior border of the ACL femoral attachment site. In some knees, it may be possible to identify a second bony ridge, the lateral bifurcate ridge which separates the attachment sites of the AM and PL bundle fibers [3, 12, 13, 20, 24, 26, 29] (Fig. 19.11). It is important to remember that because the cross-sectional area of the PL and AM bundles is variable from patient to patient, the location of the bifurcate ridge, when present, does not necessarily represent the true center of the ACL femoral attachment site.

The arthroscope is placed in the AM portal and a 90° thermal probe or motorized shaver blade is inserted into the knee joint through the AAM portal and used to remove soft tissue along the lower third of the lateral wall of the notch. The knee is positioned at 90° of flexion and the border of the inferior (posterior) articular cartilage identified. As mentioned earlier, the inferior articular cartilage border is best visualized by placing the knee in the figure-four position. The lateral intercondylar ridge is most easily identified by starting the dissection at the inferior

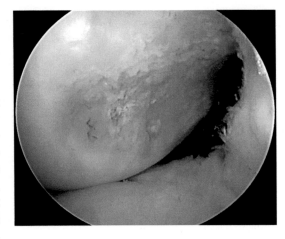

Fig. 19.11 View through the AM portal at 90° of flexion. The lateral intercondylar and bifurcate ridges are clearly seen

articular cartilage border and working in the superior (high) direction along the lateral wall of the notch. A distinct endpoint is often encountered as the tip of the thermal probe contacts the ridge. The center of the ACL femoral attachment site in the high-low direction is midway between the lateral intercondylar ridge or the superior border of the ACL footprint and the inferior articular cartilage border (Fig. 19.12). Based on anatomic studies, this distance is in the range of 7.3–8.6 mm [8, 21, 23, 28]. According to Ziegler

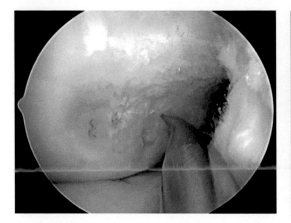

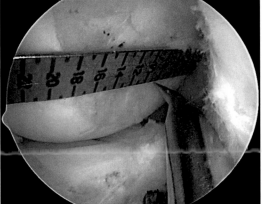

Fig. 19.12 AM portal view at 90°. The tip of the angled microfracture awl is located at the center of the ACL femoral attachment site, 2 mm deep (proximal) to the lateral bifurcate ridge, and halfway between the lateral intercondylar ridge and the inferior (posterior) articular cartilage border

Fig. 19.13 (**a**) View through the AM portal at 90° of flexion. The ACL ruler has been bent to lie flat along the lateral wall of the intercondylar notch. The ruler is inserted through the AL portal and the lower edge is positioned to lie parallel to the wall of the notch just below the lateral intercondylar ridge. In this case, the distance from the deep to shallow articular cartilage margin measures 19 mm. The tip of the microfracture awl is positioned at the 9-mm mark which is 0.5 mm deeper than the calculated 50 % distance (9.5 mm)

et al., the center of the ACL femoral tunnel in the shallow-deep (proximal-distal) direction is 1.7 mm deep (proximal) to the lateral bifurcate ridge [26]. When the lateral bifurcate ridge is not present or visualized, the shallow-deep position of the ACL femoral tunnel can be determined using an ACL ruler as described below.

19.6.3   ACL Ruler

Use of an ACL ruler allows the knee surgeon to individualize the location of the ACL femoral tunnel based on the specific anatomy of the patient. This approach allows for "a la carte" or patient-specific surgery to be performed versus the "one size fits all" approach associated with the use of offset ACL femoral aimers. This technique is particularly useful for revision ACL reconstructive surgery where there are usually no remnants of the native ACL present and the bony landmarks may have been destroyed by prior notchplasty or the previous ACL femoral bone tunnel. The knee is placed at 90° of flexion and the ACL femoral attachment site viewed through the AM portal using a 30° arthroscope. The malleable ACL ruler is bent at approximately a 45° angle at the 24-mm mark to allow it to lie flat along the lateral wall of

the notch. The ACL ruler is inserted into the intercondylar notch through either the AL or the AAM portal (Fig. 19.13). Inserting the ruler through the AL portal allows an angled microfracture awl to be inserted through the AAM portal, making it possible for the surgeon to measure and simultaneously mark the ACL femoral attachment site. However, due to the height of the AL portal above the lateral joint line, in some knees, it may be difficult to position the ACL ruler lower down the lateral wall of the notch at the location of the lateral intercondylar ridge. This limitation can often be overcome by flexing the knee to 120° and or placing the knee in the figure-four position. If these maneuvers are unsuccessful, then the ruler should be inserted into the notch through the AAM portal. The lower position of the AAM portal allows the ruler to be easily positioned along the ACL femoral attachment site.

In the situation where there are no remnants of the native ACL present, position the lower edge of the ruler parallel to and just above the lateral intercondylar ridge. This approach allows the entire ACL femoral attachment site to be visualized which aids in determining the high-low position of the ACL femoral tunnel. Alternatively, the upper edge of the ruler can be positioned parallel to and just below the lateral intercondylar ridge. Insert the ruler along the lateral wall of the notch until the tip is positioned at the deep (proximal) border of the articular cartilage. This point represents the zero reference point for the ruler. Note that this position is different than the commonly referenced "over-the-top" position which lies higher and deeper in the notch. It is important to resect enough soft tissue from the lateral sidewall of the notch to clearly visualize this point. It is helpful to place the tip of an angled microfracture awl at this location and slide the ruler into the notch until tip of the ruler contacts the tip of the microfracture awl. This step will accurately align the ruler at the correct starting point. The length of the sidewall of the notch is measured to the point where the ACL ruler touches the shallow margin of the articular cartilage (Fig. 19.13).

Insert an angled microfracture awl through the AAM portal and use it to mark the location of the ACL femoral tunnel. The center of the ACL femoral tunnel should be located at a shallow-deep position that is 45–50 % of the measured distance from the deep (proximal) articular cartilage border to the shallow articular cartilage border. This point has been validated by Bird et al. as a close approximation to the center of the ACL femoral attachment site [43]. Anatomic studies have revealed that the high-low position of the center of the ACL femoral attachment site is located 7.3–8.6 mm above the inferior articular cartilage border [21, 28, 44]. This position can be achieved by positioning the tip of the microfracture awl midway between the lateral intercondylar ridge or the superior border of the ACL footprint and the inferior (posterior) articular cartilage border.

Note that it is important to avoid positioning the ACL femoral tunnel too shallow in the notch as this will result in the ACL replacement graft experiencing higher forces in extension. The zero starting point of the ruler must be accurately identified and if in doubt the 50 % measured distance reduced by 1–2 mm to avoid positioning the ACL graft too shallow in the notch. Figure 19.14 demonstrates the anatomy of the ACL femoral attachment.

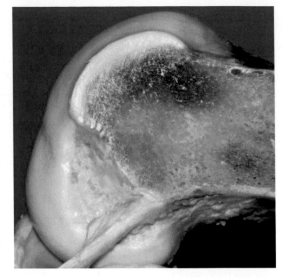

Fig. 19.14 Right knee, human cadaver. The medial femoral condyle has been removed, allowing the ACL femoral attachment site to be visualized. The lateral intercondylar ridge is clearly seen. Note that the shallow fibers of the native ACL do not completely extend to the shallow articular cartilage margin

19.7   Use of Intraoperative Fluoroscopy

At the present time, interoperative fluoroscopy is the most accurate method to determine and evaluate ACL femoral tunnel placement [45–47]. Fluoroscopy gives the surgeon the ability to precisely measure and if needed change the ACL femoral tunnel position during the surgical procedure. Fluoroscopy is especially valuable in revision cases where there are usually no remnants of the native ACL present and the bony anatomy of the ACL femoral attachment site has been altered or destroyed by prior notchplasty and the previous ACL femoral tunnel. Fluoroscopy is also extremely helpful when attempting to preserve remnants of the torn ACL or performing an augmentation technique for a partial ACL tear. In these situations, identification of the lateral intercondylar and bifurcate ridges is not feasible as this would require resection of intact ACL fibers to expose the lateral wall of the notch. The ruler technique is also not possible since the intact ACL fibers prevent accurate positioning of the ruler along the lateral wall

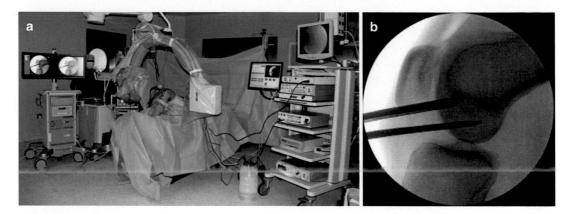

Fig. 19.15 (**a**) Intraoperative fluoroscopy. (**b**) The angled microfracture awl is positioned at the center of the ACL femoral attachment site

of the notch. Using fluoroscopy, the proper placement of the ACL femoral tunnel can be easily accomplished without the need to rely on remnants of the native ACL, measurements along the lateral wall of the notch, or the bony anatomy of the ACL femoral attachment site.

The knee is positioned at 90° of flexion and an angled microfracture awl is positioned at the chosen ACL femoral tunnel location. A sterile-draped digital c-arm is used to take a true lateral radiograph of the knee (Fig. 19.15a). A true lateral radiograph is one in which the inferior (posterior) and deep (proximal) borders of the medial and lateral femoral condyles overlap (Fig. 19.15b). Due to the size difference between the medial and lateral femoral condyles, it is often difficult to achieve a perfect overlap of the shallow (distal) borders of both condyles. However, it is not necessary to achieve a perfect overlap of the distal condylar borders to obtain reliable information.

The grid system described by Bernard and Hertel is used to locate the center of the ACL femoral attachment site [45]. This method is easy to use, is reproducible, and has been shown to be independent of the knee size, shape, and the distance between the x-ray tube and the patient. The Bernard-Hertel grid is drawn in the following way:

1. Draw a tangent to the roof of the intercondylar notch (Blumensaat's line). Draw two lines perpendicular to that line, one at the intersection of the tangent line with the shallow border of the lateral femoral condyle and the other with the intersection of the tangent line and the deep border of the lateral femoral condyle. The lateral femoral condyle can be identified by an indentation at the distal margin (Grant's notch) and the fact that the medial femoral condyle extends more distal.

2. Draw another line parallel to Blumensaat's line and tangent to the inferior border of the condyles. Measurements are made as percentages along Blumensaat's line (t), which represents the maximum sagittal diameter of the lateral femoral condyle, and line (h), which represents the maximum intercondylar notch height (Fig. 19.16).

The Bernard-Hertel grid has been used to locate the centers of the PL and AM bundle in human cadaveric specimens [19, 25, 28, 38, 44, 45, 48–50]. A summary of these studies is shown in Table 19.1.

Using data from these studies, a weighted average position for the center of the ACL femoral attachment site can be calculated. This calculation reveals that the center of the ACL femoral attachment site is located at a point which is 27 % along Blumensaat's line and 34 % of the height of the intercondylar notch (Fig. 19.17).

Commercially available software (Smith & Nephew ACUFEX Director Application Anatomic Guide) can be used to plot the Bernard and Hertel grid from the intraoperative c-arm image

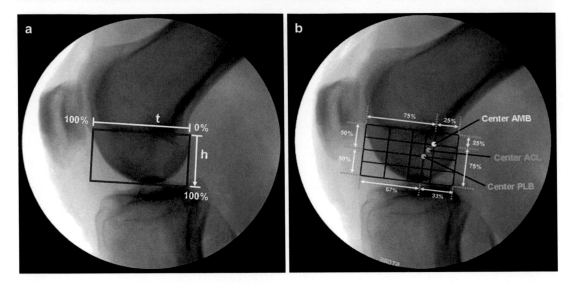

Fig. 19.16 (**a**) Bernard-Hertel grid method, (t) represents measurement along Blumensaat's line and (h) the height of the intercondylar notch. (**b**) The centers of the AM and PL bundles are shown according to the data of Columbet et al. [19]. In this study, the center of the AM bundle was found to lie at a point 25 % along Blumensaat's line (t) and 25 % along line (h). The center of the PL bundle was located at a point 33 % along line (t) and 50 % along line (h)

Table 19.1 Published anatomic studies using the Bernard-Hertel grid to locate the centers of the AMB and PLB

Summary of radiographic grid measurements						
Study	AMB depth	PLB depth	Av 50 % depth	AMB height	PLB height	Av 50 % height
Bernard-Hertel (1997) [45], $n=10$			24.8			28.5
Yamamoto (2004) [38], $n=10$	25	29	27	16	42	29
Colombet (2006) [19], $n=7$	26.4	32.3	29.4	25.3	47.6	36.5
Zantop (2008) [28], $n=20$	18.5	29.3	23.9	22.3	53.6	38.0
Tsukada (2008) [25], $n=36$	25.9	34.8	30.4	17.8	42.1	30.0
Lorenz (2009) [50], $n=12$	21	27	24	22	45	34
Forsythe (2010) [48], $n=8$	21.7	35.1	28.4	33.2	55.3	44.3
Pietrini (2011) [44], $n=12$	21.6	28.9	25.3	14.6	42.3	28.5
Iriuchishima (2010) [49], $n=15$	15	32	23.5	26	52	39
Weighted averages	22.0	31.6	26.7	21.0	46.8	33.5

(Fig. 19.18). Alternatively, the images can be saved to an image capture unit and the grid applied later as a quality control check. The microfracture awl position is adjusted under arthroscopic and fluoroscopic guidance until the desired position is obtained.

Using any or all of the above guidelines eliminates the need to use an offset ACL femoral aimer and referencing off the "over-the-top" position to determine ACL femoral tunnel placement. ACL femoral offset aimers can constrain the location of the femoral guide pin and can lead to nonanatomic placement of the ACL femoral tunnel. The above guidelines allow the surgeon to select and verify the location of the ACL femoral tunnel position using established anatomic and radiographic landmarks.

19.8 Drilling the ACL Femoral Tunnel

The 30° arthroscope is placed in the AM portal and the angled microfracture awl inserted into the notch through the AAM portal. The tip of the

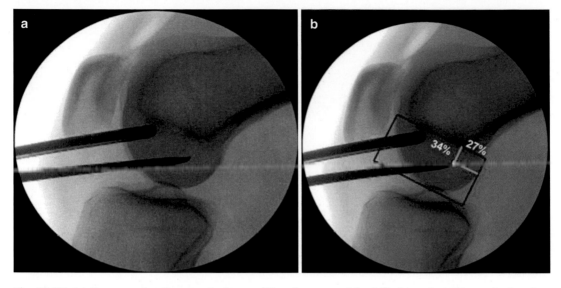

Fig. 19.17 (**a**) Intraoperative fluoroscopic image. (**b**) Bernard-Hertel grid. The tip of the angled microfracture awl is located at the 27 %/34 % location, which represents the center of the ACL femoral attachment site based on the calculated weighted average from published anatomic studies [19, 25, 28, 38, 44, 45, 48–50]

angled microfracture awl is positioned at the center of the ACL femoral attachment and the knee slowly flexed to a minimum of 120°. Flexion above 120° is often helpful in achieving longer femoral tunnel lengths. The knee is stabilized in hyperflexion by locking the foot of the operative leg under the most proximal foot post. One criticism about viewing the ACL femoral attachment site through the AM portal is that the view is compromised by the need to work in the notch with the knee flexed to 120° or higher. Due to the rotation of the ACL femoral attachment site that occurs when the knee is flexed beyond 90°, it is our experience that an excellent view of the ACL femoral attachment site, particularly the inferior and deep aspects, can be obtained (Fig. 19.19). As a result, we have not found it necessary to use a 70° arthroscope or switch the arthroscope to the AL portal.

Hyperflexion of the knee results in a loss of joint distension due to external compression of the knee joint capsule by the soft tissues of the thigh. This can result in bleeding and a loss of joint visualization due to encroachment of the fat pad into the notch. One solution to maintain adequate joint distension and visualization while working in the notch with the knee in

hyperflexion is to increase the pump fluid pressure up to 120 mm Hg. The pump pressure is decreased back to the normal setting after drilling the ACL femoral tunnel and the knee has been extended back to 90°. If increasing the fluid pressure does not solve the problem and the fat pad still limits visualization, limited resection of the fat pad should be performed using a motorized shaver blade inserted through the AAM or AL portal.

The microfracture awl is removed from the knee and a 0° ACL femoral offset aimer inserted in the notch through the AAM. The offset femoral aimer is advanced to the site of the mark left by the microfracture awl. If there is an inadequate view of the ACL femoral attachment site or loss of the microfracture awl occurs, the knee is brought back to the 90° position and further soft tissue resected using a motorized shaver blade. A drill-tip-graduated guide pin is passed into the notch through the 0° ACL offset femoral aimer and placed into the divot mark left by microfracture awl. The drill-tip guide pin is tapped into the bone using a small mallet. Keeping the tip of the drill-tip guide pin in the divot, the handle of the 0° offset aimer is slowly moved in a lateral direction, and the guide pin is

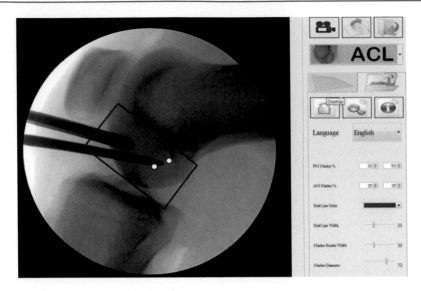

Fig. 19.18 The Smith & Nephew ACUFEX Director Application Anatomic Guide software was used to plot the location of the AM and PL bundles (*white circles*) based on the data of Columbet et al. [19]. The software also allows other data for the centers of the AM and PM bundles to be selected. In this example, the tip of the microfracture awl is positioned halfway between the centers of the AM and PL bundles (*white circles*). This location would position the ACL femoral tunnel in the center of the ACL femoral attachment site

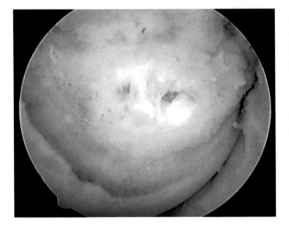

Fig. 19.19 View through the AAM portal with the knee in hyperflexion. The inferior and deep (proximal) aspects of the ACL femoral attachment site are well visualized. The ACL femoral tunnel position has been previously marked with a microfracture awl using the ACL ruler method. The marked location can be clearly seen to lie at the center of the ACL attachment site

tapped into the attachment site until the drill-tip part of the pin is fully buried into the bone. This maneuver increases the obliquity of the guide pin relative to the lateral wall of the notch, resulting in a longer femoral tunnel length and a more elliptically shaped tunnel aperture (Fig. 19.20).

An elliptically shaped tunnel covers more of the ACL femoral attachment site and more closely reproduces the anatomy of the native ACL attachment site versus a circular-shaped femoral tunnel [42]. Slowly drill the drill-tip-graduated guide pin through the lateral femoral condyle until the resistance of the lateral femoral cortex is encountered. Note the depth mark on the graduated drill-tip passing pin at the point of maximum resistance. This distance will provide a good estimate of the ACL femoral tunnel length. If the resulting ACL femoral tunnel length is less than desired, it is often possible to increase the femoral tunnel length by reversing the guide pin back to the entry point, angling the offset aimer more laterally, and increasing the knee flexion angle. These maneuvers can often redirect the drill-tip guide pin more proximally up the femoral shaft, producing a longer femoral tunnel length.

Depending on the intended graft fixation method, final drilling of the femoral tunnel is variable but essentially involves using a drill bit which is sized to the measured diameter of the ACL replacement graft. When using a cortical suspensory fixation technique such as the

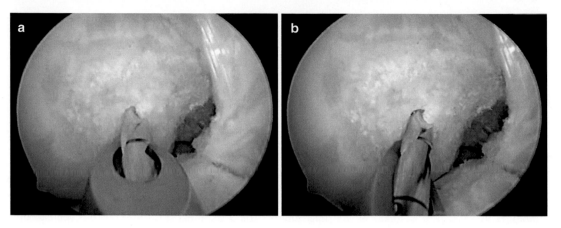

Fig. 19.20 AM portal view in hyperflexion. (**a**) The femoral drill-tip guide pin is oriented perpendicular to ACL femoral attachment site. This guide pin orientation will result in a short femoral tunnel length and a more circular shape of the ACL femoral tunnel aperture. (**b**) The 0° offset aimer has been angled laterally which results in the guide pin being oriented more obliquely to ACL femoral attachment site. A more oblique orientation of the guide pin will increase the length of the ACL femoral tunnel and produce a more elliptically shaped femoral tunnel aperture

ENDOBUTTON CL (Smith & Nephew, London, UK), it is necessary to drill a 4.5-mm tunnel through the lateral cortex of the femur. The 4.5-mm ENDOBUTTON drill bit can be used to measure the tunnel length by hooking the 10-mm drill portion on the lateral cortex and subtracting this distance from the measured length noted arthroscopically. Alternatively, the femoral tunnel length is measured using a depth gauge. During drilling of the ACL femoral tunnel, fluid flow and visualization in the notch can be facilitated by inserting a motorized shaver blade through the AL portal. The suction on the shaver can be used to maintain fluid flow and to suction bone debris created during the drilling of the ACL femoral tunnel, thus maintaining a clear visual field. The shaver can also be used to resect any portions of the fat pad restricting passage of the endoscopic reamer or obstructing visualization in the notch.

The 4.5-mm ENDOBUTTON (or equivalent) drill bit is removed from the knee joint and the appropriate size endoscopic reamer advanced over the guide pin to the ACL femoral attachment site (Fig. 19.21). The depth of the femoral socket is determined by the measured length of the femoral tunnel. For the ENDOBUTTON fixation device, the depth of the ACL femoral socket must equal the length of the ACL graft to

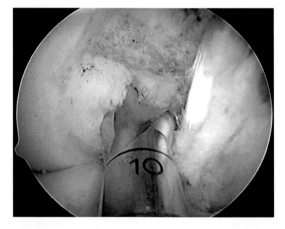

Fig. 19.21 AM portal view in hyperflexion. The endoscopic drill bit is inserted into the knee joint through the AAM portal. The ACL femoral footprint is clearly visible and the drill bit is seen to lie at the center of the ACL femoral attachment site

be inserted into the socket plus an additional minimum distance of 6 mm, to allow the ENDOBUTTON to exit the femoral tunnel and flip on the lateral femoral cortex. When femoral fixation of the ACL graft is performed with an interference screw, the femoral socket can be drilled to the length of the bone block so that the desired length of graft can be inserted into the femoral socket. The reamer is removed from the knee joint and a number 2 polyester suture threaded through the eyelet of the guide pin. The free ends of the suture are pulled out through the lateral soft tissue, leaving the loop of the suture in the femoral socket.

19.9 Assessment of the Femoral Tunnel

A motorized shaver blade is inserted into the femoral tunnel through the AAM portal and used to remove bony debris from inside the femoral tunnel. The knee is positioned at 90° and the ACL femoral tunnel inspected. A minimum 2-mm wall should remain inferiorly (posterior) and the aperture of the tunnel should be elliptically shaped rather than circular, thereby more closely restoring the shape of the native ACL femoral attachment site and maximizing the femoral tunnel surface area (Fig. 19.22).

19.10 Alternatives and Variations to This Technique

The surgical technique described in this chapter has outlined several methods for creating an anatomic ACL femoral tunnel. The principal goal of all of these methods is to create an elliptically shaped ACL femoral tunnel at the center of the native ACL femoral attachment site. Alternative techniques for creating the ACL femoral tunnel include:

1. Instead of using two medial portals, the ACL femoral attachment site can be viewed through the AL portal and the femoral tunnel drilled through an AM or AAM portal. This technique may be advantageous in small knees where instrument crowding may occur when using two medial portals. The scope can be temporarily placed into the AM portal to fully evaluate the anatomy of the ACL attachment site and to locate the center of the ACL femoral attachment site. Once this has been accomplished, the arthroscope is moved back to the AL portal and the ACL femoral tunnel drilled through the AM or AAM portal.

2. The ACL femoral tunnel can be drilled using flexible reamers, in which case, it is not necessary to hyperflex the knee.

3. The ACL femoral tunnel can be drilled using an outside-in technique. In this situation, the exit point of the guide wire within the notch can still be determined by the methods described in this chapter.

> **Memory**
> The ACL femoral attachment site is defined by two bony ridges, the lateral intercondylar and the lateral bifurcate ridges. The lateral intercondylar ridge is an important

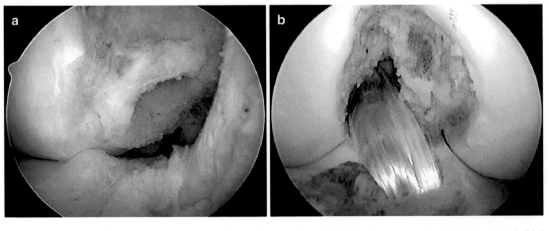

Fig. 19.22 (**a**) AM portal view at 90°. The elliptically shaped aperture of the ACL femoral tunnel is centered in the ACL femoral footprint. (**b**) 5-stranded hamstring ACL graft positioned at the center of native femoral and tibial attachment sites

anatomic landmark during surgery since the native ACL always attaches inferior (posterior) to it. The center of the ACL femoral attachment site is 1.7 mm deep (proximal) to the bifurcate ridge and 7.3–8.5 mm superior (anterior) to the inferior (posterior) articular cartilage border of the lateral femoral condyle. For anatomic single-bundle ACL reconstruction, the center of the ACL femoral attachment site is chosen as the location for the ACL femoral tunnel. This recommendation is based on biomechanical studies demonstrating that an ACL replacement graft placed at the center of the ACL femoral attachment site is more effective in controlling anterior tibial translation and the combined motions of anterior tibial translation and internal tibial rotation (simulated pivot shift test) compared to an "isometric" ACL femoral tunnel placement or femoral tunnel placements that have traditionally restored predominantly the anteromedial bundle fibers. The ACL femoral attachment site is best visualized by viewing the lateral wall of the intercondylar notch through the anteromedial portal. Anatomic placement of the ACL femoral tunnel is facilitated by drilling the femoral tunnel through an accessory anteromedial portal. Drilling the ACL femoral tunnel through the AAM portal allows acceptable femoral tunnel lengths to be obtained. The center of the ACL femoral attachment site can be located using the following methods: the native ACL footprint, the lateral intercondylar and bifurcate ridges, an ACL ruler, and intraoperative fluoroscopy.

References

1. Hussein M, van Eck CF, Cretnik A et al (2012) Prospective randomized clinical evaluation of conventional single-bundle, anatomic single-bundle, and anatomic double-bundle anterior cruciate ligament reconstruction. 281 cases with 3- to 5-year follow-up. Am J Sports Med 40:512–520

2. Kamath GV, Redfern JC, Greis PE, Burks RT (2011) Revision anterior cruciate ligament reconstruction. Am J Sports Med 39:199–217
3. Karlsson J, Irrgang JJ, van Eck CF, Samuelsson K, Mejia HA, Fu FH (2011) Anatomic single- and double-bundle anterior cruciate ligament reconstruction, part 2. Clinical application of surgical technique. Am J Sport Med 39:2016–2026
4. Lind M, Menhert F, Pedersen AB (2012) Incidence and outcome after revision anterior cruciate ligament reconstruction: results from the Danish registry of knee ligament reconstructions. Am J Sports Med 40:1551–1557
5. Marchant B, Noyes F, Barber-Westin S, Fleckenstein C (2010) Prevalence of nonanatomical graft placement in a series of failed anterior cruciate ligament reconstruction. Am J Sports Med 38:1987–1996
6. Sadoghi P, Kröpfl A, Jansson V et al (2011) Impact of tibial and femoral tunnel position on clinical results after anterior cruciate ligament reconstruction. Arthroscopy 27:355–364
7. Sommer C, Friederich NF, Müller W (2000) Improperly placed anterior cruciate ligament graft: correlation between radiological parameters and clinical results. Knee Surg Sports Traumatol Arthrosc 8:207–213
8. Trojani C, Sbihi A, Dijan P et al (2011) Causes for failure of ACL reconstruction and influence of meniscectomies after revision. Knee Surg Sports Traumatol Arthrosc 19:196–201
9. Wetzler MJ, Getelman MH, Friedman MJ, Bartolozzi AF (1998) Revision anterior cruciate ligament surgery: etiology of failures. Oper Tech Sports Med 6:64–69
10. Whitehead TS (2013) Failure of anterior cruciate ligament reconstruction. Clin Sports Med 32:177–204
11. Wright RW, Huston LJ, Spindler KP et al (2010) Descriptive epidemiology of the multicenter ACL revision study (MARS) cohort. Am J Sports Med 38:1979–1986
12. van Eck CF, Lesniak BP, Schreiber VM, Fu FH (2010) Anatomic single- and double-bundle anterior cruciate ligament reconstruction flowchart. Arthroscopy 26:258–268
13. Yasada K, van Eck CF, Hoshino Y, Fu FH, Tashman S (2011) Anatomic single- and double-bundle anterior cruciate ligament reconstruction, part 1, Basic science. Am J Sport Med 39:1789–1799
14. Amis AA, Jakob RP (1998) Anterior cruciate ligament graft positioning, tensioning and twisting. Knee Surg Sports Traumatol Arthrosc 6(Suppl 1):S2–S12
15. Bylski-Austrow DL, Grood ES, Hefsy MS (1993) Anterior cruciate ligament replacements: a mechanical study of femoral attachment location, flexion angle of tensioning, and initial tensioning. J Orthop Res 8:522–531
16. Grood ES (1992) Placement of knee ligament grafts. In: Finerman GA, Noyes FR (eds) Biology and biomechanics of the traumatized synovial joint: the knee

as a model. American Academy of Orthopaedic Surgeons, Rosemont

17. Hefzy MS, Grood ES (1986) Sensitivity of insertion locations on the length patterns of anterior cruciate ligament fibers. J Biomech Eng 108:73–82

18. Hefzy MS, Grood ES, Noyes FR (1989) Factors affecting the region of most isometric femoral attachments. Part II: Anterior cruciate ligament. Am J Sports Med 17:208–216

19. Columbet P, Robinson J, Christel P, Franceschi J-P et al (2006) Morphology of anterior cruciate ligament attachments for anatomic reconstruction: a cadaveric dissection and radiographic study. Arthroscopy 22:984–992

20. Ferretti M, Ekdahl M, Shen W, Fu F (2007) Osseous landmarks of the femoral attachment of the anterior cruciate ligament: an anatomic study. Arthroscopy 23:1218–1225

21. Kaseta MK, DeFrate LE, Charnock BL, Sullivan RT, Garrett WE (2008) Reconstruction technique affect femoral tunnel placement in ACL reconstruction. Clin Orthop Relat Res 466:1467

22. Kopf S, Musahl V, Tashman S, Szczodry M, Shen W, Fu FH (2009) A systematic review of the femoral origin and tibial insertion morphology of the ACL. Knee Surg Sports Traumatol Arthrosc 17:213–219

23. Purnell ML, Larson AI, Clancy W (2008) Anterior cruciate ligament insertions on the tibia and femur and their relationships to critical bony landmarks using high-resolution volume-rendering computed tomography. Am J Sports Med 36:2083–2090

24. Sasaki N, Ishibashi Y, Tsuda E, Yamamoto Y et al (2012) The femoral insertion of the anterior cruciate ligament: discrepancy between macroscopic and histological observations. Arthroscopy 28:1135–1146

25. Tsukada H, Ishibashi Y, Tsuda E, Furaka A, Toh S (2008) Anatomical analysis of the anterior cruciate ligament femoral and tibial footprints. J Orthop Sci 13:122–129

26. Ziegler CG, Pietrini SD, Westerhaus BD, Anderson CJ et al (2011) Arthroscopically pertinent landmarks for tunnel positioning in single-bundle and double-bundle anterior cruciate ligament reconstructions. Am J Sports Med 39:743–752

27. Shino K, Suzuki T, Iwahashi T, Mae T et al (2010) The resident's ridge as an arthroscopic landmark for anatomical femoral tunnel drilling in ACL reconstruction. Knee Surg Sports Traumatol Arthrosc 18:1164–1168

28. Zantop T, Wellman M, Fu FH, Peterson W (2008) Tunnel positioning of anteromedial and posterolateral bundles in anatomic anterior cruciate ligament reconstruction. Anatomic and radiographic findings. Am J Sports Med 36:65–72

29. van Eck CF, Morse KR, Lesniak BP, Kropf EJ et al (2010) Does the lateral intercondylar ridge disappear in ACL deficient patients? Knee Surg Sports Traumatol Arthrosc 18:1184–1188

30. Kato Y, Ingham SJM, Kramer S et al (2010) Effect of tunnel position for anatomic single-bundle ACL reconstruction on knee biomechanics in a porcine model. Knee Surg Sports Traumatol Arthrosc 18:2–10

31. Kato Y, Maeyama A, Lertwanich P, Wang JH et al (2013) Biomechanical comparison of different graft positions for single-bundle anterior cruciate ligament reconstruction. Knee Surg Sports Traumatol Arthrosc 21:816–823

32. Kondo E, Merican AM, Yasuda K, Amis AA (2011) Biomechanical comparison of anatomic double-bundle, anatomic single-bundle, and nonanatomic single-bundle anterior cruciate ligament reconstruction. Am J Sports Med 39:279–287

33. Bedi A, Musahl V, Steuber V, Kendoff D, Choi D, Allen AA, Pearle AD, Altchek DW (2011) Transtibial versus anteromedial portal reaming in anterior cruciate ligament reconstruction: an anatomic and biomechanical evaluation of surgical technique. Arthroscopy 27:380–390

34. Driscoll MD, Isabell GP, Conditt MA, Ismaily BS et al (2012) Comparison of 2 femoral tunnel locations in anatomic single-bundle anterior cruciate ligament reconstruction: a biomechanical study. Arthroscopy 28:1481–1489

35. Loh JC, Fukuda Y, Tsuda E, Steadman RJ, Fu FH, Woo SL (2003) Knee stability and graft function following anterior cruciate ligament reconstruction: comparison between the 11 o'clock and 10 o'clock femoral tunnel placement. Arthroscopy 19: 297–304

36. Musahl V, Plakseychuk A, VanScyoc AH et al (2005) Varying femoral tunnels between the anatomical footprint and isometric positions. Effect on kinematics of the anterior cruciate ligament-reconstructed knee. Am J Sports Med 33:712–718

37. Scopp JM, Jasper LE, Belkoff SM, Moorman CT (2004) The effect of oblique femoral tunnel placement on rotational constraint of the knee reconstructed using patellar tendon autografts. Arthroscopy 20:294–299

38. Yamamoto Y, Hsu WH, Woo SL, Van Scyoc A et al (2004) Knee stability and graft function after anterior cruciate ligament reconstruction: a comparison of a lateral and an anatomical femoral tunnel placement. Am J Sports Med 32:1825–1832

39. Araujo PH, van Eck CF, Macalena JA, Fu FH (2011) Advances in the three-portal technique for single- or double-bundle ACL reconstruction. Knee Surg Sports Traumatol Arthrosc 19:1239–1242

40. Cohen SB, Fu FH (2007) Three-portal technique for anterior cruciate ligament reconstruction: use of a central medial portal. Arthroscopy 23:325.e1–325.e4

41. Tompkins M, Milewski MD, Carson EW et al (2013) Femoral tunnel length in primary anterior cruciate ligament reconstruction using an accessory medial portal. Arthroscopy 29:238–243

42. Hensler D, Working Z, Illingworth K, Thorhauer E, Tashman S, Fu F (2011) Medial portal drilling: effects on the femoral tunnel aperture morphology during anterior cruciate ligament reconstruction. J Bone Joint Surg Am 93:2063–2071

43. Bird J, Carmont M, Dhillon M, Smith N, Brown C, Thompson P, Spalding T (2011) Validation of a new technique to determine midbundle femoral tunnel position in anterior cruciate ligament reconstruction using 3-D computed tomography analysis. Arthroscopy 27:1259–1267

44. Pietrini SD, Ziegler CG, Anderson CJ, Wijdicks CA et al (2011) Radiographic landmarks for tunnel positioning in double-bundle ACL reconstructions. Knee Surg Sports Traumatol Arthrosc 19:792–800

45. Bernard M, Hertel P, Hornung H, Cierpinski T (1997) Femoral insertion of the ACL. Radiographic quadrant method. Am J Knee Surg 10:14–22

46. Lobenhoffer P, Bernard M, Agneskirchner J (2003) Quality assurance in cruciate ligament surgery. Arthroscopie 16:202–208 (German)

47. Passler H, Hoher J (2004) Intraoperative quality control of the placement of bone tunnels for the anterior cruciate ligament. Unfallchirurg 107:263–272 (in German)

48. Forsythe B, Kopf S, Wong AK, Martins CA-Q et al (2010) The location of femoral and tibial tunnels in anatomic double-bundle anterior cruciate ligament reconstruction analyzed by three-dimensional computed tomography models. J Bone Joint Surg Am 92-A:1418–1429

49. Iriuchishima T, Ingham SJM, Tajima G, Horaguchi T et al (2010) Evaluation of the tunnel placement in the anatomical double-bundle ACL reconstruction: a cadaver study. Knee Surg Sports Traumatol Arthrosc 18:1226–1231

50. Lorenz S, Elser F, Mitterer M, Obst T, Imhoff AB (2009) Radiographic evaluation of the insertion sites of the 2 functional bundles of the anterior cruciate ligament using 3-dimensional computed tomography. Am J Sports Med 37:2368–2376

Fluoroscopy for Bone Tunnel Placement

20

Rainer Siebold and Hans H. Pässler

Contents

R. Siebold (✉)
Institute for Anatomy and Cell Biology,
Ruprecht-Karls University Heidelberg,
Im Neuenheimer Feld 307, Heidelberg
69120, Germany

HKF: Center for Specialised Hip-Knee-Foot Surgery,
ATOS Hospital Heidelberg, Bismarckstr. 9-15,
Heidelberg 69115, Germany
e-mail: rainer.siebold@atos.de

Hans H. Pässler
HKF: Center for Specialised Hip-Knee-Foot Surgery,
ATOS Hospital Heidelberg, Bismarckstr. 9-15,
Heidelberg 69115, Germany

20.1   Introduction

The most important requirement for anatomical ACL reconstruction is correct bone tunnel placement. However, arthroscopic control of exact bone tunnel placement is difficult. Especially on the femoral side, arthroscopic identification of anatomical bone tunnel positioning is unfavourable. But even when changing the camera to the anteromedial portal, femoral bone tunnel placement might be vague due to a lack of clear bony or soft tissue landmarks. On the tibial side fluoroscopy is important to avoid anterior intercondylar notch impingement.

20.2   Intraoperative Fluoroscopy

In 2004, Paessler and Hoeher [4] have shown that fluoroscopy is a reliable tool to control intraoperative tibial and femoral bone tunnel placement before drilling in ACL reconstruction (see also Sect. 24.4 and Chap. 19) (Fig. 20.1). Radiographic positions of the femoral and tibial ACL insertion sites are well defined [1–3, 5, 6].

On the tibial side it is important to avoid anterior intercondylar notch impingement. Therefore a K-wire is positioned in the tibial ACL insertion site using a tibial aimer. A spacer (e.g., Richard Wolf, Germany) with an 8 mm diameter head is inserted through the medial portal and placed around the K-wire. The knee is extended, and the lateral fluoroscopy is performed (Fig. 20.2) to

R. Siebold et al. (eds.), *Anterior Cruciate Ligament Reconstruction*,
DOI 10.1007/978-3-642-45349-6_20, © ESSKA 2014

Fig. 20.1 The use of the C-arm during ACL reconstruction for control of tibial and femoral bone tunnel placement. Setting in the OR

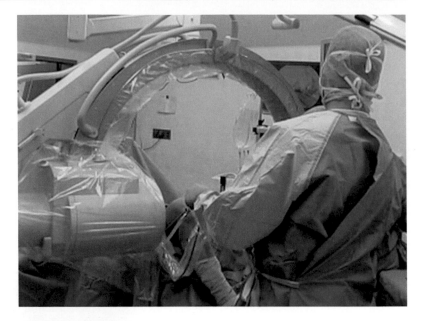

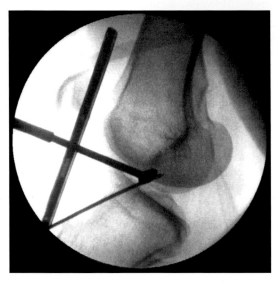

Fig. 20.2 Tibial bone tunnel placement: lateral tibial fluoroscopy to exclude an anterior intercondylar notch impingement

exclude anterior notch impingement (too anterior K-wire placement). In case of impingement, the K-wire is positioned more posterior at the tibial insertion site.

Femoral bone tunnel positioning and drilling is done through a low anteromedial portal. The knee is placed on the table in 90° of flexion. A microfracture awl is brought in place at the aimed tunnel position in the ACL insertion at the lateral intercondylar notch wall (Fig. 20.3a). The lateral fluoroscopy is performed to reconfirm correct positioning (Fig. 20.3b). In case of nonanatomical placement of the microfracture awl, the position has to be corrected before drilling.

Anatomical bone tunnel positioning is performed just posterior and along the intercondylar ridge. The ridge is an extension of the posterior cortex of the lateral distal femur and the lateral femoral condyle. An imaginary line can be drawn during surgery on the lateral fluoroscopy to estimate the intercondylar ridge, the femoral ACL footprint and correct tunnel positioning. Radiographs with tip of microfracture awl in position for SB, DB (Fig. 20.4a) or partial ACL reconstruction of AM (Fig. 20.4b) or PM (Fig. 20.4c). After marking with the microfracture awl, a K-wire is introduced and bone tunnel drilling is performed.

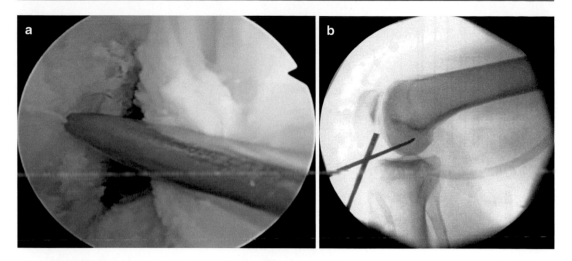

Fig. 20.3 (**a**, **b**) Femoral bone tunnel placement: lateral femoral fluoroscopy to exclude wrong femoral bone tunnel placement

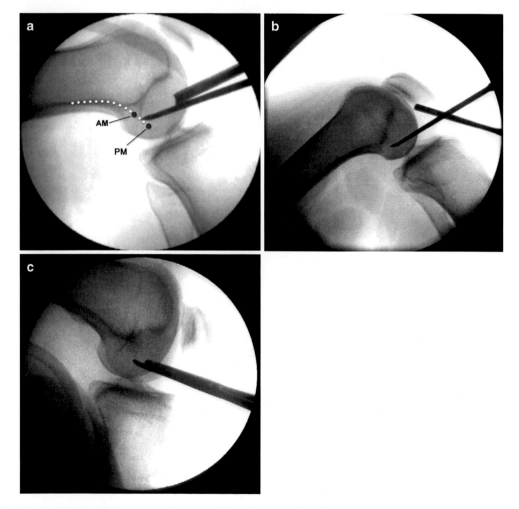

Fig. 20.4 (**a–c**) Femoral bone tunnel placement. Microfracture awl in place

References

1. Hughes AW, Dwyer AJ, Govindaswamy R et al (2012) The use of intra-operative fluoroscopy for tibial tunnel placement in anterior cruciate ligament reconstruction. Bone Joint Res 1(10): 234–237
2. Larson BJ, DeLange L (2008) Fluoroscopically-assisted hamstring ACL reconstruction. Orthopedics 31(7):657–662
3. Moloney G, Araujo P, Rabuck S et al (2013) Use of a fluoroscopic overlay to assist arthroscopic anterior cruciate ligament reconstruction. Am J Sports Med 41(8):1794–1800
4. Passler HH, Hoher J (2004) Intraoperative quality control of the placement of bone tunnels for the anterior cruciate ligament. Unfallchirurg 107(4):263–272
5. Pietrini SD, Ziegler CG, Anderson CJ et al (2011) Radiographic landmarks for tunnel positioning in double-bundle ACL reconstructions. Knee Surg Sports Traumatol Arthrosc 19(5):792–800
6. Snyder GM, Johnson DL (2011) Anatomic graft placement in ACL surgery: plain radiographs are all we need. Orthopedics 34(2):116–118

Bone Tunnel Drilling

21

Wolf Petersen, Rainer Siebold,
Bertrand Sonnery-Cottet, Jacopo Conteduca,
Pooler Archbold, Mathieu Thaunat,
and Pierre Chambat

Contents

21.1 Anteromedial Portal Technique

Wolf Petersen

21.1.1 Introduction

The anteromedial drilling technique is an important feature of anatomic ACL reconstruction (Fig. 21.1). For decades, the conventional transtibial technique has been regarded as the gold standard for femoral tunnel drilling. Transtibial endoscopic ACL reconstruction techniques, however, are associated with the risk to result in vertical graft orientation [8]. Biomechanical studies have shown that a vertical graft ensures not as good against the anterior translation and a simulated pivot shift than an anatomically positioned graft [19, 45]. A vertical femoral tunnel has been cited as one of the most common causes of clinical failure

W. Petersen, MD (✉)
Orthopädie und Unfallchirurgie, Martin Luther
Krankenhaus, Berlin,
Caspar Theyss Strasse 27-34,
Berlin D-14193, Germany
e-mail: w.petersen@mlk-berlin.de

R. Siebold, MD (✉)
Institute for Anatomy and Cell Biology,
Ruprecht-Karls University Heidelberg,
Im Neuenheimer Feld 307,
Heidelberg 69120, Germany

HKF: Center for Spezialised Hip-Knee-Foot Surgery,
ATOS Hospital Heidelberg,
Bismarckstr. 9-15, Heidelberg 69115, Germany
e-mail: rainer.siebold@atos.de

B. Sonnery-Cottet, MD (✉) • J. Conteduca, MD
M. Thaunat, MD • P. Chambat, MD
Centre Orthopédique Santy,
24 Avenue Paul Santy, 69008 Lyon, France
e-mail: sonnerycottet@aol.com

P. Archbold, MD
Musgrave Park Hospital,
Stockmans Lane, Belfast BT9 7JB, Northern Ireland

R. Siebold et al. (eds.), *Anterior Cruciate Ligament Reconstruction*,
DOI 10.1007/978-3-642-45349-6_21, © ESSKA 2014

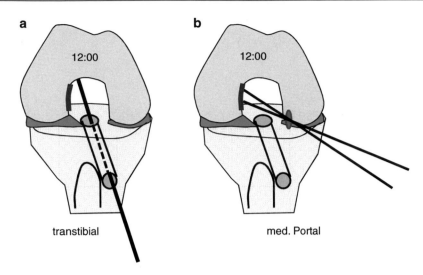

Fig. 21.1 Schematic drawing showing the transtibial (**a**) and anteromedial portal drilling technique (**b**). The anteromedial portal drilling technique allows a more accurate positioning of the femoral socket because the femoral tunnel is not determined by the tibial tunnel

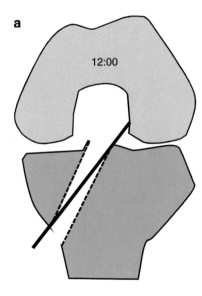
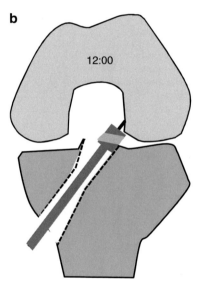

Fig. 21.2 (**a**) Schematic drawing showing that the transtibial drilling technique may be associated with iatrogenic tunnel widening due to eccentric K-wire positioning in the tibial tunnel. (**b**) Drilling through the eccentric placed K-wire may cause damage at the intra- and extra-articular tunnel aperture

after ACL reconstruction with 15–31 % of athletes complaining of pain and persistent instability [6, 42, 43].

Another downside of the transtibial drilling technique is that an eccentric K-wire positioning in the tibial tunnel may result in iatrogenic rereaming of the tibial tunnel and tibial aperture expansion with femoral tunnel preparation (Fig. 21.2).

The anteromedial drilling technique is a solution to overcome these disadvantages. Several studies have shown that the anteromedial portal drilling technique allows an accurate positioning of the femoral socket in the center of the native footprint, resulting in secondary improvement in time-zero control of tibial translation with Lachman and pivot-shift testing compared with conventional

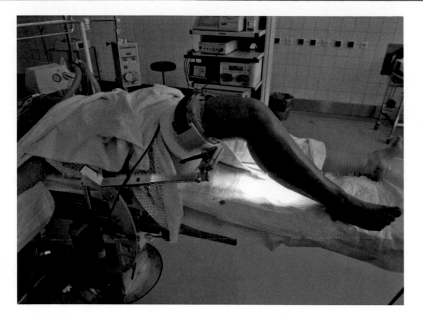

Fig. 21.3 For anteromedial portal drilling, the knee must be flexed to more than 110°. A movable leg holder facilitates anteromedial portal drilling

transtibial ACL reconstruction [8, 10, 32]. Bedi and Altchek [7] stated that endoscopic transtibial offset guides that reference the back wall are difficult to position through the anteromedial portal and should be avoided. Behrendt and Richter [9] have shown in a cadaver study that when a conventional offset guide was used through the anteromedial portal, the K-wire did not reach the middle of the ACL footprint length in any of the specimens. To overcome the disadvantages of conventional transtibial offset guides, we developed a specific offset guide, which was designed for the use via the anteromedial portal (anteromedial portal guide [MPA guide, Karl Storz, Tuttlingen]).

Despite the potential advantages of anteromedial portal reaming, a steep learning curve may exist when transitioning from conventional transtibial ACL reconstruction techniques [7]. Lubowitz [25] reported several pitfalls which may be associated with anteromedial portal drilling, such as posterior tunnel wall blowout, critically short sockets (less than 20 mm), inferior exit of the guidewire from the lateral thigh approaching critical neurovascular structures, iatrogenic injury to the medial femoral condyle with reamer passage, difficulty with visualization and instrumentation in the requisite hyperflexed position,

bending of a rigid guidewire in the hyperflexed position, and difficulty with graft passage and fixation.

Aim of this chapter is to present the technique for anteromedial portal drilling in ACL reconstruction.

21.1.2 Patient Positioning

For anatomical ACL reconstruction with the anteromedial portal drilling technique, the patient is positioned in prone position. The use of a movable leg holder facilitates the operation (Fig. 21.3). A fixed leg holder is not recommended because for anteromedial tunnel drilling the knee needs to be flexed for up to 120°.

21.1.3 Anteromedial Portal Placement

For this drilling technique, the exact placement of the anteromedial portal is essential. The intra-articular aperture of the portal should be directly above the base of the medial meniscus. A needle is always used to simulate the portal (Fig. 21.4).

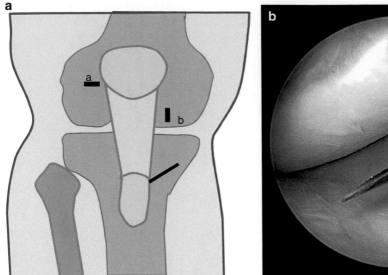

Fig. 21.4 (**a**) Schematic drawing showing both needed for anatomical ACL reconstruction (*a*. high anterolateral portal, *b*. deep anteromedial drilling portal). (**b**) A cannula is always used to simulate the portal. If the portal is placed too far medial, there is a risk that the drill bit damages the cartilage at the medial femoral condyle; if the portal is too far lateral, a posterior blowout of the tunnel wall may occur

If the portal is placed too far medially, there is a risk that the drill bit damages the cartilage at the medial femoral condyle. On the other hand, if the portal is placed laterally, a posterior blowout of the tunnel wall may occur.

The anteromedial portal is created with the knee in 90° of flexion.

21.1.4 "Medial Portal View" and Anatomical Landmarks

Due to the resident's ridge, the femoral insertion cannot be accurately visualized with the arthroscope in the anterolateral portal. A much better visualization of the femoral ACL insertion zone is possible when the arthroscope is switched to the anteromedial portal.

The "anteromedial portal view" is an essential feature of anatomical ACL reconstruction procedures because in a previous study, we have shown that the complete femoral ACL footprint can only be visualized with the arthroscope in the antero-medial portal [33].

From the medial portal, the most important landmarks for femoral tunnel placement can be visualized: the intercondylar line and the cartilage border [33, 44]. The transition between both lines marks the AM bundle insertion (Fig. 21.5).

21.1.5 Tunnel Placement

Tunnel placement starts with placement of the guide pin in the center of the femoral ACL insertion. A recent biomechanical study has shown that in situ force of the ACL graft was most closely restored with an anatomic mid-position single-bundle reconstruction and the in situ force was the highest in a so-called AM-AM reconstruction at each knee flexion angle [22].

For anteromedial portal drilling, the knee should be flexed for more than 110°. The guide pin should be placed in the center of the femoral insertion with or without the use of aiming devices. We prefer to place the guide pin (2.4 mm) with the help of a specific anteromedial portal

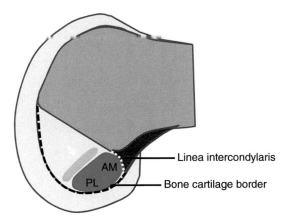

Fig. 21.5 (**a**) Schematic drawing of the femoral insertion of the anterior cruciate ligament. The *dashed line marks* the cartilage border. The *dotted line marks* the intercondylar line. (**b**) Arthroscopic presentation of the femoral ACL insertion via the anteromedial portal

aimer (medial portal aimer, Karl Storz, Tuttlingen, Germany). This guide is an offset guide, which was especially designed for the use via the anteromedial portal (Fig. 21.6). According to Bedi and Altchek [7], the use of a conventional transtibial offset guide might be a pitfall of the anteromedial portal drilling technique, because these guides tend to place the guidewire too far posterior.

The medial portal aimer is used to place the K-wire in the center of the ACL insertion (Figs. 21.6a and 21.7). The K-wire position should always be checked via the anteromedial portal (Fig. 21.8). Figure 21.6b shows a drawing of the femoral insertion zone of the ACL with both landmarks.

When the K-wire is placed centrally within the femoral insertion, the femoral tunnel is drilled with the knee flexed to more than 110° (Fig. 21.9). The technique of tunnel preparation depends on the fixation technique. For button fixation, a 4.5 mm drill is used to drill through the lateral cortex. The length of the whole tunnel varies between 30 and 45 mm. A longer tunnel might be a sign for a high noon position. Then

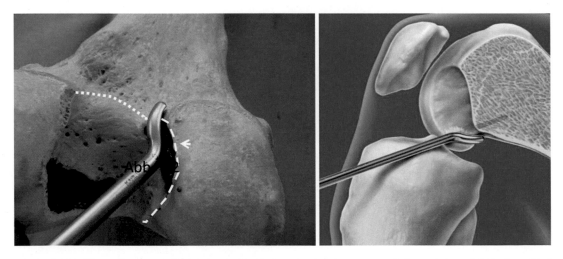

Fig. 21.6 (**a**) The medial portal aimer is hooked behind the intercondylar line in a cadaver specimen. The K-wire is placed in the center of the ACL insertion. (**b**) Drawing

showing the anteromedial portal aimer (MPA aimer, Karl Storz, Tuttlingen, Germany)

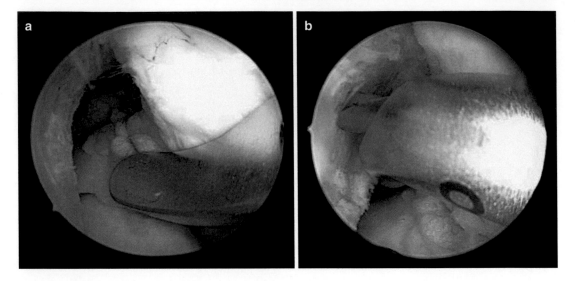

Fig. 21.7 (**a**) The medial portal aimer is introduced via the anteromedial portal (**b**) and the hook is placed behind the intercondylar line

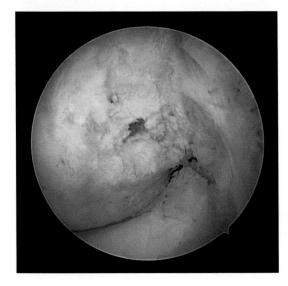

Fig. 21.8 Drill hole of the guidewire checked with the arthroscope in the anteromedial portal

with the use of dilators (Fig. 21.9). The use of dilators minimizes also the risk of cartilage damage at the medial femoral condyle caused by the sharp drill heads. In every case, the final position of the tunnel is controlled and documented with the arthroscope in the anteromedial portal (Fig. 21.10).

a blind tunnel with a diameter according to the size of the graft is drilled with up to a length of 25–30 mm depending of the length of the total tunnel. A gentle tunnel preparation is possible

> **Memory**
> The anteromedial drilling technique allows accurate bone tunnel positioning in the center of the native ACL footprint. The technique overcomes the risk of high femoral tunnel positioning with transtibial drilling. Specific aimers are available to accomplish that goal. A low anteromedial portal is essential for exact femoral tunnel drilling, and a medial portal view is recommended to identify important femoral landmarks for tunnel placement.

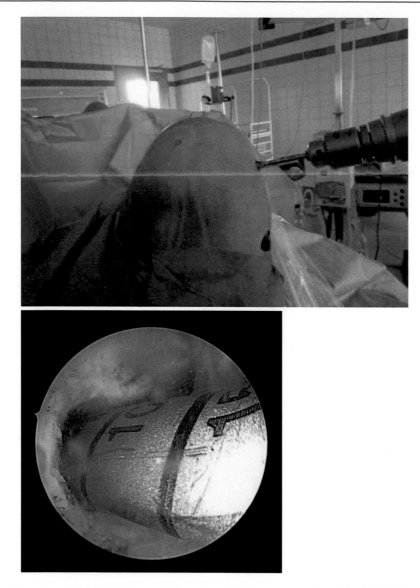

Fig. 21.9 (a) For anteromedial portal drilling, the knee should be flexed to more than 110°. (b) With the use of dilators, a gentle tunnel preparation is possible

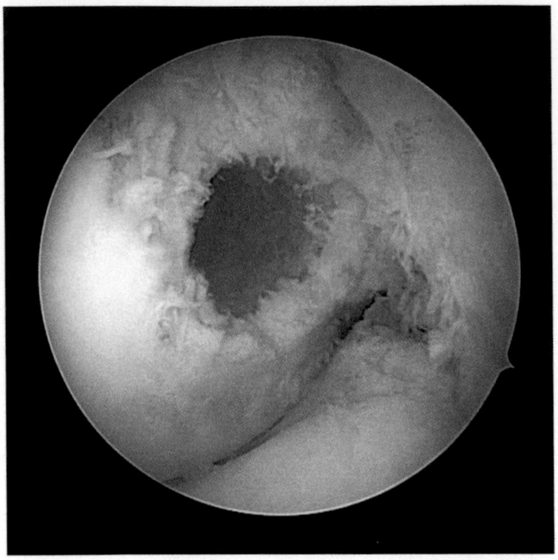

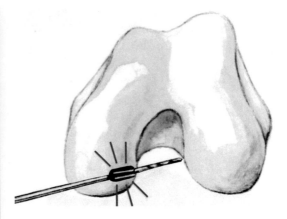

Fig. 21.11 Mechanism of intraoperative articular cartilage damage on the medial femoral condyle

Fig. 21.10 Anatomical femoral tunnel placed in the center of the femoral ACL insertion

21.2 Tips and Tricks for Anteromedial Portal Technique to Avoid Articular Cartilage Damage in ACL Reconstruction

Rainer Siebold

The exact incidence of surgical associated articular cartilage damage caused by bone tunnel drilling in ACL reconstruction is unknown. However, articular cartilage damage may significantly influence the degree of satisfaction with the surgery, the function and activity level, as well as the development of osteoarthritis. This article presents tips and tricks to avoid it [38].

21.2.1 Introduction

As reported by many surgeons [18, 21, 23, 25, 29, 34, 37], the use of the anteromedial portal technique for femoral bone tunnel drilling provides more flexibility in accurate anatomic bone tunnel positioning compared to the transtibial technique. However, anteromedial portal drilling needs a learning curve, is technically demanding, and bears

a risk for articular cartilage damage to the medial femoral condyle [18, 25]. Low flexion angles while drilling the femoral tunnel may also damage the articular cartilage or the subchondral bone plate of the lateral femoral condyle [25, 27, 46] or the posterolateral soft tissue structures [25, 27, 28].

Tibial bone tunnel drilling is also not free of intraoperative pitfalls. When drilled in a flat angle to the tibial plateau and from far medial reaming might damage the articular cartilage of the concave medial tibial plateau close to the medial tibial spine.

21.2.2 Anteromedial Portal Technique

In order to avoid an articular cartilage damage to the medial femoral condyle (Fig. 21.11), the following surgical sequence may be used: under arthroscopic control and in approximately 90° of knee flexion, a long spinal needle is inserted at the intended place of the low anteromedial portal. The needle is advanced into the joint to the intended bone tunnel position in the center of the femoral ACL insertion. The distance between the spinal needle and the articular cartilage of the medial femoral condyle is assessed in order to ensure a safe distance to accommodate the reamer's head. If ensured, the low anteromedial portal is established under arthroscopic control to avoid damage to the anterior horn of the medial meniscus by the surgical blade.

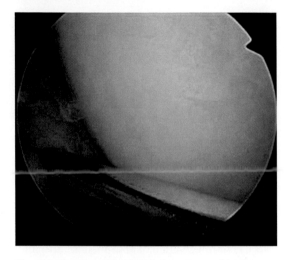

Fig. 21.12 The guide pin has been inserted in the anatomical center of the femoral AM insertion site through a low accessory anteromedial portal. The distance between the articular cartilage of the medial femoral condyle and the guide pin is too small to accommodate a reamer without significant risk to damage the cartilage

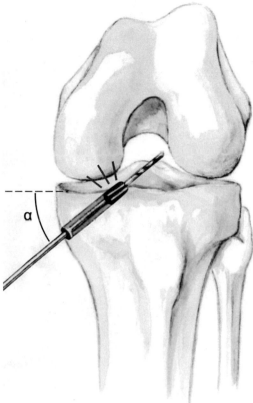

Fig. 21.14 Mechanism of intraoperative articular cartilage damage on the medial tibial plateau

32–40 mm and to avoid damage to the posterolateral soft tissue structures [25, 27, 28]. Now the cannulated reamer is carefully inserted over the guide pin into the joint passing the articular cartilage of the medial femoral condyle in a safe distance (Fig. 21.13), and the final diameter of the femoral bone tunnel is achieved [38].

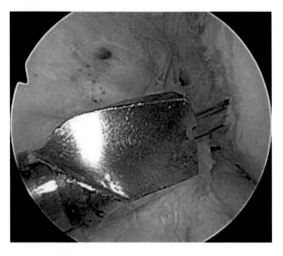

Fig. 21.13 The guide pin is reinserted into its existing 4.5 mm femoral bone tunnel, and the final diameter is established with the reamer

21.2.3 Tibial Bone Tunnel Drilling

Following, the tip of the guide pin is positioned through the low anteromedial portal into the center of the femoral ACL insertion. The distance to the medial femoral condyle is re-ensured to avoid damage to the articular cartilage [25, 27, 46] (Fig. 21.12). When safe, the knee is flexed to 130°, and the guide pin is advanced through the lateral femoral condyle to create a constant femoral bone tunnel length of approximately

The articular cartilage of the medial tibial plateau may also be damaged by bone tunnel drilling, especially when the tibial bone tunnel is drilled in a flat angle to the tibial plateau below 45° and from far medial (Fig. 21.14). From such direction, the guide pin passes very close to the articular cartilage of the concave medial tibial plateau. A reamer with a large diameter may exceed the subchondral base plate and may elevate and damage the articular cartilage of the medial tibial plateau while traveling along the guide pin.

In order to avoid this complication, we recommend higher drill angles for tibial bone tunnel drilling. In SB ACL reconstruction, the drill guide may be set to 60° starting from approximately 2 cm next to the tibial tuberosity. In DB ACL reconstruction, the tibial AM bone tunnel may be drilled in 60° to the medial tibial plateau approximately 1.5 cm medial to the tibial tuberosity, while for the tibial PM bone tunnel, the drill guide is set to 65° and approximately 2.5–3 cm medial to the tibial tuberosity. This creates a safe distance between the articular cartilage and the reamer in all cases.

> **Memory**
> Many surgeons adopt new ways of bone tunnel drilling to perform an anatomical tibial and femoral bone tunnel placement. Especially the anteromedial portal technique has a learning curve and does increase the risk for intraoperative articular cartilage damage to the medial femoral condyle. The medial tibial plateau is at risk, too. Potential pitfalls may be avoided by small modifications to the surgical technique.

21.3 Outside-In with Tips and Tricks

Bertrand Sonnery-Cottet, Jacopo Conteduca, Mathieu Thaunat, Pooler Archbold, and Pierre Chambat

This chapter describes a reproducible and simple method that allows correct femoral tunnel placement without the need for aggressive notch debridement. This outside-in technique has a number of advantages over the more conventional in-out femoral tunnel placement via the anteromedial portal. By avoiding the need to place the knee in deep flexion, it allows preservation of the ACL remnant in partial and remnant preserving reconstructions. This may be biologically advantageous. The technique can be applied for single-, double-bundle and augmentation procedures.

21.3.1 Introduction

Recently, the single-incision technique through the medial portal has been developed so that the femoral insertion of the ACL can be reached more easily when compared to the transtibial technique. Nevertheless, the in-out femoral tunnel has a number of limitations with respect to a two-incision technique. These include difficulty in reproducible anatomic positioning of the femoral tunnel as it is drilled in full flexion. There are other recognized potential pitfalls, including graft tunnel mismatch, interference screw fixation divergence, and possible blowout of the posterior cortical wall of the tunnel [15]. Moreover, this technique needs a more aggressive notch debridement to visualize the ACL femoral insertion in full flexion.

In this article, we present our technique for anatomic reconstruction of the ACL using the two-incision approach. This technique allows the surgeon to preserve the remnant and perform an augmentation procedure in partial ACL tears. It is also an easy and reproducible way for ACL revision.

21.3.2 Surgical Setup

The patient is placed in the supine position with a lateral post just proximal to the knee, in level with a padded tourniquet and a foot roll helping to keep the hip from externally rotating and the knee flexion at 90°. This allows the knee to be moved freely through its full range of motion (Fig. 21.15). Standard arthroscopic draping is used.

21.3.3 Arthroscopic Portal

The lateral portal is performed at the highest position possible just off the lateral edge of the

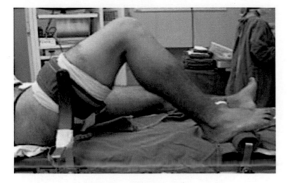

Fig. 21.15 Patient positioning

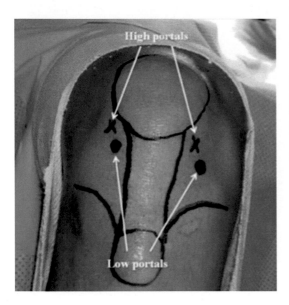

Fig. 21.16 Classic portals and high portals

patellar tendon and just off the inferior border of the patella (Fig. 21.16). This position allows the surgeon to avoid the infrapatellar fat pad and ensures an excellent wide view of the intra-articular structures [41] especially the intercondylar notch.

Arthroscopic exploration includes a complete articular assessment and meticulous exploration of the ACL lesion. The complete or incomplete nature of the ACL tear is observed. By placing the knee in the figure of four positions, the two bundles of the ACL are observed from their femoral to their tibial insertions [39]. The ACL tear can therefore be analyzed to see whether it involves one or two bundles.

21.3.4 Femoral Guide Placement

The femoral tunnel is drilled using a similar outside-in technique as described previously [15].

The knee must be at 90° of flexion to visualize the femoral insertion site of the ACL. The femoral ACL insertion is minimally debrided. Notchplasty should be avoided in order to keep the ACL femoral footprint. A specific femoral drill guide (Phusis, Saint-Ismier, France) is positioned under arthroscopic control through the anteromedial portal (Fig. 21.17).

One arm of the guide is introduced into the knee by the anteromedial portal, passing between the PCL and the medial wall of the lateral condyle. This guide is hooked on the proximal border of the lateral femoral condyle (Fig. 21.17a).

> **Tricks and Pearl**
> Introduce the femoral guide in a "vertical" orientation in order to pass it easily through the arthroscopic portal and between the PCL and the medial wall of the lateral condyle. When the hook of the guide is deep in the notch, "screw" the guide laterally to hook the guide on the proximal border of the lateral femoral condyle.

The external arm of the femoral guide lies on the lateral aspect of the lower part of the thigh. A lateral skin incision of 2 cm is made along the lateral aspect of the distal femur the point is dictated by the femoral guide. The incision is straight to the bone; the iliotibial band is split longitudinally. The boundaries inferior and posterior to the incision on the lateral femur is represented by the proximal insertion of the lateral collateral ligament and posterolateral complex thus determining a tunnel, starting at the level of distal metaphysis of the femur (Fig. 21.17b).

> **Tricks and Pearl**
> Once the femoral guide is in the correct position in the notch, push the external arm of the guide so it contacts the skin in order to mark it. Make the skin incision by centering it on the skin mark.

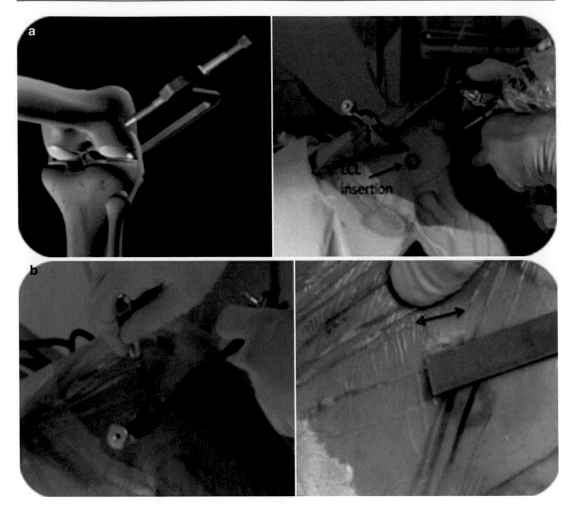

Fig. 21.17 Femoral guide placement (**a**) and lateral incision (**b**)

Once in place, the femoral guide allows placement of the guidewire 7 mm distal to the proximal border of the lateral femoral condyle in a very posterior and proximal location (Fig. 21.18). Our landmark for anatomic femoral tunnel placement is the native ACL AM bundle as recommended by other authors [35].

Another option for drilling the femoral tunnel is use of a femoral guide with a specific shape which can be introduced through the anterolateral portal to allow guide pin placement under anteromedial vision. A 8 mm ring target on the guide is positioned in the AM bundle area, with the limit of the ring just distal to the outlet of the notch and just superior to the inferior cartilaginous limit (Fig. 21.19).

The guide pin is drilled with a slight oblique direction from front to back and from high to low. A curet is used to cup the tip of the guidewire to avoid inadvertent advancement of the guidewire, causing damage to the articular surface or other intra-articular structures.

The intra-articular position of the guidewire and its relation to the anatomical footprint is then checked through the anteromedial portal. The tunnel is drilled under arthroscopic control in millimeter increments from 6 mm to at least the diameter of the graft. The edge of the tunnel, at its entrance

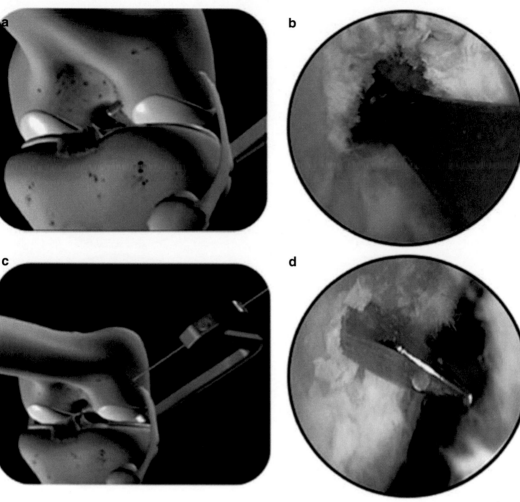

Fig. 21.18 The tip of the guide is hooked on the proximal border of the lateral femoral condyle (**a**). Arthroscopic aspect of the guide in the notch (**b**). A guide pin is placed from outside to inside (**c**). Arthroscopic aspect of the guide pin (**d**)

into the joint, is chamfered with a curet to prevent abrasion of the graft as it exits through the femoral tunnel. The proximal edge of the tunnel is located just distal to the proximal border of the lateral femoral condyle and its posterior edge, just superior to the inferior limit of the cartilage (Fig. 21.20).

> By playing with the drill while enlarging the femoral tunnel in 1 mm increments, minor adjustments of the intra-articular position of the femoral tunnel can be made.

Tricks and Pearls
To improve the visualization of the position that the drill exits within the notch, the scope is placed into the AM arthroscopic portal.

The debris from the reaming is evacuated with a synovial shaver to minimize the inflammatory response of the fat pad.

The graft is tensioned on the femoral side after several flexion-extension cycles and fixed with interference screw. A fixation device of the same

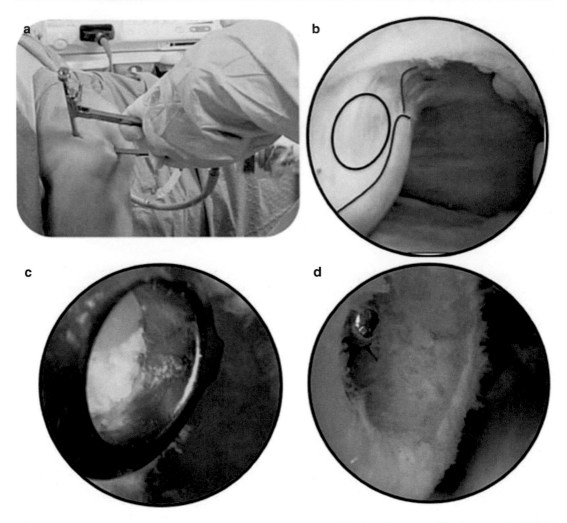

Fig. 21.19 Specific guide through AL portal (**a**). Arthroscopic landmark with the camera through AM portal: *black line* ring, target of the guide; *red line*, proximal border of the lateral condyle; *blue line*, anterior-inferior cartilaginous limit (**b**). An 8 mm ring target guide (**c**). Femoral tunnel (**d**) (Courtesy F Buscayret)

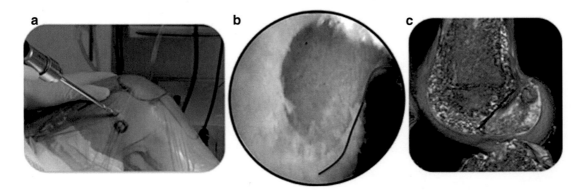

Fig. 21.20 Outside-in drilling process (**a**), arthroscopic aspect of the femoral tunnel; *red line*, proximal border of the lateral condyle, and *blue line*, anterior-inferior cartilaginous limit (**b**), 3D CT scan demonstrating femoral tunnel placement (**c**)

diameter as the tunnel is inserted in the femoral tunnel in an "outside-in" manner through the lateral incision to avoid damaging the graft at its intra-articular outlet.

> **Avoids Pitfalls**
> As the femoral tunnel is drilled at 90° and insertion of the femoral screw is performed at 30° of flexion, the iliotibial band can obstruct the entrance of the femoral tunnel leading to difficulty in insertion of the screw and potential screw breakage. This can be avoided by placing the guide pin of the screw into the femoral tunnel with the knee at 90° of flexion and advancement of the femoral interference screw to contact with the femoral tunnel entrance. The knee is then gently placed at 30° of flexion to begin and complete the interference screw insertion.
> Check the position of the interference femoral screw by placing the scope in the femoral tunnel in order to avoid a "protruding" screw which can cause iliotibial band irritation.

21.3.5 Rationale of the Out-In Technique

The knowledge of the anatomy of the ACL and in particular its femoral attachment is mandatory for successful ACL surgery. According to many authors [2, 3, 5 12, 14, 16, 17], anatomical single- or double-bundle reconstruction using a two-incision technique seems to be an easy and reproducible way to accurately position the femoral tunnel. It can be achieved with minimal notch debridement. The beneficial role of preserving the ACL remnant has already been demonstrated for ACL augmentation procedures [1, 11, 30, 36, 40]. Studies on scar patterns in ACL tears showed that the ACL remnant induces a mechanical restraint to anterior tibial translation [13, 24, 31] and that it is to improve advantageous graft integration due

to the intact vascular support of the synovial sheath [4, 20, 26].

This technique is particularly indicated for ACL revision. It allows creation of independent tunnels, especially if the primary reconstruction has been made with an in-out technique. The surgeon is not limited by the previous tunnel when placing the new femoral tunnel. In our experience of more than 100 ACL revisions/year, we never needed to perform a two stage procedure because the bone stock or the previous femoral tunnel was no a problem using the out-in technique.

> **Memory**
> The out-in technique is relatively simple, safe, reliable, and reproducible with only minimal increased morbidity. It facilitates femoral bone tunnel placement in an anatomic position and avoids damage of the ACL remnants. It can be used for single-bundle, double-bundle, augmentation, and revision surgery.

References

1. Adachi N, Ochi M, Uchio Y, Sumen Y (2000) Anterior cruciate ligament augmentation under arthroscopy. A minimum 2-year follow-up in 40 patients. Arch Orthop Trauma Surg 120:128–133
2. Aglietti P, Giron F, Cuomo P, Losco M, Mondanelli N (2007) Single-and double-incision double-bundle ACL reconstruction. Clin Orthop Relat Res 454: 108–113
3. Anderson AF, Snyder RB, Lipscomb AB Jr (2001) Anterior cruciate ligament reconstruction. A prospective randomized study of three surgical methods. Am J Sports Med 29:272–279
4. Arnoczky SP, Tarvin GB, Marshall JL (1982) Anterior cruciate ligament replacement using patellar tendon. An evaluation of graft revascularization in the dog. J Bone Joint Surg Am 64:217–224
5. Aune AK, Holm I, Risberg MA, Jensen HK, Steen H (2001) Four strand hamstring tendon autograft compared with patellar tendon-bone autograft for anterior cruciate ligament reconstruction. A randomized study with two-year follow-up. Am J Sports Med 29: 722–728
6. Battaglia TC, Miller MD (2005) Management of bony deficiency in revision anterior cruciate ligament

reconstruction using allograft bone dowels: surgical technique. Arthroscopy 21(6):767

7. Bedi A, Altchek DW (2009) The "footprint" anterior cruciate ligament technique: an anatomic approach to anterior cruciate ligament reconstruction. Arthroscopy 25(10):1128–1138

8. Bedi A, Musahl V, Steuber V, Kendoff D, Choi D, Allen AA, Pearle AD, Altchek DW (2011) Transtibial versus anteromedial portal reaming in anterior cruciate ligament reconstruction: an anatomic and biomechanical evaluation of surgical technique. Arthroscopy 27(3):380–390

9. Behrendt S, Richter J (2010) Anterior cruciate ligament reconstruction: drilling a femoral posterolateral tunnel cannot be accomplished using an over-the-top step-off drill guide. Knee Surg Sports Traumatol Arthrosc 18(9):1252–1256

10. Bowers AL, Bedi A, Lipman JD, Potter HG, Rodeo SA, Pearle AD, Warren RF, Altchek DW (2011) Comparison of anterior cruciate ligament tunnel position and graft obliquity with transtibial and anteromedial portal femoral tunnel reaming techniques using high-resolution magnetic resonance imaging. Arthroscopy 27(11):1511–1522

11. Buda R, Ferruzzi A, Vannini F, Zambelli L, Di Caprio F (2006) Augmentation technique with semitendinosus and gracilis tendons in chronic partial lesions of the ACL: clinical and arthrometric analysis. Knee Surg Sports Traumatol Arthrosc 14:1101–1107

12. Cain EL Jr, Clancy WG Jr (2002) Anatomic endoscopic anterior cruciate ligament reconstruction with patella tendon autograft. Orthop Clin North Am 33:717–725

13. Crain EH, Fithian DC, Paxton EW, Luetzow WF (2005) Variation in anterior cruciate ligament scar pattern: does the scar pattern affect anterior laxity in anterior cruciate ligament–deficient knees? Arthroscopy 21:19–24

14. Flik KR, Bach BR (2005) Anterior cruciate ligament reconstruction using the two-incision arthroscopy-assisted technique with patellar tendon autograft. Tech Orthop 20:372–376

15. Garofalo R, Mouhsine E, Chambat P, Siegrist O (2006) Anatomic anterior cruciate ligament reconstruction: the two-incision technique. Knee Surg Sports Traumatol Arthrosc 14:510–516

16. Gill TJ, Steadman JR (2002) Anterior cruciate ligament reconstruction the two incision technique. Orthop Clin North Am 33:727–735

17. Giron F, Cuomo P, Edwards A, Bull AM, Amis AA, Aglietti P (2007) Double-bundle "anatomic" anterior cruciate ligament reconstruction: a cadaveric study of tunnel positioning with a transtibial technique. Arthroscopy 23:7–13

18. Harner CD, Honkamp NJ, Ranawat AS (2008) Anteromedial portal technique for creating the anterior cruciate ligament femoral tunnel. Arthroscopy 24(1):113–115

19. Herbort M, Lenschow S, Fu FH, Petersen W, Zantop T (2010) ACL mismatch reconstructions: influence of different tunnel placement strategies in single-bundle ACL reconstructions on the knee kinematics. Knee Surg Sports Traumatol Arthrosc 18(11):1551–1558

20. Howell SM, Knox KE, Farley TE, Taylor MA (1995) Revascularization of a human anterior cruciate ligament graft during the first 2 years of implantation. Am J Sports Med 23:42–49

21. Jarvela T (2007) Double-bundle versus single-bundle anterior cruciate ligament reconstruction: a prospective, randomize clinical study. Knee Surg Sports Traumatol Arthrosc 15(5):500–507

22. Kato Y, Maeyama A, Lertwanich P, Wang JH, Ingham SJ, Kramer S, Martins CQ, Smolinski P, Fu FH (2013) Biomechanical comparison of different graft positions for single-bundle anterior cruciate ligament reconstruction. Knee Surg Sports Traumatol Arthrosc 21(4):816–823

23. Kondo E, Yasuda K, Ichiyama H et al (2007) Radiologic evaluation of femoral and tibial tunnels created with the transtibial tunnel technique for anatomic double-bundle anterior cruciate ligament reconstruction. Arthroscopy 23(8):869–876

24. Liu W, Maitland ME, Bell GD (2002) A modeling study of partial ACL injury: simulated KT 2000 tests. J Biomech Eng 124:294–301

25. Lubowitz JH (2009) Anteromedial portal technique for the anterior cruciate ligament femoral socket: pitfalls and solutions. Arthroscopy 25:95–101

26. Murray MM, Martin SD, Martin TL, Spector M (2000) Histological changes in the human anterior cruciate ligament after rupture. J Bone Joint Surg Am 82:1387–1397

27. Nakamura M, Deie M, Shibuya H et al (2009) Potential risks of femoral tunnel drilling through the far anteromedial portal: a cadaveric study. Arthroscopy 25(5):481–487

28. Neven E, D'Hooghe P, Bellemans J (2008) Double-bundle anterior cruciate ligament reconstruction: a cadaveric study on the posterolateral tunnel position and safety of the lateral structures. Arthroscopy 24(4):436–440

29. Nishimoto K, Kuroda R, Mizuno K et al (2009) Analysis of the graft bending angle at the femoral tunnel aperture in anatomic double bundle anterior cruciate ligament reconstruction: a comparison of the transtibial and the far anteromedial portal technique. Knee Surg Sports Traumatol Arthrosc 17(3): 270–276

30. Ochi M, Adachi N, Uchio Y, Deie M, Kumahashi N, Ishikawa M, Sera S (2009) A minimum 2-year follow-up after selective anteromedial or posterolateral bundle anterior cruciate ligament reconstruction. Arthroscopy 25:117–122

31. Panisset JC, Duraffour H, Vasconcelos W, Colombet P, Javois C, Potel JF, Dejour D, Société française d'arthroscopie (2008) Clinical, radiological and arthroscopic analysis of the ACL tear. A prospective study of 418 cases. Rev Chir Orthop Reparatrice Appar Mot 94(8 Suppl):362–368

32. Pascual-Garrido C, Swanson BL, Swanson KE (2012) Transtibial versus low anteromedial portal drilling for anterior cruciate ligament reconstruction: a radiographic study of femoral tunnel position. Knee Surg Sports Traumatol Arthrosc 21(4):846–850

33. Petersen W, Zantop T (2007) Anatomy of the anterior cruciate ligament with regard to its two bundles. Clin Orthop Relat Res 454:35–47

34. Pinczewski LA, Lyman J, Salmon LJ et al (2007) A 10-year comparison of anterior cruciate ligament reconstructions with hamstring tendon and patellar tendon autograft: a controlled, prospective trial. Am J Sports Med 35(4):564–574

35. Purnell ML, Larson AI, Clancy W (2008) Anterior cruciate ligament insertions on the tibia and femur and their relationships to critical bony landmarks using high-resolution volume-rendering computed tomography. Am J Sports Med 36:2083–2090

36. Siebold R, Fu F (2008) Assessment and augmentation of symptomatic anteromedial or posterolateral bundle tears of the anterior cruciate ligament. Arthroscopy 24:1289–1298

37. Siebold R, Webster KE, Feller JA et al (2006) Anterior cruciate ligament reconstruction in females: a comparison of hamstring tendon and patellar tendon autografts. Knee Surg Sports Traumatol Arthrosc 14(11):1070–1076

38. Siebold R, Benetos IS, Sartory N et al (2010) How to avoid the risk of intraoperative cartilage damage in anatomic four tunnel double bundle anterior cruciate ligament reconstruction. Knee Surg Sports Traumatol Arthrosc 18(1):64–67

39. Sonnery-Cottet B, Chambat P (2007) Arthroscopic identification of the anterior cruciate ligament posterolateral bundle: the figure of four position. Arthroscopy 23:1128.e1–3

40. Sonnery-Cottet B, Lavoie F, Ogassawara R, Scussiato RG, Kidder JF, Chambat P (2010) Selective anteromedial bundle reconstruction in partial ACL tears: a series of 36 patients with mean 24 months follow-up. Knee Surg Sports Traumatol Arthrosc 18:47–51

41. Sonnery-Cottet B, Archbold P, Zayni R, Thaunat M, Bortolletto J, Fayard JM, Chambat P (2011) High lateral portal for sparing the infrapatellar fat-pad during ACL reconstruction. Orthop Traumatol Surg Res 97:870–873

42. Trojani C, Sbihi A, Djian P, Potel JF, Hulet C, Jouve F, Bussière C, Ehkirch FP, Burdin G, Dubrana F, Beaufils P, Franceschi JP, Chassaing V, Colombet P, Neyret P (2011) Causes for failure of ACL reconstruction and influence of meniscectomies after revision. Knee Surg Sports Traumatol Arthrosc 19(2):96–201

43. Zantop T, Petersen W (2011) Arthroscopic filling of misplaced and wide bone tunnels after reconstruction of the anterior cruciate ligament with bone graft in patients with recurrent instability. Oper Orthop Traumatol 23(4):337–350

44. Zantop T, Petersen W, Sekiya JK, Musahl V, Fu FH (2006) Anterior cruciate ligament anatomy and function relating to anatomical reconstruction. Knee Surg Sports Traumatol Arthrosc 14(10):982–992

45. Zantop T, Herbort M, Raschke MJ, Fu FH, Petersen W (2007) The role of the anteromedial and posterolateral bundles of the anterior cruciate ligament in anterior tibial translation and internal rotation. Am J Sports Med 35(2):223–227

46. Zantop T, Haase AK, Fu FH et al (2008) Potential risk of cartilage damage in double bundle ACL reconstruction: impact of knee flexion angle and portal location on the femoral PL bundle tunnel. Arch Orthop Trauma Surg 128(5):509–513

ACL-Footprint Reconstruction with Insertion Site Table

22

Rainer Siebold and Peter Schuhmacher

Contents

The purpose of this article is to give surgical guidelines to restore the direct tibial C-shaped and the direct femoral "straight" insertion site of the ACL.

22.1   Introduction

Anatomical footprint restoration requires assessment of the length, width, and orientation of the direct tibial and femoral ACL insertion sites. Both SB and DB ACL reconstructions may achieve a wide range of area and geometric restoration of the individual ACL footprint. While SB ACL reconstruction may be best used for insertion sites up to 13 mm in length, DB ACL reconstruction has the potential to be more anatomical restoring narrow and long footprints up to 21 mm. The width of the restored area depends on the drill bit diameter(s) and is usually larger for SB. In larger footprints DB can replicate up to 63 % more area and 37 % more length than SB ACL reconstruction. The "Direct Insertion Site Table" resumes the concept for orientation during surgery.

22.2   Concept of Footprint Reconstruction

The concept of complete footprint restoration for anatomical ACL reconstruction was introduced recently to restore the individual ACL footprint in order to achieve a maximum of biomechanical stability and function [18, 21]. It is based on the hypothesis that the restored biomechanical

R. Siebold (✉)
Institute for Anatomy and Cell Biology, INF,
Ruprecht-Karls University Heidelberg,
Heidelberg, Germany

HKF: Center for Spezialised Hip-Knee-Foot Surgery,
ATOS Hospital Heidelberg,
Bismarckstr. 9-15, Heidelberg 69115, Germany
e-mail: rainer.siebold@atos.de

P. Schuhmacher
HKF: Center for Spezialised Hip-Knee-Foot Surgery,
ATOS Hospital Heidelberg,
Bismarckstr. 9-15, Heidelberg 69115, Germany

R. Siebold et al. (eds.), *Anterior Cruciate Ligament Reconstruction*,
DOI 10.1007/978-3-642-45349-6_22, © ESSKA 2014

envelope of the knee is a function of the amount of reconstructed insertion site area. The article defined indications for single-bundle (SB) and double-bundle (DB) ACL reconstruction of the anteromedial (AM) and posteromedial (PM) fibers using hamstrings based on the percentage of restored individual insertion site length. The authors recommended SB ACL reconstruction for "small" and "intermediate" footprints up to 14 mm in length and DB ACL reconstruction for "longer" insertion sites of 15 mm in length or more [18]. Similar recommendations were given by Eck et al. [23] who presented a flow chart for ACL reconstruction.

The geometrical individuality of the C-shaped tibial and femoral direct ACL insertions is defined not only by the anatomical length of its insertion site, which is in the range of 9–21 mm, but also by its anatomical width. According to new anatomical findings, it is not as wide as reported before [1–11, 13, 15, 16, 19, 22, 24] but only between 3.5 mm to 4.5 mm (see Chaps. 1, 2, 3, 4, and 5). Therefore the concept of anatomical footprint restoration mostly requires considering the length of both direct insertion sites to restore a maximum amount of insertion site *area.* A perfect restoration of the insertion site length on the tibia and femur may not automatically achieve a maximum of *area* restoration of both insertion sites.

This article gives guidelines for restoring the individual geometry and area of the tibial "C-shaped" and femoral "straight" direct ACL insertion sites. It introduces a "Direct Insertion Site Table" for individual size-matched SB and DB ACL reconstruction using hamstrings. Combinations of drill bit diameters and sagittal drill angles are given to achieve a maximum

of individual tibial and femoral ACL footprint reconstruction.

22.3 Direct Insertion Site Table

The "*Direct* Insertion Site Table" (Table 22.1) is based on the concept of "complete footprint restoration" [18]. For anatomical reasons (see Chaps. 1, 2, 3, 4, and 5), this table focuses on the restored direct insertion site length rather than the restored (very narrow) width. For each intraoperative measured tibial and femoral insertion site length from 8 to 21 mm, the table highlights the techniques (SB/DB) with the longest footprint reconstruction and the highest amount of area restoration. Graft bit diameters of 5–11 mm as well as drill angles of 50–65° were considered for calculation. Smaller drill angles were excluded since they have been considered technically difficult. A drill bit diameter of 11 mm is very large and was only included to demonstrate the upper limit of area restoration with SB ACL reconstruction.

The surface area of all possible tibial SB and DB bone tunnels was calculated. In SB ACL reconstruction, the restored area was calculated as an ellipse (P=length/2 (l/2) × width/2 (w/2) × π) and in DB ACL reconstruction as two ellipses including a 2 mm bone bridge P1(AM) = 1/2 × (l/2 × w/2 × π) + P2(AM + bone bridge) = w × (l/2 + 2) + P3(PM) = w × l/2 + P4(PM) = 1/2 × (l/2 × w/2 × π). In DB ACL reconstruction, only drill bit combinations for AM to PM areas between 50:50 and 60:40 were considered anatomical and were therefore included in the calculations [2, 11, 16, 19] (Table 22.1).

Guidelines for anatomical tibial and femoral ACL footprint restoration for SB and DB ACL reconstruction based on the restored insertion site length and area

SB ACL reconstruction: left column: intraoperatively measured length of tibial insertion site. Second column from left: matched drill diameter and drill angle to achieve a maximum of length reconstruction (second column from right) and area reconstruction (right column)

DB ACL reconstruction: left column: intraoperatively measured length of tibial insertion site. Second column from left: AM = anteromedial bone tunnel, "°" = sagittal drill angle, PM = posteromedial bone tunnel, length = combined reconstruction of AM + PM + 2 mm bone bridge, area = restored area

Table 22.1   Direct Insertion Site Table for ACL footprint restoration

Measured Insertion site length [mm]	Drill diameter [mm] & drill angle		Reconstructed insertion site length [mm] + [%]		Reconstructed insertion area [mm²]
SINGLE-BUNDLE					
8	6.5	55°	7.9	99	41
	6	50°	7.8	98	37
9	7.5	60°	8.7	97	51
	7	55°	8.6	96	47
10	8.5	60°	9.8	98	66
	8	55°	9.8	98	61
11	9.5	60°	11	100	82
	9	55°	11	100	78
	8.5	55°	10.4	95	69
12	10	60°	11.6	97	91
	9.5	55°	11.6	97	87
	9	50°	11.8	98	83
13 to 15	10	50°	13.1	101	103

DOUBLE-BUNDLE USING HAMSTRINGS

13	AM °	5 / 65	5.5 / 65	5 / 65	4.5 / 50						
	PM °	5 / 65	4.5 / 65	4.5 / 55	4.5 / 60						
	Length	13	13	13	13						
	Area	59	59	56	54						
14	AM °	5.5 / 60	6 / 65	5 / 50	5 / 50	5.5 / 65	4.5 / 50				
	PM °	5 / 65	4.5 / 65	5 / 65	4.5 / 55	4.5 / 50	4.5 / 50				
	Length	13.9	13.6	14	14	13	13.8				
	Area	66	64	64	60	59	56				
15	AM °	7 / 60	6 / 60	6.5 / 65	6.5 / 60	6 / 60	5.5 / 60	6 / 50	5.5 / 50	5.5 / 50	5 / 50
	PM °	4.5 / 65	5.5 / 65	5 / 60	4.5 / 55	5 / 55	5.5 / 60	4.5 / 60	5 / 60	4.5 / 50	5 / 50
	Length	15	15	15	15	15	14.7	15	15	15	15
	Area	80	78	77	75	74	73	72	71	68	68
16	AM °	7 / 65°	6,5 / 65°	6,5 / 55°	6 / 55°	6,5 / 60°	6 / 55°	6 / 50°	5,5 / 50°	5,5 / 50°	5 / 50°
	PM °	5,5 / 60°	6 / 65°	5,5 / 65°	6 / 65°	5 / 50°	5,5 / 55°	5 / 55°	5,5 / 55°	5 / 50°	5 / 50°
	Length	16.11	15.8	16	16	16	16	15.9	15.9	15.7	15.1
	Area	94	90	89	87	86	84	81	79	75	68
17	AM °	7 / 65°	7 / 60°	6,5 / 60°	7 / 65°	6,5 / 55°	6,5 / 55°	6 / 50°	6 / 50°	6,5 / 60°	6 / 50°
	PM °	6,5 / 65°	6 / 60°	6,5 / 60°	5,5 / 50°	6 / 60°	5,5 / 55°	6 / 60°	5,5 / 50°	5 / 50°	5 / 50°
	Length	16.9	17	17	16.9	16.9	16.7	16.8	17	16	16.4
	Area	104	102	100	98	96	92	91	89	86	83
18	AM °	8 / 65°	7,5 / 65°	7,5 / 60°	7 / 60°	7,5 / 60°	7 / 55°	7 / 50°	6,5 / 50°	7 / 55°	6,5 / 50°
	PM °	6,5 / 65°	7 / 65°	6,5 / 65°	7 / 65°	6 / 55°	6,5 / 60°	6 / 60°	6,5 / 60°	5,5 / 50°	6 / 55°
	Length	18	18	17.8	17.8	18	18.1	18.1	18	17.7	17.8
	Area	121	119	115	113	112	111	108	106	103	102
19	AM °	8 / 60°	7,5 / 60°	8 / 65°	7,5 / 55°	7,5 / 55°	8 / 65°	7 / 55°	7,5 / 55°	7 / 50°	7 / 50°
	PM °	7 / 65°	7,5 / 65°	6,5 / 55°	7 / 65°	6,5 / 55°	6 / 50°	7 / 55°	6 / 50°	6,5 / 55°	6 / 50°
	Length	19	18.9	18.8	18.9	19.1	18.7	19.1	19	19.1	19
	Area	130	128	125	125	122	121	121	118	117	113

22.4 Surgical Steps

In contrast to the usual order of surgical steps, the concept of complete footprint restoration requires assessment of the geometry of the tibial and femoral ACL insertion site prior to graft preparation. First, the length and the width of both direct insertions sites are measured intraoperatively using a ruler. Then the surgical technique (SB or DB ACL reconstruction) with the specific drill bit diameter(s) and sagittal drill angle(s) is assessed from the "Direct Insertion Site Table." Next, the hamstring, patella tendon, or quadriceps tendon graft is harvested and prepared according to the recommended diameter(s). The bone tunnel(s) is drilled, respectively (Table 22.1), and the ACL reconstruction is completed as usual.

The maximum length that can be technically restored with a SB ACL reconstruction using a 10 mm drill bit in a 50° sagittal drill angle is 13 mm and the maximum area 103 mm². However, the majority of tibial and femoral ACL insertion sites are longer than 13 mm (12–18 mm) and only between 3.5 mm to 4.5 mm wide (see Chaps. 1, 2, 3, 4, and 5). Hence most insertion site reconstructions using SB are too short but also too wide. Therefore a SB technique using hamstrings may only be recommended for shorter insertion sites up to 13 mm and drill diameters of 7–8 mm (Table 22.1).

22.5 Discussion

The concept aims to restore a maximum amount and shape of the tibial and femoral ACL insertion sites to achieve a maximum of biomechanical function and stability of the ACL reconstruction [18, 21]. Instead of only considering the length of the tibial insertion site to decide for the tibial footprint reconstruction, the "Direct Insertion Site Table" displays the maximum amount of area restoration for each individual (measured) insertion site length. The insertion site width was estimated to be between 3.5 mm to 4.5 mm based on recent anatomical insertion site studies showing a straight direct insertion site along the intercondylar ridge and a C-shaped tibial insertion site along the medial tibial spine [14, 20].

The maximum length that can be technically restored with a SB ACL reconstruction using a 10 mm drill bit in a 50° sagittal drill angle is 13.1 mm and the maximum area 103 mm². However, the majority of tibial and femoral ACL insertion sites are longer than 13 mm (12–18 mm) and only between 3.5 mm to 4.5 mm wide (see Chaps. 1, 2, 3, 4, and 5). Hence most insertion site reconstructions using SB are too short but also too wide. Therefore a SB technique using hamstrings may only be recommended for shorter insertion sites up to 13 mm and drill diameters of 7–8 mm (Table 22.1).

From **14 mm** insertion site length, it may be better to use a DB technique for ACL reconstruction when reconstructing with hamstrings. When choosing 5.5 mm for AM and 5.0 mm for PM, the reconstructed insertion site length will be exactly 14 mm and the width 5–5.5 mm, which is more anatomical than using a larger diameter SB ACL reconstruction.

For an insertion site length of, e.g., **17 mm**, a 10 mm SB ACL reconstruction could theoretically achieve a similar amount of area restoration as a 7 mm AM (65°) combined with a 6.5 mm PM (65°)-bundle DB ACL reconstruction (103 mm² vs. 104 mm²). However, the reconstructed surface geometry is completely different between both techniques: the 10 mm SB ACL reconstruction leads to a 10-mm-wide (nonanatomical) but only 13.1-mm-(too)-short footprint restoration, whereas the combination of a 7 mm AM- and a 6.5 mm PM-bundle DB ACL reconstruction creates a much more anatomical 6.5–7-mm-wide and 16.9-mm-long footprint restoration of the 17 mm ACL footprint. It is therefore recommended to choose a DB ACL reconstruction for longer insertion sites.

A patient with a long insertion site of, e.g., **18 mm** may be reconstructed in a SB technique with a large 11 mm SB bone tunnel (50°) resulting in an area restoration of 124 mm² but a reconstructed length of only 14.4 mm. Again, to avoid such large (nonanatomical) SB bone tunnels, DB ACL reconstruction may be preferred. The combination of an 8 mm AM (65°) with a 6.5 mm for PM (65°) fibers restores an area of 121 mm². The geometry of this restored area is characterized by a width of 6.5–8 mm and a length of 18 mm.

For patients with even longer insertion sites up to 21 mm, the geometry of the individual footprint can also be best restored using a DB ACL reconstruction (see Table 22.1).

Sahasrabudhe et al. [17] evaluated 38 patients after DB ACL reconstruction using three-dimensional computed tomography. They reported that the AP length of the reconstructed tibial footprint was as large as 17.1 ± 1.9 mm. This cannot be achieved using a SB ACL reconstruction. The AM and PM drill bit diameters are usually smaller compared to SB ACL reconstruction. The shorter the tibial footprint, the smaller the DB drill bit diameters and the width of the restored insertion site area compared to SB ACL reconstruction – and vice versa (Table 22.1). This makes it necessary to intraoperatively measure both the length and the width of the tibial footprint to adapt the ACL reconstruction accordingly. It also has to be considered which graft (diameter) fits the width of the insertion site and also the width of the intercondylar notch in order to achieve a maximized reconstruction but to avoid overstuffing and/or notch impingement.

The long axis of the reconstructed ellipse(s) has to be parallel to the long axis of the tibial insertion site. This can be achieved by changing the transverse drill angle of the tibial bone tunnel in the coronal plane.

Functional considerations are also important when deciding for a SB or DB ACL reconstruction. Activities of daily living as well as sports, work, the degree of osteoarthritis, etc. are all important [18, 21, 23]. Any alternative technique or graft may be adequate to achieve the purpose of complete footprint reconstruction. Especially for large SB bone tunnels but also for any DB bone tunnels, a graft with bone block(s) may be used to fill up large bony defects from the tunnel(s). In case of a patellar tendon or a quadriceps tendon graft, the geometrical shape of the graft may not be round but flat, so the concept has to be adapted accordingly.

> **Memory**
> Anatomical footprint restoration requires assessment of the length, width, and orientation of the direct tibial and femoral ACL insertion sites. Both SB and DB ACL reconstructions may achieve a wide range of area and geometric restoration of the individual ACL footprints. While SB ACL reconstruction may be best used for short insertion sites up to 13 mm in length, DB ACL reconstruction has the potential to be more anatomical restoring narrow and long footprints up to 21 mm. The "Direct Insertion Site Table" resumes the concept for orientation during surgery.

References

1. Arnoczky SP (1983) Anatomy of the anterior cruciate ligament. Clin Orthop Relat Res (172):19–25
2. Baer GS, Ferretti M, Fu FH (2008) Anatomy of the ACL. In: Fu FH, Cohen SB (eds) Current concepts in ACL reconstruction. SLACK, Thorofare, pp 21–32
3. Colombet P, Robinson J, Christel P et al (2006) Morphology of anterior cruciate ligament attachments for anatomic reconstruction: a cadaveric dissection and radiographic study. Arthroscopy 22(9): 984–992
4. Dodds JA, Arnoczky SP (1994) Anatomy of the anterior cruciate ligament a blueprint for repair and reconstruction. Arthroscopy 10(2):132–139
5. Duthon VB, Barea C, Abrassart S et al (2006) Anatomy of the anterior cruciate ligament. Knee Surg Sports Traumatol Arthrosc 14(3):204–213
6. Edwards A, Bull AM, Amis AA (2007) The attachments of the anteromedial and posterolateral fibre bundles of the anterior cruciate ligament: Part 1: tibial attachment. Knee Surg Sports Traumatol Arthrosc 15(12):1414–1421
7. Ferretti M, Levicoff EA, Macpherson TA et al (2007) The fetal anterior cruciate ligament: an anatomic and histologic study. Arthroscopy 23(3):278–283
8. Girgis FG, Marshall JL, Monajem A (1975) The cruciate ligaments of the knee joint. Anatomical, functional and experimental analysis. Clin Orthop Relat Res (106):216–231
9. Hamner DL, Brown CH Jr, Steiner ME et al (1999) Hamstring tendon grafts for reconstruction of the anterior cruciate ligament: biomechanical evaluation of the use of multiple strands and tensioning techniques. J Bone Joint Surg Am 81(4):549–557
10. Hara K, Mochizuki T, Sekiya I et al (2009) Anatomy of normal human anterior cruciate ligament attachments evaluated by divided small bundles. Am J Sports Med 37(12):2386–2391
11. Harner CD, Baek GH, Vogrin TM et al (1999) Quantitative analysis of human cruciate ligament insertions. Arthroscopy 15(7):741–749

12. Kopf S, Martin DE, Tashman S et al (2010) Effect of tibial drill angles on bone tunnel aperture during anterior cruciate ligament reconstruction. J Bone Joint Surg Am 92(4):871–881

13. Kopf S, Musahl V, Tashman S et al (2009) A systematic review of the femoral origin and tibial insertion morphology of the ACL. Knee Surg Sports Traumatol Arthrosc 17(3):213–219

14. Mochizuki T, Fujishiro H, Nimura A et al (2013) Anatomic and histologic analysis of the mid-substance and fan-like extension fibres of the anterior cruciate ligament during knee motion, with special reference to the femoral attachment. Knee Surg Sports Traumatol Arthrosc 22(2):336–344

15. Odensten M, Gillquist J (1985) Functional anatomy of the anterior cruciate ligament and a rationale for reconstruction. J Bone Joint Surg Am 67(2):257–262

16. Petersen W, Zantop T (2007) Anatomy of the anterior cruciate ligament with regard to its two bundles. Clin Orthop Relat Res 454:35–47

17. Sahasrabudhe A, Christel P, Anne F et al (2010) Postoperative evaluation of tibial footprint and tunnels characteristics after anatomic double-bundle anterior cruciate ligament reconstruction with anatomic aimers. Knee Surg Sports Traumatol Arthrosc 18(11):1599–1606

18. Siebold R (2011) The concept of complete footprint restoration with guidelines for single- and double-bundle ACL reconstruction. Knee Surg Sports Traumatol Arthrosc 19(5):699–706

19. Siebold R, Ellert T, Metz S et al (2008) Tibial insertions of the anteromedial and posterolateral bundles of the anterior cruciate ligament: morphometry, arthroscopic landmarks, and orientation model for bone tunnel placement. Arthroscopy 24(2): 154–161

20. Siebold R, Schuhmacher P (2012) Restoration of the tibial ACL footprint area and geometry using the Modified Insertion Site Table. Knee Surg Sports Traumatol Arthrosc 20(9):1845–1849

21. Siebold R, Zantop T (2009) Anatomic double-bundle ACL reconstruction: a call for indications. Knee Surg Sports Traumatol Arthrosc 17(3):211–212

22. Tallay A, Lim MH, Bartlett J (2008) Anatomical study of the human anterior cruciate ligament stump's tibial insertion footprint. Knee Surg Sports Traumatol Arthrosc 16(8):741–746

23. van Eck CF, Lesniak BP, Schreiber VM et al (2010) Anatomic single- and double-bundle anterior cruciate ligament reconstruction flowchart. Arthroscopy 26(2):258–268

24. Zantop T, Petersen W, Sekiya JK et al (2006) Anterior cruciate ligament anatomy and function relating to anatomical reconstruction. Knee Surg Sports Traumatol Arthrosc 14(10):982–992

Tensioning of Grafts: Any Evidence?

23

Sven U. Scheffler

Contents

23.1 Introduction

It has always been a matter of debate whether graft tensioning at the time of fixation plays an important role for long-term function of the knee joint following reconstruction of the anterior cruciate ligament (ACL). Conceptionally, it is easily understood that an ACL must not be loose at the time of fixation. However, there is no agreement on the ideal loads for graft tensioning. The following chapter will summarize the current knowledge on the impact of graft tensioning at the time of reconstruction on the clinical and functional outcome after ACL reconstruction.

23.2 Basic Principles

The intact ACL shows a non-isometric tensioning behavior throughout the range of knee motion, which is determined by the anatomic locations of its tibiofemoral insertion sites, the bony anatomy of the articulating femur and tibia, the passive capsular and ligamentous restraints of the knee joint, and the forces acting upon the ACL initiated by muscle activity of the lower limb and body weight [1, 2, 20, 24]. The ultimate goal of ACL reconstruction is to fully restore this tensioning behavior. It is believed that tensioning of an ACL graft at the time of fixation will aid in achieving this goal.

Graft tension can be manually adjusted right before final graft fixation. However, the true tension of the graft maintained immediately after

S.U. Scheffler (✉)
Department of Orthopaedic Surgery,
COPV – Chirurgisch Orthopädischer PraxisVerbund,
Breitenbachplatz 8, Berlin 14195, Germany
e-mail: sven.scheffler@gmx.com

R. Siebold et al. (eds.), *Anterior Cruciate Ligament Reconstruction*,
DOI 10.1007/978-3-642-45349-6_23, © ESSKA 2014

final fixation is also determined by the position of tibiofemoral tunnel placement [15, 21], type of graft fixation [10, 20], position of the knee joint at time of fixation [1, 19], and graft choice [2, 11]. Also, all grafts undergo biological remodeling after ACL reconstruction, which alters the in situ tension of the graft over time [13, 27]. It has been tried to separately analyze the impact of these various confounding variables, but their importance, interaction, and influence for ACL graft function are not fully understood until today.

Two different approaches are widely accepted in today's clinical practice for graft tensioning. One concept aims to modify graft tension to restore anterior-posterior laxity of the reconstructed knee to the uninjured contralateral side. The other concept assumes that stretching of the graft occurs during postoperative remodeling. Therefore, high graft tension is initially applied, overconstraining the knee joint, to compensate for this expected loss of knee stability [2, 18, 22]. However, there has been no agreement on the ideal force magnitude required for this tensioning approach. Also, there has been no consensus about superiority of one of the two concepts.

23.3   Basic Science Studies

Several cadaveric studies examined the influence of different force magnitudes for graft tensioning on knee kinematics and tibiofemoral contact forces [5, 10–12, 20].

Mae et al. found that 44 N tensioning of a quadrupled hamstring tendon graft led to restoration of normal ap-laxity after ACL reconstruction in human cadaveric knees. A preload of 88 N resulted into overconstraining the knee joint, pushing the tibia into a posterior, externally rotated, and valgus position. The in situ tension of the ACL graft was significantly higher than in the normal knee at all flexion angles from 0° to 90° at 44 N and even more at 88 N of graft tension. The authors concluded that a graft tension of 88 N would result into significantly increased tibiofemoral contact pressure, rendering the articular cartilage to the possibility of future damage.

Fleming et al. [12] compared laxity and force-based tensioning techniques, measuring tibiofemoral contact forces using bone-patellar-tendon bone (BPTB) grafts for ACL reconstruction. They found that force magnitudes of 87 N were required to restore ap-laxity to normal at 20° of flexion, which resulted into a twofold increase in tibiofemoral contact forces, while force-based graft tensioning with 25 and 50 N returned tibiofemoral contact forces to normal but was not able to restore normal ap-laxity. The authors concluded that clinical studies would be warranted to examine possible cartilage wear after applying high initial graft tension before recommending its safe use in order to restore intact ap-laxity at time zero.

While the aforementioned studies only looked at the impact of graft tensioning at time of fixation, the following studies investigated the effect of cyclic loading of an ACL reconstruction on preserving the initial graft tensioning loads [4]. Such analyses are crucial, since soft tissue grafts undergo physiologic length changes under cyclic loading or reduction of their in situ forces when kept at a constant length [16]. Such reversible viscoelastic changes also apply to fixation materials but have to be separated from viscoplastic non-recoverable length changes, i.e., knot loosening or suture stretch out of the fixation site [16]. All these factors have to be taken into account when deciding on the appropriate loads for graft tensioning.

Boylan et al. [4] found that cyclic loading of an ACL hamstring graft reconstruction, using suture/post fixation in human cadaveric knees, led to a 50 % decrease of the initial graft tensioning load of 68 and 45 N after 1,000 cycles. They found that initial graft tensioning of 68 N was required to restore anterior laxity to the ACL intact knee but that about 2 mm of increased laxity was observed at the end of cyclic loading. Lower initial graft tensioning of 45 N resulted into a significant increase of 2 mm before to even 4.5 mm after cyclic loading, possibly rendering the knee joint to functional instability. Other studies pointed out that this loss in graft tension resulted only partially from viscoelastic changes of the graft itself but that the majority originated from viscoplastic changes of the suture/post fixation, i.e., knot loosening and stretch out of the suture materials [16, 23]. Numerous studies documented differences in ACL graft construct stiffness depending on the respective fixation method [6, 9, 23, 29]. Therefore, the effect of initial graft tensioning strongly depends on the fixation method of the ACL graft. Its particular material and mechanical properties must be fully understood when choosing the appropriate tensioning force.

Identical concepts apply to graft choice. Mechanical and viscoelastic properties vary between current graft types, such as hamstring and patellar tendon grafts [8, 14]. This results into different graft lengthening under repetitive loading, as it can be expected during activities after ACL reconstruction. A BPTB graft provides higher graft stiffness and shows less loss in graft tension than a doubled hamstring tendon graft [8] and similar stiffness to a quadriceps or quadrupled hamstring tendon graft [7, 9, 25]. Therefore, overall ACL reconstruction stiffness is a result of its graft and fixation technique. A stiffer reconstruction requires less graft tensioning to restore normal ACL laxity, while a less stiff fixation necessitates higher graft tensioning loads. This must be fully understood when choosing the appropriate load to tension the ACL graft construct.

Finally, it has been shown that a delicate relationship exists between biological remodeling of an ACL graft and its in situ tension at time of fixation. Katsuragi et al. [17] found that overtensioning of an intact canine ACL with 20 N resulted into significant changes of its biological composition, which led to deterioration of its mechanical properties up to 12 weeks of healing compared to a physiologically tensioned ACL. They concluded that the in situ forces of an ACL graft construct after fixation must be known to avoid overconstraining the graft and concurrent impairment of graft healing.

Varying graft tension forces at magnitudes that will not overload the graft construct to superphysiological ACL forces after fixation might only have little effect on long-term ACL function. Fu et al. [13] noticed in their rabbit ACL reconstructions that graft tensioning with 4 N restored knee laxity significantly better than with 2 N at time zero, which also preserved better knee stability at 2 weeks of healing. However, these effects completely disappeared after 6 weeks with no differences in knee stability. Similar observations were made by Yoshiya et al. [31] in a dog model with graft pretensioning of 1 versus 39 N of a patellar tendon ACL reconstruction. The higher preload resulted into significant lower anterior knee laxity at time zero in the high-tensioning group, but no differences at 3 months of healing. Also, high ACL graft tensioning resulted into significantly higher graft degeneration and impaired revascularization at 3 months, prompting the authors to conclude that very high pretensioning, i.e., overconstraining, of the graft must be avoided.

Conversely, underconstraining the graft also impairs long-term mechanical function. Tohyama et al. [26] found for a canine patellar tendon ACL reconstruction that undertensioning an ACL graft (graft elongation >95 % confidence limits of the intact ACL) led to significantly higher knee laxity at 18 months post reconstruction than in an ACL graft that was tightened to elongate within the 95 % confidence interval of the intact ACL at time of fixation.

In summary of current in vivo animal studies, it was shown that optimal knee stability was achieved after mid- and long-term healing when elongation behavior of the intact ACL [26] and anterior knee stability [17] were restored at time of fixation, neither under- or overconstraining the knee joint.

23.4   Clinical Studies

Very few studies exist that have analyzed the effect of graft tensioning on the clinical outcome after ACL reconstruction [3, 18, 22, 28, 30, 32]. All published studies have only examined the impact of different force magnitudes. None have compared the influence of different graft types and fixation techniques on the efficacy of graft tensioning to improve clinical results after ACL reconstruction.

The group of Yoshiya et al. [32] pretensioned a BPTB graft with either 25 or 50 N in a prospective randomized trial of ACL reconstruction using interference screw fixation. Both preloads overconstrained anterior tibial translation by 2 mm without significant differences between the groups at time of fixation. At 3 months, anterior knee laxity returned to contralateral intact ACL values, with a further nonsignificant increase at 6 months and no changes at 1 and 2 years. There were no differences in anterior knee stability between both study groups at any time point of the study.

van Kampen et al. [28] prospectively followed 38 patients after pretensioning a bone-patellar tendon bone graft with either 20 or 40 N prior to interference screw fixation. At their follow-up from 6 to 52 weeks, no differences were found between the groups for clinical evaluation (Lysholm, Lachman Test, IKDC, radiographs), concluding that lower tensioning forces might suffice without the risk of overconstraining the knee joint.

In a prospective randomized double-blind clinical trial of Nicholas et al. [22] BPTB grafts were preloaded with either 90 or 45 N. No information was given on the type of graft fixation. Authors found significant lower anterior knee laxity in the high-tension group 1 week after surgery, while no differences were found at final follow-up at an average of 20 months. No differences were found for clinical scores (KOS); however, all five patients with abnormal side-to-side differences >5 mm in KT-1000 measurements were in the low-tension group. The authors concluded that lower preloads of 45 N might not be sufficient to restore long-term stability after ACL reconstruction.

Bastian et al. [3] chose a different approach for preloading their BPTB grafts in ACL reconstruction. In their retrospective case series of 28 patients, no specific loads were chosen, but the anterior knee laxity was reduced to the intact contralateral knee at time of fixation. No intraoperative measurements of the required forces were reported. Baseline anterior-posterior translation increased from 6 ± 1 mm (values for intact and reconstructed knee) to 6.8 ± 1.1 mm at 3 months and to 7.5 ± 1.1 mm at 12 months, which was statistically significant. A further significant increase up to 9.0 ± 1.9 mm was observed between 12 months and final follow-up at an average of 5.3 years. Patients scored "normal" or "nearly normal," respectively, in 79 % (IKDC) and 4 (3–9) points (Tegner; median, range) or 89 ± 9 points (Lysholm; mean $\pm$ SD). Radiological evaluation showed no, minimal, or moderate joint degeneration in 5, 20, and 75 % of patients, respectively. MRI confirmed intact ACL transplants in all patients. The authors concluded that the approach to pretension a BPTB graft to restore normal AP translation allowed for satisfactory clinical outcome at midterm healing, but could not prevent a small loss of anterior-posterior stability and onset of degenerative changes in the reconstructed knee joints.

Two prospective randomized clinical studies looked at the effect of different pretensioning loads of hamstring tendons in ACL reconstruction [18, 30]. Yasuda et al. [30] pretensioned their doubled semitendinosus and gracilis tendons connected to polyester tapes with either 20, 40, or 80 N in 70 patients. Grafts were fixed at the femoral and tibial tunnel exits with staples. At a minimum of 2 years, significant higher anterior knee laxity was found in the lowest-tension group compared to the highest-tension group, in which anterior knee laxity was reduced to within 1 mm of the intact contralateral knee. There were no differences in subjective outcome (Noyes scores), range of motion, knee stability, or muscle strength at final follow-up between any of the groups. Kim et al. [18] used a similar ACL reconstruction technique as Yasuda, with staple fixation of a quintupled semitendinosus tendon connected to polyester tapes. They compared functional and clinical outcome after preloads of 80, 120, and 150 N at a minimum of 1 year postoperatively. They were not able to detect any differences in subjective outcome, anterior knee stability, recovery of muscle strength, and range of motion between the groups. In conclusion of these studies, hamstring tendon grafts using staple fixation away from the joint line seem to require higher preloads of around 80 N to restore long-term stability and knee function close to the ACL intact knee joint.

Memory

Currently, no clear general recommendations can be given on the ideal graft tensioning force of an ACL reconstruction at time of fixation. The ideal tensioning force has to be adapted to a specific graft and fixation type. No current studies exist that have examined these details and have pointed out differences between the various grafts and fixation techniques that are currently available in clinical practice. Overconstrainment of a graft must be avoided, which is rather dependent on anatomic tunnel positioning and position of the knee joint at time of fixation than on the actual tensioning force applied during graft fixation. The pretensioning concept of restoring intact anterior-posterior knee stability seems to be the safest approach to prevent overconstraining the knee joint, but will not assure unchanged knee stability over time. As of today's scientific knowledge, it is valid to state that the concept of pretensioning a soft tissue graft has only limited importance among the factors for successful ACL reconstruction, such as anatomic tunnel placement, proper graft fixation, or postoperative rehabilitation.

References

1. Amis AA, Jakob RP (1998) Anterior cruciate ligament graft positioning, tensioning and twisting. Knee Surg Sports Traumatol Arthrosc 6(Suppl 1):S2–S12
2. Arneja S, McConkey MO, Mulpuri K et al (2009) Graft tensioning in anterior cruciate ligament reconstruction: a systematic review of randomized controlled trials. Arthroscopy 25(2):200–207
3. Bastian JD, Tomagra S, Schuster AJ, Werlen S, Jakob RP, Zumstein MA (2013) ACL reconstruction with physiological graft tension by intraoperative adjustment of the anteroposterior translation to the uninjured contralateral knee. Knee Surg Sports Traumatol Arthrosc 21(5):1226–33
4. Boylan D, Greis PE, West JR, Bachus KN, Burks RT (2003) Effects of initial graft tension on knee stability after anterior cruciate ligament reconstruction using hamstring tendons: a cadaver study. Arthroscopy 19(7):700–705
5. Brady MF, Bradley MP, Fleming BC, Fadale PD, Hulstyn MJ, Banerjee R (2007) Effects of initial graft tension on the tibiofemoral compressive forces and joint position after anterior cruciate ligament reconstruction. Am J Sports Med 35(3):395–403
6. Brown CH, Wilson DR, Hecker AT, Ferragamo M (2004) Graft-bone motion and tensile properties of hamstring and patellar tendon anterior cruciate ligament femoral graft fixation under cyclic loading. Arthroscopy 20(9):922–935
7. Burks RT, Leland R (1988) Determination of graft tension before fixation in anterior cruciate ligament reconstruction. Arthroscopy 4(4):260–266
8. Ciccone WJ, Bratton DR, Weinstein DM, Elias JJ (2006) Viscoelasticity and temperature variations decrease tension and stiffness of hamstring tendon grafts following anterior cruciate ligament reconstruction. J Bone Joint Surg Am 88(5):1071–1078
9. Dargel J, Koebke J, Brüggemann G-P, Pennig D, Schmidt-Wiethoff R (2009) Tension degradation of anterior cruciate ligament grafts with dynamic flexion-extension loading: a biomechanical model in porcine knees. Arthroscopy 25(10):1115–1125
10. Eagar P, Hull ML, Howell SM (2004) How the fixation method stiffness and initial tension affect anterior load–displacement of the knee and tension in anterior cruciate ligament grafts: a study in cadaveric knees using a double-loop hamstrings graft. J Orthop Res 22(3):613–624
11. Elias JJ, Rai SP, Ciccone WJ (2008) In vitro comparison of tension and stiffness between hamstring tendon and patella tendon grafts. J Orthop Res 26(11):1506–1511
12. Fleming BC, Brady MF, Bradley MP, Banerjee R, Hulstyn MJ, Fadale PD (2008) Tibiofemoral compression force differences using laxity- and force-based initial graft tensioning techniques in the anterior cruciate ligament-reconstructed cadaveric knee. Arthroscopy 24(9):1052–1060
13. Fu S-C, Cheng W-H, Cheuk Y-C et al (2013) Effect of graft tensioning on mechanical restoration in a rat model of anterior cruciate ligament reconstruction using free tendon graft. Knee Surg Sports Traumatol Arthrosc
14. Graf BK, Vanderby R, Ulm MJ, Rogalski RP, Thielke RJ (1994) Effect of preconditioning on the viscoelastic response of primate patellar tendon. Arthroscopy 10(1):90–96
15. Herbort M, Lenschow S, Fu FH, Petersen W, Zantop T (2010) ACL mismatch reconstructions: influence of different tunnel placement strategies in single-bundle ACL reconstructions on the knee kinematics. Knee Surg Sports Traumatol Arthrosc 18(11):1551–1558
16. Höher J, Scheffler SU, Withrow JD et al (2000) Mechanical behavior of two hamstring graft constructs for reconstruction of the anterior cruciate ligament. J Orthop Res 18(3):456–461

17. Katsuragi R, Yasuda K, Tsujino J, Keira M, Kaneda K (2000) The effect of nonphysiologically high initial tension on the mechanical properties of in situ frozen anterior cruciate ligament in a canine model. Am J Sports Med 28(1):47–56

18. Kim S-G, Kurosawa H, Sakuraba K, Ikeda H, Takazawa S (2005) The effect of initial graft tension on postoperative clinical outcome in anterior cruciate ligament reconstruction with semitendinosus tendon. Arch Orthop Trauma Surg 126(4): 260–264

19. Mae T, Shino K, Nakata K, Toritsuka Y, Otsubo H, Fujie H (2008) Optimization of graft fixation at the time of anterior cruciate ligament reconstruction. Part II: effect of knee flexion angle. Am J Sports Med 36(6):1094–1100

20. Mae T, Shino K, Nakata K, Toritsuka Y, Otsubo H, Fujie H (2008) Optimization of graft fixation at the time of anterior cruciate ligament reconstruction: part I: effect of initial tension. Am J Sports Med 36(6):1087–1093

21. Markolf KL, Hame S, Hunter DM et al (2002) Effects of femoral tunnel placement on knee laxity and forces in an anterior cruciate ligament graft. J Orthop Res 20(5):1016–1024

22. Nicholas SJ, D'Amato MJ, Mullaney MJ, Tyler TF, Kolstad K, McHugh MP (2004) A prospectively randomized double-blind study on the effect of initial graft tension on knee stability after anterior cruciate ligament reconstruction. Am J Sports Med 32(8):1881–1886

23. Scheffler SU, Südkamp NP, Göckenjan A, Hoffmann RFG, Weiler A (2002) Biomechanical comparison of hamstring and patellar tendon graft anterior cruciate ligament reconstruction techniques: the impact of fixation level and fixation method under cyclic loading. Arthroscopy 18(3):304–315

24. Sherman SL, Chalmers PN, Yanke AB et al (2012) Graft tensioning during knee ligament reconstruction:

principles and practice. J Am Acad Orthop Surg 20(10):633–645

25. Stapleton TR, Curd DT, Baker CL (1999) Initial biomechanical properties of anterior cruciate ligament reconstruction autografts. J South Orthop Assoc 8(3):173–180; discussion 180

26. Tohyama H, Beynnon BD, Johnson RJ, Renström PA, Arms SW (1996) The effect of anterior cruciate ligament graft elongation at the time of implantation on the biomechanical behavior of the graft and knee. Am J Sports Med 24(5):608–614

27. Tohyama H, Yasuda K (1998) Significance of graft tension in anterior cruciate ligament reconstruction. Basic background and clinical outcome. Knee Surg Sports Traumatol Arthrosc 6(Suppl 1):S30–S37

28. van Kampen A, Wymenga AB, van der Heide HJ, Bakens HJ (1998) The effect of different graft tensioning in anterior cruciate ligament reconstruction: a prospective randomized study. Arthroscopy 14(8): 845–850

29. Yamanaka M, Yasuda K, Tohyama H, Nakano H, Wada T (1999) The effect of cyclic displacement on the biomechanical characteristics of anterior cruciate ligament reconstructions. Am J Sports Med 27(6): 772–777

30. Yasuda K, Tsujino J, Tanabe Y, Kaneda K (1997) Effects of initial graft tension on clinical outcome after anterior cruciate ligament reconstruction. Autogenous doubled hamstring tendons connected in series with polyester tapes. Am J Sports Med 25(1):99–106

31. Yoshiya S, Andrish JT, Manley MT, Bauer TW (1987) Graft tension in anterior cruciate ligament reconstruction. An in vivo study in dogs. Am J Sports Med 15(5):464–470

32. Yoshiya S, Kurosaka M, Ouchi K, Kuroda R, Mizuno K (2002) Graft tension and knee stability after anterior cruciate ligament reconstruction. Clin Orthop Relat Res 394:154–160

Fixation

24

Giuseppe Milano, Wolf Petersen, Juergen Hoeher,
Hans H. Paessler, Ralph Akoto, Vincenzo Campana,
Maristella F. Saccomanno, and Rainer Siebold

Contents

24.1 Fixation with Implants: An Overview of Fixation Systems and Strengths

Maristella F. Saccomanno, Vincenzo Campana,
and Giuseppe Milano

24.1.1 Introduction

Anterior cruciate ligament (ACL) graft fixation is
one the most investigated topics in sports medicine
literature and has been proposed to be the major

G. Milano (✉) • V. Campana • M.F. Saccomanno
Department of Orthopaedics, Catholic University,
Largo A. Gemelli, 8, Rome 00168, Italy
e-mail: giuseppe.milano@rm.unicatt.it

W. Petersen (✉)
Department of Orthopaedic and Trauma Surgery,
Martin Luther Hospital, Berlin Grunewald,
Caspar Theyss Strasse 27-34, Berlin D-14193, Germany
e-mail: w.petersen@mlk-berlin.de

J. Hoeher (✉)
Clinic for Sports Traumatology at Cologne Merheim
Medical Center, Ostmerheimer Staße 200,
Cologne 51109, Germany
e-mail: jhoeher@t-online.de

H.H. Paessler • R. Siebold
Institute for Anatomy and Cell Biology,
Ruprecht-Karls University Heidelberg,
Im Neuenheimer Feld 307,
Heidelberg 69120, Germany

HKF: Center for Specialized Hip-Knee-Foot Surgery,
ATOS Hospital Heidelberg, Bismarckstr. 9-15,
Heidelberg 69115, Germany
e-mail: hanspaessler@me.com

R. Akoto
Department of Trauma and Orthopedic Surgery,
University of Witten/Herdecke, Cologne Merheim
Medical Center, Ostmerheimer Straße 200,
Cologne 51109, Germany

R. Siebold et al. (eds.), *Anterior Cruciate Ligament Reconstruction*,
DOI 10.1007/978-3-642-45349-6_24, © ESSKA 2014

factor influencing the graft's mechanical properties in the immediate postoperative period; therefore, it is believed to be a decisive factor in the timing of the rehabilitation program and the return of patients to desired activity levels [25, 26, 84, 127].

There are two landmark studies on ACL graft fixation. In 1984 Noyes et al. [136] subjected various ligament graft tissues to high strain-rate failure tests to determine their strength and elongation properties and, then, the results were compared with the mechanical properties of normal ACL. They showed that the structural properties of bone–patellar tendon–bone (BPTB) graft were superior to soft tissue grafts (fascia lata, single hamstring tendon, or multiple hamstring tendons) and provided an estimation of the ACL in vivo loading during "normal activity," on average, of 454 N. Three years later, Kurosaka et al. [108] conducted the first biomechanical study on ACL graft fixation. They showed better mechanical properties on BPTB grafts fixed with titanium interference screw than staples or sutures tied over buttons. However, the authors concluded that the fixation site was the weakest link of ACL reconstruction, a statement that has probably had the single most striking influence on the field in terms of generating further research.

Later studies [79, 81, 184] demonstrated that doubled semitendinosus and gracilis tendon graft is the strongest and stiffest autograft available for biological ACL reconstruction even if several biomechanical studies have shown that fixation of DSTG can be weaker than that of patellar tendon graft, depending on the fixation technique that is used [7, 25, 26, 30, 84, 161, 179].

Nowadays, many different fixation devices are available for soft tissue grafts or bone–tendon–bone (BTB) grafts, and several studies made a comparison between them. Although some laboratory studies showed significant differences between various methods, excellent clinical results may be demonstrated with a wide range of options [43, 55, 80, 168, 169].

Therefore, recent studies shifted the attention from ACL graft fixation methods to anatomical reconstruction and proper tunnel placement, as it seems to be the major cause related to ACL reconstruction failure [116].

We will now summarize the main properties of available ACL graft fixation devices.

24.1.2 Graft Fixation Mechanisms

Before talking about fixation devices, we should understand how the femur–graft–tibia system is composed. We will consider three different units: femoral fixation-site unit, tendon unit (graft), and tibial fixation-site unit. The type of graft will influence the choice of the best fixation device, and especially in case of soft tissue graft, we might use different fixation devices for femoral and tibial side.

Main characteristics of graft fixation are strength and stiffness. Graft fixation to bone has to be:

- Strong enough to avoid failure
- Stiff enough to restore load displacement response and allow biological incorporation of the graft into the bone tunnels
- Secure enough to resist slippage (or stretch) under cyclic loading

ACL graft fixation mechanisms can be classified according to the amount, application site and distribution of forces that resist graft pullout. Variables which determine the magnitude, application, and distribution of resistance to pullout force are graft (soft tissue or BTB grafts), hardware design, and bone density.

Regardless of the type of graft, ACL fixation methods can be divided into two key types:

- Aperture or intratunnel fixation (interference screw and cross pins)
- Extra-articular fixation (cortical fixation devices, femoral loops, and tibial cortical fixation).

Otherwise, we can describe graft fixation as anatomical (aperture or joint line fixation), non-anatomical, and semi-anatomical, according to the location of fixation in relation to the joint line. Therefore, graft fixation directly at the joint line (site of the insertion of the native ACL) is considered anatomical; extra-articular fixation could be considered nonanatomical (staple, buttons) or semi-anatomical (transfixation devices, distal interference fixation).

Additionally, indirect and direct fixation should be distinguished. Direct fixation means that the graft is anchored to the tunnel without using any additional material except the fixation device itself; indirect fixation means that there is a linkage material between graft and fixation device.

Several fixation devices are now available according to soft tissue or BTB grafts. Several biomechanical and clinical studies have been conducted in order to find out the ideal graft fixation construct: it should be similar in strength and stiffness to the native human anterior cruciate ligament. Actually, the majority of these generally exceed the 450-N safe early physiological loading threshold proposed by Noyes et al. [136].

Biomechanical studies are usually performed in vitro or ex vivo using animal models (porcine or bovine knees) or human cadavers. Two types of biomechanical tests are commonly used to evaluate the mechanical behavior of ACL graft fixation techniques [19, 40, 200]: single-cycle load-to-failure and cyclic loading test. The former is the most commonly used, and it allows to determine the structural properties of the bone–graft–fixation device complex, such as ultimate failure load, yield load, linear stiffness, and displacement at failure. Advantages of this type of test are that the weak link in the fixation complex can be easily identified, such as the mode and site of the fixation failure and upper limit of the strength of the construction. Cycling loading test evaluates the ability of the bone-graft-fixation device complex to resist elongation or slippage under repetitive submaximal loads over time. Actually, a comparison of mechanical properties of various fixation constructs is very difficult. First, the use of different research models and biomechanical testing protocols make it difficult to compare the results of one study with another. Second, human cadaveric specimens in the age range of patients typically undergoing ACL reconstruction are generally not available; therefore, specimens from older

donors are often used, and it has been demonstrated that fixation strength of fixation devices could be underestimated in that condition [29]. Otherwise, porcine bones is still the prevailing practice in ACL graft fixation studies, although it's well documented that they are not suitable for this purpose [137]. Finally, in vitro biomechanical studies provided the only evaluation of certain parameters (such as ultimate failure load, yield point, stiffness, displacement to failure and mode of failure) at time zero, prior to biological fixation of ACL graft. Limited information is available regarding how such parameters change during the process of biological incorporation, when probably the weak link shifts from the ACL graft fixation–bone tunnel interface to the intra-articular part of ACL graft [95, 127]

24.1.3 Bone–Tendon–Bone Graft Fixation

Patellar tendon or other allograft tendon with bone plugs is generally used.

In ACL reconstruction with BTB grafts, bone block healing is reported to occur between 4 and 12 weeks after surgery [45, 140]. Until biological fixation has occurred, high fixation strength is necessary. During the last decades, many different fixation methods have been proposed.

We can classify BTB fixation methods as follows:

- *Interference compression: interference screw.* Fixation properties of interference screw fixation of BTB grafts depend on the generation of friction between the bone block and bone tunnel wall and the engagement of the screw threads into the bone block and bone tunnel wall.
- *Transverse compression: transcondylar screw.* Fixation is achieved with a blunt-nosed transverse screw that enters the femoral tunnel from the lateral cortex, pushing the bone plug against the medial tunnel wall (Fig. 24.1).
- *Transverse suspension.* It consists of one or more cross pins that pass transversally through

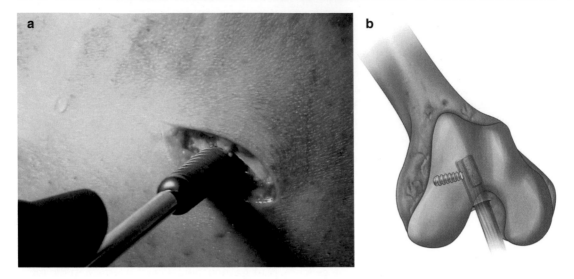

Fig. 24.1 Transcondylar screw for femoral fixation of BTB graft. (**a**) A blunt-nose setscrew is introduced through a small incision on the lateral aspect of the distal femur. (**b**) A line drawing illustrates the mechanism of fixation

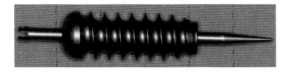

Fig. 24.2 The Cross-Press Fix (Arthrex) guarantees femoral fixation of BTB graft by a combination of compression and suspension fixation mechanism

the bone plug, such as Rigid-fix (DePuy Mitek, Raynham, Massachusetts) and Bio-Transfix T3 (Arthrex, Naples, Florida).
- *Hybrid system.* It is a combination of compression and suspension fixation mechanism (Cross-Press Fix, Arthrex) (Fig. 24.2).
- *Press-fit.* It consists of using autologous bone previously harvested or a beta-tricalcium phosphate (β-TCP) plug filled in either tibial or femoral tunnel without any other fixation devices.

24.1.3.1 Interference Screws

Interference screw fixation of BTB graft is the most widely used and is considered the gold standard.

Fixation strength of interference screw can be affected by several variables, such as:
- *Screw diameter and gap size.* Although it has been demonstrated that there are no

differences in fixation strength between 7 and 9 mm screws [92, 103, 165], the influence of screw diameter is probably most relevant when a significant discrepancy exists between the bone block and the bone tunnel wall. Generally, bone block size has to match the diameter of the bone tunnel in order to achieve a solid fixation [37], and the greater is the interference gap, the larger should be the screw diameter [32].
- *Screw divergence.* It means that the direction of the interference screw is not parallel to the bone block and the axis of the bone tunnel. On the femoral side, screw divergence of more than 15° from the orientation of the bone plug dramatically decreases the fixation strength of the construct [28, 32, 64, 75, 97, 139, 146, 155, 159].
- *Screw length.* Biomechanical studies did not show any significant influence on initial fixation properties [20, 28, 148].
- *Bone mineral density.* Bone mineral density (BMD) is probably the most important variable that influences initial fixation strength and stiffness and resistance to slippage during cyclic loading. It is already known that BMD in humans decreased with age and BMD of females is lower than that of males. However,

focusing on ACL reconstruction, recent studies on the evaluation of the BMD around the fixation area stated two important landmarks: BMD of the femoral tunnel is higher than that of the tibial tunnel, so that implies that a proportional larger diameter interference screw should be used for fixation in the proximal tibia than that used for fixation on the distal femur [183]; and the anteromedial area of the tibia is the most acceptable in the interference screw fixation [110].

Nowadays, different types of interference screws are available: metal, biodegradable, and biocomposite.

Metal interference screw represented the traditional fixation for ACL reconstruction for many years. This fixation technique has been shown to provide high initial fixation strength while promoting early osseous integration [31, 69, 92]. Despite favorable reports on metal interference screws, concerns exist regarding damage of bone–tendon junction during screw placement [120], violation of the posterior cortex [74], presence of intra-articular hardware [164, 171], the distortion on postoperative magnetic resonance imaging (MRI) evaluation, and the requirement for hardware removal during revision surgery [9, 24, 59, 119, 125, 167, 177, 186]. As a consequence, developments in bioengineering and biomaterials field stated that the ideal implant should be biocompatible, biomimetic, and biodegradable. Therefore, biodegradable screws have been proposed. Biodegradable interference screws can be divided into fast- and slow-degradable screws. Fast-degradable screws might have a higher incidence of soft tissue reactions [104, 124, 196]. Commonly used biodegradable screws consist of polyglycolic acid (PGA), poly-p-dioxanone and copolymers of polyglycolic acid/polylactic acid (PGA/PLA) as well as various stereoisomers of the lactic acid molecule: poly-l-lactic acid (PLLA) and poly-D-lactic acid (PDLA). Each polymer has its material-specific properties, and an implant created from a single type of polymer is naturally limited by those properties; therefore, copolymer blending combines the desired properties of

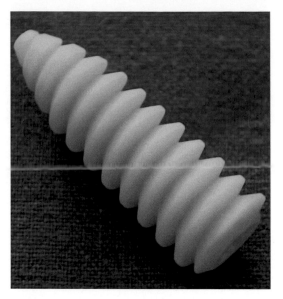

Fig. 24.3 Biocomposite interference screw (PLA and β-TCP)

different polymers and overcome limitations of single-type polymers.

More recently, biocomposite materials have been introduced; these materials are composed of a combination of the previously listed polymers and osteoconductive materials, such as beta-tricalcium phosphate (β-TCP) or hydroxyapatite (Fig. 24.3). Particularly, β-TCP as part of a composite implant seems to offer good ultrastructural properties for cell adhesion [18].

Biocomposite implants are designed to degrade over time. Unlike biodegradable implants, however, biocomposite implants degrade more quickly, while their osteoconductive properties promote faster graft incorporation and faster new bone formation [8, 10].

Bone xenograft interference screws were also proposed, but fixation seems to be less secure than that obtained with metallic screws [54].

Several biomechanical studies showed that primary fixation of BTB graft achieved with biodegradable or biocomposite screws is as strong and stiff as that obtained with metallic screws [25, 29, 33, 96, 103, 108, 158].

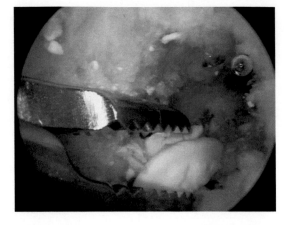

Fig. 24.4 Large degraded fragments of an interference screw are removed during arthroscopy performed for persistent joint effusions 4 months after ACL reconstruction

Concerns associated with the use of biodegradable interference screws include:

- Intraoperative or early postoperative screw breakage [77]
- Inflammatory reaction mediated by the presence of large amounts of acidic particles produced during implant degradation [2] (Fig. 24.4). This often manifests as an aseptic effusion, synovitis, or the presence of a cyst at the orifice of the tibial tunnel [6, 11, 22, 70, 73, 142, 168, 169, 180, 192, 193]
- Screw migration with further damage (articular or not) [166]: it can be asymptomatic or mimic meniscus injuries [24, 113], cause pain and swelling [77, 107, 164, 166], mechanical complaints [111, 201], wound dehiscence [160], and sometimes it can appear like a palpable mass [77, 160]
- The increased cost over metallic screws [142]
- The potential for bone tunnel widening [48, 180]

24.1.3.2 Transverse Fixation

Transverse compression and transverse suspension have been proposed in order to avoid complications related to interference screws, but, actually, there are no many studies in literature about mechanical behavior and clinical results of these fixation devices [36, 115, 129, 198, 207]. The advantages of these devices are mainly related to the fact that they do not interfere with bone-graft healing, since they are placed transversally to the bone plug, fixing the graft with a suspension (pins) or lateral compression (set-screw) mechanism; therefore, the contact area between the device and plug is reduced compared to the interference screw, allowing an early biological fixation and a more complete bone regrowth into the tunnel [115]. Furthermore, transcondylar screws can be easily removed without leaving a wide tunnel, which might complicate immediate graft replacement during revision surgery. Finally, they can be considered as a salvage procedure because they guarantee a stable fixation even when the posterior cortex of the femoral tunnel is blown out.

However, transverse femoral fixation devices have also some potential disadvantages. First, the orientation of the femoral tunnel has to be rather vertical to allow the placement of the fixation device perpendicularly to the bone plug of the graft, without violating the femoral insertion of the lateral collateral ligament [68, 129, 150]. This reproduces a nonanatomical placement of the femoral insertion of the graft. Second, graft fixation is not performed under direct visualization, as occurs with interference screws [206]. Despite caution in graft harvest, grafts are not perfect cylinders and double pins may be placed eccentrically. The eccentricity of these pins might bring less stable fixation and a probable delay in bone-graft healing.

Biomechanical studies comparing the difference between interference screw and transverse screw or absorbable cross pin did not show any significant differences in failure load and stiffness [36, 129, 198, 207].

Finally, in order to avoid disadvantages related to any fixation device, a hardware-free press-fit fixation technique has been developed. Animal studies showed that press-fit fixation with microporous pure beta-TCP plugs of BTB grafts or patellar tendon grafts without bone blocks for ACL reconstruction leads to primary stability comparable with that achieved by fixation with metal interference screws in case of BTB grafts [122, 123]. In order to enhance initial fixation strength of press-fit ACL graft fixation, dilating a femoral tunnel that is underdrilled by 1 mm appears to be a reasonable technical procedure [47]. Advantages of the bone–patellar tendon–bone (BPTB) press-fit fixation include unlimited bone-to-bone healing, cost effectiveness, avoidance of disadvantages associated with hardware and ease for revision surgery. On the other hand, fixation strength completely depends on bone quality.

24.1.3.3 Clinical Studies

Several clinical studies compared biodegradable and metal interference screws according to residual anterior laxity evaluated using clinical tests and a KT arthrometer measurement and most used subjective and objective functional outcome assessment questionnaires, such as Lysholm Knee scoring scale and IKDC score. Despite biomechanical differences, no clinical differences were detected [9, 17, 50, 51, 60, 98, 125, 147].

Furthermore, no significant differences were also found comparing interference screws and cross-pin fixation [58, 117]. Even considering major complications associated with cross-pin fixation, such as fracture, posterior transcortical breach, migration, resorption, and lateral prominence of the device, clinical results are not affected [181].

Good clinical results are also reported on press-fit fixation technique [57, 76, 202]. A recent study [102], comparing autogenous bone plug versus bioabsorbable interference screws for the tibial tunnel, showed no differences on clinical assessment, but a reduction of tibial tunnel widening at MRI evaluation and a reduction of the complication rate using an autogenous bone plug.

24.1.4 Soft Tissue Graft Fixation

The most used soft tissue graft is autologous-doubled semitendinosus and gracilis tendon graft.

Soft tissue graft–bone tunnel integration generally takes longer time than BTB graft incorporation. On the basis of animal studies, it occurs between 6 and 12 weeks after surgery [154]. Therefore, it can be assumed that primary fixation of soft tissue graft is crucial for a longer time.

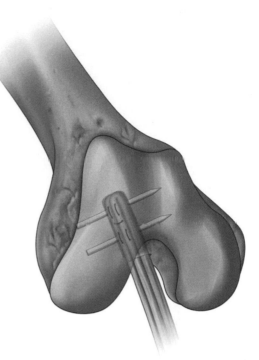

Fig. 24.5 A line drawing illustrates the mechanism of fixation of RigidFix (DePuy Mitek)

Because of variability related to surgical techniques, graft geometry, and bone density, we will analyze femoral and tibial fixation separately.

24.1.4.1 Femoral Fixation

Three different fixation mechanisms are available:
- *Compression: interference screws*. As above-mentioned, they can be metal or biodegradable. Compressive loads are oriented transversely to the longitudinal axis of the graft and are shared along three interfaces: bone–screw, screw–tendon, and tendon–bone.
- *Expansion*. It consists of one or more cross pins that pass through the graft and femoral tunnel, producing a bulging of the graft, such as RigidFix (DePuy, Mitek) and Bio-Transfix T3 (Arthrex) (Fig. 24.5). This fixation is based on an initial press-fit of the graft into the bone tunnel. As the pins are inserted transversely to the femoral tunnel, they increase the volume of the graft and therefore cause a pressure

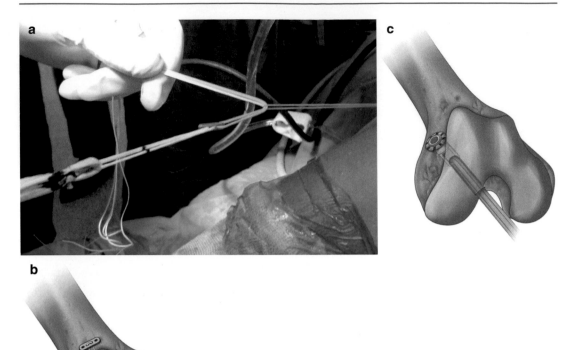

Fig. 24.6 Cortical suspension devices for femoral fixation of soft tissue graft. (**a**) The graft is passed into the loop of a TightRope (Arthrex). (**b**) A line drawing illustrates the mechanism of fixation of metal plates with suture loops. (**c**) A line drawing illustrates the mechanism of fixation of all-metal devices

effect against the tunnel walls; this pressure is directed in a centrifugal way with respect to the insertion point of the pins. Expansion fixation depends on some variables, such as initial press-fit of the graft, bone density and, above all, correct placement of the pins. Indeed, an eccentric placement of the pins inside the tunnel would produce a nonhomogeneous load distribution at the bone–tendon interface and would impair fixation strength.

- *Suspension.* This mechanism is further subdivided into:
  - (a) Cortical: metal plates with suture loops, such as EndoButton (Smith & Nephew, Andover, Massachusetts), RetroButton (Arthrex), ToggleLoc (Biomet, Warsaw, Indiana), TightRope (Arthrex), XO Button (Conmed Linvatec, Largo, Florida), and FlipTack (Karl Storz, Tuttlingen, Germany), or all metal, such as Swing-Bridge (Citieffe, Bologna, Italy), EZLoc (Biomet), and EndoButton Direct (Smith & Nephew). This fixation mechanism consists of a hardware placed over the anterior-lateral cortex of the distal femur, which suspends the graft into the femoral tunnel (Fig. 24.6). In this type of fixation, resistance vectors are parallel and opposite to pullout forces and are focused on the cortical bone of the distal femur, at the bone–

hardware interface. Therefore, the smaller is the contact surface of the fixation device, the greater is load concentration. The contact surface of the fixation device can vary, depending on the design of the device.

(b) Cancellous: the graft is suspended to a screw or a press-fit anchor, which is fixed into the cancellous bone of the femoral metaphysis, such as Linx-HT (DePuy, Mitek) and AporFix (Cayenne Medical, Scottsdale, Arizona) (Fig. 24.7). In this fixation, resistance is due to transverse compressive forces at the cancellous bone–hardware interface.

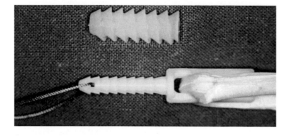

Fig. 24.7 Cancellous suspension devices for femoral fixation of soft tissue graft (Linx-HT, DePuy Mitek). The graft (*bottom*) is suspended to a screw (*top*), which is fixed into the femoral tunnel

(c) Cortical-cancellous: transepicondylar fixation systems that are based on the use of a transverse suspension bar that is perpendicular to pullout forces, such as Bone Mulch Screw (Biomet), Crosspin (Stryker, Kalamazoo, Michigan), TransFix (Arthrex), AXL Cross Pin (Biomet), Biosteon Cross-Pin (Stryker), Pinn-ACL (ConMed Linvatec), and Bio-Transfix (Arthrex) (Fig. 24.8). In this type of fixation, resistance is distributed along the contact surface between hardware and bone, and it depends on bone density and length of the lever arms with respect to the point of application of pullout forces (i.e., graft suspension point).

There is no consensus on the best method for achieving soft tissue graft fixation.

Interference screw fixation can be used also for soft tissue grafts, but it is affected by different variables on the femoral or tibial side. Fixation properties of interference screw fixation of soft tissue graft depend on the friction generated by the compression of the soft tissue graft against the bone tunnel wall. Therefore, BMD still remains the most important variable that influences initial fixation. Other factors strictly linked to the screw

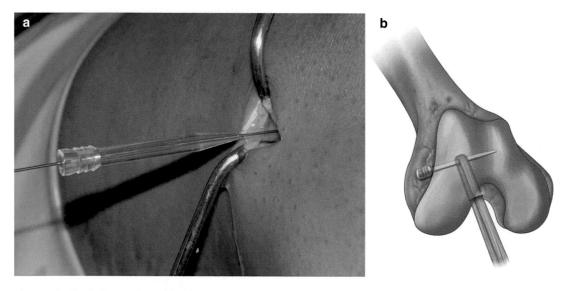

Fig. 24.8 Cortical-cancellous suspension devices for femoral fixation of soft tissue graft. (**a**) A transverse suspension bar (Bio-Transfix, Arthrex) is introduced through a small incision on the lateral aspect of the distal femur. (**b**) A line drawing illustrates the mechanism of fixation

design and screw placement in the femoral tunnel are the following:

- *Screw geometry.* Few studies have examined the influence of screw diameter on the initial fixation properties of soft tissue ACL graft. One of the major concerns associated with metallic interference screws is the risk of graft laceration or rotation during fixation. Indeed, using screws smaller than tunnel diameter increases the risk of graft slippage, while larger screws might lead to graft damage [208]. For this reason, a hybrid femoral fixation technique with extracortical button and undersized interference screw has been proposed [85, 199]. Nowadays, the newest biodegradable screw generations are sharply threaded just at the tip for easy starting conditions of the screw, followed by blunt threading to prevent tissue laceration. Thus, precise matching of the graft and tunnel diameters can easily be performed.
- *Tendon fit.* Steenlage et al. [178] demonstrated that four-strand hamstring tendon graft fixed in a distal femur with a bioabsorbable screw resulted in a significant higher ultimate failure load if the bone tunnel was sized within 0.5 mm of the graft diameter versus within 1 mm of the measured size of the graft.
- *Screw placement.* On the femoral site, screw position generally is anterior to the graft to allow anatomical posterior placement of the graft in the tunnel. Screw divergence of more than 15° decreases the fixation strength of the construct. Therefore, in order to decrease screw divergence, several studies suggested that the screw should be placed through the tibial tunnel or using intraoperative fluoroscopy [27, 38, 39, 134, 162].

Biomechanical studies comparing bioabsorbable and metallic interference screws showed that primary fixation of soft tissue graft achieved with biodegradable screws is as strong and stiff as that obtained with metallic screws [7, 34, 71, 194].

The advantages of intratunnel soft tissue graft fixation using interference screws compared with extratunnel fixation methods are the following:

- Anatomical and direct fixation. Interference screw fixation near the joint line aperture has been shown to enhance soft tissue graft–bone healing, tendon-to-bone integration, and fixation strength [197].
- Reduced graft "working length." If an extratunnel fixation device is used, the greater distance between the location of the fixation and the native ACL insertion may create a "bungee-cord" [156] or a "windshield-wiper" effect resulting in bone tunnel widening [63, 89]. The bungee-cord effect is an elastic longitudinal deformation of the graft, while the windshield-wiper effect is described as a sagittal intratunnel graft motion. Recently, Cheung et al. [41], in an in vivo study, demonstrated that femoral tunnel widening was greater in femoral cross-pin fixation than bioabsorbable interference screw fixation, probably related to the windshield-wiper and bungee-cord effects.
- High stiffness. In case of extratunnel fixation, the long distance between the femoral and tibial fixation device could result not only in a graft-tunnel motion but also in a low-construct stiffness.

On the contrary, biological and mechanical advantages promoted by using cortical fixation devices over intratunnel fixation are:

- Better healing because of the longer tunnel. It allowed more bone surface area to the tendon to heal.
- Circumferential healing of all sides of the graft to the tunnel wall.
- The ability to completely fill the bone tunnel.
- The ability to grip cortical bone instead of cancellous bone. Cortical bone is 30 times stronger than cancellous bone and is not as affected by other variables such as BMD, gender, age, alcohol, and smoking [90].

Several biomechanical studies on porcine models compared intratunnel and extratunnel fixation devices. They showed superior mechanical properties using extratunnel fixation devices [3, 128, 175, 209].

Several studies also compared different extratunnel fixation devices, without demonstrating clinically relevant differences between them in terms of structural properties under load-to-failure or cyclic loading conditions [16, 45, 61, 99, 145, 168, 169].

24.1.4.2 Clinical Studies on Femoral Fixation

Despite biomechanical studies showed some differences between different devices, two recent reviews [55, 168, 169] comparing biodegradable and metal interference screws, including BTB and soft tissue grafts, showed no differences neither in anterior laxity nor respect to IKDC, Lysholm, or Tegner activity score, although the incidence of knee effusion was higher in the biodegradable screw group [168, 169].

Moreover, also two recent literature reviews comparing intratunnel versus extratunnel fixation showed no clinical differences [43, 80].

Clinical studies comparing extratunnel fixation devices such as EndoButton and Transfix [149, 205], RigidFix and EndoButton [13], or RigidFix and Transfix [78] did not show any significant difference in functional outcomes.

As we mentioned before, tunnel widening is one of the major concern regarding extratunnel fixation devices. In particular, EndoButton seemed to be associated with femoral tunnel enlargement already Detectable 3 months after surgery [14, 110, 172]. However, clinical results are not affected. A recent study [133] showed that ACL reconstruction using a transfemoral fixation device and an additional bone plug augmentation of the femoral tunnel aperture provides significantly higher degree of graft filling at MRI evaluation. The same authors [132] recently reported clinical and MRI evaluation after ACL reconstruction using hamstring and transfemoral fixation at 5-year follow-up. They observed that hamstring graft integrity and signal intensity scores were significantly higher in patients with deformed, broken, or dislocated pins as compared to patients with fully or mainly intact pins. The authors concluded that biodegradable fixation pins lose structural integrity in a way that suggests continuous loading of the pin/graft construct, thereby questioning osseous incorporation of the graft. However, no significant clinical differences were detected.

24.1.4.3 Tibial Fixation

Tibial fixation is generally considered more challenging than femoral fixation for at least two

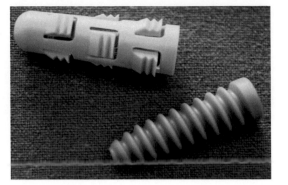

Fig. 24.9 Expansion device for tibial fixation of soft tissue graft (GraftBolt, Arthrex): it consists of an expandable ridged sheath and a tapered expansion screw

main reasons: BMD is significantly lower than that of the distal femur and tibial fixation devices must resist tension applied parallel to the axis of the tibial bone tunnel [25, 26, 114, 179]. Potential pitfalls in tibial fixation include graft slippage or micromotion, which can produce residual laxity and tunnel widening. For these reasons, tibial fixation represents the weak link of femur–graft–tibia complex right after an ACL reconstruction with soft tissue grafts.

Tibial fixation devices can be distinguished as follows:

- *Compression devices:* interference screws.
- *Expansion devices*: they consist of an expandable four-channel, ridged sheath and a tapered expansion screw. The four channels individually capture and grip each of the four strands of the hamstring tendon graft into separate compartments and directly compress each of the graft strands against the cancellous bone in order to maximize bony integration. This family of devices includes Intrafix (DePuy Mitek), AperFix II (Cayenne Medical), BIOSURE SYNC (Smith & Nephew), ExoShape (MedShape, Atlanta, Georgia), and GraftBolt (Arthrex) (Fig. 24.9).
- *Cortical anchoring devices*: staples, sutures over post, screws, and spiked washers.
- *Hybrid fixation*: it is a combination of compression and cortical fixation devices.

Less innovation has been made regarding tibial fixation compared to femoral fixation, and

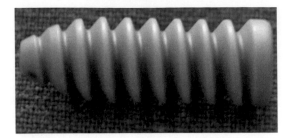

Fig. 24.10 PEEK interference screw (Arthrex)

variations in interference screws have prevailed. Besides metallic, biodegradable, and biocomposite devices, plastic implants made up of polyether ether ketone (PEEK) and polyethylene terephthalate (PET) are becoming popular. They do not resorb, but are inert, and do not interfere with imaging studies. Moreover, they can be overdrilled in cases of ACL revision (Fig. 24.10).

Factors affecting initial fixation properties of interference screws on the tibial side are different from the femoral side and are the following:

- *Screw geometry*. Length has a greater influence at the tibial side because the area over which friction is generated between the bone tunnel wall and soft tissue graft is determined by the screw length. Several studies showed that a long screw (28–35 mm) significantly increases ultimate failure load and reduces slippage if the screw head engages the tibial cortex [83, 163, 195, 196]. A recent study [86] on porcine tibias using biocomposite wedge interference screws of different lengths and diameters showed that longer and wider screws provide high strength and no slippage. In fact, it is generally recommended that the diameter of the screw at the tibial side should be 1 mm larger than the diameter of the tunnel, especially if a hybrid system is not used.

- *Tunnel dilation*. Biomechanical studies [52, 53, 174] reported conflicting results on the efficacy of serial dilation versus extraction drilling. Previous studies [52, 53], conducted on porcine tibias, showed that tunnel dilation does not enhance soft tissue tendon graft fixation strength in healthy bone. On the contrary, a recent study [174], which performed a radiostereometric analysis on 40 patients to evaluate migration of the graft in the bone tunnels and knee laxity, found less slippage in the serial dilated group compared to the extraction drilling group.

- *Screw placement*. Soft tissue graft may be fixed by inserting the screw on the side (eccentrically) or down to the center (concentrically) of the graft strands. Concentric screw placement maximizes contact between the graft strands and bone tunnel wall, providing a greater surface area for healing, even if actually, no differences have been detected [170, 173]. Screw divergence is also important at the tibial side. Even if it is rare, it has been demonstrated that screw divergence of $\geq 15°$ significantly reduces soft tissue tendon graft–bone tunnel fixation [5, 52, 53].

- *Bone mineral density*. As previously discussed, BMD at the tibial side is the most important variable [110, 183].

Recent biomechanical studies comparing tibial fixation devices often showed conflicting results.

A study [152, 153] conducted on human cadavers, compared anterograde Delta Screw (Arthrex) and retrograde RetroScrew (Arthrex). The authors demonstrated that the Delta Screw had a higher maximum insertion torque and exhibited a larger increase in intra-articular graft tension as compared to the RetroScrew. However, the same authors also showed no significant difference between the two devices on osteoporotic bones [153, 153]. A recent study conducted on 20 bovine tibias confirmed no differences between the devices [191].

Kousa et al. [106] tested six different tibial fixation devices in porcine tibias and showed that expansion device (Intrafix) provided stronger fixation than interference and cortical fixation. Subsequently, two cadaver studies [35, 190] compared Intrafix and biodegradable screws, showing conflicting results.

Aga et al. [1] in porcine model using bovine tendons recently compared metal, biodegradable, and PEEK interference screws and five 5 expansion devices. The authors showed that although the highest ultimate failure loads and least amounts of cyclic displacement were observed for expansion devices, group comparisons of screw and expansion devices did not result in any significant differences for ultimate failure load and cyclic displacement.

Cortical tibial fixation devices can provide secure initial fixation [114], but the implants are often prominent and can cause local skin irritation and pain [25, 26].

In order to improve the strength of the graft fixation and reduce the risk of slippage, hybrid fixation systems have been developed and compared with standard non-augmented fixation. The following hybrid combinations were tested: screw and washer with bone dowel [91], screw and washer with interference screw [204], interference screw with staple [56], interference screw with double spike plate [182], interference screw with autograft bone augmentation [157, 185], and interference screw with Bio-Tenodesis Screw [189]. All these studies demonstrated better mechanical properties for hybrid fixation systems, even in osteoporotic bone [157].

24.1.4.4 Clinical Studies on Tibial Fixation

No clinical differences were found out using metal or biodegradable screws [55, 168, 169].

However, biodegradable screws are associated with a great risk of cyst formation [6, 70, 73] and bone tunnel widening at the tibial side [42, 49, 112, 187]. Particularly, these problems are mostly reported in studies involving PLLA-based screws, maybe because this polymer is the most frequently used [24, 77, 107, 111, 142, 160, 164, 166, 201].

Studies comparing interference screws, cortical fixations, and screw with sheath did not show any significant clinical differences [66, 82, 94].

A recent study [135] compared clinical outcomes of tibial fixation between a biodegradable interference screw and hybrid fixation (screw and post-fixation). They showed a significant difference at Lachman test evaluation in favor of the biodegradable interference screw supplemented by a post-tie using a screw washer.

Memory

Several different devices are available for BTB and soft tissue grafts. Despite biomechanical differences, clinical results seem to be acceptable with most fixation techniques. The best fixation method has not yet been defined. The majority of the devices tested exceed the physiological load of the healthy ACL proposed by Noyes et al. [136]. Biodegradable interference screws are actually the gold standard for BTB graft fixation. New biocomposite screws can also improve osteointegration. On the other hand, in case of soft tissue graft fixation, suspension devices seem to offer the best mechanical properties on the femoral side, while biodegradable interference screw still remains the most used fixation device at the tibial side.

24.2 Press-Fit Fixation Using the Patellar Tendon

Wolf Petersen

24.2.1 Introduction

Due to the development of the cost in healthcare, an increasing interest in ACL press-fit fixation was noted during the recent years. Press-fit fixation allows direct bone-to-bone healing and reduces the number of disadvantages associated with hardware fixation, such as graft laceration, bone resorption, chronic synovitis, or allergic reactions [202]. Another important feature of this fixation technique is easier revision of ACL reconstruction.

One biomechanical study has shown that the ultimate load for the press-fit fixation was significantly lower than that for the interference screw fixation [131]; others have shown that there is no difference in the fixation strength between press-fit fixation and interference screw fixation [46, 121, 141]. Clinical studies reported encouraging results after BPTB press-fit ACL reconstruction in the medium and long term [88].

The aim of this article is to present a technique for femoral BPTB press-fit fixation (Fig. 24.11). We use this technique in young high-level athletes, in revisions, and in patients who wish to get a BPTB graft.

24.2.2 Technique

In most press-fit fixation techniques, the diameter of the bone block is 0.5–1 mm smaller than the diameter of the tunnel. Therefore, bone block and tunnel preparation are crucial for this surgical technique.

24.2.2.1 Graft Harvesting

For graft harvesting, we use a 6-cm longitudinal incision starting at the distal aspect of the patella running distally ending at the tibial tuberosity. A 9–10-mm wide medial strip of the patellar tendon was excised. The graft is harvested with one bone block from the tibial tuberosity and one bone block from the patella. The bone block from the tibial tuberosity is formed to a trapezoid shape by using an oscillating saw. Normally, the tibial bone block is used for femoral graft fixation, and the patellar block is used for tibial press-fit fixation. If a tibial press-fit fixation is desired, the patellar bone block is formed as a wedge.

The trapezoid-shaped bone block has a diameter of 0.5 mm larger than the bone tunnel and a graft sizer (Karl Storz, Tuttlingen) is used to ensure that it can be completely passed through the appropriate template. The bone block is then tapered with the rongeur in a fashion that its distal 5 mm had the same size as the bone tunnel (Fig. 24.12).

24.2.2.2 Tunnel Preparation

For the femoral tunnel, an anteromedial drilling technique is used because biomechanical and anatomical studies have shown that tunnels created by the anteromedial portal drilling technique match the ACL footprint much closer than tunnels created with the transtibial technique.

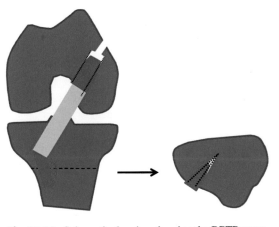

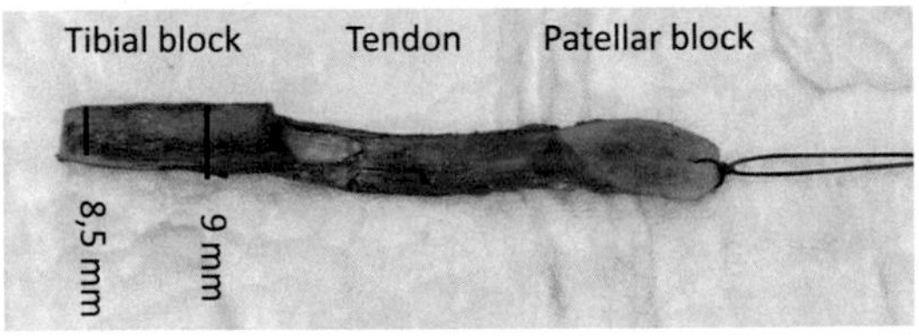

Fig. 24.11 Schematic drawing showing the BPTP press-fit technique

Fig. 24.12 Bone–patellar tendon–bone autograft prepared for press-fit fixation

For placement of the guide wire, a specific anteromedial portal aimer is used. This guide is an offset guide, which was especially designed to be used via the anteromedial portal. The Medial Portal Aimer is used to place the guide wire in the center of the ACL insertion. The K-wire position has to be visualized via the anteromedial portal. Anatomical landmarks for a correct tunnel placement are the intercondylar line and the cartilage border as described by Petersen and Zantop [143].

When the K-wire is placed centrally within the femoral insertion, the femoral tunnel is drilled with a 4.5-mm drill. The length of the whole tunnel varies between 30 and 45 mm. Then a blind tunnel is drilled with a 6-mm drill up to a length of 25–30 mm depending of the length of the total tunnel. For further preparation, dilatators are used (Karl Storz, Tuttlingen, Germany). The tunnel is dilated to a diameter 0.5 to 1 mm smaller than the tibial graft cylinder (Fig. 24.13a–c).

In every case the final position of the tunnel is controlled and documented with the arthroscope via the anteromedial portal.

An alternative for femoral tunnel preparation is the use of a special reamer as described by Hertel and Behrend [87]. Then, the harvested bone block can be used to fill the femoral tunnel.

For tibial tunnel placement, a specific guide is used as well. In 45° of flexion aiming and drilling of the tibial tunnel is performed. For anatomical tunnel placement, the tibial stump of the ACL should be left in situ. In cases with no remnants, the anterior horn of the lateral meniscus is used as landmark. Anatomical studies have shown that the posterior border of the anterior horn of the lateral meniscus corresponds with the middle of the tibial ACL insertion [143]. The K-wire is placed in the center of the tibial ACL footprint. Then, the tunnel is drilled 0.5 mm larger than the tibial bone block.

24.2.2.3 Graft Passage and Fixation

First, a guide wire with a suture loop is passed into the femoral bone tunnel. Then, the suture loop is pulled out of the femoral tunnel. This

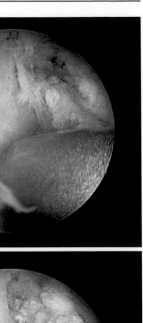

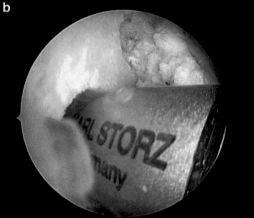

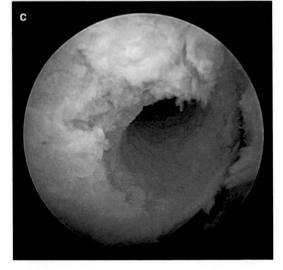

Fig. 24.13 (**a**) The medial portal aimer is introduced via the medial portal and the guide wire is placed in the center of the femoral insertion. (**b–c**) A careful tunnel preparation can be archived with help of dilators

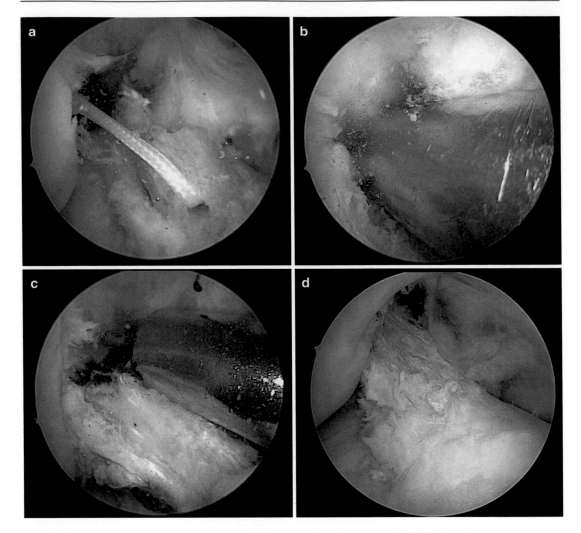

Fig. 24.14 (**a–d**) Patellar tendon bone graft is pulled into the femoral bone tunnel, (**d**) final result

suture loop serves to pull the graft into the joint. With the tibial bone block running first, the graft is introduced through the tibial tunnel into the joint. Thus, the bone block can easily slide into the femoral bone tunnel to half of its length (Fig. 24.14a–d).

Holding tension on the femoral sutures and keeping the knee flexed to 110–120°, a straight impactor is introduced into the joint through the anteromedial portal. Under arthroscopic control, the bone block can be gently tapped into the femoral tunnel until the bone block lied flush with the entrance of the femoral bone tunnel. Then, stabil-

ity of the fixation was tested by pulling at the distal holding suture of the graft with maximal manual power.

At the tibia, a small groove is created with a chisel at the distal end of the tunnel. The straight impactor is used to hammer the patellar bone block with the sharp side first into this groove to archive a tibial press-fit fixation. Then, the space between tibial tunnel wall and graft may be filled with autologous bone cylinder gained from tunnel preparation. When drills and dilators were used, a bone substitute made of tricalcium phosphate (Synthricer, Karl Storz) can be used.

24.2.3 Results and Discussion

The technique described in this article is an arthroscopic modification of the press-fit technique described by Hertel et al. [88]. This technique is practiced in the Martin Luther Hospital for more than 20 years. Hertel et al. [88] published 10-year results after mini-open BPTB press-fit fixation. In this retrospective cohort study, there were no reruptures and osteoarthritic changes were only mild. The majority of patient presented with excellent or good results after the follow-up of 10 years after surgery. This mini-open technique is an anatomical technique because the femoral tunnel is drilled via the medial arthrotomy [87]. The surgical principles of this technique have already been published [144]: portal drilling, portal view, and foot print reconstruction. We expect that the same results can be achieved with the arthroscopic technique because this arthroscopic technique is also an anatomical technique [144].

Other authors described also encouraging clinical results after BPTB press-fit fixation ([57, 72, 202]; Boszotta and Anderl 1997). Therefore, we believe that press-fit fixation is a good alternative to interference screw or cross-pin fixation in BPTB ACL reconstruction. Press-fit fixation has several advantages. The technique is cost effective. Other advantages are direct bone-to-bone healing without interfering implants, no graft laceration as seen in interference screw fixation, and no bone resorption, chronic synovitis, or allergic reactions due to resorption of the implant.

24.3 Press-Fit Fixation Using Quadriceps Tendon

Juergen Hoeher and Ralph Akoto

24.3.1 Why Quadriceps Tendon Autograft?

The use of the quadriceps tendon (QT) autograft for ACL reconstruction was first described by Marshall et al. [118]. Other pioneers using the

QT autograft were Blauth, Staeubli, Fulkerson, and others [21, 65, 176]. In the past the QT was less frequently used than other grafts. However, more recently the QT graft has gained interest by many ACL surgeons [49, 188] mostly because of its good biomechanical and biological characteristics [151] and its low donor-side morbidity [130].

Patients involved in high-demand valgus stress sports or martial arts (e.g. judo) (Fig. 24.15) or patients with chronic MCL deficiency may particularly benefit from keeping hamstring function intact as the hamstring reflex has been shown to be an important factor for dynamic knee joint stability [62, 126]. For this group of patients, another advantage for QT could be its lesser donor-side morbidity as compared to a patellar tendon autograft [67, 101].

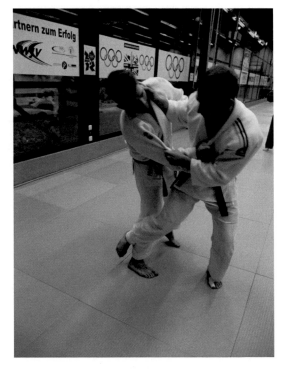

Fig. 24.15 Judo athlete with typical action, resulting in high valgus stress of the knee joint, dynamic hamstring activity is required for stabilization of the knee

24.3.2 Press-Fit Fixation in ACL Surgery

Implant-free press-fit fixation avoiding the use of interference screws has been introduced by several authors in the past using various grafts [23, 88, 138] as it appears to be a more biological approach. Press-fit fixation has been shown to provide good biomechanical fixation strength [46] and good clinical results [57, 88, 138]. Huber developed an implant-free press-fit technique for a quadriceps tendon autograft using a transtibial approach [12]. However, several studies have suggested that the transtibial approach may result in a nonanatomical femoral tunnel placement [15, 105]. We therefore have developed a modification of the Huber technique in our institution using a QT autograft with implant-free press-fit fixation in anteromedial portal technique with good clinical results [4].

24.3.3 What We Need

The equipment needed for ACL reconstruction using QT graft with press-fit fixation is listed in Fig. 24.16.

24.3.4 Surgical Technique

The patient is positioned supine on a standard operating table with a tourniquet at the upper thigh. A roll at the inferior part of the table allows to position the leg in 90° and 120° of knee flexion. A leg holder attached to the table is used to stabilize the thigh on the lateral side (Fig. 24.17a, b).

At surgery a routine diagnostic arthroscopy is performed, and if necessary, meniscus surgery is performed via standard meniscus portals. Then, with the knee flexed to 90°, a low anteromedial portal is placed 1 cm medial to the patellar tendon and close to the superior tibial edge. The orientation of the portal is checked with a spinal needle, and care is taken to reach the femoral footprint of the ACL. This portal is then slightly enlarged to be used as the "working" anteromedial portal (Fig. 24.18).

24.3.4.1 Graft Harvesting

A 4–5 cm longitudinal incision is made from the proximal aspect of the patella extending proximally and centered over the quadriceps tendon. A 50 mm long and 10 mm wide strip of the tendon is excised, while care is taken to leave the suprapatellar pouch of the joint intact (Fig. 24.19a–e). The proximal end of the graft is sutured in "whipstitch-technique" with a high-strength polyethylene suture (Fig. 24.19f, g). The sutured end of the graft is then threaded through the hollow burr, which is attached to an oscillating compression drill (Fig. 24.19h–j). Two-thirds of the circumference of this specific hollow burr has sharp teeth, while the other one-third is blunt (Fig. 24.19k). Using the hollow burr with an inner diameter of 9.4 mm, a cylindrical bone cylinder of 20 mm length will be harvested from the proximal aspect of the patella. Thus, a graft with a total length of 7 cm is created consisting of a 50 mm strip of tendon and a 20 mm cylindrical bone block. Finally, the tendon defect is closed with a running suture.

> **Pitfall**
> When harvesting the bone block of the quadriceps tendon, the hollow burr must be guided parallel to the cortex of the patella. It should be avoided to penetrate the cortical bone with the blunt part of the hollow burr, as it may lead to heat development or the hollow burr may get stuck. The hollow burr should be cooled with water while harvesting the patellar bone block.

Due to the size of the customized burr, the cylindrical bone block has a diameter of exactly 9.4 mm, which may be confirmed using an appropriate graft sizer (Fig. 24.20a).

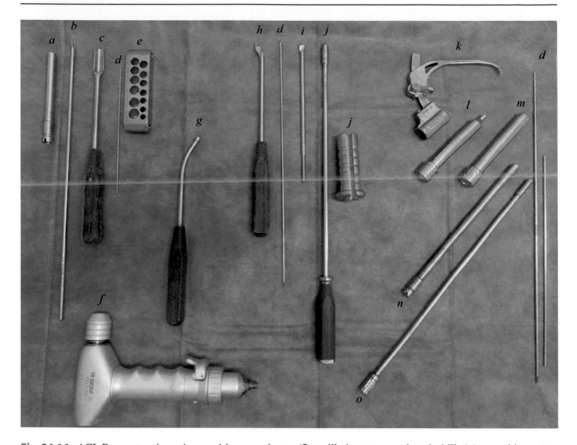

Fig. 24.16 ACL Reconstruction using quadriceps tendon graft and press-fit fixation. Instrumentation required (Richard Wolf, Knittlingen, Germany): (**a**) specific hollow burr (inner diameter 9.4 mm) with two-thirds of the circumference carrying sharp teeth, and one-third of circumference being blunt; (**b**) thread puller; (**c**) bone elevator; (**d**) 1.8 and 2.5 mm K-wires; (**e**) graft sizer template; (**f**) oscillating compression air drill; (**g**) curved impactor; (**h**) femoral offset guide; (**i**) 8 mm cannulated reamer; (**j**) 9 mm compactor and retracting sleeve; (**k**) tibial drill guide (device "Heidelberg"); (**l**) tibial K-wire drill guide; (**m**) tibial hollow burr drill guide; (**n**) hollow burr (outer diameter 9.5 mm) with full circumference carrying sharp teeth; (**o**) strait impactor

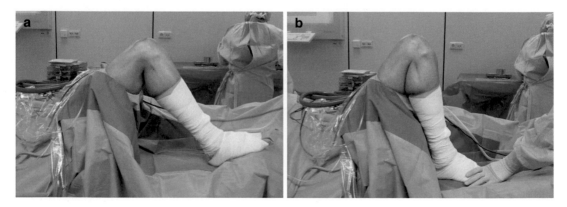

Fig. 24.17 Positioning: The patient is positioned supine using a lateral leg holder, an upper thigh tourniquet, and a leg role at the inferior part of the table that allows to position the leg in (**a**) 90° and (**b**) 120° of knee flexion

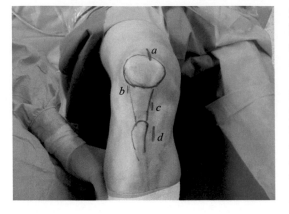

Fig. 24.18 Skin incisions and arthroscopic portals (right knee): (*a*) Incision for quadriceps tendon graft harvesting. (*b*) High anterolateral portal. (*c*) Low anteromedial portal. (*d*) Incision for tibial tunnel preparation

For graft preparation, the bone block is tapered with the ronguer in a fashion that its distal half (1 cm) just fits into a 9.0 mm template (Fig. 24.20b). Then, a 1.6 mm hole is drilled through the bone block and a polyester suture is introduced for later graft passage. Finally, a second high-strength polyethylene suture is whip-stitched to the proximal tendon end (Fig. 24.21).

> **Tips and Pearls**
> The bone block of the graft should not be longer than 20 mm; otherwise it may be difficult to pass the bone block through the joint easily and to direct it into the femoral bone tunnel

24.3.4.2 Tunnel Placement and Preparation

A femoral drill guide with a 7 mm offset hook is introduced through the anteromedial portal at 90° of knee flexion. The offset hook is placed in the over-the-top position and the knee is gently bent to 120° of flexion. After passing a 2.5 mm guide wire through the drill guide into the lateral femoral condyle, an 8.0 mm cannulated reamer is used to create a socket into the femur of

20 mm in length (Fig. 24.22a, b). The femoral bone tunnel is further impacted with a 9.0 mm compactor to a depth of approximately 22 mm (Fig. 24.22c).

For the tibial tunnel, a tibial drill guide is introduced through the anteromedial portal and placed with the alignment hook into the center of the tibial footprint of the ACL. A 2–3 cm longitudinal skin incision is made on the medial aspect of the tibia so that the drill guide can be placed on the anteromedial aspect of the tibia. A 2.5 mm guide wire is then introduced into the joint through the drill guide (Fig. 24.23a). Then, the guide wire is replaced by a drill sleeve, so that a 9.5 mm hollow burr can be used for creating the tibial tunnel (Fig. 24.23b, c). Thus, a cylindrical bone block can be retrieved from the tibial bone (Fig. 24.24a).

> **Pitfall**
> The tibial bone block is usually still connected to the tibial plateau via the tibial ACL remnants. The bone block should be freed with an electric hook before retrieving the hollow burr with the bone block inside out of the tibial tunnel.

A cortical bone bridge of about 1 cm length is created distal to the exit of the tibial tunnel and a suture loop is passed around it for later graft fixation.

24.3.4.3 Preparation of the Bone Plug Retrieved from the Tibia

On the back table, the bone cylinder retrieved from the tibia is divided into three parts. Additionally, the proximal bone plug of about two cm in length is longitudinally split so that it can be used as a wedge for compressing the graft tissue in the bone tunnel. The middle part of the bone plug may be used to fill up the bony defect in the patella, while the distal part will be used to fill up the tibial tunnel distally at the end of surgery (Fig. 24.24b).

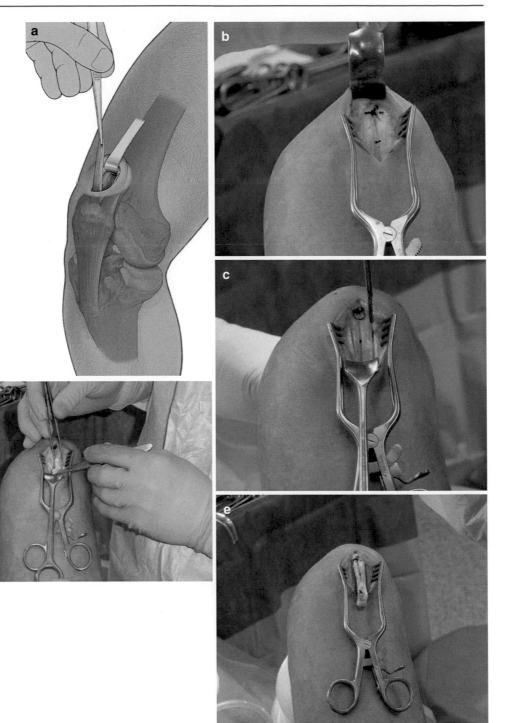

Fig. 24.19 Harvesting the quadriceps tendon graft. (**a–e**) A 50 mm long and 10 mm wide strip of the tendon is excised; care is taken to leave the suprapatellar pouch intact; (**f–g**) Proximal end of graft whipstitched using a high-strength polyethylene suture; (**h–j**) the sutured end of the graft is threaded through a hollow burr, which is attached to an oscillating compression air drill; (**k**) the cutting edge of a 9.4 mm hollow burr for graft harvesting. Two-thirds of the circumference of this specific hollow burr has sharp teeth, while the other one-third is blunt

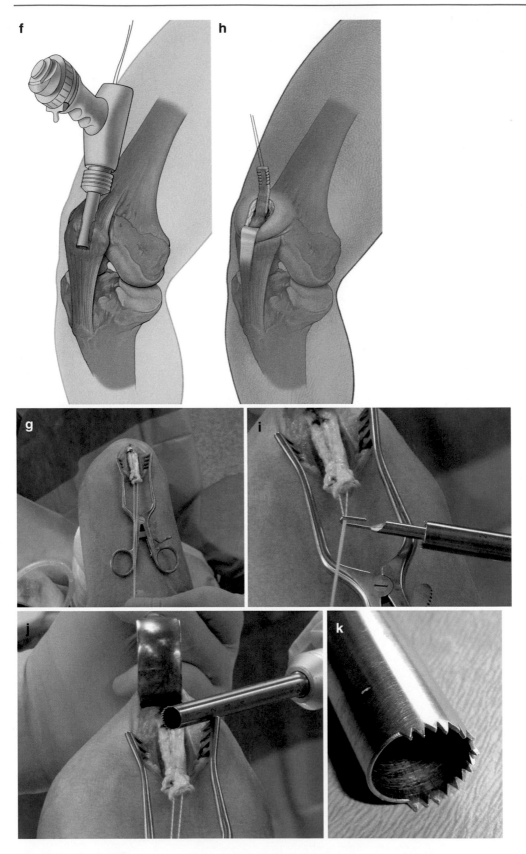

Fig. 24.19 (continued)

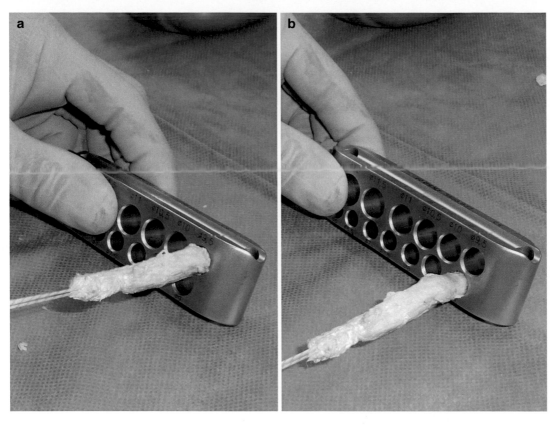

Fig. 24.20 Graft preparation. (**a**) The cylindrical 20 mm bone block with a diameter of 9.4 mm. It is confirmed that the entire bone block can be passed through a 9.5 mm template. (**b**) After bone block preparation using a rongeur, half of the bone block fits easily in a 9.0 mm template. The entire bone block may not pass this template

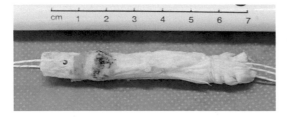

Fig. 24.21 QT graft after preparation: total length 7 cm consisting of a 50 mm tendon strip and a 20 mm cylindrical bone plug being armed with a high-strength polyester sutures

24.3.4.4 Graft Placement and Graft Fixation

With the bone block running first, the graft is introduced through the tibial tunnel into the joint in a common fashion. Thus, the bone block can easily slide into the femoral bone tunnel to half of its length.

> **Tips and Pearls**
> The bone block of the graft should be rotated as such that the tendon insertion is located away from the camera. Then, the probe may be used to better direct the bone block into the right position in the femoral bone tunnel.

Holding tension on the femoral sutures and keeping the knee flexed to 120°, a straight impactor is now introduced into the joint through the anteromedial portal. Under arthroscopic control, the bone block can now gently be tapped into the femoral tunnel until the bone block lies flush with the entrance of the femoral bone tunnel (Fig. 24.25a–c). Bringing the knee towards extension, the graft is pulled distally with the sutures

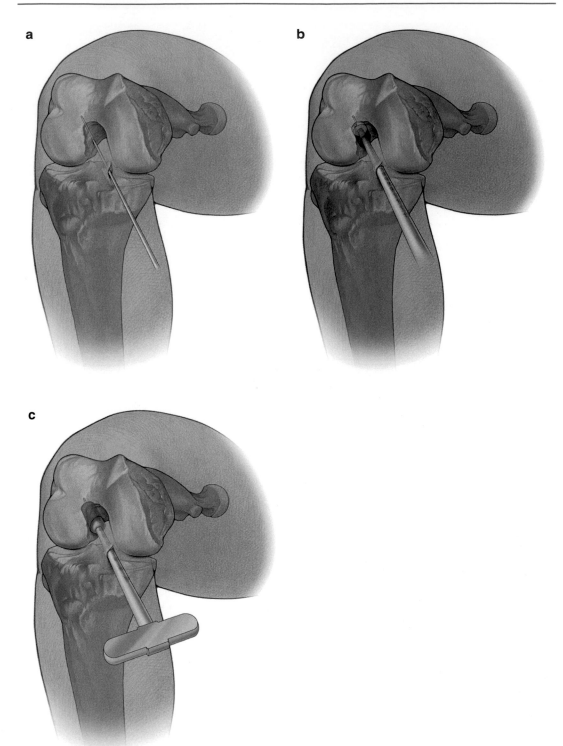

Fig. 24.22 Preparation of the femoral tunnel. (**a**) At 120° of knee flexion a 2.5 mm guide wire is introduced into the lateral femoral condyle through the anteromedial portal. (**b**) An 8.0 mm cannulated reamer is used to create a socket into the femoral ACL footprint of 20 mm in length. (**c**) The femoral tunnel is impacted with 9.0 mm cannulated compactor

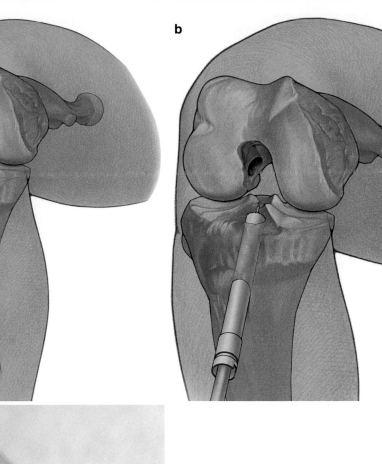

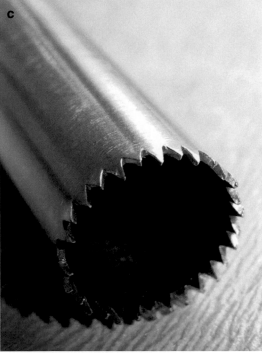

Fig. 24.23 Creating the tibial tunnel. (**a**). The alignment hook of the tibial drill guide is introduced through the anteromedial portal and is placed into the center of the tibial footprint. A 2.5 mm guide wire is introduced into the tibial footprint of the ACL. (**b**) A 9.5 mm hollow burr is drilled over the guide wire, thus harvesting an 8.5 mm cancellous bone plug from the tibial tunnel. (**c**) The cutting edge of a 9.5 mm hollow burr for the tibial tunnel preparation. The entire circumference of this hollow burr has sharp teeth

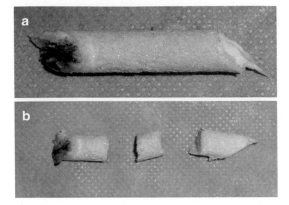

Fig. 24.24 Cylindrical-free bone block retrieved from the tibia with a hollow burr: (**a**) Total cylindrical bone block. (**b**) The tibial bone cylinder divided into three parts: the proximal bone plug of about two cm is used as a wedge for compressing the graft tissue in the bone tunnel. The middle part of the bone plug may be used to fill up the bony defect in the patella, while the distal part will be used to fill up the tibial tunnel distally at the end of surgery

exiting the tibial tunnel to ensure press-fit fixation and absolute stability of the bone block on the femoral side. After moving the knee through the range of motion, half of the exiting sutures distally are passed through the additional cortical hole so that sutures can sequentially be tied over the bone bridge at about 30° of knee flexion. Then, the shimmed, split bone plug can be introduced onto the anterior aspect of the tendon tissue in the tibial tunnel. Now, it can gently be tapped proximally alongside the graft tissue up to the joint line, thus providing compression of the graft against the tibial bone tunnel wall (Fig. 24.26a–c). The distal bone plug retrieved from the tibia is used to fill up the distal part of the tibial tunnel (Fig. 24.26d). Any remaining bone material is used to fill up the bony defect in the patella. Subsequentially, the wounds are closed in a common fashion.

We recommend a standardized rehabilitation protocol with partial weight bearing for 3 weeks. A CT scan 3 months after surgery is suitable to evaluate the amount of bone loss and the tunnel healing quality (Fig. 24.27). We have used this technique in more than 100 patients over the past 2 years. Clinical studies to compare this surgical technique to standardized techniques using hamstring tendons are under way and will be important to further define the benefit of this surgical approach.

Memory

The quadriceps tendon (QT) autograft as a substitute for a ruptured ACL has gained popularity in recent years because of its good biomechanical properties and its low donor-side morbidity. Among various surgical techniques, the use of an implant-free press-fit fixation technique has shown good biomechanical and clinical results. This chapter describes an arthroscopic ACL reconstruction technique with a quadriceps tendon autograft using press-fit fixation and an anteromedial portal technique. A 5 cm quadriceps tendon graft is harvested with an adjacent 2 cm bone block. The femoral tunnel is created through a low anteromedial portal in its anatomical position. The tibial tunnel is created with a hollow burr, thus acquiring a free cylindrical bone block. The graft is then passed through the tibial tunnel, and the bone block, customized at its tip, is tapped into the femoral tunnel through the anteromedial portal to provide press-fit fixation. The graft is tensioned distally and sutures are tied over a bone bridge at the distal end of the tibial tunnel. From the cylindrical bone block harvested from the tibia, the proximal end is customized and gently tapped next to the graft tissue into the tibial tunnel to assure press fitting of the graft in the tibial tunnel. The distal part of the tibial tunnel is filled up with the remaining bone.

This technique may be an alternative particularly for patients who benefit from preserving hamstring function as an active valgus stabilizer, like high-demand valgus stress sports (martial arts, judo, etc.) or in chronic medial collateral ligament (MCL) insufficiency.

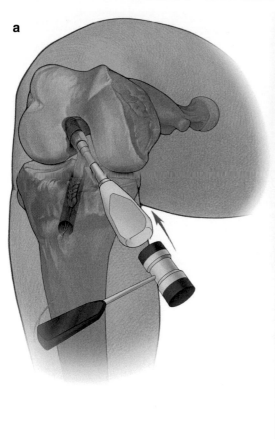

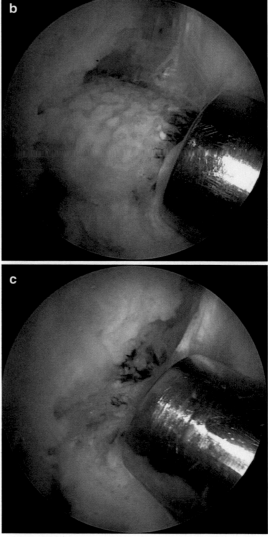

Fig. 24.25 Femoral graft fixation. (**a**) With the knee flexed to 120°, the cylindrical bone plug of the QT graft is pulled into the femoral tunnel to about 1 cm of length of the bone block. Using an impactor introduced through the anteromedial portal, the bone block is gently tapped into the femoral tunnel until the bone lock is flush with the femoral cortex; (**b**) Arthroscopic view: The cylindrical bone plug of the QT stuck halfway in the femoral tunnel is gently tapped into the bone tunnel using a straight impactor placed to the end of the bone block to achieve press-fit fixation; (**c**) Arthroscopic view: After tapping the cylindrical bone plug in the femoral tunnel, it is flush with the tunnel entrance and press-fit fixation is achieved

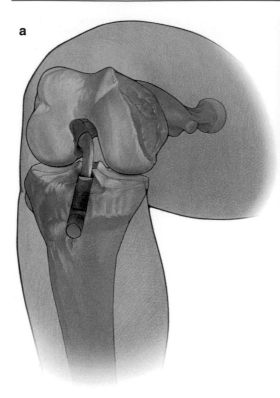

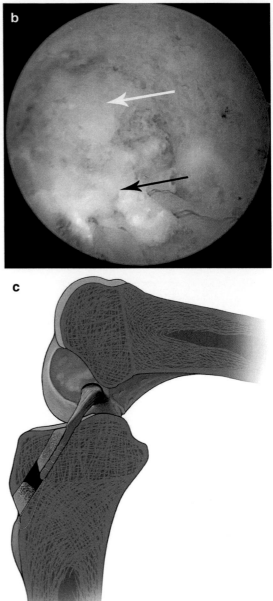

Fig. 24.26 Tibial graft fixation. (**a**) Using a shaped bone wedge harvested from the tibia, the graft is compressed against the bone tunnel wall close to the joint line, additionally the graft is secured with sutures tied over a bone bridge; (**b**) arthroscopic "tunnel" view: the graft (*black arrow*) and the shaped bone wedge (*white arrow*). (**c**) The remaining part of the harvested bone plug is stuffed into the tibial tunnel like a cork to close the bone tunnel distally

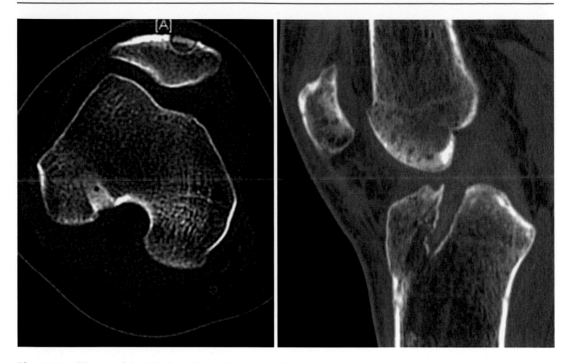

Fig. 24.27 CT scan of the right knee 3-month postoperatively

24.4   Hamstring Press-Fit Fixation Without Hardware

Hans H. Paessler and Rainer Siebold

24.4.1 Introduction

A variety of fixation devices are used for anterior cruciate ligament reconstruction (ACL) with hamstring tendon grafts. These devices increase costs and can present artifacts in magnetic resonance imaging as well as complications in revision surgery.

The technique uses press-fit fixation of hamstring grafts closes to the anatomical ACL insertion, thus eliminating both the bungee and windshield-wiper effects and the need for any implant. Basically, the semitendinosus and the gracilis tendon are formed to a loop by knotting both ends together to a simple knot, which is secured by nonabsorbable sutures. A bottle neck-like tunnel is created on the femoral side,

in which the knot of the tendon loop is firmly secured just proximal the cortical thickness of the notch wall to the anatomical insertion (Fig. 24.28).

24.4.2 Surgical Technique

24.4.2.1 Graft Preparation

The semitendinosus and gracilis tendons are harvested from the pes anserinus in a standard fashion and cleaned from soft tissue. On the workstation the ends of each tendon are tied together by a simple knot. The knots are maximally tightened under cyclic manual load and secured with 4 diverging U-shaped Ethibond 2 sutures (Fig. 24.29). One end of the graft now has a tendon knot and the other a tendon loop. With the help of a Mersilene tape (or similar), the tendon loops are pulled one after the other through a measuring template in 0.5 mm steps in order to find the smallest diameter of both loops. The diameter of the knots should be 4 mm more than

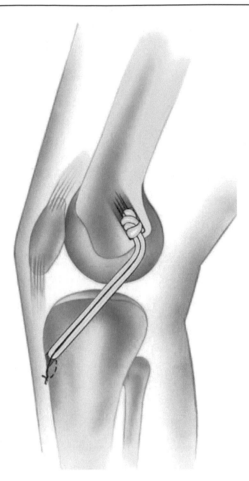

Fig. 24.28 Anterior cruciate ligament reconstruction using hamstrings in press-fit technique without hardware

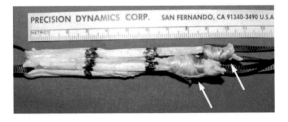

Fig. 24.29 The ends of the thus prepared tendons are tied together to a knot to form a closed loop (the length of the semitendinosus loop being about 7.5 cm without the knot and that of the gracilis loop being 8.5 cm)

the diameter of the loops in order to prevent later knot slipping.

The lengths of the loops should be a total of 75 mm for the semitendinosus tendon and 85 mm for the gracilis tendon. This includes about

5–6 mm in the femoral cortical bone tunnel (plus 1 cm of tendon knot), about 30 mm intra-articular graft length and a length of the tibial tunnel at 45° of about 40 mm. The gracilis loop must be longer because the knot of the gracilis tendon will later be positioned proximal to the semitendinosus knot on the femoral side. Two tapes are pulled through each of the ST and GT loop, one proximal at the knot, the other at the end of the loop. To distinguish between the ST and GT loop, the two tapes are used in 2 colors. The semitendinosus graft will be first pulled into the femoral tunnel from proximal to distal followed by the thinner gracilis graft.

Finally, the intra-articular portion of the graft is marked. A second mark is made 3 cm beyond the first mark. This mark should be seen at the intra-articular entrance of the tibial tunnel, when both grafts are inserted completely into the tunnels. Each loop is held by a separate tape. The lengths of the loops and the diameters of their knots are measured with a precision of up to 0.5 mm.

24.4.2.2 Femoral Tunnel

Under arthroscopic visualization, interfering ACL remnants are removed with a shaver, and a careful notchplasty is performed if it is necessary to enlarge the notch roof, especially in case of osteophytes. Next, the femoral tunnel is prepared. The C-arm was initially positioned at the upper end of the table. It is now moved to the joint for positioning of the tip of the K-wire. The tip of a K-wire is inserted into the cortex to a depth of 1–2 mm at the anatomical center of the original ACL insertion, just in between the center of the anteromedial and posterolateral fibers.

The ideal position of the tip is on an imaginary line continuing from the posterior cortex of the femur distal, about 5–7 mm inferior to Blumensaat's line (Fig. 24.30). A hard copy of this fluoroscopic image is added to the patient's chart, to complement the set of arthroscopic images. Its correct position may be measured using the method of Bernard and Hertel.

The knee is then flexed to 120° and the K-wire is advanced through the lateral condyle.

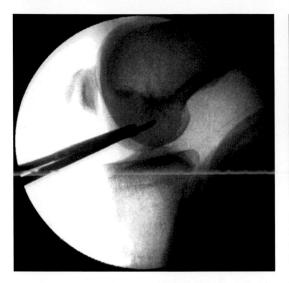

Fig. 24.30 A 4 mm offset femoral drill guide is applied via the medial portal. Femoral C-arm control of position of K-wire tip

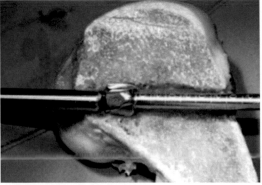

Fig. 24.31 An impactor with a diameter corresponding to the one of the drill is inserted 12 mm deep into the femoral tunnel. A K-wire is inserted through the impactor, perforating the skin at the lateral thigh. A skin incision of 12–15 mm is made at the point where the K-wire perforates it. Using a cannulated drill, a tunnel is drilled along the K-wire. The diameter of the drill corresponds to the diameter of the tendon knot

Using a cannulated drill, a tunnel, as thick as the loops (7.0–9.0 mm), is drilled all the way through the femur. A cannulated compactor with a diameter of 7.0 mm is introduced into the femoral tunnel from the joint to a depth of 10 mm with the 10 mm long-stepped leading nose. It serves as a stop for the subsequent drilling operation from outside-in (Fig. 24.31).

The K-wire is advanced to the level of the skin on the lateral thigh. A 12 mm incision is made over the pointing wire tip, and the underlying fascia is split longitudinally.

The K-wire is advanced and overdrilled down to the compactor with a drill bit of 11 mm, matching the knot diameter of the semitendinosus graft, using the compactor as a drill centering aid (Fig. 24.31). Next, the drill is replaced by the stepped compactor, which is driven in, under arthroscopic vision, until its graduated 10 mm long-stepped leading nose is seen in the tunnel entrance into the notch. In this process, the remaining cancellous bone is compacted against the cortex. This manifests itself in a change to a higher pitch of the blows driving in the compactor. This results in the tunnel having a 4 mm step (bottleneck principle).

The edge of the femoral tunnel is contoured. A Mersilene tape holding suture is passed through the joint with the aid of a K-wire. If there are any doubts about a possible posterior blow out, the arthroscope may be inserted through the lateral side into the tunnel to visualize the posterior wall.

24.4.2.3 Tibial Tunnel

The knee is flexed to 90°, and preparation of the tibial tunnel is performed. The tibial tunnel is predrilled with a K-wire using a drill guide. Positioning is halfway between the medial tibial tubercle and the anterior inner border of the lateral meniscus.

The tibial drill guide is inserted with the knee in 90° degree of flexion. A 2.5 mm drill bit is then inserted. Its position is again confirmed by C-arm imaging. An impingement probe is mounted over the 2.5 mm drill bit. The knee is placed in full extension. On the X-ray image on the C-arm monitor, the impingement probe should have 2 mm of clearance to the notch roof (Fig. 24.32). After confirmation of correct placement of the 2.5 mm drill bit, the tibial cortex is pierced with a 6.5 mm or a 7 mm reamer (depending on the diameter of the semitendinosus plus gracilis tendon loop). This is followed by compaction drilling with a dilator of the same diameter, to compact the cancellous bone surrounding the

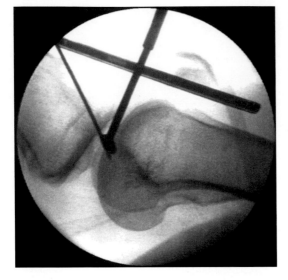

Fig. 24.32 Lateral fluoroscopy view of the tibial impingement probe. The knee is in hyperextension

tibial tunnel. The cortex of the tibial plateau is drilled under arthroscopic visualization. Any tissue remnants anterior to the tunnel mouth are removed to prevent formation of a cyclops lesion postoperatively.

24.4.2.4 Graft Implantation
The Mersilene tapes on the two grafts are pulled in from femoral to tibial in an outside-in fashion. The gracilis loop with the thinner knot follows after the semitendinosus loop. The two loops are firmly pulled. A sudden jerk indicates that the semitendinosus and the gracilis tendon knot have reached the step in the tunnel – the bottleneck. The knee is taken through its range of motion, to ensure that there is no impingement. A probe is then passed into the tibial tunnel to reconfirm the graft's position. The knee is fully flexed. With both hands, maximum traction is applied to both loops, and the knee is taken through a full range of motion at least 20 times. This allows the knots to snug themselves down.

24.4.2.5 Distal Graft Fixation
For tibial fixation, a 4.5 mm drill bit is used to pierce the cortex 1 cm distal to the tibial tunnel exit. A curved forceps is passed through the underlying cancellous bone, from distal to

proximal and from proximal to distal to fashion a bony bridge. A passer is used to pull a traction suture below the bone bridge. This suture is placed through one end of each Mersilene tape, to railroad the tapes through the bone bridge, in a distal direction.

With the knee flexed to about 10°, maximum traction is exerted on the Mersilene tapes, and the ends of the semitendinosus tape are first tied with a simple knot. Then, the knee is brought into full extension and the second knot is tight, followed by 3 knots. Stability is confirmed manually and then the tapes of the gracilis loop are tied in the same way (Fig. 24.33).

24.4.3 Biomechanical Testing

In cooperation with Weiler and Kandziora, Unfallchirurgische Klinik, Charité, Berlin (Director: Prof. Dr. Haas), biomechanical pull out tests on pig knees have shown that under cyclic loading (100×300 N, 100×400 N, 100×500 N, 100×600 N, and 100×700 N) the bottleneck technique demonstrated to be twofolds stronger than the "gold standard" BTB fixed with interference screws.

In a further experimental study, Kilger et al. [100] tested eight fresh-frozen cadaveric knees (52 ± 7 years) using a robotic/universal force-moment sensor testing system. The knee kinematics of the intact, ACL-deficient, EndoButton-reconstructed, and knot/press-fit-reconstructed knee in response to both a 134-N anterior tibial load and a combined rotatory load at multiple knee flexion angles was determined. Differences between the four knee states were evaluated with a 2-factor repeated-measures analysis of variance ($P < .05$). Results: In response to an anterior tibial load, the anterior tibial translation for the knot/press-fit reconstruction was found to be not significantly different from that of the intact ACL as well as that of the EndoButton reconstruction ($P > .05$). In response to a combined rotatory load, neither reconstruction procedure could effectively reduce the coupled anterior tibial translation to that of the intact knee and no significant difference between the two

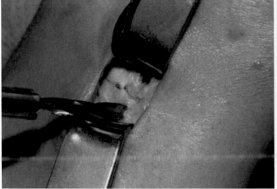 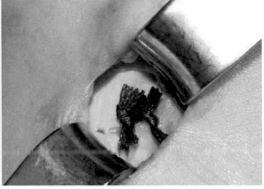

Fig. 24.33 A 1 cm distally to the tibial end of the tunnel a drill hole of 4.5 mm is made and a bone bridge is created by under-tunneling it with a curved clip. The first strips of the Mersilene tapes are pulled through the help of a Deschamp and tied to the second strips after repeated maximal loading. This is done with the knee close to full extension (5–10°)

reconstructions could be detected ($P > .05$). The stiffness of the knot/press-fit complex was found to be 37.8 ± 9.6 N/mm, and the load at failure was 540 ± 97.7 N, which is equal to other devices published in the literature. The authors concluded that the knot/press-fit technique restores knee kinematics as well as the EndoButton CL fixation and has similar biomechanical properties as other devices published in the literature.

Jagodzinski et al. [93] recently published a study on tibial press-fit fixation for ACL reconstruction. The authors used hamstring tendons of 21 human cadavers (age: 41.9 ± 13.1 years). A press-fit fixation with looped semitendinosus and gracilis tendons secured by a tape (T) over a bone bridge, or by a baseball-stitched suture (S), was compared with degradable interference screw fixation (I) in 21 porcine tibiae. The constructs were cyclically strained and subsequently loaded to failure. The maximum load to failure, stiffness, and elongation during cyclical loading were measured. The maximum load to failure was highest for the T-fixation at 970 ± 83 N, followed by the I-fixation with 544 ± 109 N, and the S-fixation with 402 ± 78 N ($P < 0.03$). Stiffness of the constructs averaged 78 ± 13 N/mm for T, 108 ± 18 N/mm for S, and 162 ± 27 N/mm for I ($P < 0.03$). Elongation during initial cyclical loading was 2.0 ± 0.6 mm for T, 3.3 ± 1.1 mm for S, and 1.4 ± 0.5 mm for I (S inferior to I and T, $P < 0.05$). Elongation between the 20th and 1,500th loading cycle was lower for T (2.2 ± 0.7 mm) compared

with I (4.1 ± 2.7 mm) and S (4.8 ± 0.7 mm; $P < 0.001$). The T-fixation technique exhibited a significantly higher failure load than the S- and I-techniques. All techniques exhibited larger elongation during initial cyclical loading than is reported in the literature for grafts with bone blocks. Only one technique (T) showed satisfactory elongation behavior during long-term cyclic loading. Interference screw fixation demonstrated significantly higher stiffness. The authors concluded that only the tape fixation technique seemed to exhibit adequate mechanical properties necessary for early aggressive rehabilitation programs.

24.4.4 Prospective and Randomized Study

In an own clinical study, ACL reconstruction with hamstrings was compared to ACL reconstruction with BTB. Sixty-two ACL-insufficient patients (31 BPT and 31 HT) were included. Surgical procedures were performed without any implants using an anteromedial portal- and a press-fit technique by the senior author as described above for the hamstrings. At 8.8 years after reconstruction, 53 patients (28 BPT and 25 HT) were examined by different clinical and functional tests, and bilateral MRI scans were performed. Results: The ICKD was significantly better in the HT group. The clinical examination including range of motion, KT-1000 test (MEDmetric, San Diego, CA), and pivot-shift test showed no significant differences. On isokinetic testing, the mean quadriceps strength was close to normal (96 %) in both groups, but the hamstring strength was lower in the HT group (100.3 %/95.1 %). Kneeling (1.5/1.1, P _ .002), knee walking (1.72/1.14, P _ .002), and single-leg hop test (95.8 %/99.1 %, P _ .057) were better in the HT group. The MRI findings about the mean degree of cartilage lesion (ICRS) of the operated (2.1/2.1) and nonoperated (1.4/1.8) knee showed no significant differences. No significant difference was found in the grade of medial or lateral meniscal lesion or the number of patients having meniscal lesions when the operated and nonoperated knees were compared. Tunnel measurements, Caton Index, and the sagittal ACL angle were similar.

The authors concluded that the implant-free press-fit technique for ACL reconstruction is a reliable technique to preserve the cartilage and meniscal status without significant differences between the operated and nonoperated knees in the long term. Significantly, less anterior knee pain was noted in the hamstring group, when testing for kneeling and knee walking [203].

Memory

The advantages of above technique are (Fig. 24.28):

1. The knot is close to the anatomical site of the proximal insertion of the ACL preventing the "bungee effect."
2. The intensive contact between the bony wall of the tunnel and graft collagen along a long distance may accelerate graft incorporation.
3. Broad-based contact under pressure between the graft and the bone (as opposed to suspending fixation from the lateral cortical bone).
4. No implants are utilized for fixation which prevents hardware discomfort and eventually surgical removal, facilitates revision surgery, avoids metal artifacts on MRI and lowers overall costs.

References

1. Aga C, Rasmussen MT, Smith SD et al (2013) Biomechanical comparison of interference screws and combination screw and sheath devices for soft tissue anterior cruciate ligament reconstruction on the tibial side. Am J Sports Med 41:841–848
2. Agarwal CM, Athanasiou KA (1997) Technique to control pH in vicinity of biodegrading PLA-PGA implants. J Biomed Mater Res 38:105–114
3. Ahmad CS, Gardner TR, Groh M et al (2004) Mechanical properties of soft tissue femoral fixation devices for anterior cruciate ligament reconstruction. Am J Sports Med 32:635–640
4. Akoto R, Hoeher J (2012) Anterior cruciate ligament (ACL) reconstruction with quadriceps tendon autograft and press-fit fixation using an anteromedial portal technique. BMC Musculoskelet Disord 13:161. doi:10.1186/1471-2474-13-161
5. Almazan A, Herrera JP, Chaidez C et al (2009) A complication of soft tissue graft tibial fixation with the IntraFix device. Med Sci Monit 15:CS19–CS21
6. Apostolopoulos A, Nikolopoulos D, Polyzois I et al (2012) Pretibial cyst formation after anterior cruciate ligament reconstruction with poly-L acid screw fixation: a case report presentation and review of the literature. J Surg Orthop Adv 21:151–156
7. Aune AK, Ekeland A, Cawley PW (1998) Interference screw fixation of hamstring versus patellar tendon graft for anterior cruciate ligament reconstruction. Knee Surg Sports Traumatol Arthrosc 6:99–102
8. Barber FA, Dockery WD (2008) Long-term absorption of beta-tricalcium phosphate poly-L-lactic acid interference screws. Arthroscopy 24:441–447
9. Barber FA, Elrod BF, McGuire DA et al (1995) Preliminary results of an absorbable interference screw. Arthroscopy 11:537–548
10. Barber FA, Dockery WD, Hrnack SA (2011) Long-term degradation of a poly-lactide co-glycolide/β--tricalcium phosphate biocomposite interference screw. Arthroscopy 27:637–643
11. Barfod G, Svendsen RN (1992) Synovitis of the knee after intra-articular fracture fixation with Biofix. Acta Orthop Scand 63:680–681
12. Barie A, Kargus S, Huber J, Schmitt H, Streich NA (2010) Anterior cruciate ligament reconstruction using quadriceps tendon autograft and press-fit fixation. Unfallchirurg 113(8):629–634. doi:10.1007/s00113-010-1854-0
13. Basad E, Kipper A, Wüsten OA et al (2010) Comparative study after hamstring ACL plasty with RigidFix (pin fixation) and EndoButton (anchor fixation). Z Orthop Unfall 148:276–281
14. Baumfeld JA, Diduch DR, Rubino LJ et al (2008) Tunnel widening following anterior cruciate ligament reconstruction using hamstring autograft: a comparison between double cross-pin and suspensory graft fixation. Knee Surg Sports Traumatol Arthrosc 16:1108–1113

15. Bedi A, Musahl V, Steuber V, Kendoff D, Choi D, Allen AA, Pearle AD, Altchek DW (2011) Transtibial versus anteromedial portal reaming in anterior cruciate ligament reconstruction: an anatomic and biomechanical evaluation of surgical technique. Arthroscopy 27(3):380–390. doi:10.1016/j.arthro.2010.07.018

16. Bellisari GE, Kaeding CC, Litsky AS (2010) Mechanical evaluation of cross pins used for femoral fixation of hamstring grafts in ACL reconstructions. Orthopedics 33:722

17. Benedetto KP, Fellinger M, Lim TE et al (2000) A new bioabsorbable interference screw: preliminary results of a prospective, multicenter, randomized clinical trial. Arthroscopy 16:41–48

18. Bernstein A, Tecklenburg K, Südkamp P et al (2012) Adhesion and proliferation of human osteoblast-like cells on different biodegradable implant materials used for graft fixation in ACL-reconstruction. Arch Orthop Trauma Surg 132:1637–1645

19. Beynnon BD, Amis AA (1998) In vitro testing protocols for the cruciate ligaments and ligament reconstructions. Knee Surg Sports Traumatol Arthrosc 6:S70–S76

20. Black KP, Saunders MM, Stube KC et al (2000) Effects of interference fit screw length on tibial tunnel fixation for anterior cruciate ligament reconstruction. Am J Sports Med 28:846–849

21. Blauth W (1984) 2-strip substitution-plasty of the anterior cruciate ligament with the quadriceps tendon. Unfallheilkunde 87(2):45–51

22. Böstman O, Pihlajamäki H (2000) Adverse tissue reactions to bioabsorbable fixation devices. Clin Orthop Relat Res 371:216–227

23. Boszotta H (1997) Arthroscopic anterior cruciate ligament reconstruction using a patellar tendon graft in press-fit technique: surgical technique and follow-up. Arthroscopy 13:332–339

24. Bottoni CR, DeBerardino TM, Fester EW et al (2000) An intra-articular bioabsorbable interference screw mimicking an acute meniscal tear 8 months after an anterior cruciate ligament reconstruction. Arthroscopy 16:395–398

25. Brand J Jr, Weiler A, Caborn DN et al (2000) Graft fixation in cruciate ligament reconstruction. Am J Sports Med 28:761–774

26. Brand JC Jr, Pienkowski D, Steenlage E et al (2000) Interference screw fixation strength of a quadrupled hamstring tendon graft is directly related to bone mineral density and insertion torque. Am J Sports Med 28(5):705–710

27. Brodie JT, Torpey BM, Donald GD 3rd et al (1996) Femoral interference screw placement through the tibial tunnel: a radiographic evaluation of interference screw divergence angles after endoscopic anterior cruciate ligament reconstruction. Arthroscopy 12:435–440

28. Brown CH Jr, Hecker AT, Hipp JA et al (1993) The biomechanics of interference screw fixation of patellar tendon anterior cruciate ligament grafts. Am J Sports Med 21:880–886

29. Brown GA, Peña F, Grøntvedt T et al (1996) Fixation strength of interference screw fixation in bovine, young human, and elderly human cadaver knees: influence of insertion torque, tunnel-bone block gap, and interference. Knee Surg Sports Traumatol Arthrosc 3:238–244

30. Brown CH Jr, Wilson DR, Hecker AT et al (2004) Graft–bone motion and tensile properties of hamstring and patellar tendon anterior cruciate ligament femoral graft fixation under cyclic loading. Arthroscopy 20:922–935

31. Bryan JM, Bach BR Jr, Bush-Joseph CA et al (1996) Comparison of "inside-out" and "outside-in" interference screw fixation for anterior cruciate ligament surgery in a bovine knee. Arthroscopy 12:76–81

32. Butler JC, Branch TP, Hutton WC (1994) Optimal graft fixation – the effect of gap size and screw size on bone plug fixation in ACL reconstruction. Arthroscopy 10:524–529

33. Caborn DN, Urban WP Jr, Johnson DL et al (1997) Biomechanical comparison between BioScrew and titanium alloy interference screws for bone-patellar tendon-bone graft fixation in anterior cruciate ligament reconstruction. Arthroscopy 13:229–232

34. Caborn DN, Coen M, Neef R et al (1998) Quadrupled semitendinosus-gracilis autograft fixation in the femoral tunnel: a comparison between a metal and a bioabsorbable interference screw. Arthroscopy 14:241–245

35. Caborn DN, Brand JC Jr, Nyland J et al (2004) A biomechanical comparison of initial soft tissue tibial fixation devices: the Intrafix versus a tapered 35-mm bioabsorbable interference screw. Am J Sports Med 32:956–961

36. Camillieri G, McFarland EG, Jasper LE et al (2004) A biomechanical evaluation of transcondylar femoral fixation of anterior cruciate ligament grafts. Am J Sports Med 32:950–955

37. Cassim A, Lobenhoffer P, Gerich T, Tscherne H (1993) The fixation strength of the interference screw in anterior cruciate ligament replacement as a function of technique and experimental setup. Trans Ortho Res Soc 18:31

38. Chan YS, Wang CJ (2006) Femoral interference screw placement through the tibial tunnel: a novel method without graft damage. Arthroscopy 22:1251.e1–1251.e4

39. Chan YS, Lo YP, Lien LC et al (2009) Improved divergence angles with femoral interference screw placement through the tibial tunnel as measured by multiplanar reconstruction computed tomography. Arthroscopy 25:54–61

40. Chen NC, Brown CH (2008) Biomechanics of intra-tunnel anterior cruciate ligament graft fixation. In: Prodromos CC (ed) The anterior cruciate ligament. Reconstruction and basic science, 1st edn. Elsevier, Philadelphia

41. Cheung P, Chan WL, Yen CH et al (2010) Femoral tunnel widening after quadruped hamstring anterior cruciate ligament reconstruction. J Orthop Surg 18:198–202

42. Choi NH, Lee JH, Son KM et al (2010) Tibial tunnel widening after anterior cruciate ligament reconstructions with hamstring tendons using Rigidfix femoral fixation and Intrafix tibial fixation. Knee Surg Sports Traumatol Arthrosc 18:92–97

43. Colvin A, Sharma C, Parides M et al (2011) What is the best femoral fixation of hamstring autografts in anterior cruciate ligament reconstruction?: a meta-analysis. Clin Orthop Relat Res 469:1075–1081

44. Conner CS, Perez BA, Morris RP et al (2010) Three femoral fixation devices for anterior cruciate ligament reconstruction: comparison of fixation on the lateral cortex versus the anterior cortex. Arthroscopy 26:796–807

45. Corsetti JR, Jackson DW (1996) Failure of anterior cruciate ligament reconstruction: the biologic basis. Clin Orthop Relat Res 325:42–49

46. Dargel J, Schmidt-Wiethoff R, Schneider T, Bruggemann GP, Koebke J (2006) Biomechanical testing of quadriceps tendon-patellar bone grafts: an alternative graft source for press-fit anterior cruciate ligament reconstruction? Arch Orthop Trauma Surg 126(4):265–270. doi:10.1007/s00402-005-0048-7

47. Dargel J, Schmidt-Wiethoff R, Brüggemann GP et al (2007) The effect of bone tunnel dilation versus extraction drilling on the initial fixation strength of press-fit anterior cruciate ligament reconstruction. Arch Orthop Trauma Surg 127:801–807

48. Dave LY, Leong OK, Karim SA, Chong CH (2014) Tunnel enlargement 5 years after anterior cruciate ligament reconstruction: a radiographic and functional evaluation. Eur J Orthop Surg Traumatol 24:217–223

49. DeAngelis JP, Fulkerson JP (2007) Quadriceps tendon – a reliable alternative for reconstruction of the anterior cruciate ligament. Clin Sports Med 26(4):587–596. doi:10.1016/j.csm.2007.06.005

50. Drogset JO, Grontvedt T, Tegnander A (2005) Endoscopic reconstruction of the anterior cruciate ligament using bone-patellar tendon-bone grafts fixed with bioabsorbable or metal interference screws: a prospective randomized study of the clinical outcome. Am J Sports Med 33:1160–1165

51. Drogset JO, Straume LG, Bjørkmo I et al (2011) A prospective randomized study of ACL-reconstructions using bone-patellar tendon-bone grafts fixed with bioabsorbable or metal interference screws. Knee Surg Sports Traumatol Arthrosc 19:753–759

52. Duffee AR, Brunelli JA, Nyland J et al (2007) Bioabsorbable screw divergence angle, not tunnel preparation method influences soft tissue tendon graft-bone tunnel fixation in healthy bone. Knee Surg Sports Traumatol Arthrosc 15:17–25

53. Dunkin BS, Nyland J, Duffee AR et al (2007) Soft tissue tendon graft fixation in serially dilated or extraction-drilled tibial tunnels: a porcine model study using high-resolution quantitative computerized tomography. Am J Sports Med 35:448–457

54. Efe T, Bauer J, Herdrich S et al (2010) Comparison between bovine bone and titanium interference screws for implant fixation in ACL reconstruction: a biomechanical study. Arch Orthop Trauma Surg 130:993–999

55. Emond CE, Woelber EB, Kurd SK (2011) A comparison of the results of anterior cruciate ligament reconstruction using bioabsorbable versus metal interference screws: a meta-analysis. J Bone Joint Surg Am 93:572–580

56. Fabbriciani C, Mulas PD, Ziranu F et al (2005) Mechanical analysis of fixation methods for anterior cruciate ligament reconstruction with hamstring tendon graft. An experimental study in sheep knees. Knee 12:135–138

57. Felmet G (2010) Implant-free press-fit fixation for bone-patellar tendon-bone ACL reconstruction: 10-year results. Arch Orthop Trauma Surg 130(8):985–992. doi:10.1007/s00402-010-1050-2

58. Fernandes TL, Protta TR, Fregni F et al (2012) Isokinetic muscle strength and knee function associated with double femoral pin fixation and fixation with interference screw in anterior cruciate ligament reconstruction. Knee Surg Sports Traumatol Arthrosc 20:275–280

59. Fineberg MS, Zarins B, Sherman OH (2000) Practical considerations in anterior cruciate ligament replacement surgery. Arthroscopy 16:715–724

60. Fink C, Benedetto KP, Hackl W et al (2000) Bioabsorbable polyglyconate interference screw fixation in anterior cruciate ligament reconstruction: a prospective computed tomography-controlled study. Arthroscopy 16:491–498

61. Flanigan DC, Kanneganti P, Quinn DP et al (2011) Comparison of ACL fixation devices using cadaveric grafts. J Knee Surg 24:175–180

62. Friemert B, Franke S, Gollhofer A, Claes L, Faist M (2010) Group I afferent pathway contributes to functional knee stability. J Neurophysiol 103(2):616–622. doi:10.1152/jn.00172.2009

63. Fu FH, Bennett CH, Lattermann C et al (1999) Current trends in anterior cruciate ligament reconstruction. Part I: biology and biomechanics of reconstruction. Am J Sports Med 27:821–830

64. Fu FH, Bennett CH, Ma CB, Menetrey J et al (2000) Current trends in anterior cruciate ligament reconstruction. Part II. Operative procedures and clinical correlations. Am J Sports Med 28:124–130

65. Fulkerson JP, Langeland R (1995) An alternative cruciate reconstruction graft: the central quadriceps tendon. Arthroscopy 11(2):252–254

66. Gaweda K, Walawski J, Węgłowski R et al (2009) Comparison of bioabsorbable interference screws and posts for distal fixation in anterior cruciate ligament reconstruction. Int Orthop 33:123–127

67. Geib TM, Shelton WR, Phelps RA, Clark L (2009) Anterior cruciate ligament reconstruction using

quadriceps tendon autograft: intermediate-term outcome. Arthroscopy 25(12):1408–1414. doi:10.1016/j.arthro.2009.06.004

68. Gelber PE, Reina F, Torres R (2010) Effect of femoral tunnel length on the safety of anterior cruciate ligament graft fixation using cross-pin technique: a cadaveric study. Am J Sports Med 38:1877–1884

69. Gerich TG, Cassim A, Lattermann C et al (1997) Pullout strength of tibial graft fixation in anterior cruciate ligament replacement with a patellar tendon graft: interference screw versus staple fixation in human knees. Knee Surg Sports Traumatol Arthrosc 5:84–88

70. Ghazikhanian V, Beltran J, Nikac V et al (2012) Tibial tunnel and pretibial cysts following ACL graft reconstruction: MR imaging diagnosis. Skeletal Radiol 41:1375–1379

71. Giurea M, Zorilla P, Amis AA et al (1999) Comparative pull-out and cyclic-loading strength tests of anchorage of hamstring tendon grafts in anterior cruciate ligament reconstruction. Am J Sports Med 27:621–625

72. Gobbi A, Diara A, Mahajan S, Zanazzo M, Tuy B (2002) Patellar tendon anterior cruciate ligament reconstruction with conical press-fit femoral fixation: 5-year results in athletes population. Knee Surg Sports Traumatol Arthrosc 10:73–79

73. Gonzalez-Lomas G, Cassily RT, Remotti F et al (2011) Is the etiology of pretibial cyst formation after absorbable interference screw use related to a foreign body reaction? Clin Orthop Relat Res 469:1082–1088

74. Graf B, Uhr F (1988) Complications of intra-articular cruciate reconstruction. Clin Sports Med 7:835–848

75. Hackl W, Benedetto KP, Hoser C et al (2000) Is screw divergence in femoral bone-tendon-bone graft fixation avoidable in anterior cruciate ligament reconstruction using a single-incision technique? A radiographically controlled cadaver study. Arthroscopy 16:640–647

76. Halder AM (2010) Arthroscopic reconstruction of anterior cruciate ligament with press-fit technique. Unfallchirurg 113:635–640

77. Hall MP, Hergan DM, Sherman OH (2009) Early fracture of a bioabsorbable tibial interference screw after ACL reconstruction with subsequent chondral injury. Orthopedics 32:208

78. Hamid M, Majid M (2012) Anterior cruciate ligament reconstruction using autologous hamstring single-bundle Rigidfix technique compared with single-bundle Transfix technique. Adv Biomed Res 1:32

79. Hamner DL, Brown CH, Steiner ME et al (1999) Hamstring tendon graft for reconstruction of anterior cruciate ligament: biomechanical evaluation of the use of multiple strands and tensioning techniques. J Bone Joint Surg Am 81:549–557

80. Han DL, Nyland J, Kendzior M et al (2012) Intratunnel versus extratunnel fixation of hamstring autograft for anterior cruciate ligament reconstruction. Arthroscopy 28:1555–1566

81. Handl M, Drzík M, Cerulli G et al (2007) Reconstruction of the anterior cruciate ligament: dynamic strain evaluation of the graft. Knee Surg Sports Traumatol Arthrosc 15(3):233–241

82. Harilainen A, Sandelin J (2009) A prospective comparison of 3 hamstring ACL fixation devices (Rigidfix, BioScrew, and Intrafix) randomized into 4 groups with 2 years of follow-up. Am J Sports Med 37:699–706

83. Harvey AR, Thomas NP, Amis AA (2003) The effect of screw length and position on fixation of four-stranded hamstring grafts for anterior cruciate ligament reconstruction. Knee 10:97–102

84. Harvey A, Thomas NP, Amis AA (2005) Fixation of the graft in reconstruction of the anterior cruciate ligament. J Bone Joint Surg Br 87:593–603

85. Herbort M, Weimann A, Zantop T et al (2007) Initial fixation strength of a new hybrid technique for femoral ACL graft fixation: the bone wedge technique. Arch Orthop Trauma Surg 127:769–775

86. Herrera A, Martínez F, Iglesias D et al (2010) Fixation strength of biocomposite wedge interference screw in ACL reconstruction: effect of screw length and tunnel/screw ratio. A controlled laboratory study. BMC Musculoskelet Disord 11:139

87. Hertel P, Behrend H (2010) Implant-free anterior cruciate ligament reconstruction with the patella ligament and press-fit double bundle technique. Unfallchirurg 113(7):540–548

88. Hertel P, Behrend H, Cierpinski T, Musahl V, Widjaja G (2005) ACL reconstruction using bone-patellar tendon-bone press-fit fixation: 10-year clinical results. Knee Surg Sports Traumatol Arthrosc 13(4):248–255. doi:10.1007/s00167-004-0606-5

89. Hoher J, Livesay GA, Ma CB et al (1999) Hamstring graft motion in the femoral bone tunnel when using titanium button/polyester tape fixation. Knee Surg Sports Traumatol Arthrosc 7:215–219

90. Howell SM (2008) High-stiffness, slippage resistant cortical fixation has many advantages over intratunnel fixation. In: Prodromos CC (ed) The anterior cruciate ligament. Reconstruction and basic science, 1st edn. Elsevier, Philadelphia

91. Howell SM, Roos P, Hull ML (2005) Compaction of a bone dowel in the tibial tunnel improves the fixation stiffness of a soft tissue anterior cruciate ligament graft: an in vitro study in calf tibia. Am J Sports Med 33:719–725

92. Hulstyn M, Fadale PD, Abate J et al (1993) Biomechanical evaluation of interference screw fixation in a bovine patellar bone-tendon-bone autograft complex for anterior cruciate ligament reconstruction. Arthroscopy 9:417–424

93. Jagodzinski M, Scheunemann K, Knobloch K et al (2006) Tibial press-fit fixation of the hamstring tendons for ACL-reconstruction. Knee Surg Sports Traumatol Arthrosc 14(12):1281–1287

94. Jagodzinski M, Geiges B, von Falck C et al (2010) Biodegradable screw versus a press-fit bone plug

fixation for hamstring anterior cruciate ligament reconstruction: a prospective randomized study. Am J Sports Med 38:501–508

95. Järvinen TL, Alami GB, Karlsson J (2010) Anterior cruciate ligament graft fixation – a myth busted? Arthroscopy 26:681–684

96. Johnson LL, vanDyk GE (1996) Metal and biodegradable interference screws: comparison of failure strength. Arthroscopy 12:452–456

97. Jomba NM, Raso VJ, Leung P (1993) Effect of varying angles on the pullout strength of interference screw fixation. Arthroscopy 9:580–583

98. Kaeding C, Farr J, Kavanaugh T et al (2005) A prospective randomized comparison of bioabsorbable and titanium anterior cruciate ligament interference screws. Arthroscopy 21:147–151

99. Kamelger FS, Onder U, Schmoelz W et al (2009) Suspensory fixation of grafts in anterior cruciate ligament reconstruction: a biomechanical comparison of 3 implants. Arthroscopy 25:767–776

100. Kilger RH, Thomas M, Hanford S et al (2005) The effectiveness of reconstruction of the anterior cruciate ligament using the novel knot/press-fit technique: a cadaveric study. Am J Sports Med 33(6):856–863

101. Kim SJ, Kumar P, Oh KS (2009) Anterior cruciate ligament reconstruction: autogenous quadriceps tendon-bone compared with bone-patellar tendon-bone grafts at 2-year follow-up. Arthroscopy 25(2):137–144. doi:10.1016/j.arthro.2008.09.014

102. Kim SJ, Bae JH, Song SH et al (2013) Bone tunnel widening with autogenous bone plugs versus bioabsorbable interference screws for secondary fixation in ACL reconstruction. J Bone Joint Surg Am 95:103–108

103. Kohn D, Rose C (1994) Primary stability of interference screw fixation. Influence of screw diameter and insertion torque. Am J Sports Med 22:334–338

104. Konan S, Haddad FS (2009) The unpredictable material properties of bioabsorbable PLC interference screws and their adverse effects in ACL reconstruction surgery. Knee Surg Sports Traumatol Arthrosc 17:293–297

105. Kopf S, Forsythe B, Wong AK, Tashman S, Irrgang JJ, Fu FH (2012) Transtibial ACL reconstruction technique fails to position drill tunnels anatomically in vivo 3D CT study. Knee Surg Sports Traumatol Arthrosc 20(11):2200–2207. doi:10.1007/s00167-011-1851-z

106. Kousa P, Järvinen TL, Vihavainen M et al (2003) The fixation strength of six hamstring tendon graft fixation devices in anterior cruciate ligament reconstruction. Part II: tibial site. Am J Sports Med 31:182–188

107. Krappel FA, Bauer E, Harland U (2006) The migration of a BioScrew as a differential diagnosis of knee pain, locking after ACL reconstruction: a report of two cases. Arch Orthop Trauma Surg 126:615–620

108. Kurosaka M, Yoshiya S, Andrish JT (1987) A biomechanical comparison of different surgical techniques of graft fixation in anterior cruciate ligament reconstruction. Am J Sports Med 15:225–229

109. Kuskucu SM (2008) Comparison of short-term results of bone tunnel enlargement between EndoButton CL and cross-pin fixation systems after chronic anterior cruciate ligament reconstruction with autologous quadrupled hamstring tendons. J Int Med Res 36:23–30

110. Lee YS, Nam SW, Hwang CH et al (2012) Computed tomography based evaluation of the bone mineral density around the fixation area during knee ligament reconstructions: clinical relevance in the choice of fixation method. Knee 19:793–796

111. Lembeck B, Wulker N (2005) Severe cartilage damage by broken poly-L-lactic acid (PLLA) interference screw after ACL reconstruction. Knee Surg Sports Traumatol Arthrosc 13:283–286

112. Lind M, Feller J, Webster KE (2009) Tibial bone tunnel widening is reduced by polylactate/hydroxyapatite interference screws compared to metal screws after ACL reconstruction with hamstring grafts. Knee 16:447–451

113. Macdonald P, Arneja S (2003) Biodegradable screw presents as a loose intra-articular body after anterior cruciate ligament reconstruction. Arthroscopy 19(6):E22–E24

114. Magen HE, Howell SM, Hull ML (1999) Structural properties of six tibial fixation methods for anterior cruciate ligament soft tissue grafts. Am J Sports Med 27:35–43

115. Mariani PP, Camillieri G, Margheritini F (2001) Transcondylar screw fixation in anterior cruciate ligament reconstruction. Arthroscopy 17:717–723

116. Markatos K, Kaseta MK, Lallos SN et al (2013) The anatomy of the ACL and its importance in ACL reconstruction. Eur J Orthop Surg Traumatol 23:747–752, Accessed 22 Sep 2012

117. Marks P, O'Donnell S, Yee G (2008) A pilot clinical evaluation comparing the Mitek bone-tendon-bone cross pin and bioabsorbable screw in anterior cruciate ligament reconstruction fixation, a randomized double blind controlled trial. Knee 15:168–173

118. Marshall JL, Warren RF, Wickiewicz TL, Reider B (1979) The anterior cruciate ligament: a technique of repair and reconstruction. Clin Orthop Relat Res 143:97–106

119. Marti C, Imhoff AB, Bahrs C (1997) Metallic versus bioabsorbable interference screw fixation of bone-patellar tendon-bone autograft in arthroscopic anterior cruciate ligament reconstruction. A preliminary report. Knee Surg Sports Traumatol Arthrosc 5:217–221

120. Matthews LS, Soffer SR (1989) Pitfalls in the use of interference screws for anterior cruciate ligament reconstruction: brief report. Arthroscopy 5:225–226

121. Mayr HO, Beck T, Hube R, Jäger A, von Eisenhart-Rothe R, Bernstein A, Plitz W, Hein W (2005) Axial load in case of press-fit fixation of the

ACL graft – a fundamental study. Z Orthop Ihre Grenzgeb 143(5):556–560

122. Mayr HO, Hube R, Bernstein A et al (2007) Betatricalcium phosphate plugs for press-fit fixation in ACL reconstruction. A mechanical analysis in bovine bone. Knee 14:239–244

123. Mayr HO, Dietrich M, Fraedrich F et al (2009) Microporous pure beta-tricalcium phosphate implants for press-fit fixation of anterior cruciate ligament grafts: strength and healing in a sheep model. Arthroscopy 25:996–1005

124. Mayr R, Rosenberger R, Agraharam D et al (2012) Revision anterior cruciate ligament reconstruction: an update. Arch Orthop Trauma Surg 132:1299–1313

125. McGuire DA, Barber FA, Elrod BF et al (1999) Bioabsorbable interference screws for graft fixation in anterior cruciate ligament reconstruction. Arthroscopy 15:463–473

126. Melnyk M, Gollhofer A (2007) Submaximal fatigue of the hamstrings impairs specific reflex components and knee stability. Knee Surg Sports Traumatol Arthrosc 15(5):525–532. doi:10.1007/s00167-006-0226-3

127. Milano G, Mulas PD, Sanna-Passino E et al (2005) Evaluation of bone plug and soft tissue anterior cruciate ligament graft fixation over time using transverse femoral fixation in a sheep model. Arthroscopy 21:532–539

128. Milano G, Mulas PD, Ziranu F et al (2006) Comparison between different femoral fixation devices for ACL reconstruction with doubled hamstring tendon graft: a biomechanical analysis. Arthroscopy 22:660–668

129. Milano G, Mulas PD, Ziranu F et al (2007) Comparison of femoral fixation methods for anterior cruciate ligament reconstruction with patellar tendon graft: a mechanical analysis in porcine knees. Knee Surg Sports Traumatol Arthrosc 15:733–738

130. Mulford JS, Hutchinson SE, Hang JR (2012) Outcomes for primary anterior cruciate reconstruction with the quadriceps autograft: a systematic review. Knee Surg Sports Traumatol Arthrosc. doi:10.1007/s00167-012-2212-2

131. Musahl V, Abramowitch SD, Gabriel MT, Debski RE, Hertel P, Fu FH, Woo SL (2003) Tensile properties of an anterior cruciate ligament graft after bone-patellar tendon-bone press-fit fixation. Knee Surg Sports Traumatol Arthrosc 11(2):68–74

132. Nebelung S, Deitmer G, Gebing R et al (2012) Anterior cruciate ligament reconstruction using biodegradable transfemoral fixation at 5-year follow-up: clinical and magnetic resonance imaging evaluation. Knee Surg Sports Traumatol Arthrosc 20:2279–2286

133. Nebelung S, Deitmer G, Gebing R et al (2013) Improved outcomes after anterior cruciate ligament reconstruction with quadrupled hamstring autografts and additional bone plug augmentation at five year follow-up. Int Orthop 37:399–405

134. Ninomiya T, Tachibana Y, Miyajima T et al (2011) Fixation strength of the interference screw in the femoral tunnel: the effect of screw divergence on the coronal plane. Knee 18:83–87

135. Noh JH, Yang BG, Yi SR et al (2012) Hybrid tibial fixation for anterior cruciate ligament reconstruction with Achilles tendon allograft. Arthroscopy 28:1540–1546

136. Noyes FR, Butler DL, Grood ES et al (1984) Biomechanical analysis of human ligament grafts used in knee-ligament repairs and reconstructions. J Bone Joint Surg Am 66:344–352

137. Nurmi JT, Sievänen H, Kannus P et al (2004) Porcine tibia is a poor substitute for human cadaver tibia for evaluating interference screw fixation. Am J Sports Med 32:765–771

138. Paessler HH, Mastrokalos DS (2003) Anterior cruciate ligament reconstruction using semitendinosus and gracilis tendons, bone patellar tendon, or quadriceps tendon-graft with press-fit fixation without hardware. A new and innovative procedure. Orthop Clin North Am 34(1):49–64

139. Pandey V, Acharya K, Rao S et al (2011) Femoral tunnel-interference screw divergence in anterior cruciate ligament reconstruction using bone-patellar tendon-bone graft: a comparison of two techniques. Indian J Orthop 45:255–260

140. Panni AS, Milano G, Lucania L et al (1997) Graft healing after anterior cruciate ligament reconstruction in rabbits. Clin Orthop Relat Res 343:203–212

141. Pavlik A, Hidas P, Czigány T, Berkes I (2004) Biomechanical evaluation of press-fit femoral fixation technique in ACL reconstruction. Knee Surg Sports Traumatol Arthrosc 12(6):528–533

142. Pereira HM, Correlo VM, Silva-Correia J et al (2013) Migration of "bioabsorbable" screws in ACL repair. How much do we know? A systematic review. Knee Surg Sports Traumatol Arthrosc 21:986–994

143. Petersen W, Zantop T (2007) Anatomy of the anterior cruciate ligament with regard to its two bundles. Clin Orthop Relat Res 454:35–47

144. Petersen W, Forkel P, Achtnich A, Metzlaff S, Zantop T (2013) Technique of anatomical footprint reconstruction of the ACL with oval tunnels and medial portal aimers. Arch Orthop Trauma Surg. 133(6):827–33

145. Petre BM, Smith SD, Jansson KS et al (2013) Femoral cortical suspension devices for soft tissue anterior cruciate ligament reconstruction: a comparative biomechanical study. Am J Sports Med 41:416–422

146. Pierz K, Baltz M, Fulkerson J (1995) The effect of Kurosaka screw divergence on the holding strength of bone-tendon-bone grafts. Am J Sports Med 23:332–335

147. Płomiński J, Borcz K, Kwiatkowski K et al (2008) Fixation of patellar tendon bone graft in reconstruction of patellar ligaments. Comparison of bioabsorbable and metal interference screws – results of treatment. Ortop Traumatol Rehabil 10:44–53

148. Pomeroy G, Baltz M, Pierz K et al (1998) The effects of bone plug length and screw diameter on the holding strength of bone-tendon-bone grafts. Arthroscopy 14:148–152

149. Price R, Stoney J, Brown G (2010) Prospective randomized comparison of endobutton versus cross-pin femoral fixation in hamstring anterior cruciate ligament reconstruction with 2-year follow-up. ANZ J Surg 80:162–165

150. Pujol N, David T, Bauer T et al (2006) Transverse femoral fixation in anterior cruciate ligament (ACL) reconstruction with hamstrings grafts: an anatomic study about the relationships between the transcondylar device and the posterolateral structures of the knee. Knee Surg Sports Traumatol Arthrosc 14:724–729

151. Rabuck SJ, Musahl V, Fu FH, West RV (2013) Anatomic anterior cruciate ligament reconstruction with quadriceps tendon autograft. Clin Sports Med 32(1):155–164. doi:10.1016/j.csm.2012.08.014

152. Rhee PC, Levy BA, Stuart MJ et al (2011) A biomechanical comparison of the Delta screw and RetroScrew tibial fixation on initial intra-articular graft tension. Knee Surg Sports Traumatol Arthrosc 19:781–786

153. Rhee PC, Dahm DL, Stuart MJ et al (2011) Delta screw versus RetroScrew tibial fixation for ACL reconstruction. Knee Surg Sports Traumatol Arthrosc 19:S94–S100

154. Rodeo SA, Arnoczky SP, Torzilli PA et al (1993) Tendon-healing in a bone tunnel. A biomechanical and histological study in the dog. J Bone Joint Surg Am 75:1795–1803

155. Rodin D, Levy IM (2003) The use of intraoperative fluoroscopy to reduce femoral interference screw divergence during endoscopic anterior cruciate ligament reconstruction. Arthroscopy 19:314–317

156. Rork PE (2000) Bungee cord effect in hamstring tendon ACL reconstruction. Orthopedics 23:184

157. Roy S, Fernhout M, Stanley R et al (2010) Tibial interference screw fixation in anterior cruciate ligament reconstruction with and without autograft bone augmentation. Arthroscopy 26:949–956

158. Rupp S, Krauss PW, Fritsch EW (1997) Fixation strength of a biodegradable interference screw and a press-fit technique in anterior cruciate ligament reconstruction with a BPTB graft. Arthroscopy 13:61–65

159. Sabat D, Arora S (2011) Femoral tunnel-interference screw divergence in anterior cruciate ligament reconstruction using bone-patellar tendon-bone graft: a comparison of two techniques. Indian J Orthop 45(6):583–584

160. Sassmannshausen G, Carr CF (2003) Transcutaneous migration of a tibial bioabsorbable interference screw after anterior cruciate ligament reconstruction. Arthroscopy 19:E133–E136

161. Scheffler SU, Südkamp NP, Göckenjam A et al (2002) Biomechanical comparison of hamstring and patellar tendon graft anterior cruciate ligament reconstruction techniques: the impact of fixation level and fixation method under cyclic loading. Arthroscopy 18:304–315

162. Schroeder FJ (1999) Reduction of femoral interference screw divergence during endoscopic anterior cruciate ligament reconstruction. Arthroscopy 15:41–48

163. Selby JB, Johnson DL, Hester P et al (2001) Effect of screw length on bioabsorbable interference screw fixation in a tibial bone tunnel. Am J Sports Med 29:614–619

164. Shafer BL, Simonian PT (2002) Broken poly-L-lactic acid interference screw after ligament reconstruction. Arthroscopy 18:E35

165. Shapiro JD, Jackson DW, Aberman HM et al (1995) Comparison of pullout strength for seven- and nine-millimeter diameter interference screw size as used in anterior cruciate ligament reconstruction. Arthroscopy 11:596–599

166. Sharma V, Curtis C, Micheli L (2008) Extra-articular extraosseous migration of a bioabsorbable femoral interference screw after ACL reconstruction. Orthopedics 31

167. Shellock FG, Mink JH, Curtin S et al (1992) MR imaging and metallic implants for anterior cruciate ligament reconstruction: assessment of ferromagnetism and artifact. J Magn Reson Imaging 2:225–228

168. Shen C, Jiang SD, Jiang LS et al (2010) Bioabsorbable versus metallic interference screw fixation in anterior cruciate ligament reconstruction: a meta-analysis of randomized controlled trials. Arthroscopy 26:705–713

169. Shen HC, Chang JH, Lee C et al (2010) Biomechanical comparison of Cross-pin and Endobutton-CL femoral fixation of a flexor tendon graft for anterior cruciate ligament reconstruction – a porcine femur-graft-tibia complex study. J Surg Res 161:282–287

170. Shino K, Pflaster DS (2000) Comparison of eccentric and concentric screw placement for hamstring graft fixation in the tibial tunnel. Knee Surg Sports Traumatol Arthrosc 8:73–75

171. Sidhu DS, Wroble RR (1997) Intraarticular migration of a femoral interference fit screw. A complication of anterior cruciate ligament reconstruction. Am J Sports Med 25:268–271

172. Silva A, Sampaio R, Pinto E (2010) Femoral tunnel enlargement after anatomic ACL reconstruction: a biological problem? Knee Surg Sports Traumatol Arthrosc 18:1189–1194

173. Simonian PT, Sussmann PS, Baldini TH et al (1998) Interference screw position and hamstring graft location for anterior cruciate ligament reconstruction. Arthroscopy 14:459–464

174. Sørensen OG, Larsen K, Jakobsen BW et al (2011) Serial dilation reduces graft slippage compared to extraction drilling in anterior cruciate ligament reconstruction: a randomized controlled trial using radiostereometric analysis. Knee Surg Sports Traumatol Arthrosc 19:347–354

175. Speirs A, Simon D, Lapner P (2010) Evaluation of a new femoral fixation device in a simulated anterior cruciate ligament reconstruction. Arthroscopy 26:351–357

176. Staeubli HU, Bollmann C, Kreutz R, Becker W, Rauschning W (1999) Quantification of intact quadriceps tendon, quadriceps tendon insertion, and suprapatellar fat pad: MR arthrography, anatomy, and cryosections in the sagittal plane. AJR Am J Roentgenol 173(3):691–698

177. Stählin AC, Weiler A, Rufenacht H et al (1997) Clinical degradation and biocompatibility of different bioabsorbable interference screws: a report of six cases. Arthroscopy 13:238–244

178. Steenlage E, Brand JC Jr, Johnson DL (2002) Correlation of bone tunnel diameter with quadrupled hamstring graft fixation strength using a biodegradable interference screw. Arthroscopy 18:901–907

179. Steiner ME, Hecher AT, Brown CH et al (1994) Anterior cruciate ligament graft fixation comparison of hamstring and patellar tendon grafts. Am J Sports Med 22:240–246

180. Stener S, Ejerhed L, Sernert N et al (2010) A long-term, prospective, randomized study comparing biodegradable and metal interference screws in anterior cruciate ligament reconstruction surgery: radiographic results and clinical outcome. Am J Sports Med 38:1598–1605

181. Studler U, White LM, Naraghi AM et al (2010) Anterior cruciate ligament reconstruction by using bioabsorbable femoral cross pins: MR imaging findings at follow-up and comparison with clinical findings. Radiology 255:108–116

182. Tetsumura S, Fujita A, Nakajima M et al (2006) Biomechanical comparison of different fixation methods on the tibial side in anterior cruciate ligament reconstruction: a biomechanical study in porcine tibial bone. J Orthop Sci 11:278–282

183. Tie K, Wang H, Wang X et al (2012) Measurement of bone mineral density in the tunnel regions for anterior cruciate ligament reconstruction by dual-energy X-ray absorptiometry, computed tomography scan, and the immersion technique based on Archimedes' principle. Arthroscopy 28:1464–1471

184. To JT, Howell SM, Hull ML (1999) Contribution of femoral fixation methods to the stiffness of anterior cruciate ligament replacement at the implantation. Arthroscopy 15:379–387

185. Tomihara T, Ohashi H, Yo H (2007) Comparison of direct and indirect interference screw fixation for tendon graft in rabbits. Knee Surg Sports Traumatol Arthrosc 15:26–30

186. Tuompo P, Partio EK, Jukkala-Partio K et al (1996) Strength of the fixation of patellar tendon bone grafts using a totally absorbable self-reinforced poly-L-lactide expansion plug and screw. An experimental study in a bovine cadaver. Arthroscopy 12:422–427

187. Uzumcugil O, Yalcinkaya M, Ozturkmen Y et al (2012) Effect of PEEK polymer on tunnel widening after hamstring ACL reconstruction. Orthopedics 35:e654–e659

188. van Eck CF, Illingworth KD, Fu FH (2010) Quadriceps tendon: the forgotten graft. Arthroscopy 26(4):441–442. doi:10.1016/j.arthro.2010.02.021; author reply 442–443

189. Walz B, Nyland J, Fisher B et al (2012) Supplemental bio-tenodesis improves tibialis anterior allograft yield load in extremely low density tibiae. Arch Orthop Trauma Surg 132:343–347

190. Wang JL, Liu YJ, Wang AY et al (2009) Biomechanical evaluation of tendon graft fixation at the tibial site in anterior cruciate ligament reconstruction with Intrafix and bioabsorbable interference screw. Zhonghua Yi Xue Za Zhi 89:886–889

191. Wang RY, Arciero RA, Obopilwe E et al (2012) Comparison of the retro screw and standard interference screw for ACL reconstruction. J Knee Surg 25:227–235

192. Warden WH, Chooljian D, Jackson WD (2008) Ten-year magnetic resonance imaging follow-up of bioabsorbable poly-L-lactic acid interference screws after anterior cruciate ligament reconstruction. Arthroscopy 24:370.e1–370.e3

193. Weiler A, Helling HJ, Kirch U et al (1996) Foreign-body reaction and the course of osteolysis after polyglycolide implants for fracture fixation: experimental study in sheep. J Bone Joint Surg Br 78:369–376

194. Weiler A, Hoffmann RF, Stähelin AC et al (1998) Hamstring tendon fixation using interference screws: a biomechanical study in calf tibial bone. Arthroscopy 14:29–37

195. Weiler A, Hoffmann RF, Siepe CJ et al (2000) The influence of screw geometry on hamstring tendon interference fit fixation. Am J Sports Med 28:356–359

196. Weiler A, Hoffmann RF, Stahelin AC et al (2000) Biodegradable implants in sports medicine: the biological base. Arthroscopy 16:305–321

197. Weiler A, Hoffmann RF, Bail HJ et al (2002) Tendon healing in a bone tunnel. Part II: histologic analysis after biodegradable interference fit fixation in a model of anterior cruciate ligament reconstruction in sheep. Arthroscopy 18:124–135

198. Weimann A, Zantop T, Rummler M et al (2003) Primary stability of bone–patellar tendon–bone graft fixation with biodegradable pins. Arthroscopy 19:1097–1102

199. Weimann A, Zantop T, Herbort M et al (2006) Initial fixation strength of a hybrid technique for femoral ACL graft fixation. Knee Surg Sports Traumatol Arthrosc 14:1122–1129

200. Weiss JA, Paulos LE (1999) Mechanical testing of ligament fixation devices. Tech Orthop 14:14–21

201. Werner A, Wild A, Ilg A, Krauspe R (2002) Secondary intraarticular dislocation of a broken bioabsorbable interference screw after anterior cruciate ligament reconstruction. Knee Surg Sports Traumatol Arthrosc 10:30–32

202. Widuchowski W, Widuchowska M, Koczy B, Dragan S, Czamara A, Tomaszewski W, Widuchowski J

(2012) Femoral press-fit fixation in ACL reconstruction using bone-patellar tendon-bone autograft: results at 15 years follow-up. BMC Musculoskelet Disord 13:115. doi:10.1186/1471-2474-13-115

203. Wipfler B, Donner S, Zechmann CM et al (2011) Anterior cruciate ligament reconstruction using patellar tendon versus hamstring tendon: a prospective comparative study with 9-year follow-up. Arthroscopy 27(5):653–665

204. Yoo JC, Ahn JH, Kim JH et al (2006) Biomechanical testing of hybrid hamstring graft tibial fixation in anterior cruciate ligament reconstruction. Knee 13:455–459

205. Yosmaoğlu HB, Baltacı G, Kaya D et al (2011) Comparison of functional outcomes of two anterior cruciate ligament reconstruction methods with hamstring tendon graft. Acta Orthop Traumatol Turc 45:240–247

206. Zantop T, Welbers B, Weimann A (2004) Biomechanical evaluation of a new cross-pin technique for the fixation of different sized bone-patellar tendon-bone grafts. Knee Surg Sports Traumatol Arthrosc 12:520–527

207. Zantop T, Ruemmler M, Welbers B et al (2005) Cyclic loading comparison between biodegradable interference screw fixation and biodegradable double cross pin fixation of human bone–patellar tendon–bone grafts. Arthroscopy 21:934–941

208. Zantop T, Weimann A, Schmidtke R et al (2006) Graft laceration and pullout strength of soft-tissue anterior cruciate ligament reconstruction: in vitro study comparing titanium, poly-d, l-lactide, and poly-d, l-lactide-tricalcium phosphate screws. Arthroscopy 22:1204–1210

209. Zantop T, Weimann A, Wolle K et al (2007) Initial and 6 weeks postoperative structural properties of soft tissue anterior cruciate ligament reconstructions with cross-pin or interference screw fixation: an in vivo study in sheep. Arthroscopy 23:14–20

Remodeling of Hamstring Tendon Grafts After ACL Reconstruction

25

Rob P.A. Janssen and Sven U. Scheffler

Contents

R.P.A. Janssen, MD, PhD (✉)
Department of Orthopaedic Surgery,
Orthopaedic Center Máxima, Máxima Medical Center,
Ds. Th. Fliednerstraat 1, 5631 BM Eindhoven,
The Netherlands
e-mail: r.janssen@mmc.nl

S.U. Scheffler, PD Dr. med.
Department of Orthopaedic Surgery,
COPV – Chirurgisch Orthopädischer Praxis Verbund,
Breitenbachplatz 8, 14195 Berlin, Germany

25.1   Introduction

Anterior cruciate ligament (ACL) reconstruction techniques have been improved over the last 10 years, but graft failure is not uncommon: 0.7–10 % [1, 2]. Successful ACL reconstruction requires understanding of several factors: anatomical graft placement, mechanical properties of the selected graft tissue, mechanical behavior and fixation strength of fixation materials, as well as the biological processes that occur during graft remodeling, maturation, and incorporation. They influence directly the mechanical properties of the knee joint after ACL reconstruction and, therefore, determine the rehabilitation and time course until normal function of the knee joint can be expected [2–10]. Even though substantial research efforts have been published on various aspects of ACL reconstruction, there is limited knowledge on the biology of the human ACL graft [2, 4–8, 11–21]. Graft healing after ACL reconstruction occurs at two different sites: intra-tunnel graft incorporation [22, 23] and intra-articular graft remodeling, often referred to as "ligamentization" [2, 5, 6, 8, 9, 12, 20, 24, 25]. This chapter presents the current knowledge on intra-articular remodeling of ACL grafts with special focus on human hamstring autografts.

25.2   Phases of Remodeling

Animal and human in vitro and in vivo research have demonstrated three characteristic stages of graft healing after ACL reconstruction: an early

R. Siebold et al. (eds.), *Anterior Cruciate Ligament Reconstruction*,
DOI 10.1007/978-3-642-45349-6_25, © ESSKA 2014

graft healing phase with central graft necrosis and hypocellularity and no detectable revascularization of the graft tissue, followed by a phase of proliferation, the time of most intensive remodeling and revascularization, and, finally, a ligamentization phase with characteristic restructuring of the graft towards the properties of the intact ACL [2, 5, 6, 17, 21, 24, 26–29]. However, a full restoration of either the biological or mechanical properties of the intact ACL is not achieved [6, 24, 28].

25.2.1 Early Graft Healing Phase

This phase is defined as the period from the time of anterior cruciate ligament reconstruction until the fourth postoperative week. It is marked by increasing necrosis, mainly in the center of the graft and hypocellularity [6, 24, 28, 30–32]. An influx of host cells can be seen into the graft's periphery between the first and second week [29, 32]. The source of these cells is thought to be the synovial fluid, cells from the stump of the native ACL or bone marrow elements originating from drilling the tunnels. Preservation of the ACL stump and Hoffa fat pad may be beneficial for graft healing in this phase [10, 16, 30]. At the same time, no graft revascularization can be observed [29, 30, 33, 34]. Even though beginning disintegration of collagen fibrils and their orientation can be observed as early as 3 weeks after reconstruction [35], the graft's overall collagen structure and crimp pattern are maintained [24, 28]. This explains the slow decrease in the mechanical properties of the graft in this early healing phase [6, 33, 36]. During this early healing phase, between 2 and 4 weeks, the lack of sufficient biological graft incorporation is the weak site of the reconstruction with consistent failure by graft pullout [35–38], therefore requiring and relying on appropriate mechanical graft fixation. A shift towards the intra-articular graft region becoming the weak link is noted during the proliferation healing phase when the maximum remodeling activity seems to interfere with the mechanical strength of the healing graft [14, 35, 36].

25.2.2 Proliferation Phase of Graft Healing

The proliferation phase is defined as the period between 4 and 12 weeks after ACL reconstruction.

This phase is characterized by maximum cellular activity and changes of the extracellular matrix, which are paralleled by the lowest mechanical properties of the reconstructed ACL graft. Graft necrosis leads to a release of growth factors, which stimulate cell migration and proliferation as well as extracellular matrix synthesis and revascularization [31, 34, 39–41]. An increased number of specific fibroblasts, so-called myofibroblasts, appear. They are responsible for the restoration of the in situ tension that is required for the later ligamentization phase [6, 42–44]. At the end of the proliferation phase, cell density is still increased but recedes towards the intact ACL's cellularity [2, 6, 31, 38, 45–47]. Revascularization of the graft starts from the fourth postoperative week [6, 14, 30, 47], progressing from the periphery of the graft to the entire graft diameter at 12 weeks [47, 48].

Animal studies have shown that the mechanical properties of the graft are at its weakest at 6–8 weeks. Three factors contribute to the decline in the grafts' mechanical properties: (a) increased revascularization and extracellular infiltration, (b) loss of regular collagen orientation and crimp pattern, and (c) decrease in collagen fibril density, followed by increased collagen synthesis with a shift from large diameter collagen fibrils to small diameter fibrils [6, 14, 23, 29, 31, 35, 38, 45, 46, 49–52]. Furthermore, increased collagen III synthesis (with lower mechanical strength than type I collagen) may further explain why a full restoration of the mechanical strength of the intact ACL has not been observed in any in vivo model even after 2 years of healing [3, 6, 48, 51].

The reduced mechanical properties of healing grafts in animal models seem to contradict the successful clinical outcomes after ACL reconstruction with immediate aggressive rehabilitation in humans. Significant differences were found in biopsy studies between the remodeling activity of human ACL grafts during the first 3 months and the healing graft in animal models. The complete loss and replacement of all intrinsic graft has not been observed in human biopsy studies [26, 53]. The excessive graft necrosis in animals could not be confirmed in humans, where necrosis or degeneration never involved more than 30 % of the graft's biopsies [1, 26, 53]. Neovascularization was not as excessive in humans [53]. Large areas of human healing graft stay unchanged displaying tendinous structure with normal collagen alignment and crimp pattern [53]. Loss of collagen organization was only detected in areas of neovascularization in human biopsies, which corresponds to the findings in animal studies [2, 6]. However, human biopsy studies confirm the remodeling cascade of (limited) graft necrosis, recellularization, revascularization, and changes in collagen crimp and composition during the early healing and proliferation phases, suggesting that also the human ACL graft might have its lowest mechanical strength around 6–8 weeks postoperatively [17, 26]. Loading of the graft must be high enough to stimulate graft cells to produce cellular and extracellular components for preservation of graft stability, but without compromising graft integrity, which might result into an early stretch-out of the ACL reconstruction [6].

25.2.3 Ligamentization Phase of Graft Healing

The ligamentization phase involves the continuous remodeling of the healing graft towards morphology and mechanical strength of the intact ACL from 12 weeks onwards. A clear end point is not known for certain changes still occur even years after reconstruction. In animal models, cellularity slowly returns to values of the intact ACL between 3 and 6 months postoperatively [6, 14, 47, 48]. Vascularity throughout the graft decreases and returns to values of the intact ACL between 6 and 12 months, when vessels become evenly distributed throughout the entire graft [6, 14, 30, 47]. Collagen fibers regain their organization, which microscopically resembles

the appearance of the intact ACL around 6–12 months after reconstruction [6, 43]. However, the initial loss in collagen crimp and strict parallel alignment of the proliferation phase is only partially restored [6, 43]. The heterogenous composition of collagen fibers of varying diameter of the intact ACL is never restored [38, 46, 54, 55]. It has been shown that the mechanical properties of the ACL-reconstructed knee joint improve substantially during the phase of ligamentization and reach their maximum properties at around 1 year. However, not a single animal study has demonstrated that the structural properties (e.g., failure load, stiffness) of the healing graft could surpass 50–60 % of the intact ACL [6, 14, 23, 35, 36, 45, 46, 52, 56, 57]. While human biopsy studies showed substantial differences from animal models during the proliferation phase, the ligamentization phase is rather similar in both models in terms of biological progression. However, the timeline of these biological changes is different: studies in humans have shown a prolonged remodeling process compared to animal models [2, 4–6, 8, 12, 17, 20, 21, 25, 26].

25.3 Remodeling of Human Hamstring Autografts After ACL Reconstruction

When interpreting animal data with regard to changes occurring in human autografts, important clinical factors such as graft isometricity, anatomical positioning, patient compliance, healing response, vascularity, biomechanical strength, and postoperative rehabilitation must be considered. These factors are difficult to control in animal models. Nevertheless, the results of animal studies are important, because human research has been limited to postmortem and second-look arthroscopic evaluation [5]. Research on remodeling of human hamstring autografts after ACL reconstruction can be divided into MRI and biopsy studies [2, 4, 5, 7, 8, 12, 13, 16, 19–21, 58]. The current knowledge on remodeling of human hamstring ACL grafts and rehabilitation will be presented in the next Sections.

25.3.1 MRI Studies of Human Hamstring ACL Grafts

MRI studies have examined the revascularization of human hamstring autografts after ACL reconstruction [7, 13, 16, 19]. In a gadolinium-enhanced MRI study, Howell et al. did not demonstrate any discernible blood supply in an unimpinged 4-strand hamstring ACL graft during the 2 years of implantation. The graft retained the same hypovascular appearance as the normal posterior cruciate ligament. In contrast, the periligamentous soft tissues were richly vascularized and covered the graft by 1 month. They postulated that the viability of an unimpinged human hamstring ACL graft may depend more on synovial diffusion than on revascularization [13]. This is in contrast to findings in animal studies, where gadolinium-enhanced MRI showed significant upregulated neovascularization during the first 3 postoperative months [14]. This underlines the differences in remodeling between humans and animal models. Although human biopsy studies have shown that neovascularization of the hamstring graft occurs, the extent of vascularity in humans might be below the threshold detectable with gadolinium-enhanced MRI [6]. Gohil et al. investigated the effect of minimal debridement of the stump of the ruptured ACL on revascularization of 4-strand human hamstring ACL autografts. They concluded that minimal debridement led to earlier revascularization within the midsubstance of the ACL graft at 2 months, but found no evidence that the minimal debridement accelerated the recovery of graft strength [16]. Other authors examined the effect of autologous platelet concentrate on remodeling of 4-strand human hamstring ACL autografts with a standardized accelerated rehabilitation protocol. Vogrin et al. used contrast-enhanced MRI and found that revascularization of the graft only started at 4–6 weeks after ACL reconstruction [7]. Autologous platelet concentrate did not influence intra-articular remodeling of hamstring grafts [7, 19]. The revascularization of the human hamstring graft at 4–6 weeks correlates with the proliferation phase of graft healing.

25.3.2 Biopsy Studies of Human Hamstring ACL Grafts

Human biopsy studies have examined the remodeling process of the hamstring tendon autograft at various time intervals after clinically successful ACL reconstruction [2, 4, 5, 8, 12, 19–21, 58]. The human hamstring autograft remains viable after reconstruction and shows typical stages of remodeling: early phase graft healing, a proliferation phase, and a ligamentization phase [2, 4, 8, 20]. Graft integrity is much less compromised during the early healing and proliferation phase in human ACL grafts, which might allow for the assumption that the mechanical properties are also substantially higher than in animal models during the first 3 postoperative months [6, 8, 53].

Focus of human hamstring biopsy studies has been the proliferation and ligamentization phases of graft healing, as most biopsies were taken at second-look arthroscopies from 4 months onwards after ACL reconstruction. Janssen et al. examined 67 patients who underwent retrieval of midsubstance biopsies after clinically successful 4-strand hamstring autograft ACL reconstruction with a standardized accelerated rehabilitation program. Cellular and vascular densities were increased up to 24 months after ACL reconstruction. Especially the strong increase in myofibroblast density, from 13 up to 24 months, indicated an active remodeling process from 1 to 2 years (Fig. 25.1). Furthermore, vessel density increased over 24 months, whereas cell and myofibroblast density decreased but stayed higher than native hamstring and ACL controls. Collagen orientation did not return to normal in the study period (up to 117 months after ACL reconstruction) [2].

Human biopsy studies that analyzed changes of the extracellular matrix observed changes that are in line with the findings of animal models. Marumo et al. found that the collagen cross-links of hamstring tendon autografts had changed from

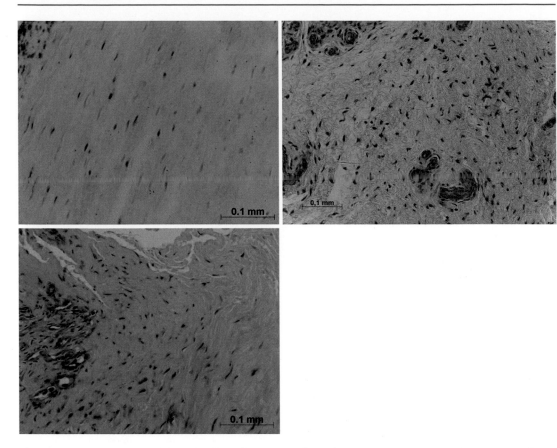

Fig. 25.1 Alpha-smooth staining biopsies of human hamstring ACL graft showing a moderate number of myofibroblasts 6–12 months (*top left*) compared to 13–24 months (*top right*) and over 24 months (*bottom left*) after ACL reconstruction. Note an increased number of myofibroblasts and vessels in biopsies at 13–24 months and over 24 months after ACL reconstruction (Reproduced with permission from Janssen et al. [2])

time zero, when they were significantly different from the intact ACL, to 1 year postoperatively, when both grafts had acquired cross-link ratios that were identical to the intact ACL, confirming the ligamentization process found in animal models. Interestingly, biopsy specimens taken at 6 months still showed significantly different cross-link ratios of the healing grafts compared to the intact ACL, which is different from the earlier cross-link restoration found in animal models [5, 6, 12]. This also confirms the different timelines of the remodeling of human ACL grafts. Zaffagnini et al. confirmed the observations in animal models [14, 39, 55] that human hamstring ACL grafts showed a replacement of large by small diameter fibrils, which did not change even after more than 2 years [21]. Sanchez et al. showed that use of

platelet-rich plasma preparation rich in growth factors (PRGF) in hamstring ACL autografts resulted in temporal histological changes during the 6- to 24-month postoperative period in comparison to non-PRGF-treated grafts [20]. Biopsies were taken from the periphery of the hamstring autograft, and the authors question whether these ACL substitutes entirely replicate the full mechanical properties of the intact ACL [20]. A better understanding of the graft biology in human ACL reconstruction will depend on the possibility to obtain core biopsy samples of the grafts [8].

In summary, human hamstring ACL autografts undergo a process of adaptation rather than full restoration of the intact ACL's biological properties, which takes at least 1 year after reconstruction.

25.3.3 Human Hamstring Remodeling and Accelerated Rehabilitation

Knowledge about the duration of the remodeling process of ACL grafts may influence and improve rehabilitation protocols [2, 5, 6]. It is agreed that ACL graft healing can only progress if mechanical loading occurs; however, the most adequate magnitude at the varying phases of healing is still not clarified [1, 6, 49, 59]. Patients who return quickly to high-risk activities with accelerated rehabilitation achieved earlier normal function of the knee [60–62]. Patients can return to even most strenuous activities after primary ACL reconstruction at 6 months [6]. Arthroscopic findings and clinical results after hamstring ACL reconstruction are found to be satisfactory with both accelerated and less aggressive rehabilitation programs [2, 5, 61–64]. However, some authors found that early return to vigorous physical activity may increase the risk of greater knee laxity after ACL reconstruction [1, 65]. It is crucial to understand what rehabilitation activities might lead to excessive ACL tensioning and therefore must be avoided during the first three postoperative months.

Human hamstring ACL graft remodeling takes at least 1 year after ACL reconstruction and is prolonged compared to animal models, on which current rehabilitation protocols are based after ACL reconstruction [2, 4–6, 12, 14, 20–23, 38, 43, 44, 47, 58, 66]. Janssen et al. question whether accelerated rehabilitation is to be recommended after nonanatomic 4-strand hamstring ACL reconstruction [2]. No final conclusions can be drawn on the mechanical strength of healing ACL grafts in humans with no available techniques for in vivo measurement of their mechanical properties. Even though it is not fully understood what the exact mechanisms are that guide the remodeling process, it seems to be important that physiological knee joint mechanics are restored to provide the same mechanical stimulus to the healing ACL graft as to the intact ACL. This guides adequate remodeling that will maintain initial graft integrity and (partial) cell viability while initiating cellular and extracellular proliferation and differentiation to adapt the graft to its new biological and mechanical environment.

> **Memory**
> Hamstring tendon grafts remain viable after ACL reconstruction. The graft undergoes three characteristic stages of graft healing after ACL reconstruction: an early graft healing phase with limited graft necrosis and hypocellularity and no detectable revascularization of the graft tissue, followed by a phase of proliferation, the time of most intensive remodeling and revascularization, and, finally, a ligamentization phase with characteristic restructuring of the graft towards the properties of the intact ACL. An adaptation of the healing graft towards the intact ACL occurs without a full restoration of either the biological or mechanical properties of the intact ACL. Future research will have to be directed to (a) optimizing cruciate ligament reconstructions to fully restore the anatomy and function while providing the mechanical strength of the intact cruciate ligaments, (b) developing biological treatment options that impact on graft healing especially during the early and proliferation phase to optimize extracellular matrix remodeling and avoid excessive remodeling activity that might impair mechanical integrity of the healing graft, and (c) better differentiate the "good" from the "bad" remodeling changes, so that the time to return to full activity without any restrictions can be reduced.

References

1. Ménétrey J, Duthon VB, Laumonier T et al (2008) "Biological failure" of the anterior cruciate ligament graft. Knee Surg Sports Traumatol Arthrosc 16: 224–231
2. Janssen RP, van der Wijk J, Fiedler A et al (2011) Remodelling of human hamstring autografts after anterior cruciate ligament reconstruction. Knee Surg Sports Traumatol Arthrosc 19:1299–1306
3. McFarland EG (1993) The biology of anterior cruciate ligament reconstructions. Orthopedics 16: 403–410
4. Falconiero RP, Distefano VJ, Cook TM (1998) Revascularization and ligamentization of autogenous

anterior cruciate ligament grafts in humans. Arthroscopy 14:197–205

5. Marumo K, Saito M, Yamagishi T et al (2005) The "ligamentization" process in human anterior cruciate ligament reconstruction with autogenous patellar and hamstring tendons. Am J Sports Med 33:1166–1173

6. Scheffler SU, Unterhauser FN, Weiler A (2008) Graft remodeling and ligamentization after cruciate ligament reconstruction. Knee Surg Sports Traumatol Arthrosc 16:834–842

7. Vogrin M, Rupreht M, Dinevski D et al (2010) Effects of a platelet gel on early graft revascularization after anterior cruciate ligament reconstruction: a prospective randomized, double-blind, clinical trial. Eur Surg Res 45:77–85

8. Claes S, Verdonk P, Forsyth R et al (2011) The "ligamentization" process in anterior cruciate ligament reconstruction: what happens to the human graft? A systematic review of the literature. Am J Sports Med 39:2476–2483

9. Mayr HO, Stoehr A, Dietrich M et al (2012) Graft-dependent differences in the ligamentization process of anterior cruciate ligament grafts in a sheep trial. Knee Surg Sports Traumatol Arthrosc 20: 947–956

10. Papalia R, Franceschi F, Vasta S et al (2012) Sparing the anterior cruciate ligament remnant: is it worth the hassle? Br Med Bull 104:91–111. doi:10.1093/bmb/ldr053

11. Xu Y, Ao Y (2009) Histological and biomechanical studies of inter-strand healing in four-strand autograft anterior cruciate ligament reconstruction in a rabbit model. Knee Surg Sports Traumatol Arthrosc 17: 770–777

12. Lane JG, McFadden P, Bowden K et al (1993) The ligamentization process: a 4 year case study following ACL reconstruction with a semitendinosus graft. Arthroscopy 9:149–153

13. Howell SM, Knox KE, Farley TE et al (1995) Revascularization of a human anterior cruciate ligament graft during the first two years of implantation. Am J Sports Med 23:42–49

14. Weiler A, Peters G, Mäurer J et al (2001) Biomechanical properties and vascularity of an anterior cruciate ligament graft can be predicted by contrast-enhanced magnetic resonance imaging. A two-year study in sheep. Am J Sports Med 29: 751–761

15. Scheffler SU, Scherler J, Pruss A et al (2005) Biomechanical comparison of human bone-patellar tendon-bone grafts after sterilization with peracetic acid ethanol. Cell Tissue Bank 6:109–115

16. Gohil S, Annear PO, Breidahl W (2007) Anterior cruciate ligament reconstruction using autologous double hamstrings: a comparison of standard versus minimal debridement techniques using MRI to assess revascularization. J Bone Joint Surg Br 89-B:1165–1171

17. Zaffagnini S, De Pasquale V, Marchesini Reggiani L et al (2007) Neoligamentization process of BTPB used for ACL graft: histological evaluation from 6 months to 10 years. Knee 14:87–93

18. Scitz H, Menth-Chiari WA, Lang S et al (2008) Histological evaluation of the healing potential of the anterior cruciate ligament by means of augmented and non-augmented repair: an in vivo animal study. Knee Surg Sports Traumatol Arthrosc 16:1087–1093

19. Figueroa D, Melena P, Calco R et al (2010) Magnetic resonance imaging evaluation of the integration and maturation of semitendinosus-gracilis graft in anterior cruciate ligament reconstruction using autologous platelet concentrate. Arthroscopy 26:1318–1325

20. Sanchez M, Anitua E, Azofra J et al (2010) Ligamentization of tendon grafts treated with an endogenous preparation rich in growth factors: gross morphology and histology. Arthroscopy 26: 470–480

21. Zaffagnini S, De Pasquale V, Marchesini Reggiani L (2010) Electron microscopy of the remodelling process in hamstring tendon used as ACL graft. Knee Surg Sports Traumatol Arthrosc 18:1052105–1052108

22. Weiler A, Hoffmann RF, Bail HJ et al (2002) Tendon healing in a bone tunnel. Part II: histological analysis after biodegradable interference fit fixation in a model of anterior cruciate ligament reconstruction in sheep. Arthroscopy 18:124–135

23. Weiler A, Peine R, Pahminez-Azar A et al (2002) Tendon healing in a bone tunnel. Part I: biomechanical results after biodegradable interference fit fixation in a model of anterior cruciate ligament reconstruction in sheep. Arthroscopy 18:113–123

24. Amiel D, Kleiner JB, Roux RD et al (1986) The phenomenon of "ligamentization": anterior cruciate ligament reconstruction with autogenous patellar tendon. J Orthop Res 4:162–172

25. Stener S, Ejerhed L, Movin T et al (2012) The reharvested patellar tendon has the potential for ligamentization when used for anterior cruciate ligament revision surgery. Knee Surg Sports Traumatol Arthrosc 20:1168–1174

26. Rougraff BT, Shelbourne KD (1999) Early histologic appearance of human patellar tendon autografts used for anterior cruciate ligament reconstruction. Knee Surg Sports Traumatol Arthrosc 7:9–14

27. Amiel D, Frank C, Harwood F et al (1984) Tendons and ligaments: a morphological and biochemical comparison. J Orthop Res 1:257–265

28. Amiel D, Kleiner JB, Akeson WH (1986) The natural history of the anterior cruciate ligament autograft of patellar tendon origin. Am J Sports Med 14: 449–462

29. Kleiner JB, Amiel D, Harwood FL et al (1989) Early histological, metabolic, and vascular assessment of anterior cruciate ligament autografts. J Orthop Res 7:235–242

30. Arnoczky SP, Tarvin GB, Marshall JL (1982) Anterior cruciate ligament replacement using patellar tendon. An evaluation of graft revascularization in the dog. J Bone Joint Surg 64-A:217–224

31. Shino K, Kawasaki T, Hirose H et al (1984) Replacement of the anterior cruciate ligament by an allogeneic tendon graft. An experimental study in the dog. J Bone Joint Surg 66-B:672–681

32. Kleiner JB, Amiel D, Roux RD et al (1986) Origin of replacement cells for the anterior cruciate ligament autograft. J Orthop Res 4:466–474

33. Shino K, Horibe S (1991) Experimental ligament reconstruction by allogeneic tendon graft in a canine model. Acta Orthop Belg 57(Suppl 2):44–53

34. Yoshikawa T, Tohyama H, Katsura T (2006) Effects of local administration of vascular endothelial growth factor on mechanical characteristics of the semitendinosus tendon graft after anterior cruciate ligament reconstruction in sheep. Am J Sports Med 34:1918–1925

35. Goradia VK, Rochat MC, Grana WA et al (2000) Tendon-to-bone healing of a semitendinosus tendon autograft used for ACL reconstruction in a sheep model. Am J Knee Surg 13:143–151

36. Papageorgiou CD, Ma CB, Abramowitch SD et al (2001) A multidisciplinary study of the healing of an intra-articular anterior cruciate ligament graft in a goat model. Am J Sports Med 29:620–626

37. Grana WA, Egle DM, Mahnken R et al (1994) An analysis of autograft fixation after anterior cruciate ligament reconstruction in a rabbit model. Am J Sports Med 22:344–351

38. Weiler A, Förster C, Hunt P et al (2004) The influence of locally applied platelet-derived growth factor-BB on free tendon graft remodeling after anterior cruciate ligament reconstruction. Am J Sports Med 32:881–891

39. Jackson JR, Minton JA, Ho ML et al (1997) Expression of vascular endothelial growth factor in synovial fibroblasts is induced by hypoxia and interleukin 1beta. J Rheumatol 24:1253–1259

40. Kuroda R, Kurosaka M, Yoshiya S et al (2000) Localization of growth factors in the reconstructed anterior cruciate ligament: immunohistological study in dogs. Knee Surg Sports Traumatol Arthrosc 8:120–126

41. Kawamura S, Ying L, Kim HJ et al (2005) Macrophages accumulate in the early phase of tendon-bone healing. J Orthop Res 23:1425–1432

42. Murray MM, Martin SD, Martin TL et al (2000) Histological changes in the human anterior cruciate ligament after rupture. J Bone Joint Surg 82-A:1387–1397

43. Weiler A, Unterhauser FN, Bail HJ et al (2002) Alpha-smooth muscle actin is expressed by fibroblastic cells of the ovine anterior cruciate ligament and its free tendon graft during remodeling. J Orthop Res 20:310–317

44. Unterhauser FN, Bosch U, Zeichen J et al (2004) Alpha-smooth muscle actin containing contractile fibroblastic cells in human knee arthrofibrosis tissue. Winner of the AGA-DonJoy Award 2003. Arch Orthop Trauma Surg 124:585–591

45. Ballock RT, Woo SL, Lyon RM et al (1989) Use of patellar tendon autograft for anterior cruciate ligament reconstruction in the rabbit: a long-term histologic and biomechanical study. J Orthop Res 7:474–485

46. Jackson DW, Grood ES, Goldstein JD et al (1993) A comparison of patellar tendon autograft and allograft used for anterior cruciate ligament reconstruction in the goat model. Am J Sports Med 21:176–185

47. Unterhauser FN, Bail HJ, Höher J et al (2003) Endoligamentous revascularization of an anterior cruciate ligament graft. Clin Orthop Relat Res 414:276–288

48. Petersen W, Wildemann B, Pufe T et al (2003) The angiogenic peptide pleiotrophin (PTN/HB-GAM) is expressed in fracture healing: an immunohistochemical study in rats. Arch Orthop Trauma Surg 124:603–607

49. Tohyama H, Yasuda K (2002) The effect of increased stress on the patellar tendon. J Bone Joint Surg 84-B:440–446

50. Jackson DW, Grood ES, Cohn BT et al (1991) The effects of in situ freezing on the anterior cruciate ligament. An experimental study in goats. J Bone Joint Surg 73-A:201–213

51. Spindler KP, Andrish JT, Miller RR et al (1996) Distribution of cellular repopulation and collagen synthesis in a canine anterior cruciate ligament autograft. J Orthop Res 14:384–389

52. Blickenstaff KR, Grana WA, Egle D (1997) Analysis of a semitendinosus autograft in a rabbit model. Am J Sports Med 25:554–559

53. Johnson LL (1993) The outcome of a free autogenous semitendinosus tendon graft in human anterior cruciate reconstructive surgery: a histological study. Arthroscopy 9:131–142

54. Abe S, Kurosaka M, Iguchi T et al (1993) Light and electron microscopic study of remodeling and maturation process in autogenous graft for anterior cruciate ligament reconstruction. Arthroscopy 9:394–405

55. Liu SH, Yang RS, al-Shaikh R et al (1995) Collagen in tendon, ligament, and bone healing. A current review. Clin Orthop Relat Res 318:265–278

56. Ng GY, Oakes BW, Deacon OW et al (1995) Biomechanics of patellar tendon autograft for reconstruction of the anterior cruciate ligament in the goat: three-year study. J Orthop Res 13:602–608

57. Ng GY, Oakes BW, Deacon OW et al (1996) Long-term study of the biochemistry and biomechanics of anterior cruciate ligament-patellar tendon autografts in goats. J Orthop Res 14:851–856

58. Scranton PE Jr, Lanzer WL, Ferguson MS et al (1998) Mechanisms of anterior cruciate ligament neovascularization and ligamentization. Arthroscopy 14:702–716

59. Ohno K, Yasuda K, Yamamoto N et al (1993) Effects of complete stress-shielding on the mechanical properties and histology of in situ frozen patellar tendon. J Orthop Res 11:592–602

60. Shelbourne KD, Nitz P (1990) Accelerated rehabilitation after anterior cruciate ligament reconstruction. Am J Sports Med 18:292–299

61. Howell SM, Taylor MA (1996) Brace–free rehabilitation, with early return to activity, for knees

reconstructed with a double-looped semitendinosus and gracilis graft. J Bone Joint Surg 78-A:814–825

62. Beynnon BD, Johnson RJ, Naud S et al (2011) Accelerated versus nonaccelerated rehabilitation after anterior cruciate ligament reconstruction: a prospective, randomized, double blind investigation evaluating knee joint laxity using stereophotogrammetric analysis. Am J Sports Med 39:2536–2548

63. Beynnon BD, Uh BS, Johnson RJ et al (2005) Rehabilitation after anterior cruciate ligament reconstruction: a prospective, randomized, double-blind comparison of programs administered over 2 different time intervals. Am J Sports Med 33:347–359

64. Janssen RP, Du Mée AW, van Valkenburg J et al (2012) Anterior cruciate ligament reconstruction with hamstring tendons and accelerated rehabilitation: a 10-year prospective study on clinical results, knee osteoarthritis and its predictors. Knee Surg Sports Traumatol Arthrosc 21:1977–1988. doi:10.1007/s00167-012-2234-9

65. Fujimoto E, Sumen Y, Urabe Y et al (2004) An early return to vigorous activity may destabilize anterior cruciate ligaments reconstructed with hamstring grafts. Arch Phys Med Rehabil 85:298–302

66. Dustmann M, Schmidt T, Gangey I et al (2008) The extracellular remodeling of free-soft-tissue autografts and allografts for reconstruction of the anterior cruciate ligament: a comparison study in sheep model. Knee Surg Sports Traumatol Arthrosc 16:360–369

Semitendinosus and Gracilis Tendon Regeneration Following Harvest

Martina Åhlén, Mattias Lidén, and Jüri Kartus

Contents

26.1 Background

Studies have shown that the semitendinosus (ST) and gracilis (G) tendons are able to regenerate after harvest, and probably they are the only known tendons in the human body that can regenerate after harvest of the whole tendon from the musculotendinous junction all the way to the insertion. This chapter will focus on the existing knowledge about the ST and G tendon regeneration frequency, quality of the regenerated tendon, level of insertion, cross-sectional area and weakness in flexion and internal rotation of the knee after harvest.

26.2 What the Diagnostic Methods Have Shown: The Regeneration Rate and Morphology

In 1992 Cross et al. [6] were the first to report that the ST and G tendons could regenerate after examining patients with magnetic resonance imaging (MRI). These findings have subsequently been verified using MRI [2, 5, 7, 9, 13, 18, 28, 30, 33], computed tomography [19, 21] and ultrasonography [27] after both ST and G tendon harvests. However, the reported regeneration rates differ from 46 % [33] to 95 % [2] (Figs. 26.1 and 26.2). Likewise, the insertion place of the regenerated tendons differs. Studies [2, 5, 8, 19] have concordantly reported a nearly

M. Åhlén, MD • J. Kartus, MD, PhD (✉)
Department of Orthopedics, NU-Hospital Group,
Trollhättan/Uddevalla, Sweden
e-mail: juri.kartus@vgregion.se

M. Lidén, MD, PhD
Department of Plastic Surgery, Sahlgrenska
University Hospital, Göteborg, Sweden

R. Siebold et al. (eds.), *Anterior Cruciate Ligament Reconstruction*,
DOI 10.1007/978-3-642-45349-6_26, © ESSKA 2014

Fig. 26.1 Ahlen et al. (Originally published in Ahlen et al. [2]) have reported that 95 % of the tendons regenerated after harvest of both the *ST* and *G*. Axial MRI of the operated right side demonstrates how the measurements were done. The cross-sectional area was calculated 4 cm above the centre of the joint line (*A*), and the tendons were followed until they merged on the pes anserinus (*B–E*)

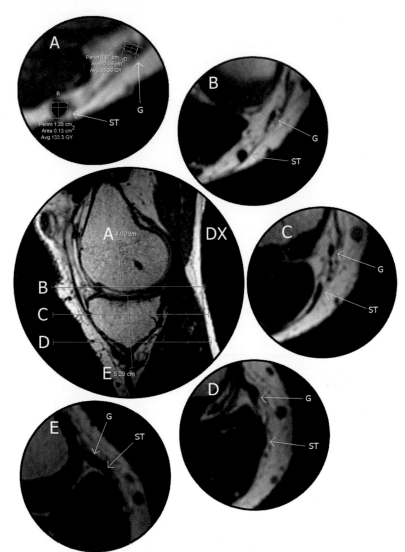

normal insertion place of the regenerated ST and G tendons compared to the initially reported more proximal [30, 36] and medial insertion [6, 27]. An explanation for this could be that only the ST tendon is harvested and the G tendon is left in place in some studies [8, 19]. However, since studies where both tendons were harvested have shown a nearly normal insertion place [2, 5], additional factors such as different time intervals between the harvesting procedure and the radiographic examination must be considered. This is supported by Nakame et al. [19] in a study using 3D CT, where they described that no patient had evidence of regeneration after 1 month, and

all but two patients out of 29 showed regenerated tendon tissue after 12 months. The tendons coursed as expected from the muscle bellies to their normal insertion site on the proximal tibia. There are reports that the regenerated tendons are hypertrophied in the early phase [36] but gradually decrease in cross-sectional area [27]. While studies with a long-term follow-up report a close to normal regenerated tendon cross-sectional area [2, 5, 27].

Another contributing factor to the inconsistency in the reported regeneration rate and insertion place could be differences in the harvesting procedure. Choi et al. [5] who performed MRI

Fig. 26.2 Axial MRI of the nonoperated left side from the same patient showing that the cross-sectional area of the tendons and the point of insertion on the pes anserinus were similar compared to the operated side (Originally published in Ahlen et al. [2]). Levels (*A–E*) correspond to the same levels as in Fig. 26.1, *ST* and *G* correspond to normal non harvested tendons, *SIN* corresponds to the left side

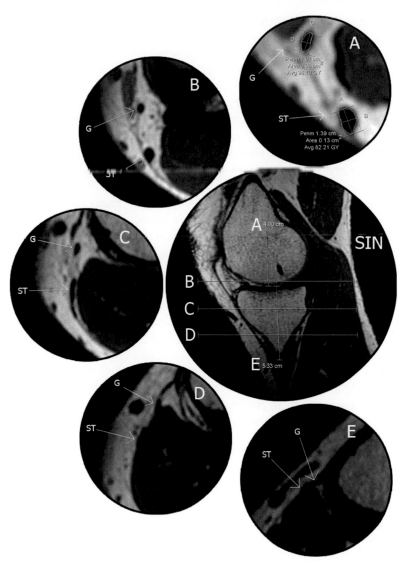

before harvest and a minimum of 2 years post harvest of both the ST and G tendons are one of the few authors who noticed a more distal insertion of the regenerated tendons than their original site. They describe that when harvesting the tendons, they used a "delicate reverse L-shaped" incision and preservation of the sartorius fascia to protect the regenerating tube. Other factors of influence could be the way of defining the insertion point, differences in the size of the study population and the female/male ratio.

There are studies with long follow-up times from harvest to tendon assessment where a few patients do not display regenerated tendon. The cause of this is not known. Too aggressive postoperative rehabilitation could rupture a weak tendon structure in the first months after harvest, and comorbidities or smoking could also influence the regeneration rate.

26.3 How Does the Tendon Regenerate?

Initially, it was suggested that the tendon regenerates in a proximal to distal direction [28], and Leis et al. [16] termed it "the lizard tail phenomenon". However, the present opinion is that the tendon matures uniformly along the harvest site. In a comprehensive review from 2005, Carofino and Fulkerson [4] suggested that the regeneration process proceeds through several stages and that it takes approximately 18 months to yield a neo-tendon that is similar to a normal tendon in structure and composition. His statement is partly based on the findings of Papandrea et al. [27] who performed serial ultrasonography in the same patients. They registered an initial haematoma followed by an oedema with gradual solidification along the entire harvest site. After 6 months they were able to detect collagen fibres, and at 18 months there was a structure with the morphology of a normal tendon at the harvest site.

Additional support for this theory was recently presented by Otoshi et al. [26], using an animal model to assess tendon regeneration in Achilles tendons. The authors describe a similar regeneration and maturation process uniformly along the length of the regenerated tendon and conclude that the haematoma scaffold enhances migration of fibroblast precursor cells from the surrounding peritendinous tissue and tendon sheath.

It has been suggested [12] that the ST tendon has a better potential of remodelling than the patellar tendon due to its significantly higher density of collagen fibrils and fibroblasts and that the surgical method "stripping" when harvesting the tendons plays an important role in the regenerative process [24] since synovial cells possess the ability to differentiate when subjected to mechanical stress. Eriksson et al. [8] proposed that the initially formed haematoma, also described by Papandrea et al. [27], that occupies the harvest defect acts as a scaffold for fibrocyte migration and the subsequent tendon regeneration.

The present opinion is that the tendon maturation occurs uniformly along the harvest defect, there is an initially formed haematoma where synovial cells differentiate and there is a gradual collagen deposition, and by approximately one and a half year, there is a structure with the morphology of a normal tendon at the harvest site.

26.4 Is the Regenerated Tendon Real Tendon or Just Scar Tissue?

There are few published studies [8, 10, 24, 38] addressing the histological appearance of the regenerated ST tendon. The studies confirm that it is essentially real tendon tissue that regenerates and not just scar tissue. Eriksson et al. [8] obtained open biopsies from the tendon in five patients, 20 months after harvest, and described that the regenerated tendons showed the features of a normal tendon, but there were focal small scar-like areas with more irregularly oriented collagen, increased fibroblastic proliferation and capillary formation compared to normal control tendon. Okahashi et al. [24] obtained surgical biopsies 1 year after ACL reconstruction in nine patients. They found that histologically and immunohistochemically, the regenerated tendon closely resembles normal tendon. However, no regularity in the cell nucleus size, shape or distribution was found in the regenerated tendon. Ferretti et al. [10] obtained open biopsies from regenerated tendon in three patients, one after 6 months and two after 2 years. In the specimens retrieved 2 years postoperatively, the central thicker portion of the specimen was occupied by well-orientated tendon-like fibres together with uniformly distributed spindle-shaped cells that had the appearance of mature tenocytes. One of the longest reported time periods, between harvest and the biopsy procedure, is still less than 2.5 years [8], and it is possible that then the postoperative maturation process is not completed yet. A long-term histological study was done by Ahlen et al. (In February 2014 yet unpublished material) where biopsies from the regenerated ST tendon were compared with normal ST tendon from the same patient. Preliminary results indicate no differences between the regenerated ST tendon compared with the normal ST tendon, but that there were some focal areas with scar tissue formation in the regenerated tendons.

To assess the final histological outcome for the entire tendon and cover the full regeneration process, the optimal would be a long-term serial study with histological examination of the entire regenerated tissue with comparisons to normal tendon.

26.5 Loss of Strength and Morbidity Following Harvest of the Tendons

The muscular function of the ST and G is important, particularly in terms of deep flexion and internal rotation of the knee. If the tendons fail to completely regenerate or if they have a more proximal insertion, it is likely that the biomechanics of the knee will change. A proximal insertion place would make the tendons' lever arms shorter and a proximal shift of the musculotendinous junction would lead to shortened muscle bellies, and the muscles' ability to flex the knee would be limited, whereas an insertion place located to the medial tibia fascia or popliteal fascia would reduce the ability to generate force in internal rotation. It is possible that weakness in internal rotation results in reduced protection ability towards pivoting and external rotation of the knee, for instance, during cutting manoeuvres.

Consequently, ST and G autografts may be less suitable for athletes dependent on strength in deep knee flexion, such as gymnasts, ballet dancers, orienteers and wrestlers. There are studies reporting that patients regain strength in knee flexion [30, 37] and internal rotation [2], but there are also reports of remaining weakness in deep flexion [2, 5, 20, 34] and internal rotation more than 2 years after harvest [3, 29, 35]. However, most of the studies reporting full recovery of the flexion strength after harvest studied the peak torque, which is known to be a less sensitive measure of ST and G strength. The peak torque is generated at low knee flexion angles (15–30°), and at those angles the biceps femoris muscle is the primary knee flexor [25]. Both Ohkoshi et al. [23] and Adachi et al. [1] found that the peak torque was generated at shallower angles after ACL reconstruction with ST or ST/G autograft indicating that muscles that are active at lower flexion angles such as biceps femoris have undergone hypertrophy. Further studies have shown that the semimembranosus and biceps femoris undergo compensatory hypertrophy after harvest of the ST/G or ST alone [7, 14, 36]. The ST/G complex is most important in deep knee flexion angles, e.g. more than 75° [25], and it has also

been suggested that the tendons play a greater role in flexion when the hip is extended [34].

Several researchers [2, 5, 19, 20, 33, 34] report a significant deficit in deep knee flexion strength, regardless of morphologic regeneration.

Both for internal rotation [29] and deep knee flexion [34], there are reports of more strength deficit after harvesting both ST and G tendons compared with only the ST tendon. Tashiro et al. [34] who are one of the few conducting a randomized prospective study reported a significant weakness up to 30 % in muscle strength at knee flexion angles greater than 70°. They compared single- and double-tendon harvest and found that the weakness could be minimized if the gracilis tendon was preserved.

Williams et al. [36] found that the muscle bellies of the ST/G remained shortened after regeneration of the tendons, and Nishino et al. [22] who studied the relationship between knee flexion torque and the morphology of the ST muscle after ACL reconstruction found that deficits in deep knee flexion were associated with atrophy and shortening of the ST muscle. This persistent shortening of the ST/G muscles in regenerated tendons was further confirmed in 2011 by Choi et al. [5]. They reported that the musculotendinous junction shifted proximally by approximately 4 cm for the ST tendon and 3 cm for the G tendon resulting in significant weakness in deep knee flexion, minimum 2 years after surgery. This is in line with the findings of Ahlen et al. [2] who reported a significant weakness in deep knee flexion 8 years after harvest, even though the tendons had regenerated and regained a nearly normal insertion position on the pes anserinus in the majority of patients.

26.6 Can the Regenerated Tendons Be Used for Revision Surgery?

One essential question is whether regenerated ST/G tendon can be used for ACL revision surgery in the same way as has been reported for the patellar tendon. MRI [15, 32] and biopsy studies [15, 31] reveal that the patellar tendon does not normalize after harvest of its central third. In spite of that, reharvested patellar tendon has been used for ACL revision surgery, but with inferior results compared to primary harvested patellar tendon autograft [17]. In animal models the biomechanical strength in regenerated ST [11, 16] and Achilles tendons [26] has been described to be inferior to normal tendon up to 1 year after harvest, but with a trend of increasing strength over time [16]. To this date there is only one report in the literature of regenerated ST tendon used for revision ACL surgery [38].

Since the ST/G tendon regeneration is unpredictable in terms of focal scarring and until studies have been done with long-term biomechanical testing in humans, it is our opinion that regenerated ST/G tendon cannot be recommended for ACL revision surgery.

Memory
- The reason why the tendons sometimes fail to regenerate needs further research. The reported regeneration frequency and insertion place differ among studies.
- Further prospective long-term studies evaluating the histology of the regenerated tendon are needed.
- Persistent weakness in deep knee flexion after harvest is present in most patients after harvest of the ST or ST/G tendons.
- If possible, harvest of only the semitendinosus should be performed since there are indications that the strength deficit in internal rotation and deep knee flexion then could diminish.
- It is the authors' opinion that until further studies have been done, regenerated ST or G tendons should not be used for revision surgery.

References

1. Adachi N, Ochi M, Uchio Y, Sakai Y, Kuriwaka M, Fujihara A (2003) Harvesting hamstring tendons for ACL reconstruction influences postoperative hamstring muscle performance. Arch Orthop Trauma Surg 123(9):460–465
2. Ahlen M, Liden M, Bovaller A, Sernert N, Kartus J (2012) Bilateral magnetic resonance imaging and functional assessment of the semitendinosus and gracilis tendons a minimum of 6 years after ipsilateral harvest for anterior cruciate ligament reconstruction. Am J Sports Med 40(8):1735–1741. doi:10.1177/0363546512449611, 0363546512449611 [pii]
3. Armour T, Forwell L, Litchfield R, Kirkley A, Amendola N, Fowler PJ (2004) Isokinetic evaluation of internal/external tibial rotation strength after the use of hamstring tendons for anterior cruciate ligament reconstruction. Am J Sports Med 32(7):1639–1643
4. Carofino B, Fulkerson J (2005) Medial hamstring tendon regeneration following harvest for anterior cruciate ligament reconstruction: fact, myth, and clinical implication. Arthroscopy 21(10):1257–1265. doi:10.1016/j.arthro.2005.07.002, S0749-8063(05)01089-3 [pii]
5. Choi JY, Ha JK, Kim YW, Shim JC, Yang SJ, Kim JG (2012) Relationships among tendon regeneration on MRI, flexor strength, and functional performance after anterior cruciate ligament reconstruction with hamstring autograft. Am J Sports Med 40(1):152–162. doi:10.1177/0363546511424134, 0363546511424134 [pii]
6. Cross MJ, Roger G, Kujawa P, Anderson IF (1992) Regeneration of the semitendinosus and gracilis tendons following their transection for repair of the anterior cruciate ligament. Am J Sports Med 20(2):221–223
7. Eriksson K, Hamberg P, Jansson E, Larsson H, Shalabi A, Wredmark T (2001) Semitendinosus muscle in anterior cruciate ligament surgery: morphology and function. Arthroscopy 17(8):808–817, S0749806301080896 [pii]
8. Eriksson K, Kindblom LG, Hamberg P, Larsson H, Wredmark T (2001) The semitendinosus tendon regenerates after resection: a morphologic and MRI analysis in 6 patients after resection for anterior cruciate ligament reconstruction. Acta Orthop Scand 72(4):379–384
9. Eriksson K, Larsson H, Wredmark T, Hamberg P (1999) Semitendinosus tendon regeneration after harvesting for ACL reconstruction. A prospective MRI study. Knee Surg Sports Traumatol Arthrosc 7(4):220–225
10. Ferretti A, Conteduca F, Morelli F, Masi V (2002) Regeneration of the semitendinosus tendon after its use in anterior cruciate ligament reconstruction: a histologic study of three cases. Am J Sports Med 30(2):204–207
11. Gill SS, Turner MA, Battaglia TC, Leis HT, Balian G, Miller MD (2004) Semitendinosus regrowth: biochemical, ultrastructural, and physiological characterization of the regenerate tendon. Am J Sports Med 32(5):1173–1181
12. Hadjicostas PT, Soucacos PN, Paessler HH, Koleganova N, Berger I (2007) Morphologic and

histologic comparison between the patella and hamstring tendons grafts: a descriptive and anatomic study. Arthroscopy 23(7):751–756. doi:10.1016/j.arthro.2007.02.002, S0749-8063(07)00139-9 [pii]

13. Hioki S, Fukubayashi T, Ikeda K, Niitsu M, Ochiai N (2003) Effect of harvesting the hamstrings tendon for anterior cruciate ligament reconstruction on the morphology and movement of the hamstrings muscle: a novel MRI technique. Knee Surg Sports Traumatol Arthrosc 11(4):223–227. doi:10.1007/s00167-003-0361-z

14. Irie K, Tomatsu T (2002) Atrophy of semitendinosus and gracilis and flexor mechanism function after hamstring tendon harvest for anterior cruciate ligament reconstruction. Orthopedics 25(5):491–495

15. Kartus J, Movin T, Papadogiannakis N, Christensen LR, Lindahl S, Karlsson J (2000) A radiographic and histologic evaluation of the patellar tendon after harvesting its central third. Am J Sports Med 28(2):218–226

16. Leis HT, Sanders TG, Larsen KM, Lancaster-Weiss KJ, Miller MD (2003) Hamstring regrowth following harvesting for ACL reconstruction: the lizard tail phenomenon. J Knee Surg 16(3):159–164

17. Liden M, Ejerhed L, Sernert N, Bovaller A, Karlsson J, Kartus J (2006) The course of the patellar tendon after reharvesting its central third for ACL revision surgery: a long-term clinical and radiographic study. Knee Surg Sports Traumatol Arthrosc 14(11):1130–1138. doi:10.1007/s00167-006-0167-x

18. Makihara Y, Nishino A, Fukubayashi T, Kanamori A (2006) Decrease of knee flexion torque in patients with ACL reconstruction: combined analysis of the architecture and function of the knee flexor muscles. Knee Surg Sports Traumatol Arthrosc 14(4):310–317. doi:10.1007/s00167-005-0701-2

19. Nakamae A, Deie M, Yasumoto M, Adachi N, Kobayashi K, Yasunaga Y, Ochi M (2005) Three-dimensional computed tomography imaging evidence of regeneration of the semitendinosus tendon harvested for anterior cruciate ligament reconstruction: a comparison with hamstring muscle strength. J Comput Assist Tomogr 29(2):241–245, 00004728-200503000-00018 [pii]

20. Nakamura N, Horibe S, Sasaki S, Kitaguchi T, Tagami M, Mitsuoka T, Toritsuka Y, Hamada M, Shino K (2002) Evaluation of active knee flexion and hamstring strength after anterior cruciate ligament reconstruction using hamstring tendons. Arthroscopy 18(6):598–602

21. Nakamura E, Mizuta H, Kadota M, Katahira K, Kudo S, Takagi K (2004) Three-dimensional computed tomography evaluation of semitendinosus harvest after anterior cruciate ligament reconstruction. Arthroscopy 20(4):360–365. doi:10.1016/j.arthro.2004.01.032, S0749806304000830 [pii]

22. Nishino A, Sanada A, Kanehisa H, Fukubayashi T (2006) Knee-flexion torque and morphology of the semitendinosus after ACL reconstruction. Med Sci Sports Exerc 38(11):1895–1900. doi:10.1249/01.mss.0000230344.71623.51, 00005768-200611000-00003 [pii]

23. Ohkoshi Y, Inoue C, Yamane S, Hashimoto T, Ishida R (1998) Changes in muscle strength properties caused by harvesting of autogenous semitendinosus tendon for reconstruction of contralateral anterior cruciate ligament. Arthroscopy 14(6):580–584

24. Okahashi K, Sugimoto K, Iwai M, Oshima M, Samma M, Fujisawa Y, Takakura Y (2006) Regeneration of the hamstring tendons after harvesting for arthroscopic anterior cruciate ligament reconstruction: a histological study in 11 patients. Knee Surg Sports Traumatol Arthrosc 14(6):542–545. doi:10.1007/s00167-006-0068-z

25. Onishi H, Yagi R, Oyama M, Akasaka K, Ihashi K, Handa Y (2002) EMG-angle relationship of the hamstring muscles during maximum knee flexion. J Electromyogr Kinesiol 12(5):399–406, S1050641102000330 [pii]

26. Otoshi K, Kikuchi S, Ohi G, Numazaki H, Sekiguchi M, Konno S (2011) The process of tendon regeneration in an achilles tendon resection rat model as a model for hamstring regeneration after harvesting for anterior cruciate ligament reconstruction. Arthroscopy 27(2):218–227. doi:10.1016/j.arthro.2010.07.012, S0749-8063(10)00691-2 [pii]

27. Papandrea P, Vulpiani MC, Ferretti A, Conteduca F (2000) Regeneration of the semitendinosus tendon harvested for anterior cruciate ligament reconstruction. Evaluation using ultrasonography. Am J Sports Med 28(4):556–561

28. Rispoli DM, Sanders TG, Miller MD, Morrison WB (2001) Magnetic resonance imaging at different time periods following hamstring harvest for anterior cruciate ligament reconstruction. Arthroscopy 17(1):2–8. doi:10.1053/jars.2001.19460, S0749-8063(01)30106-8 [pii]

29. Segawa H, Omori G, Koga Y, Kameo T, Iida S, Tanaka M (2002) Rotational muscle strength of the limb after anterior cruciate ligament reconstruction using semitendinosus and gracilis tendon. Arthroscopy 18(2):177–182

30. Simonian PT, Harrison SD, Cooley VJ, Escabedo EM, Deneka DA, Larson RV (1997) Assessment of morbidity of semitendinosus and gracilis tendon harvest for ACL reconstruction. Am J Knee Surg 10(2):54–59

31. Svensson M, Kartus J, Christensen LR, Movin T, Papadogiannakis N, Karlsson J (2005) A long-term serial histological evaluation of the patellar tendon in humans after harvesting its central third. Knee Surg Sports Traumatol Arthrosc 13(5):398–404

32. Svensson M, Kartus J, Ejerhed L, Lindahl S, Karlsson J (2004) Does the patellar tendon normalize after harvesting its central third? A prospective long-term MRI study. Am J Sports Med 32(1):34–38

33. Tadokoro K, Matsui N, Yagi M, Kuroda R, Kurosaka M, Yoshiya S (2004) Evaluation of hamstring strength and tendon regrowth after harvesting for anterior cruciate ligament reconstruction. Am J Sports Med 32(7):1644–1650

34. Tashiro T, Kurosawa H, Kawakami A, Hikita A, Fukui N (2003) Influence of medial hamstring tendon harvest on knee flexor strength after anterior cruciate

ligament reconstruction. A detailed evaluation with comparison of single- and double-tendon harvest. Am J Sports Med 31(4):522–529

35. Viola RW, Sterett WI, Newfield D, Steadman JR, Torry MR (2000) Internal and external tibial rotation strength after anterior cruciate ligament reconstruction using ipsilateral semitendinosus and gracilis tendon autografts. Am J Sports Med 28(4):552–555

36. Williams GN, Snyder-Mackler L, Barrance PJ, Axe MJ, Buchanan TS (2004) Muscle and tendon morphology after reconstruction of the anterior cruciate ligament with autologous semitendinosus-gracilis graft. J Bone Joint Surg Am 86-A(9):1936–1946, 86/9/1936 [pii]

37. Yasuda K, Tsujino J, Ohkoshi Y, Tanabe Y, Kaneda K (1995) Graft site morbidity with autogenous semitendinosus and gracilis tendons. Am J Sports Med 23(6):706–714

38. Yoshiya S, Matsui N, Matsumoto A, Kuroda R, Lee S, Kurosaka M (2004) Revision anterior cruciate ligament reconstruction using the regenerated semitendinosus tendon: analysis of ultrastructure of the regenerated tendon. Arthroscopy 20(5):532–535. doi:10.1016/j.arthro.2004.01.031, S0749806304000829 [pii]

Long-Term Outcome of ACL Reconstruction

27

Steven Claes, Rene Verdonk, Johan Bellemans and Peter C. Verdonk

Contents

27.1 Introduction

The occurrence of osteoarthritis (OA) is often thought of as a near-inevitable long-term consequence of ACL injury, with prevalences of 50–80 % reported a decade after the initial trauma [18, 36]. In this view, ACL tears are often quoted as being responsible for a large percentage of the "young patients with old knees," [18, 37] irrespective of the treatment method. Although surgical ACL reconstruction using tendon grafts has become the current standard of care to treat the functionally unstable ACL-deficient knee [36], controversy remains to exist regarding the effect of ACL reconstruction on the development of knee OA in this generally young population. Current literature contains a number of reports suggesting that the prevalence of OA remains unchanged whether or not the ACL is surgically reconstructed [14, 19], but Daniel et al. [4] even detected an increased incidence of OA in the ACL-reconstructed group. On the other end of the spectrum, some authors seem to maintain excellent results a decade after ACL reconstruction, with reported OA prevalences of 2–3 % [14, 29].

Current controversy on the occurrence of OA after ACL reconstruction has been fueled by rather small, heterogeneous, and retrospective case series and expert opinions [3, 19, 22, 23, 30, 32]. Therefore, this chapter compiles the current literature on long-term outcome after autologous ACL reconstruction while conducting a thorough meta-analysis to obtain evidence-based

S. Claes, MD, PhD (✉)
Department of Orthopedic Surgery,
Algemeen Ziekenhuis Herentals, Herentals, Belgium
e-mail: steven.claes@azherentals.be

Department of Orthopedic Surgery,
University Hospitals Leuven, Leuven, Belgium

R. Verdonk, MD, PhD
Department of Orthopaedics and Traumatology,
Jan Palfyn Ziekenhuis, Ghent, Belgium

J. Bellemans, MD
Testeltsesteenweg 24,
Langdorp, Belgium

P. C. Verdonk, MD, PhD
Antwerp Orthopedic Center,
Monica Hospitals Antwerp, Antwerp, Belgium

Faculty of Medicine, Ghent University,
Ghent, Belgium

R. Siebold et al. (eds.), *Anterior Cruciate Ligament Reconstruction*,
DOI 10.1007/978-3-642-45349-6_27, © ESSKA 2014

prevalences of (radiographic) OA. In addition, the relationship between meniscal status and the occurrence of OA in the ACL-reconstructed knee will be unraveled.

27.2 Methods

This meta-analysis was set up and reported according to the recommendations proposed by the PRISMA statement [24].

A systematic review of the literature was performed in order to identify all studies concerning the long-term outcome after autologous ACL reconstruction in the human knee. "Long-term" outcome was defined as a mean follow-up of minimum 10 years. The PubMed MEDLINE, EMBASE, and Cochrane Library databases were searched from their earliest entry points to October 2010.

Searches were limited to studies published in English and French. Studies reporting on long-term outcome after ACL reconstruction without radiographic evaluation were excluded. Reports with a mean follow-up less than 10 years were excluded as well.

Each study was evaluated for the following variables: study type; mean follow-up after ACL reconstruction; operative technique; time period of surgery; number of patients with radiographs at final follow-up; number of patients with meniscectomy prior to, at the time of, or after ACL reconstruction within this group; and number of patients with radiographic OA of operated knee. Relevant data from each included study was extracted and recorded on multiple worksheets.

The definition of OA in this chapter is exclusively based on radiological criteria, due to the obvious lack of reported data combining both clinical and radiological aspects of OA in current literature. Furthermore, the presence of different radiological classification systems for OA used in the studied reports (e.g., Kellgren and Lawrence, Ahlbäck, Fairbanks, IKDC) necessitated the development of a conversion method for the various OA scores in order to allow subsequent statistical analysis. Due to its widespread use and reliability [21], the "IKDC radiographic grading

system" [10] was chosen as the reference classification to which other scores were translated to best effort. With regard to OA, IKDC grades A and B were considered as being normal or nearly normal, while IKDC grades C and D were considered to represent OA of the knee.

Many included reports mention a subpopulation of meniscectomized patients at final follow-up. The radiographic outcome of this subset of patients was studied separately in order to evaluate the impact of meniscectomy on the prevalence of OA. Subjects treated with meniscal repair were appointed to the non-meniscectomy group, unless failure of the suture was reported during follow-up.

Meta-analyses were performed to obtain the average prevalence of OA and the difference between patients with and without meniscectomy. Considered study estimates are the log-transformed OA odds and odds ratios (and risk ratios), the latter expressing the effect of meniscectomy on OA. The random-effects approach of DerSimonian and Laird [5] was used to take into account the heterogeneity in the combination of the results of the studies. P values smaller than 0.05 are considered significant. All analyses have been performed using SAS software, version 9.2 of the SAS System for Windows (SAS Institute Inc., Cary, NC, USA).

27.3 Results

The computerized search using the aforementioned search terms delivered 211 studies describing outcome after ACL reconstruction. With regard to study selection, the PRISMA flow diagram [24] applied to all identified studies has been described in detail before [2]. Finally, only 16 reports could be included for systematic review and meta-analysis [3, 6, 7, 11, 14–16, 19, 22, 23, 27–29, 32, 34, 35], accounting for a total number of 1,554 subjects available for meta-analysis. This number represents all patients available for radiographic examination at the time of follow-up, not at inclusion. The presence or absence of associated meniscal lesions necessitating resection before, during, or after ACL reconstruction was mentioned in 11 out of 16 included articles, accounting for a total of 614 meniscectomized subjects on a total of 1,264 (48.6 %). Only 5 of the included reports were set up as a prospective study, with the remaining 11 studies being retrospective in nature.

The combined estimate for the prevalence of OA (IKDC C or D) from the random-effects meta-analysis on 1,554 included knees equaled *27.9 %* (95 % CI: 16.3–43.5 %). However when looking at the subgroups, the combined estimate for the prevalence of OA equaled *16.4 %* (95 % CI: 7.0–33.9 %) in patients *without meniscectomy* but *50.4 %* (95 % CI: 27.4–73.1 %) in patients *with meniscectomy*. The combined odds ratio therefore equaled 3.54 (95 % CI: 2.56–4.91), meaning that the odds for having OA is 3.54 times higher after meniscectomy.

27.4   Discussion

The key message of this chapter is that the *prevalence of OA after ACL reconstruction is probably lower than commonly thought*. From the early days on, ACL rupture has been linked with the occurrence of premature OA in the injured knee [9, 12, 20]. Remarkably, contemporary ACL reconstruction techniques have not been able to change this common belief. Indeed, many still consider early OA as an almost inevitable consequence of ACL reconstruction, with reported OA prevalence between 50 and 100 % [13, 17]. This first-ever meta-analysis on ACL reconstruction and OA shows that the use of this dramatically high prevalence is not justifiable on the basis of the available evidence in current literature. On the contrary, our results indicate that the prevalence of knee OA after ACL reconstruction is significantly lower than commonly perceived. Indeed, the combined estimate from the random-effects meta-analysis equals 28 %, and the upper limit of the 95 % CI for this estimate is lower than 50 % (43.5 %).

The question remains: can ACL reconstruction prevent the occurrence of early OA? To date, a direct proof to confirm or reject this statement stays difficult to deliver. One of the main issues in this debate is the lack of controlled, prospective studies on the long-term natural history of the ACL-deficient knee. The advent of modern ACL reconstruction in the 1980s was merely driven by the superior short- and mid-term results with regard to stability and knee function when compared to nonoperative treatment. However, some early reports on conservative ACL treatment had already shown unfavorable long-term results with very high rates (i.e., 60–90 %) of early OA in the ACL-deficient knee [1, 12, 33]. To the contrary, other authors have reported much better functional and radiographic results after nonoperative treatment. For example, Neumann et al. treated ACL-injured patients with activity modification and physical therapy and reported a prevalence of only 15 % OA at 15 years of follow-up [26]. The true natural history of these injuries may never be known due to the existence of asymptomatic ACL-deficient subjects or so-called copers, patient selection bias, or conservative treatment heterogeneity in published reports.

Additionally, this meta-analysis confirmed that meniscectomy should be considered as an important risk factor for developing OA after ACL reconstruction, with 42 % of patients showing radiographic OA compared to 19 % of patients with a preserved meniscal status (OR = 3.54). Recent cadaveric experiments by Musahl et al. have confirmed the secondary stabilizing effect of both the medial and lateral meniscus in the ACL-deficient knee [25]. These authors showed that the medial meniscus functions as an important secondary restraint to anterior tibial translation in the ACL-deficient knee (i.e., during the Lachman test), while the lateral meniscus has a relatively more important secondary restraining role to the combined axial and rotatory loads (i.e., during the pivot-shift examination). In this view, anterior or rotatory instability in the absence of a functional ACL results in excess shearing forces being applied at the meniscus, thus giving rise to meniscal damage, degenerative tears, and pain necessitating resection of the meniscus. Most authors have reported higher rates of subsequent meniscal injuries after conservatively managed ACL ruptures when compared to ACL-reconstructed knees, with incidences as high as 98 % in chronic ACL-deficient knees [13, 14]. Even in a recent RCT published in the New England Journal of Medicine questioning the need for prompt ACL reconstructive surgery [8], the conservatively treated cohort experienced 33 % more meniscal tears after the ACL injury. As this meta-analysis has clearly identified meniscectomy as the risk factor of utmost importance with regard to the development of early OA, the occurrence of OA can be directly related to the inability of the ACL-injured knee to protect its menisci. In other words, this meta-analysis supports the statement that "the key to lowering the risk of knee OA is decreasing the rate of meniscectomy" [31].

Memory

This meta-analysis on the relation between ACL reconstruction and the development of OA has shown that the prevalence of OA is definitely lower than commonly perceived. However, associated meniscal resection dramatically increases the risk for developing OA (OR 3.54). This finding bears the inherent consequence of attempting a repair of meniscus injuries sustained at the time of ACL tear, as well as contemplating reconstruction of the ruptured ACL in order to protect the menisci from excessive shear forces, subsequent tearing, and premature development of OA. Moreover, in an era of questioning the cost-effectiveness of surgical procedures, the results of this study have the potential to justify current clinical practice regarding ACL-injured subjects. Finally, these results should be used as a baseline for upcoming long-term outcome studies on recent ACL techniques and to counsel ACL-injured patients in an evidence-based way.

References

1. Barrack RL, Bruckner JD, Kneisl J, Inman WS, Alexander AH (1990) The outcome of nonoperatively treated complete tears of the anterior cruciate ligament in active young adults. Clin Orthop Relat Res 259:192–199

2. Claes S, Hermie L, Verdonk R, Bellemans J, Verdonk P (2013) Is osteoarthritis an inevitable consequence of anterior cruciate ligament reconstruction? A meta-analysis. Knee Surg Sports Traumatol Arthrosc 21:1967–1976

3. Cohen M, Amaro JT, Ejnisman B et al (2007) Anterior cruciate ligament reconstruction after 10 to 15 years: association between meniscectomy and osteoarthrosis. Arthroscopy 23(6):629–634

4. Daniel DM, Stone ML, Dobson BE, Fithian DC, Rossman DJ, Kaufman KR (1994) Fate of the ACL-injured patient. A prospective outcome study. Am J Sports Med 22(5):632–644

5. DerSimonian R, Laird N (1986) Meta-analysis in clinical trials. Control Clin Trials 7(3):177–188

6. Drogset JO, Grontvedt T, Robak OR, Molster A, Viset AT, Engebretsen L (2006) A sixteen-year follow-up of three operative techniques for the treatment of acute ruptures of the anterior cruciate ligament. J Bone Joint Surg Am 88(5):944–952

7. Fink C, Hoser C, Hackl W, Navarro RA, Benedetto KP (2001) Long-term outcome of operative or nonoperative treatment of anterior cruciate ligament rupture – is sports activity a determining variable? Int J Sports Med 22(4):304–309

8. Frobell RB, Roos EM, Roos HP, Ranstam J, Lohmander LS (2010) A randomized trial of treatment for acute anterior cruciate ligament tears. N Engl J Med 363(4):331–342

9. Funk FJ Jr (1983) Osteoarthritis of the knee following ligamentous injury. Clin Orthop Relat Res 172:154–157

10. Hefti F, Muller W, Jakob RP, Staubli HU (1993) Evaluation of knee ligament injuries with the IKDC form. Knee Surg Sports Traumatol Arthrosc 1(3–4):226–234

11. Hertel P, Behrend H, Cierpinski T, Musahl V, Widjaja G (2005) ACL reconstruction using bone-patellar tendon-bone press-fit fixation: 10-year clinical results. Knee Surg Sports Traumatol Arthrosc 13(4):248–255

12. Kannus P, Jarvinen M (1987) Conservatively treated tears of the anterior cruciate ligament. Long-term results. J Bone Joint Surg Am 69(7):1007–1012

13. Keays SL, Newcombe PA, Bullock-Saxton JE, Bullock MI, Keays AC (2010) Factors involved in the development of osteoarthritis after anterior cruciate ligament surgery. Am J Sports Med 38(3):455–463

14. Kessler MA, Behrend H, Henz S, Stutz G, Rukavina A, Kuster MS (2008) Function, osteoarthritis and activity after ACL-rupture: 11 years follow-up results of conservative versus reconstructive treatment. Knee Surg Sports Traumatol Arthrosc 16(5):442–448

15. Lebel B, Hulet C, Galaud B, Burdin G, Locker B, Vielpeau C (2008) Arthroscopic reconstruction of the anterior cruciate ligament using bone-patellar tendon-bone autograft: a minimum 10-year follow-up. Am J Sports Med 36(7):1275–1282

16. Lerat JL, Chotel F, Besse JL et al (1998) [The results after 10–16 years of the treatment of chronic anterior laxity of the knee using reconstruction of the anterior cruciate ligament with a patellar tendon graft combined

with an external extra-articular reconstruction]. Rev Chir Orthop Reparatrice Appar Mot 84(8):712–727

17. Li RT, Lorenz S, Xu Y, Harner CD, Fu FH, Irrgang JJ (2011) Predictors of radiographic knee osteoarthritis after anterior cruciate ligament reconstruction. Am J Sports Med 39:2595–2603

18. Lohmander LS, Englund PM, Dahl LL, Roos EM (2007) The long-term consequence of anterior cruciate ligament and meniscus injuries: osteoarthritis. Am J Sports Med 35(10):1756–1769

19. Lohmander LS, Ostenberg A, Englund M, Roos H (2004) High prevalence of knee osteoarthritis, pain, and functional limitations in female soccer players twelve years after anterior cruciate ligament injury. Arthritis Rheum 50(10):3145–3152

20. McDaniel WJ Jr, Dameron TB Jr (1980) Untreated ruptures of the anterior cruciate ligament. A follow-up study. J Bone Joint Surg Am 62(5):696–705

21. Mehta VM, Paxton LW, Fornalski SX, Csintalan RP, Fithian DC (2007) Reliability of the international knee documentation committee radiographic grading system. Am J Sports Med 35(6):933–935

22. Meuffels DE, Favejee MM, Vissers MM, Heijboer MP, Reijman M, Verhaar JA (2009) Ten year follow-up study comparing conservative versus operative treatment of anterior cruciate ligament ruptures. A matched-pair analysis of high level athletes. Br J Sports Med 43(5):347–351

23. Meystre JL, Vallotton J, Benvenuti JF (1998) Double semitendinosus anterior cruciate ligament reconstruction: 10-year results. Knee Surg Sports Traumatol Arthrosc 6(2):76–81

24. Moher D, Liberati A, Tetzlaff J, Altman DG (2009) Preferred reporting items for systematic reviews and meta-analyses: the PRISMA statement. PLoS Med 6(7):e1000097

25. Musahl V, Citak M, O'Loughlin PF, Choi D, Bedi A, Pearle AD (2010) The effect of medial versus lateral meniscectomy on the stability of the anterior cruciate ligament-deficient knee. Am J Sports Med 38(8): 1591–1597

26. Neuman P, Englund M, Kostogiannis I, Friden T, Roos H, Dahlberg LE (2008) Prevalence of tibiofemoral osteoarthritis 15 years after nonoperative treatment of anterior cruciate ligament injury: a prospective cohort study. Am J Sports Med 36(9):1717–1725

27. Oiestad BE, Holm I, Aune AK et al (2010) Knee function and prevalence of knee osteoarthritis after anterior cruciate ligament reconstruction: a prospective study with 10 to 15 years of follow-up. Am J Sports Med 38(11):2201–2210

28. Pernin J, Verdonk P, Si Selmi TA, Massin P, Neyret P (2010) Long-term follow-up of 24.5 years after intra-articular anterior cruciate ligament reconstruction with lateral extra-articular augmentation. Am J Sports Med 38(6):1094–1102

29. Pinczewski LA, Lyman J, Salmon LJ, Russell VJ, Roe J, Linklater J (2007) A 10-year comparison of anterior cruciate ligament reconstructions with hamstring tendon and patellar tendon autograft: a controlled, prospective trial. Am J Sports Med 35(4):564–574

30. Reider B (2009) Acl & Oa. Am J Sports Med 37(7):1279–1281

31. Richmond JC, Lubowitz JH, Poehling GG (2011) Prompt operative intervention reduces long-term osteoarthritis after knee anterior cruciate ligament tear. Arthroscopy 27(2):149–152

32. Salmon LJ, Russell VJ, Refshauge K et al (2006) Long-term outcome of endoscopic anterior cruciate ligament reconstruction with patellar tendon autograft: minimum 13-year review. Am J Sports Med 34(5):721–732

33. Segawa H, Omori G, Koga Y (2001) Long-term results of non-operative treatment of anterior cruciate ligament injury. Knee 8(1):5–11

34. Seon JK, Song EK, Park SJ (2006) Osteoarthritis after anterior cruciate ligament reconstruction using a patellar tendon autograft. Int Orthop 30(2):94–98

35. Shelbourne KD, Gray T (2009) Minimum 10-year results after anterior cruciate ligament reconstruction: how the loss of normal knee motion compounds other factors related to the development of osteoarthritis after surgery. Am J Sports Med 37(3):471–480

36. Spindler KP, Wright RW (2008) Clinical practice. Anterior cruciate ligament tear. N Engl J Med 359(20):2135–2142

37. Torg JS, Conrad W, Kalen V (1976) Clinical diagnosis of anterior cruciate ligament instability in the athlete. Am J Sports Med 4(2):84–93

Part V

Double Bundle ACL Reconstruction

Double-Bundle ACL Reconstruction with Hamstrings

28

Timo Järvelä and Rainer Siebold

Contents

T. Järvelä, MD, PhD (✉)
Department of Orthopaedics, Sports Clinic and Hospital Mehiläinen, Tampere, Finland

Medical Faculty, Tampere University,
Tampere, Finland
e-mail: timo.jarvela@sci.fi

R. Siebold, MD
Institute for Anatomy and Cell Biology,
Ruprecht-Karls University Heidelberg,
Im Neuenheimer Feld 307,
Heidelberg 69120, Germany

HKF: Center for Spezialised Hip-Knee-Foot Surgery,
ATOS Hospital Heidelberg,
Bismarckstr. 9-15, Heidelberg 69115, Germany
e-mail: rainer.siebold@atos.de

28.1   Indications

Different factors may influence the decision of whether to perform a single-bundle (SB) or double-bundle (DB) ACL reconstruction when using hamstrings. The size of the knee may be most important [11, 16, 18]. The smaller the knee, the more difficult it is to perform an anatomically and technically correct DB ACL reconstruction. The required ap length for DB measured at the tibial and femoral insertion sites was suggested to be 14mm or more – depending on the diameters of the two grafts [11, 16, 18]. In case of large grafts, more space is needed to perform a DB ACL reconstruction. The "insertion site table" (see Chap. 22) displays the size of the insertion site needed to perform a SB or DB ACL reconstruction. It can be measured preoperatively on MRI or – more reliable – intraoperatively using a ruler [11, 16, 18].

The width of the intercondylar notch is important too. A large and wide intercondylar notch does easily accommodate a large and wide SB ACL reconstruction. In contrast, in case of a narrow intercondylar notch, a flat ACL reconstruction, e.g., a DB ACL reconstruction using hamstrings, or a flat quadriceps- or patella-tendon ACL reconstruction may be of advantage to avoid notch impingement and graft failure. The width can also be measured preoperatively on MRI or intraoperatively.

It is recommended not to under- or oversize the anteromedial (AM) and posterolateral bundle

R. Siebold et al. (eds.), *Anterior Cruciate Ligament Reconstruction*,
DOI 10.1007/978-3-642-45349-6_28, © ESSKA 2014

Table 28.1 Suggested indications for anatomical SB versus DB ACL reconstruction

SB ACL reconstruction	DB ACL reconstruction
Small knee (no room for the DB technique)	Large enough knee
Thin hamstring tendons	Good quality of the hamstring tendons
Non-athlete or	High-level athlete
Recreational athlete	Pivoting sports
Isolated ACL injury	ACL injury combined with meniscal injury

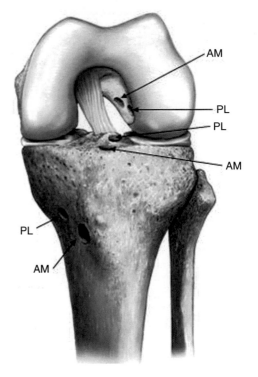

Fig. 28.1 Schematic drawing showing the bone tunnels in DB ACL reconstruction (*AM* anteromedial, *PL* posterolateral)

(PL) grafts. The diameter for the AM bundle graft is usually in the range between 6 and 7 mm and for the PL bundle between 5 and 6 mm, respectively. In case of thin and/or short hamstring tendons, the graft sizes may be too small, and a SB ACL reconstruction may be recommended instead.

The activity level of the patient may have some importance, too. Patients with a high activity level, e.g., athletes who are performing demanding pivoting sports (ball games, skiing, gymnastic, etc.), may benefit from a more anatomical and biomechanically stronger DB ACL reconstruction.

Concomitant injuries do also play a role. Musahl et al. [14] showed in their cadaveric study that the DB ACL reconstruction was able to restore intact knee kinematics during the pivot shift testing significantly better than the anatomical SB or non-anatomical SB technique after ACL transaction and concomitant medial and lateral meniscectomies. A summary of the suggested indications for anatomical SB and DB ACL reconstructions is displayed in Table 28.1.

28.2 Tibial Bone Tunnel Drilling

The DB technique described here is published originally by Järvelä [8] in 2007. The drilling of the tibial tunnels is done with a tibial drill guide. First, the tibial tunnel for the AM bundle is drilled. An ACL tibial drill guide is placed on the AM aspect of the ACL tibial footprint with the

angle set to 55°. The starting point of the AM tibial tunnel is the same as in standard ACL SB technique. Once acceptable placement of the AM tibial pin is obtained (no impingement in knee extension), the PL tibial guidewire is placed on the PL aspect of the ACL tibial footprint with the angle set to 55°. The PL tibial tunnel has a more medial starting point on the tibial cortex than a standard ACL tibial tunnel. An osseous bridge of 1 to 2 cm should be preserved on the tibial cortex between the two bone tunnels (Fig. 28.1) and at the articular side. The AM tibial tunnel is drilled first followed by the PL tunnel. The diameter of the AM tibial tunnel is typically 6–7 mm and that of the PL tunnel 5–6 mm.

New anatomical understanding of the tibial insertion site may change our way of DB ACL reconstruction. These findings suggest to place the PL bone tunnel posteromedial instead of posterolateral for anatomical reconstruction (see Chap. 1).

28.3 Femoral Bone Tunnel Drilling and Screw Fixation

The drilling of the femoral bone tunnels may be performed with special aimers or freehand. We prefer a freehand technique without a guide to achieve a better flexibility for AM and PL bone tunnel positioning.

First, the AM and PL bone tunnel positions are marked with a 30° awl. A sufficient distance between the markings for AM and PL should be kept to later preserve a bony bridge between both tunnels. We recommend controlling the position of both centers by fluoroscopy to avoid wrong intraoperative bone tunnel placement and for documentation. Both centers should be placed in continuity to the posterolateral femoral cortex at the posterior aspect of – and along – the intercondylar ridge (see Chaps. 3 and 4).

When correct center position is achieved, the AM femoral tunnel is drilled first through a low anteromedial portal. Transtibial drilling is not recommended to avoid non-anatomical bone tunnel positioning. A guide pin is placed to the marked AM position and drilled through the femoral condyle at 120° of knee flexion. The guide pin is overdrilled by a cannulated 4.5mm drill. The final diameter of the AM tunnel is drilled after harvesting and measuring the diameter of the hamstring autografts. The diameter of the AM femoral tunnel is typically between 6 and 7 mm and the depth of the tunnel between 25 and 35 mm.

The PL femoral tunnel is drilled in a similar way to AM in a flexion angle between 90° [8] and 130° [17]. The PL diameter is usually between 5 and 6 mm and the depth of the tunnel approximately 25–35 mm. The bony wall between both femoral bone tunnels should be a minimum of 1–2 mm (Fig. 28.1) to achieve good tendon-to-bone healing at the joint line.

Both grafts are inserted from distal to proximal via the tibial tunnels into the femoral tunnels. The PL graft is passed first (Fig. 28.2) followed by the AM graft.

In case of femoral inside-out fixation with two bioabsorbable interference screws (technique described by Järvelä et al. [8]), a notching of the femoral PL tunnel is performed after the PL graft

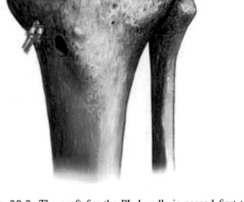

Fig. 28.2 The graft for the PL bundle is passed first to the PL tunnel

and the guide pin for the screw driver are in place (Figs. 28.3 and 28.4). The size of the PL screw is usually 6 × 25 mm. Then the AM graft is inserted and is fixed accordingly (Fig. 28.5) using a 7 × 25 mm bioresorbable interference screw. After conditioning of the AM and PL bundles, tibial fixation is achieved by two 7 × 30mm and 6 × 25mm bioresorbable interference screws in 30° and 15° of flexion. The described technique requires four implants.

28.4 Femoral Button and Tibial Bone Bridge Fixation

When using a femoral extracortical fixation [17], both grafts are fixed to a femoral button system according to the length of the femoral AM and PL bone tunnels (Fig. 28.6). A bone bridge should be preserved between the two femoral and tibial bone tunnels (Fig. 28.7a–c). The PL graft is

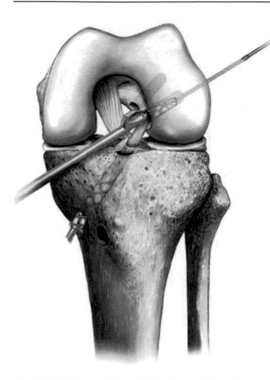

Fig. 28.3 The notching of the femoral tunnels is performed before inserting the bioabsorbable screws

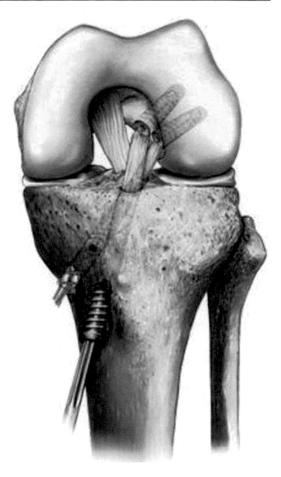

Fig. 28.5 Final result of DB ACL reconstruction fixed with 4 bioabsorbable screws

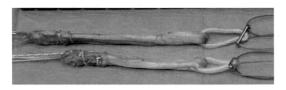

Fig. 28.6 AM and PL grafts with femoral extracortical button system

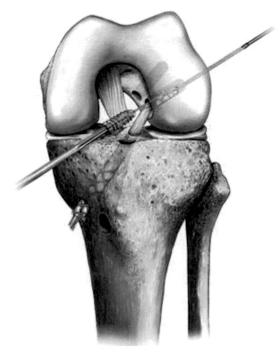

Fig. 28.4 Insertion of the bioabsorbable screw for PL graft fixation

inserted first from distal to proximal, and the button is flipped on the femoral cortex. The insertion of the bone tunnel of the AM graft is performed accordingly. After conditioning of both bundles, tibial fixation is achieved by tying the tibial no.2 non-resorbable graft sutures of AM and PL in extension over the tibial bone bridge between the two bone tunnels (Fig. 28.8). A bioresorbable interference screw, usually 8×25mm, may be inserted in the tibial AM bone tunnel. No screw is

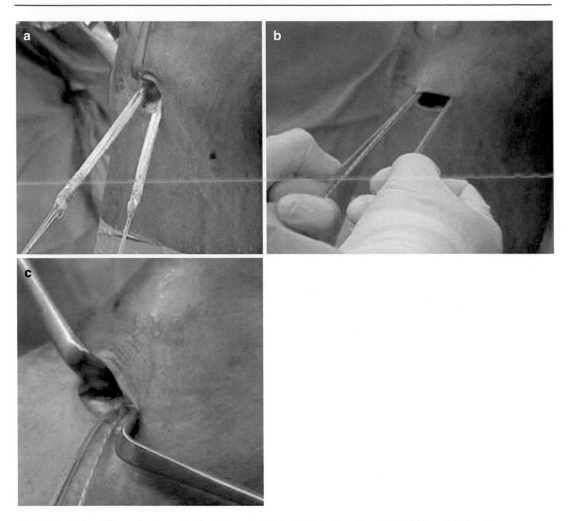

Fig. 28.7 AM and PL grafts are pulled in their tunnels (**a**). Conditioning of grafts (**b**). Tying of AM to PL sutures over the tibial cortical bone bridge (**c**)

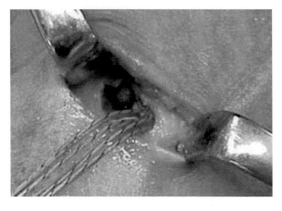

Fig. 28.8 Tibial fixation of AM and PL with non-resorbable graft sutures over bone bridge between the AM and PL bone tunnels. A bioresorbable screw is inserted into the AM bone tunnel for additional fixation

used for additional PL fixation. The described DB technique requires 2–3 implants.

28.5   Pitfalls and Complications

The risk for pitfalls is higher compared to SB. Bone tunnel placement has to be performed very carefully to avoid wrong positioning or bone tunnel communication caused by drilling. It is recommended to introduce the PL graft first for better arthroscopic view and better control of AM and PL graft handling. Especially femoral graft fixation with screws may be difficult and has to be performed without damaging the grafts or the bone bridge. The need for additional implants, a longer operation time, and a potentially higher number of pitfalls increase the costs associated with a DB ACL reconstruction. Therefore the DB technique has to be used critically and may only be recommended for experienced ACL surgeons.

## 28.6	Literature Results

According to the 21 prospective randomized studies [1–10, 12, 13, 15, 17, 19–25] found from the English literature and published so far, six studies (29 %) did not find any significant differences in the clinical results between double-bundle and single-bundle ACL reconstructions. However, 15 studies (71 %) reported significantly better results with the double-bundle technique than with the single-bundle technique. Nine of these trials reported better rotational stability, seven trials noted better anterior stability, three trials showed better objective knee scores, three trials had better subjective knee scores, four trials had fewer graft failures, one trial showed less tunnel enlargement, and one trial was found to have less degenerative changes in the knee joint with double-bundle technique compared to the single-bundle technique. In addition, none of the studies found that the single-bundle technique had better results in any of these evaluations than the double-bundle technique.

All the above randomized, controlled trials comparing double-bundle and single-bundle ACL reconstructions are summarized in Table 28.2.

Table 28.2 Randomized controlled trials comparing double-bundle (DB) and single-bundle (SB) ACL reconstruction

Authors	Year published	Number of patients	Follow-up time	Results
Adachi et al. [1]	2004	108	32 months	No difference
Aglietti et al. [2]	2007	75	2 years	Better rotational and anterior stability in DB group
Aglietti et al. [3]	2010	70	2 years	Better anterior stability and subjective and objective knee scores in DB group
Järvelä [8]	2007	65	14 months	Better rotational stability in DB group
Järvelä et al. [9]	2008	77	2 years	Better rotational stability and fewer graft failures in DB group
Järvelä et al. [10]	2008	60	2 years	Less tunnel enlargement in DB group
Yagi et al. [23]	2007	60	1 year	Better rotational stability in DB group
Muneta et al. [13]	2007	68	2 years	Better rotational and anterior stability in DB group
Streich et al. [19]	2008	50	2 years	No difference
Siebold et al. [17]	2008	70	19 months	Better rotational and anterior stability and objective knee scores in DB group
Sastre et al. [15]	2010	40	2 years	No difference
Zaffagnini et al. [25]	2008	100	3 years	Better anterior stability and objective and subjective knee scores in DB group

Table 28.2 (continued)

Authors	Year published	Number of patients	Follow-up time	Results
Zaffagnini et al. [24]	2010	79	8 years	Better functional scores and fewer graft failures and less degenerative changes in DB group
Wang et al. [22]	2009	64	10 months	No difference
Ibrahim et al. [7]	2009	218	29 months	Better rotational and anterior stability in DB group
Suomalainen et al. [21]	2011	153	2 years	Fewer graft failures in DB group
Araki et al. [4]	2011	20	1 year	No difference
Fujita et al. [5]	2011	55	2 years	No difference
Hussein et al. [6]	2011	281	51 months	Better rotational and anterior stability in DB group
Lee et al. [12]	2012	42	2 years	Better rotational stability in DB group
Suomalainen et al. [20]	2012	90	5 years	Fewer graft failures in DB group

References

1. Adachi N, Ochi M, Uchio Y et al (2004) Reconstruction of the anterior cruciate ligament. Single- versus double-bundle multistranded hamstring tendons. J Bone Joint Surg Br 86(4):515–520
2. Aglietti P, Giron F, Cuomo P et al (2007) Single-and double-incision double-bundle ACL reconstruction. Clin Orthop Relat Res 454:108–113
3. Aglietti P, Giron F, Losco M et al (2010) Comparison between single-and double-bundle anterior cruciate ligament reconstruction: a prospective, randomized, single-blinded clinical trial. Am J Sports Med 38(1):25–34
4. Araki D, Kuroda R, Kubo S et al (2011) A prospective randomised study of anatomical single-bundle versus double-bundle anterior cruciate ligament reconstruction: quantitative evaluation using an electromagnetic measurement system. Int Orthop 35(3):439–446
5. Fujita N, Kuroda R, Matsumoto T et al (2011) Comparison of the clinical outcome of double-bundle, anteromedial single-bundle, and posterolateral single-bundle anterior cruciate ligament reconstruction using hamstring tendon graft with minimum 2-year follow-up. Arthroscopy 27(7):906–913
6. Hussein M, van Eck CF, Cretnik A et al (2012) Prospective randomized clinical evaluation of conventional single-bundle, anatomic single-bundle, and anatomic double-bundle anterior cruciate ligament reconstruction: 281 cases with 3- to 5-year follow-up. Am J Sports Med 40(3):512–520
7. Ibrahim SA, Hamido F, Al Misfer AK et al (2009) Anterior cruciate ligament reconstruction using autologous hamstring double bundle graft compared with single bundle procedures. J Bone Joint Surg Br 91(10):1310–1315
8. Jarvela T (2007) Double-bundle versus single-bundle anterior cruciate ligament reconstruction: a prospective, randomize clinical study. Knee Surg Sports Traumatol Arthrosc 15(5):500–507
9. Jarvela T, Moisala AS, Paakkala T et al (2008) Tunnel enlargement after double-bundle anterior cruciate ligament reconstruction: a prospective, randomized study. Arthroscopy 24(12):1349–1357
10. Jarvela T, Moisala AS, Sihvonen R et al (2008) Double-bundle anterior cruciate ligament reconstruction using hamstring autografts and bioabsorbable interference screw fixation: prospective, randomized, clinical study with 2-year results. Am J Sports Med 36(2):290–297
11. Kopf S, Pombo MW, Szczodry M et al (2011) Size variability of the human anterior cruciate ligament insertion sites. Am J Sports Med 39(1):108–113
12. Lee S, Kim H, Jang J et al (2012) Comparison of anterior and rotatory laxity using navigation between single- and double-bundle ACL reconstruction: prospective randomized trial. Knee Surg Sports Traumatol Arthrosc 20(4):752–761
13. Muneta T, Koga H, Mochizuki T et al (2007) A prospective randomized study of 4-strand semitendinosus tendon anterior cruciate ligament reconstruction comparing single-bundle and double-bundle techniques. Arthroscopy 23(6):618–628

14. Musahl V, Bedi A, Citak M et al (2011) Effect of single-bundle and double-bundle anterior cruciate ligament reconstructions on pivot-shift kinematics in anterior cruciate ligament- and meniscus-deficient knees. Am J Sports Med 39(2):289–295

15. Sastre S, Popescu D, Nunez M et al (2010) Double-bundle versus single-bundle ACL reconstruction using the horizontal femoral position: a prospective, randomized study. Knee Surg Sports Traumatol Arthrosc 18(1):32–36

16. Siebold R (2011) The concept of complete footprint restoration with guidelines for single- and double-bundle ACL reconstruction. Knee Surg Sports Traumatol Arthrosc 19(5):699–706

17. Siebold R, Dehler C, Ellert T (2008) Prospective randomized comparison of double-bundle versus single-bundle anterior cruciate ligament reconstruction. Arthroscopy 24(2):137–145

18. Siebold R, Schuhmacher P (2012) Restoration of the tibial ACL footprint area and geometry using the Modified Insertion Site Table. Knee Surg Sports Traumatol Arthrosc 20(9):1845–1849

19. Streich NA, Friedrich K, Gotterbarm T et al (2008) Reconstruction of the ACL with a semitendinosus tendon graft: a prospective randomized single blinded comparison of double-bundle versus single-bundle technique in male athletes. Knee Surg Sports Traumatol Arthrosc 16(3):232–238

20. Suomalainen P, Jarvela T, Paakkala A et al (2012) Double-bundle versus single-bundle anterior cruciate ligament reconstruction: a prospective randomized study with 5-year results. Am J Sports Med 40(7): 1511–1518

21. Suomalainen P, Moisala AS, Paakkala A et al (2011) Double-bundle versus single-bundle anterior cruciate ligament reconstruction: randomized clinical and magnetic resonance imaging study with 2-year follow-up. Am J Sports Med 39(8):1615–1622

22. Wang JQ, Ao YF, Yu CL et al (2009) Clinical evaluation of double-bundle anterior cruciate ligament reconstruction procedure using hamstring tendon grafts: a prospective, randomized and controlled study. Chin Med J (Engl) 122(6):706–711

23. Yagi M, Kuroda R, Nagamune K et al (2007) Double-bundle ACL reconstruction can improve rotational stability. Clin Orthop Relat Res 454:100–107

24. Zaffagnini S, Bruni D, Marcheggiani Muccioli GM et al (2011) Single-bundle patellar tendon versus non-anatomical double-bundle hamstrings ACL reconstruction: a prospective randomized study at 8-year minimum follow-up. Knee Surg Sports Traumatol Arthrosc 19(3):390–397

25. Zaffagnini S, Bruni D, Russo A et al (2008) ST/G ACL reconstruction: double strand plus extra-articular sling vs double bundle, randomized study at 3-year follow-up. Scand J Med Sci Sports 18(5):573–581

"Ribbonlike" Double-Bundle ACL Reconstruction with Restoration of "C"-Shaped Tibial Insertion Site

29

Rainer Siebold

Contents

R. Siebold, MD (✉)
Institute for Anatomy and Cell Biology,
Ruprecht-Karls University Heidelberg,
Im Neuenheimer Feld 307, Heidelberg
69120, Germany

HKF: Center for Spezialised Hip-Knee-Foot Surgery,
ATOS Hospital Heidelberg, Bismarckstr. 9-15,
Heidelberg 69115, Germany
e-mail: rainer.siebold@atos.de

According to recent measurements, the dimensions at midsubstance are an average of 12.2 mm wide but only 3.6 mm flat. On the tibial side, the "C"-shaped bony insertion has an average length of 13.7 mm and a width of only 3.3 mm, and the femoral straight bony insertion along the intercondylar ridge has an average length of 16.0 mm and a width of 3.5 mm (see Chaps. 1, 2, 3, 4, and 5).

From these measurements, an anatomical flat and long footprint reconstruction may be advantageous. However, most "traditional" single-bundle (SB) ACL grafts are too wide, resulting in a too short and too wide footprint reconstruction.

For closer restoration of the flat "ribbonlike" shape, DB reconstruction may be advantageous over SB reconstruction when using hamstrings. In contrast when using a patella tendon graft or quadriceps tendon SB ACL reconstruction is sufficient, as the geometry of the graft is flat (PT) or can be harvested flat (QT). However, these grafts might be associated with a higher morbidity at the harvest site.

The aim of this chapter was to highlight a way of DB ACL reconstruction by restoring the "C"-shaped tibial and "straight" femoral ACL insertions using hamstrings.

R. Siebold et al. (eds.), *Anterior Cruciate Ligament Reconstruction*,
DOI 10.1007/978-3-642-45349-6_29, © ESSKA 2014

29.1 Surgical Technique

The hamstrings are harvested using a standard approach (see Sect. 17.1). The semitendinosus tendon is harvested first. If it is 26 cm or longer, the semitendinosus tendon is used for ACL DB reconstruction, and the gracilis tendon is left in situ. The length of the doubled semitendinosus tendon for the anteromedial (AM) graft is prepared to 7 cm and the length for the posteromedial graft (PM) to 6–7 cm. If the semitendinosus tendon is too short, the gracilis tendon is harvested too and used for PM.

Both grafts are looped over an Endobutton CL (Smith & Nephew, Andover, USA) according to the lengths of the femoral bone tunnels and are armed distally with two No. 2 nonresorbable sutures each. 1.5 cm of femoral tendon-to-bone contact is recommended when choosing the Endobutton size. The diameters of the grafts are measured for bone tunnel drilling; a press-fit situation is aimed for.

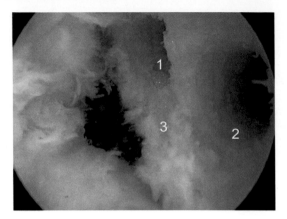

Fig. 29.1 Femoral bone tunnel placement along intercondylar ridge. Place both bone tunnels in the direct femoral insertion site of the ACL and not too far posterior (arthroscopically "inferior") in the area of the indirect femoral ACL insertion (see Chaps. 1, 2, 3, and 4). *1* AM bone tunnel, *2* PM bone tunnel, *3* indirect ACL insertion

29.2 Femoral Bone Tunnel Drilling

The length of the femoral insertion site is measured along the intercondylar ridge with the knee in approximately 110–115° of flexion. In this position, the intercondylar ridge is aligned approximately horizontally. The posterior intercondylar notch roof and the lateral intercondylar wall are cleaned from soft tissue, and the centers of both femoral bone tunnels are marked using a chondropick. ACL remnants might be kept for orientation of bone tunnel placement if present. Other landmarks on the femoral side are the intercondylar ridge (resident's ridge) and the cartilage of the lateral femoral condyle (see Chap. 19).

The two chondropicks are kept in place in the centers of the AM and PM fibers, and a lateral fluoroscopy is performed to control positioning and for documentation (see Chap. 20). After reconfirmation of positioning of the centers, the femoral AM bone tunnel is drilled first in anteromedial portal technique (or outside in) and the PM bone tunnel second (see Chap. 21). Keep a bone bridge of 1–2 mm between AM and PM

bone tunnel for better ingrowth and stability of the tendon grafts at the joint line (Fig. 29.1). The maximum size of both femoral tunnels may not exceed 7.5 for AM and 6.5 for PM. These large diameters for DB would require an insertion site length of 18 mm (see Chap. 22). Smaller grafts are more anatomical, e.g., 6 mm for AM and 5 mm for PM, as the width of the femoral and tibial direct ACL insertion does not exceed 5 mm (see Chaps. 1, 2, 3, 4, and 5).

29.3 Tibial Bone Tunnel Drilling

On the tibial side, two bone tunnels cannot anatomically restore the "C-shaped" flat insertion site (Fig. 29.2) (see Chaps. 1, 2, 3, 4, and 5). However, bone tunnels should be aligned to the "C" shape to achieve an anatomical approximation of the direct footprint. To verify the AP length of the tibial ACL insertion, a measurement is recommended (Fig. 29.3).

The AM bone tunnel is drilled first. It is placed in the anteromedial part of the "C" which is an average of 8.7 mm wide (Fig. 29.4a, b). This position would also be the place for an SB bone tunnel in ACL reconstruction. A very good landmark for anterior referencing is the anterior fibers of the lateral meniscus, which blend with the anterior part of the direct tibial insertion site (Fig. 29.2). A K-wire is placed first using a tibial aimer, which is then overdrilled by the diameter of the AM graft (Fig. 29.4b). The PM bone tunnel is drilled accordingly in the posteromedial part of the "C" which has an average AP length of 10.8 mm (range 7.6–14.5 mm) just lateral of the medial tibial spine (Fig. 29.4c).

Be careful not to damage the medial tibial spine or the medial tibial plateau. Both tibial bone tunnels should therefore be drilled from close to the tibial tuberosity and not from too far

medial (Fig. 29.5). Avoid a single-bundle bone tunnel in the center of the ACL stump ("traditional technique"), because the bony insertion of the lateral meniscus will be damaged.

After cleaning of the joint from detritus, the PM is pulled in first, followed by the AM graft (Fig. 29.6a–c). The two Endobuttons are flipped, and the grafts are conditioned by bringing the knee 20 times through a full range of motion. Tibial fixation is performed in extension by tying the nonresorbable graft sutures over the bony bridge between the AM and PM bone tunnels. One bioscrew may be bolt in the AM bone tunnel at 90° of flexion for additional tibial fixation.

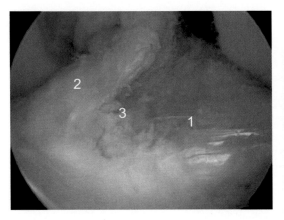

Fig. 29.2 Left knee with "C"-shaped tibial insertion of the ACL (see also Chaps. 1, 2, 3, and 4). *1* anterior horn of lateral meniscus, *2* ACL, *3* bony insertion of 1

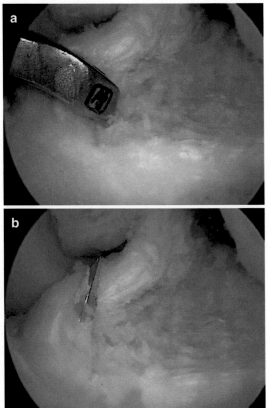

Fig. 29.4 (**a**) Tibial AM bone tunnel placement in the anteromedial aspect of the "C"-shaped insertion site. This is also the place for an SB ACL reconstruction. When the bone tunnel is placed in the center of the ACL stump ("traditional technique"), the bony insertion of the lateral meniscus will be damaged. (**b**) Tibial AM (or SB) K-wire placement. (**c**) Tibial PM K-wire placement. There is no tibial *posterolateral* ACL insertion site

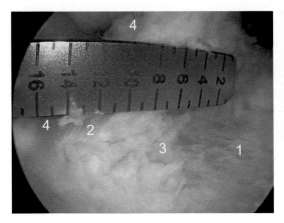

Fig. 29.3 Measurement of AP length of "C"-shaped tibial ACL insertion site along medial tibial spine to choose graft sizes for hamstring DB ACL reconstruction (see Chap. 22). *1* anterior horn of lateral meniscus, *2* ACL, *3* bony insertion of 1, *4* medial tibial spine

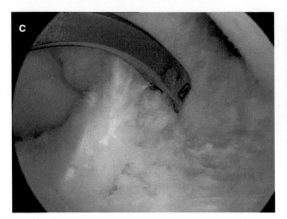

Fig. 29.4 (continued)

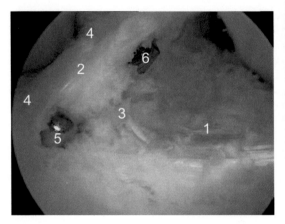

Fig. 29.5 AM and PM bone tunnel placement in antero-posterior direction along the medial tibial spine in the area of the "C"-shaped ACL insertion. Important is to preserve the medial tibial spine. *1* anterior horn of lateral meniscus, *2* ACL, *3* bony insertion of *1*, *4* medial tibial spine, *5* AM, *6* PM

It is important to control the result of the ACL reconstruction (Fig. 29.7). Therefore, after fixation, the knee is rescoped to exclude anterior impingement caused by the grafts or remnants of the ACL stump. An overlength of the tibial bio-screw is excluded, too.

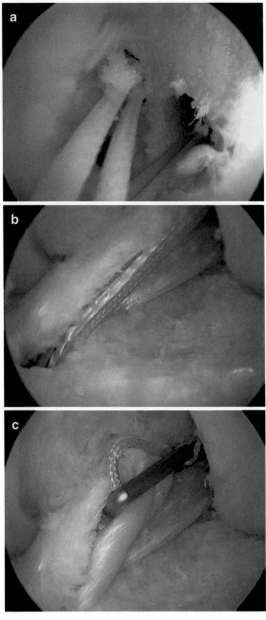

Fig. 29.6 (**a**) Sutures in place to pull the AM and PM graft into their bone tunnels. *White* AM, *green* PM. (**b**) PM graft in place, AM sutures of Endobutton. (**c**) PM graft in place, Endobutton of AM is pulled through the joint

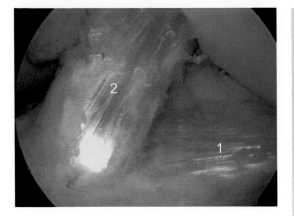

Fig. 29.7 DB ACL reconstruction with hamstrings in place. The reconstruction is flat running over the bony insertion of the lateral meniscus. *1* anterior horn of lateral meniscus, *2* AM in front of PM

Memory

The anterior and posterior border of the anterior horn of the lateral meniscus are excellent landmarks for anteroposterior

referencing of the tibial ACL insertion site. The direct tibial "C"-shaped footprint is aligned along the medial tibial spine from the Tuberculum intercondylare mediale and is curved toward the anterior border of the lateral meniscus. The anteriorly inserting ACL fibers cross over the bony insertion of the anterior root of the lateral meniscus in a "ribbonlike" manner. When using hamstrings, the geometry of the DB ACL reconstruction is more anatomical compared to SB (see Chap. 22). However, DB ACL reconstruction is more difficult to perform. The above technique for flat ACL reconstructions was used in more than 250 patients using smaller-diameter grafts. Long-term results have to prove the clinical advantage of the new technique over a "traditional" ACL reconstruction. When using PT or QT, graft geometry is more anatomical, and the DB technique is unnecessary.

Part VI

ACL Reconstruction with Extra-articular Stabilisation

ACL Reconstruction with Extra-articular Plasty

30

David Dejour, Stefano Zaffagnini,
Panagiotis G. Ntagiopoulos, Alberto Grassi,
Giulio Maria Marcheggiani Muccioli,
and Maurilio Marcacci

Contents

D. Dejour, MD (✉) • P.G. Ntagiopoulos
Department of Knee Surgery and Sports Medicine,
Lyon-Ortho-Clinic, Clinique de la Sauvegarde,
8 Ave Ben Gourion, Lyon 69009, France
e-mail: dejour@me.com

S. Zaffagnini • A. Grassi • G.M.M. Muccioli
M. Marcacci
Clinica Ortopedia e Traumatologica II, Laboratorio di
Biomeccanica ed Innovazione Tecnologica,
Istituto Ortopedico Rizzoli, Bologna, Italy

30.1 Indications for Extra-articular Plasty

Chronic anterior cruciate ligament (ACL) laxity, and in particular rotational laxity associated with a severe positive pivot-shift test (PST), has been associated to the combined damage of the ACL and the posterolateral structures of the knee [6, 26, 32]. Other authors have also recorded possible evidence of damage of these structures along with ACL tears with the presence of the "Segond fracture" that results from avulsion of the iliotibial band (ITB) or the "anterior oblique band" of the lateral collateral ligament (LCL) [8]. Further evidence of the gross instability after ACL and lateral structures damage is the lateral tibial subluxation and the subsequent "bone bruising" observed in magnetic resonance imaging [11, 37]. As Dodds and Amis have recently published, these posterolateral structures may not have been yet directly identified, but probably act as secondary restraints to the PST, supplementing the primary restraint role of the ACL in anteroposterior laxity, with emphasis on rotatory laxity and internal rotation [15]. The persistence of this rotatory laxity has been reported even after cases of uneventful ACL reconstruction, suggesting that a single-bundle intra-articular reconstruction could not be sufficient to completely restore rotational knee stability in certain patients [38].

The debate on the additional structures damaged, other than the intra-articular compound, and the need to control especially the rotation after ACL reconstruction, gave rise to the strategy to combine intra-articular ACL reconstruction with extra-articular plasty. The main arguments of the supporters of this procedure are as follows: (1) the previously mentioned evidence of the *additional structures being damaged* in ACL tears favor that there are *additional structures required to be addressed* in ACL reconstruction, (2) the strong association of the posterolateral structures in controlling internal tibial rotation, and (3) the lateral extra-articular plasty is far from the center of the knee rotation and provides a greater lever arm for controlling PST and internal rotation than the intra-articular reconstruction [15, 30]. The rationale behind extra-articular plasty is therefore to create a restraint in internal tibial rotation.

Authors who favor the supplementary extra-articular plasty to standard ACL reconstruction record reduced PST results and lateral tibial translation [14, 41], but the introduction of evidence-based inclusion criteria for any similar technique as a primary or a revision option is difficult and remains sporadical and empirically based [14, 15, 30].

In the authors' practice, extra-articular plasty is *supplementing* the *primary intra-articular ACL reconstruction* in:

1. *Challenging primary cases* where *gross PST* is recorded and high-energy sports activities are expected
2. Chronic cases of ACL laxity with an excessive anterior tibial translation and previous meniscectomy
3. *Revision* cases of ACL reconstruction, especially cases where previous graft placement was anatomic and re-rupture was the result of minimal force
4. Patients with joint *hyperlaxity* and knee recurvatum

30.2 Surgical Techniques

There are several techniques of extra-articular tenodesis described in the literature since the 1960s. The Lemaire procedure involved the dissection of an 18 cm ITB strip, which was left attached to GT and was passed under the LCL into a bone tunnel in the lateral femoral condyle and then was reattached to the GT in a second bone tunnel [24]. Macintosh described a procedure where, in short terms, a 20 cm ITB strip was dissected, turned down to Gerdy's tubercle (GT), and then looped deep into the femoral condyle near the LCL [27]. The Ellison procedure was a modification of the Macintosh procedure, where the ITB strip was detached from GT before being inserted in the femoral condyle [18]. Christel described a less invasive modification of the original Lemaire procedure, where a shorter ITB strip was twisted 180° and inserted to the lateral femoral condyle after going under the LCL [9]. Losee et al. published a technique where the ITB was slinged and "reefed" around the posterolateral corner of the knee [26]. Andrews used isometric bundles of the ITT in combination with ACL reconstruction, in order to treat anterolateral instability [3]. In the late 1990s, and differently from the previous techniques, Marcacci described a procedure of ACL reconstruction where hamstrings graft was used both for intra-articular reconstruction and lateral tenodesis, through the over-the-top position [28]. Some years later, Colombet used a single-bundle hamstrings graft passed through a tibial and femoral tunnel and fixed it to Gerdy's tubercle to perform the combined reconstruction [10]. Accordingly, Neyret proposed the combination of bone-patellar tendon-bone for intra-articular reconstruction and gracilis for extra-articular tenodesis [17].

30.2.1 ACL Reconstruction: Patellar Tendon and Extra-articular Plasty with Iliotibial Band (DD, PGN)

Extra-articular plasty technique involves the reconstruction of a lateral graft, as described by Lemaire [24] and Christel [9]. The rationale of the procedure lies on the reconstruction of an ITB graft that passes under the LCL who acts as a pulley and is fixed in the femur on the isometric point close to the lateral epicondyle. Usually, the graft preparation for the extra-articular plasty *follows* the primary graft harvesting for the ACL reconstruction (e.g., patellar tendon, hamstrings, or quadriceps tendon) and is performed *prior to* arthroscopy.

1. The knee is prepared and draped in the 90° flexed position. Key anatomical landmarks for the procedure are shown in Fig. 30.1 and involve the ITB, the GT, and the fibular head (FH).

2. Along the midline of the ITB and parallel to the direction of its fibers, a 5 cm skin incision is performed down to the GT (Fig. 30.2a). Subcutaneous tissue is dissected in order to visualize clearly the ITB (Fig. 30.2b), and especially its anterior and posterior borders (Fig. 30.2c).

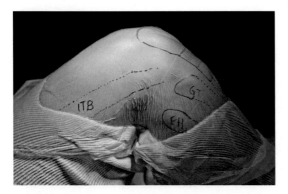

Fig. 30.1 Anatomical landmarks for the lateral plasty are the ITB, the GT, and the FH

3. With the use of a No. 15 blade, the middle third of the ITB is sharply divided in order to detach proximally a 10 mm width × 80 mm length rectangular stripe (Fig. 30.3a), while leaving its distal insertion attached to the GT (Fig. 30.3b).

4. The obtained graft is whipstitched in a standard fashion (Fig. 30.4a) and sized (Fig. 30.4b).

5. At this point, arthroscopic intra-articular ACL reconstruction follows in the surgeon's preferred technique. In the authors' practice, ACL reconstruction is performed through outside in femoral and tibial tunnels. The intra-articular ACL graft is passed through both femoral and tibial tunnels and securely fixed. The extra-articular plasty continues with the fixation of the ITB graft. It is mandatory that the knee is now flexed *more than 90°* for the rest of the procedure (Fig. 30.5).

6. This maneuver helps to easily *identify the LCL* that runs from the lateral femoral epicondyle to the FH (Fig. 30.6a). LCL is incised on its anterior and posterior borders, and a small pulley is undermined with scissors (Fig. 30.6b). With the use of a curved Kelly clamp (Fig. 30.6c), the ITB graft is passed *under the LCL* from a distal to proximal direction (Fig. 30.6d).

7. The desired insertion point of the ITB graft lies in the isometric *point just posterior to the femoral attachment of the LCL* (Fig. 30.7a). In this case, the desired point is identified with a circle (Fig. 30.7a: 2), while the pull-out

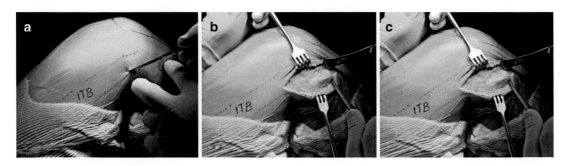

Fig. 30.2 (**a**) Perform a 5 cm skin incision down to the GT; (**b**) dissect subcutaneous tissue in order to visualize clearly the ITB and (**c**) especially its anterior and posterior borders

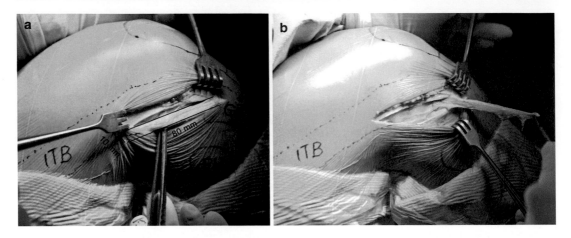

Fig. 30.3 (**a**) Detach a 10 mm width × 80 mm length rectangular stripe from the middle third of the ITB, (**b**) its distal insertion is left attached to the GT

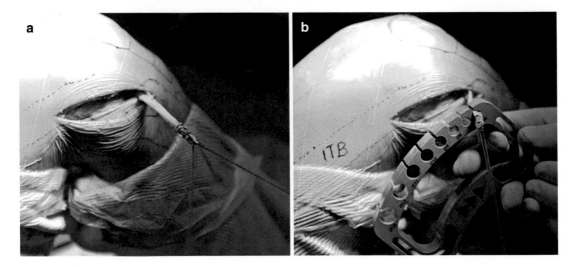

Fig. 30.4 (**a**) Whipstitch and (**b**) size the ITB graft

sutures from the intra-articular ACL graft are visible (Fig. 30.7a: 1). A K-wire is advanced to the desired location while we closely follow the LCL course (Fig. 30.7b). The direction of the K-wire should take caution not to interfere with the intra-articular femoral ACL tunnel (Fig. 30.7c).

8. A cannulated drill is gently advanced *unicortically* in a standard fashion in order not to violate the far medial cortex but long enough to accommodate the full length of the ITB graft. The ITB graft is pulled medially into the new

tunnel (Fig. 30.8a). The graft will be fixed at 70° of knee flexion, after cycling, *while the foot is positioned in neutral position.* An accordingly sized interference screw is used for the fixation of the graft, while a Kocher clamp is used medially to secure the sutures temporarily and to tighten the construct (Fig. 30.8b). Final image of the extra-articular plasty shows the ITB graft that passes under the LCL and is fixed into the femur in a separate tunnel than the intra-articular ACL graft (Fig. 30.8c: 1).

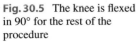 The knee is flexed in 90° for the rest of the procedure

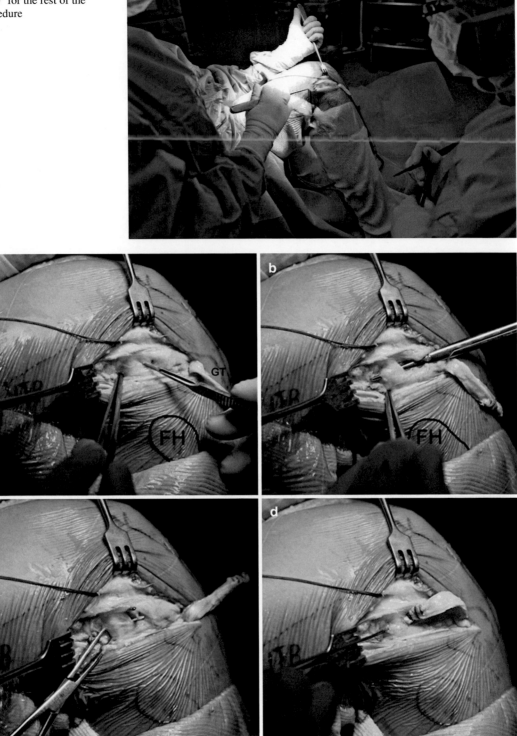

Fig. 30.6 (**a**) Identify the LCL, (**b**) incise the LCL on its anterior and posterior borders and create a small pulley under the LCL, (**c**) use a curved Kelly clamp, and (**d**) pass the graft under the LCL

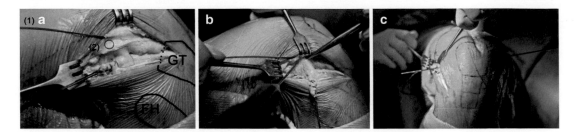

Fig. 30.7 (**a**) The insertion point of the ITB graft (*2*) is just posterior to the femoral attachment of the LCL, (*1*) the pull-out sutures from the intra-articular ACL graft, (**b**) a K-wire is advanced to the desired location, (**c**) the direction of the K-wire should take caution not to interfere with the intra-articular femoral ACL tunnel

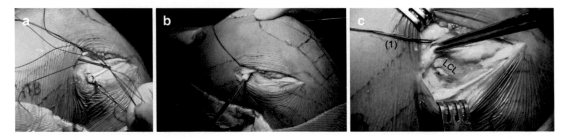

Fig. 30.8 (**a**) Pull the ITB graft medially into the tunnel; (**b**) use an interference screw to fix the graft while a Kocher clamp is securing the sutures; (**c**) final image of the extra-articular plasty with the ITB graft under the LCL in a separate femoral tunnel than (*1*) the intra-articular ACL graft

Tricks and Pearls

1. Identify properly the posterior border of the ITB and harvest the graft towards the posterior part of it.
2. Harvest sufficient length of the ITB graft (7–8 cm). It is preferable to err towards a longer graft than a shorter one, which may not reach inside the desired tunnel.
3. Identification of the LCL in order to pass the graft under it is facilitated by flexing the knee more than 90° and palpating its insertion on the fibular head.
4. In order not to interfere with the femoral tunnel of the intra-articular ACL graft and its fixation, aim the tunnel of the extra-articular plasty medially and superiorly. Position the arthroscope in the tunnel to confirm if necessary.

5. In case a longer ITB graft was harvested, make sure that the tunnel length is enough to accommodate its whole length. If not, this would lead to improper stretching and tensioning of the extra-articular plasty.
6. Tibia rotation while fixing the extra-articular plasty was originally described in external rotation by Lemaire. The associated lateral femorotibial stiffness led to change of this step. Tibia must be in neutral rotation while fixing the extra-articular plasty, to avoid stiffness of the lateral compartment.
7. During wound closure, be very meticulous in the hemostasis and the coagulation of small vessels located in the posterior aspect of the ITB. If not treated with caution, they can cause postoperative hematoma.

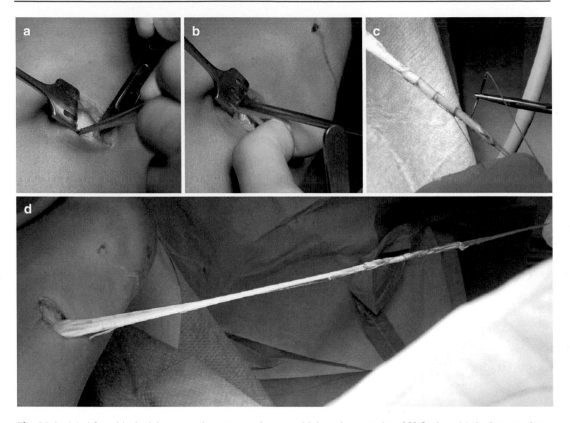

Fig. 30.9 (**a**) After skin incision over the pes anserinus and dissection of subcutaneous tissue, the fascial incision is made parallel to the orientation of the pes tendons; (**b**) both tendons are harvested using a blunt tendon stripper maintaining firm tension on the tendon distally and with knee in more than 90° flexion; (**c**) the harvested tendons are sutured together using nonabsorbable stitches at the free end; (**d**) gracilis and semitendinosus tendons are harvested maintaining intact their tibial insertion

30.2.2 ACL Reconstruction and Lateral Plasty with Hamstrings (SZ, MM)

30.2.2.1 Arthroscopic Setting

With the patient in the supine position on the operating table, a pneumatic tourniquet is placed as high as possible around the proximal part of the thigh. A support is placed laterally at the upper level of the knee to stress the joint during arthroscopic evaluation. Usually a medial supra-patellar portal is used for the water inflow, an anterolateral viewing portal, and an anteromedial working portal. Under arthroscopic control, meniscectomies or chondroplasty is performed where necessary. After confirmation of ACL lesion, the tibial insertion area and the intercondylar notch are prepared.

30.2.2.2 Graft Harvesting

With the patient's leg in a figure-4 position, the pes anserinus is located by following the hamstring tendons distally to their attachment on the anteromedial tibia. A 3 cm transverse incision is made over the pes anserinus (2 cm distal and 1 cm medial to the tibial tubercle).

Subcutaneous tissue is then dissected and the fascia is incised parallel to the orientation of the pes tendons (Fig. 30.9a). The sartorius tendon is retracted superiorly, and the gracilis and semitendinosus tendons are bluntly dissected from the surrounding soft tissue. Both tendons are harvested using a blunt tendon stripper (Acufex, Microsurgical, Mansfield, MA), while maintaining firm tension on the tendon distally and with knee in more than 90° flexion to facilitate the detachment of the tendon (Fig. 30.9b). This step

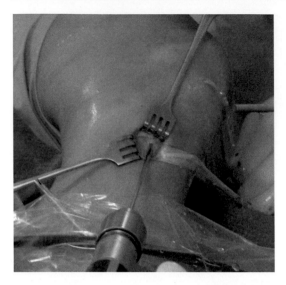

Fig. 30.10 The tibial tunnel is prepared under arthroscopic visualization inserting a guide pin on the medial aspect of the tibia through the graft harvesting incision

should be performed carefully in order to obtain the maximum length of the tendons, which is usually approximately 20 cm. The tibial insertion of both tendons is preserved to maintain their neurovascular supply. The harvested tendons are then sutured together using three nonabsorbable Flexidene No. 2 stitches (Laboratory Bruneau, Boulogne Billancourt, France), and the sutures are tightened (Fig. 30.9c), with emphasis at the free proximal tendon ends (Fig. 30.9d).

30.2.2.3 Tibial Tunnel Preparation

Preparation of the tibial tunnel is performed under arthroscopic visualization by inserting a guide pin on the medial aspect of the tibia through the graft harvesting incision (Fig. 30.10), directed to the medial posterior part of the ACL tibial insertion (Fig. 30.11a). After reaming the tibial tunnel according to ligament diameter (usually 8–9 mm), a looped wire passer is inserted from the tibial tunnel into the notch (Fig. 30.11b) and is brought out from the anteromedial portal under arthroscopic visualization (Fig. 30.11c, d).

30.2.2.4 Over-the-Top Position

With the knee positioned at 90° flexion and the foot externally rotated, a 3–5 cm longitudinal incision is made directly above the lateral femoral epicondyle (Fig. 30.12). The posterior third of the iliotibial band is divided and is retracted anteriorly. The lateral aspect of the thigh is dissected using electrocautery and scissors, in order to reach the lateral intermuscular septum, which separates the vastus lateralis muscle (above) from the lateral head of the gastrocnemius muscle (below). When the lateral intermuscular septum has been clearly identified, it is possible to reach the posterior aspect of the joint capsule by passing over this structure. If this is not possible, the septum can be divided. It is possible to determine the correct placement of the "over-the-top" position and to protect the posterior structures during the next step, by palpating the posterior tubercle of the lateral femoral condyle with a finger. A curved Kelly clamp is passed from the anteromedial portal into the notch, and its tip is placed as far proximally possible against the posterior part of the capsule. After palpating the tip of the clamp from the lateral side of the femur just posterior to the intermuscular septum (Fig. 30.13), it is pushed through the thin posterior layer of knee capsule, reaching the posterior space previously prepared. A suture loop is then placed into the tip of the clamp (Fig. 30.14), pulled anteriorly through the anteromedial portal and placed into the wire loop previously inserted in the portal. Pulling the wire from the tibial side brings the suture loop at the bottom of the tibial tunnel and out from the tibial incision.

30.2.2.5 Graft Placement and Fixation

The suture is tied on the free end of the graft (Fig. 30.15b) and is pulled through the knee joint (Fig. 30.15b), and the graft is retrieved from the lateral incision (Fig. 30.15c). A groove is made in the lateral aspect of the femur just proximally to the start of the lateral condyle (Fig. 30.16a, b), allowing the anteriorization of the grafts and the achievement of a more isometric position. Once the graft is placed in the correct position, it is tensioned and the knee cycled through a full range of motion about 20 times to check its stability. Then, the graft can be secured to the lateral femoral cortex into the groove with two metal staples (Fig. 30.17a, b)

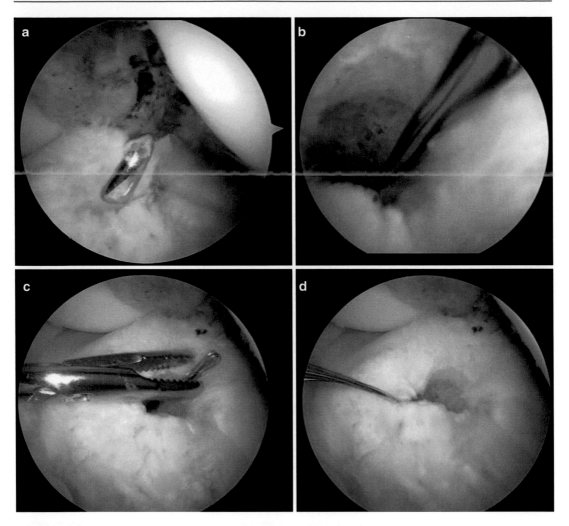

Fig. 30.11 (**a**) The guide pin is directed to the medial posterior part of the ACL tibial insertion; (**b**) the wire loop is inserted from the tibial tunnel into the notch, (**c**) grasped with a clamp, and (**d**) brought out from the anteromedial portal

while maintaining the knee at about 90° of flexion and the foot externally rotated. Putting under tension, the remaining part of the graft makes it possible to evaluate its length and whether or not it is long enough to reach GT in the anterolateral aspect of the tibia (Fig. 30.17c). If this condition is satisfied, a 1–2 cm skin and fascia incision is performed just below the GT (Fig. 30.18a). Then, a small Kelly clamp is passed under the fascia from this incision to the lateral femoral condyle (Fig. 30.18b), where the sutures at the end of the graft are placed in the tip of the clamp and pulled down (Fig. 30.18c), emerging from

the GT incision (Fig. 30.18d). The graft is tensioned and the knee is cycled again to check the isometry of the lateral tenodesis and the freedom of flexion-extension. Another metallic staple is then used to fix the graft below GT to the lateral aspect of the tibia. An intra-articular drain is threaded through the superomedial portal, and additional drains are inserted in each wound. The iliotibial tract defect is closed, taking care to prevent lateral tilt and patellar compression, while the medial fascia over the pes anserinus is not closed, in order to prevent compartment syndrome.

30.3 Pitfalls and Complications

30.3.1 Patellar Tendon and Extra-articular Lateral Plasty with Iliotibial Band

The addition of an extra-articular gesture in ACL reconstruction adds little difficulty in an already challenging procedure. Despite its popularity, ACL reconstruction remains technically demanding with a low threshold for complications. One

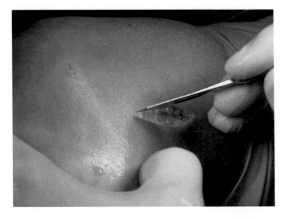

Fig. 30.12 The 3–5 cm incision to reach the over-the-top position is performed longitudinally just above the lateral femoral condyle, with the knee positioned at 90° flexion and the foot externally rotated

Fig. 30.13 A clamp is inserted in the anteromedial portal and directed to the notch; with a finger on the lateral side of the femur just posterior to the intermuscular septum, it is possible to palpate the tip of the clamp against the posterior part of the capsule

of the complications of the extra-articular plasty is the improper placement of the additional femoral tunnel, and care must be taken to avoid interference with the intra-articular femoral tunnel because this would lead to loss of primary fixation. Another drawback is the additional required skin and soft-tissue exposure for the procedure along with the donor-site morbidity of the ITB. Proper graft placement and tensioning are mandatory and malpositioning or over-tensioning the ITB graft would lead to knee stiffness. The rehabilitation program remains the same as for an isolated graft with a partial weight-bearing period of 3 weeks.

30.3.2 Hamstrings and Extra-articular Lateral Tenodesis

30.3.2.1 Graft Rupture

As the main feature for the success of this technique is the adequate length of the graft, all events that could cause a short-graft harvesting or graft rupture should be carefully avoided. A meticulous dissection of both gracilis and semitendinosus tendons from their fascial attachments is mandatory (Fig. 30.19) in order to prevent early cutting of the tendons when advancing the tendon stripper. If this event happens and

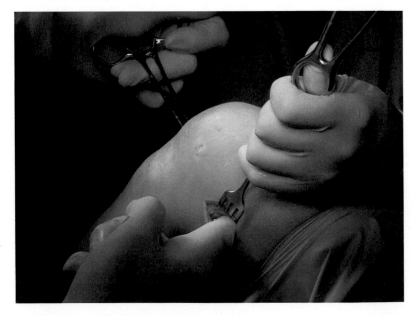

one of the two tendons is shorter, the graft could be sutured in any case, and the reconstruction should be performed according to the described technique. In most of the cases, the intra-articular graft will be formed by two strands, while the lateral plasty will be inevitably formed by a biomechanically weaker single strand.

In order to gain an additional 1 or 2 cm in length, the distal attachment of the semitendinosus to the adjacent gracilis tendon could be dissected (Fig. 30.20). Another potential danger of the graft's integrity could be the sharpness of the edges of the tibial tunnel hole, and as tension is applied to the graft when passing through the tibial tunnel, it could produce a cutting mechanism that could damage the graft. Therefore, before passing the graft through the tibial tunnel, the edges of the osseous tunnel should be accurately smoothened with a motorized shaver (Fig. 30.21a, b).

Detachment of the distal insertion of the tendons from the anteromedial tibia could be caused by excessive graft tensioning as well; therefore, the graft should be correctly tensioned with a progressive increase of the force avoiding rough stretches. In case of detachment of the distal insertion of the tendons, both the strands of the distal end of the graft could be sutured together, and the graft should be retrieved downwards through the tibial tunnel and fixed with an interference screw or metallic staple. At this point, the

possibility to perform the lateral tenodesis depends from the remaining length of the graft.

Additionally, the fixation of the graft with metallic staples, especially at the lateral femoral cortex, could be a source of graft damage, as the barb of the staple coupled with high tension applied to the graft could produce a guillotine effect. In order to avoid this drawback, the staples should be firmly fixed in the bone cortex but

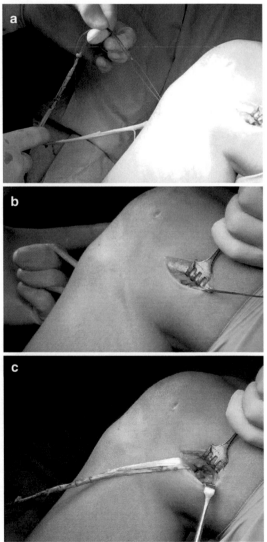

Fig. 30.15 (**a**) The suture that exits from the tibial tunnel is tied on the free end of the graft, (**b**) pulling the sutures and passage of the graft through the tibial tunnel and in the knee joint; (**c**) at the end the graft is retrieved from the lateral incision

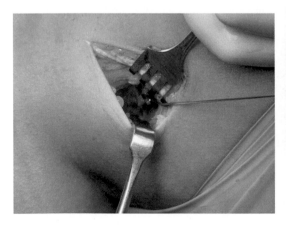

Fig. 30.14 The clamp is pushed through the thin posterior layer of knee capsule, reaching the posterior space previously prepared

Fig. 30.16 (**a**) A groove is created in the lateral aspect of the femur just proximally to the start of the lateral condyle; (**b**) final aspect of the groove where the graft should be placed to reach a more isometric position

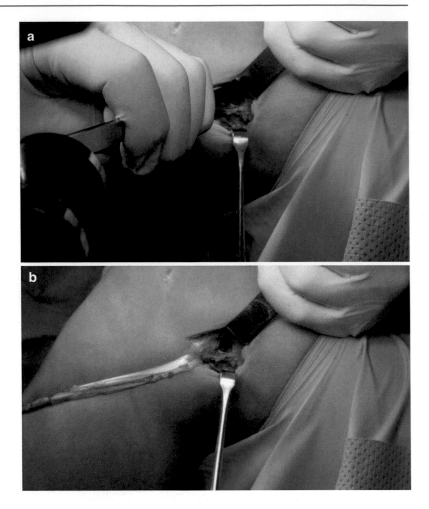

without driven too deeply. On the other hand, a not firm fixation will lead to loss of proper graft tension and almost certain failure of the reconstruction. In the case of graft rupture that does not allow the lateral tenodesis, the ACL reconstruction could be performed by maintaining only the intra-articular part, with all the limitations derived from a single-bundle nonanatomical technique.

30.3.2.2 Incorrect Graft Placement

Correct graft placement, both for intra- and extra-articular part, is mandatory in order to obtain good outcomes and avoid dangerous complications. Positioning the tibial tunnel to the postero-medial part of ACL tibial insertion, coupled with the use of the over-the-top position, guarantees the correct location of the graft, which is posteriorly enough to avoid impingement. Nevertheless,

in chronic cases, big osteophytes, especially on the medial edge of the lateral condyle, could obstruct the intercondylar notch; therefore, a true notchplasty should be performed to avoid graft impingement. Any soft tissue in the posterior part of the roof that can obstruct the "over-the-top" position must be carefully removed as well.

The incorrect placement of the extra-articular tenodesis could produce excessive tension on the graft along the range of motion, causing pain and joint stiffness. This could be avoided by fixing the graft in the isometric position. Creating a small groove in the lateral aspect of the femur allows the graft to move anteriorly, while the repeated cycling allows the construct to find its optimal placement for the distal fixation and to check the graft tension along the complete range of motion.

Fig. 30.17 (**a**) The graft is tensioned with the knee at 90° and (**b**) is secured with two metallic staples on the lateral femoral cortex; (**c**) by pulling the remaining part of the graft, it is possible to check whether or not it is long enough to reach GT in the anterolateral aspect of the tibia

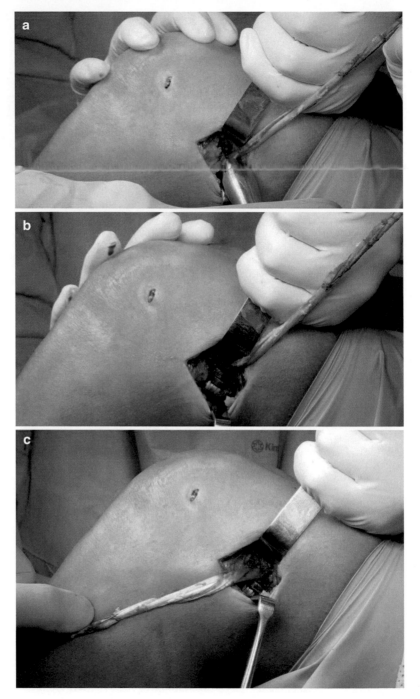

30.3.2.3 Iatrogenic Injuries

Inexpert graft harvesting could damage important anatomical structures. The infrapatellar branches of the saphenous nerve could be generally injured when performing skin incision and tendon dissection; the risk is considered higher when performing median incision for bone-patellar tendon-bone harvesting compared to hamstrings. Furthermore, this risk could be theoretically reduced by performing an oblique rather than vertical incision, according to the course of the nerve. When the infrapatellar

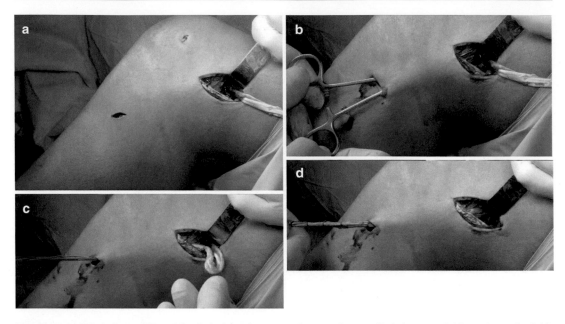

Fig. 30.18 (**a**) A 1–2 cm skin and fascia incision is performed just below GT, (**b**) a small Kelly clamp is passed below the fascia to the lateral femoral condyle, (**c**) the sutures at the end of the graft are placed in the tip of the clamp and are pulled down, and (**d**) at the end of this maneuver, the graft emerges from the GT incision where it can be secured with a metallic staple

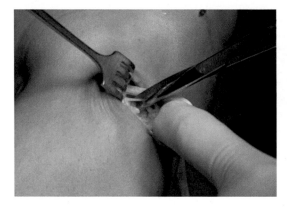

Fig. 30.19 All the fascial attachments of both gracilis and semitendinosus tendon should be dissected carefully in order to prevent early cutting of the tendons when advancing the tendon stripper

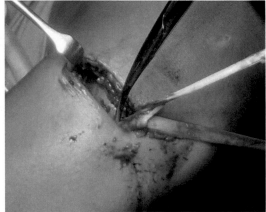

Fig. 30.20 By dissecting the distal attachment of the semitendinosus to the adjacent gracilis tendon, it is possible to gain an additional 1 or 2 cm in length

branches of the saphenous nerve are damaged, sensitivity deficit appears on the anterolateral aspect of the proximal calf. Care should also be taken when handling gracilis and semitendinosus tendons in order not to damage the superficial medial collateral ligament (MCL), as it lies immediately deep to the expansion of the pes anserinus and should not be mistaken for it.

A more dangerous and harmful complication related to this technique is the injury of the popliteal artery when approaching to the over-the-top position. Although this is a rare event, it should be considered as a vascular emergency and its treatment is beyond the scope of this chapter. But this risk is almost inconsistent, if all the steps are scrupulously followed.

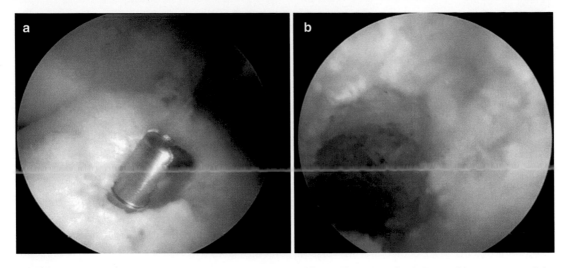

Fig. 30.21 (**a**) The sharp edges of the tibial tunnel are smoothened with a motorized shaver; (**b**) appearance of the tibial tunnel before the passage of the graft

30.4   Literature Results

30.4.1 Results of Extra-articular Plasty in ACL Reconstruction Surgery

The extra-articular plasty was initially performed without concomitant intra-articular ACL reconstruction. Evidently, the early results were promising mostly because it was controlling the pivot shift but it failed to restore anteroposterior stability, which was leading to meniscus damage and then to femorotibial degenerative changes [26, 35, 36]. The main reasons that the interest on these techniques was weakened after the first years were: the evolution of all-arthroscopic ACL reconstruction was favored over these more invasive and less cosmetic techniques, the absence of concomitant intra-articular ACL reconstruction, the donor-site morbidity, and the long rehabilitation protocols that included a 2-month period of knee immobilization [15].

When extra-articular plasty was combined with intra-articular ACL reconstruction, the results were more encouraging. Dejour et al. treated 148 patients with 11.5 years follow-up using open intra-articular ACL reconstruction with patellar tendon and extra-articular plasty with the Lemaire technique and recorded that

89 % scored "satisfied" or "very satisfied" in a subjective score [13]. Using the same technique, they treated 251 cases of chronic ACL laxity and recorded that 83 % had "good" or "excellent" functional results [12]. Jensen et al. found no significant differences between intra-articular ACL reconstruction and additional extra-articular plasty, but they recorded that extra-articular plasty reduces the feeling of "giving way" [22]. Similarly, Noyes and Barber and Lerat et al. found significant increase of stability when extra-articular plasty was added to ACL reconstruction [25, 33].

Successful results were published by Ferretti et al. in a study where the authors used an intra-articular reconstruction with doubled hamstrings graft and an extra-articular reconstruction by a modification of the Macintosh procedure for ACL revision cases [20]. Marcacci et al. reported the long-term results of their nonanatomic over-the-top ACL reconstruction combined with lateral tenodesis using hamstrings graft [29]. The authors recommended the technique for primary ACL reconstruction since they recorded that 90 % of 54 consecutive cases scored "good" or "excellent" results in IKDC after an average of 11 years [29]. Bignozzi et al. evaluated the results of the latter technique with computer-assisted navigation and found that the in vivo addition of an extra-articular procedure to single-bundle ACL reconstruction successfully controlled coupled tibial translation during the Lachman test and reduced anteroposterior laxity at 90° of flexion [4]. Buda et al. utilized the same nonanatomic over-the-top technique using allograft tendons, for multiple-revision ACL reconstruction, reporting "good" or "excellent" results in 83 % of patients and 92 % with "normal" to "nearly-normal" PST [5]. Also, Trojani et al. reported the results of ACL revision with additional lateral plasty, showing better results in terms of stability and failure rate compared to isolated intra-articular reconstruction [39].

Apart from the graft choice and its versatile course until its usual final insertion in the lateral femoral condyle, most of these authors agree that the critical point for the success of the extra-articular plasty is the point of femoral fixation [15, 30]. This has been defined to be located slightly posteriorly and proximally to the femoral insertion of the LCL [7, 16, 23]. Colombet published a technique where he uses navigation in order to facilitate the identification of this femoral insertion point [10].

30.4.2 Comparison of Intra-articular ACL Reconstruction with and Without Extra-articular Plasty

A reasonable argument in favor of supplementary extra-articular plasty is that it provides additional protection on the intra-articular reconstruction, especially in the early rehabilitation period. Even though the in vitro study of the extra-articular plasty showed that it decreases up to 43 % the forces upon the primary intra-articular construct [19], the direct clinical value of the addition of extra-articular plasty is yet to be proved [15]. The few available studies that compare the two options produce contradicting results. Earlier reports showed no clear differences between intra-articular reconstruction and the addition of extra-articular plasty and that there is no benefit from the supplementary procedure [1, 2, 22, 34–36]. On the other hand, some authors recorded benefits from the addition of

extra-articular plasty, such as better PST control [21], reduced tibial internal rotation, and better constraint of lateral tibial displacement [14, 25, 40, 41]. Monaco and Ferretti et al. recorded that the addition of extra-articular plasty significantly reduced internal tibial rotation at 30° of flexion when compared to single- or double-bundle ACL reconstruction [31]. Zaffagnini et al. compared single-bundle ACL reconstruction with and without extra-articular plasty and found superior results for the extra-articular plasty group, in terms of subjective clinical findings and time to return to sports activities [40]. More recently, the same group compared double-bundle ACL reconstruction versus single-bundle ACL reconstruction with extra-articular plasty and recorded that the latter resulted in better control of static knee laxity, reduced mediolateral instability in early flexion, and reduced rotatory instability at 90° of flexion [41].

Memory

Extra-articular techniques in the reconstruction of anterior cruciate ligament are becoming more and more popular in selected primary cases and especially in the revision setting. The rationale of extra-articular plasty lies on the possible damage of additional structures in ACL tears that need to be restored and the need to create a restraint in internal tibial torsion, especially in patients with increased recorded laxity and explosive pivot-shift test. The lateral extra-articular plasty is far from the center of the knee rotation and therefore provides a greater lever arm for controlling internal rotation than the intra-articular reconstruction. Several techniques of extra-articular plasty or tenodesis have been described. Most of them involve using the iliotibial band or the hamstrings. The two most popular techniques are described in this chapter along with surgical tips and possible pitfalls: the extra-articular plasty of Lemaire and the lateral extra-articular tenodesis with hamstrings.

References

1. Acquitter Y, Hulet C, Locker B et al (2003) Patellar tendon-bone autograft reconstruction of the anterior cruciate ligament for advanced-stage chronic anterior laxity: is an extra-articular plasty necessary? A prospective randomized study of 100 patients with five year follow-up. Rev Chir Orthop Reparatrice Appar Mot 89(5):413–422

2. Amis AA, Scammell BE (1993) Biomechanics of intra-articular and extra-articular reconstruction of the anterior cruciate ligament. J Bone Joint Surg Br 75(5): 812–817

3. Andrews JR, Sanders RA, Morin B (1985) Surgical treatment of anterolateral instability: a follow-up study. Am J Sports Med 13:112–119

4. Bignozzi S, Zaffagnini S, Lopomo N et al (2009) Does a lateral plasty control coupled translation during antero-posterior stress in single-bundle ACL reconstruction? An in vivo study. Knee Surg Sports Traumatol Arthrosc 17(1):65–70

5. Buda R, Ruffilli A, Di Caprio F (2013) Allograft salvage procedure in multiple-revision anterior cruciate ligament reconstruction. Am J Sports Med 41(2): 402–410

6. Bull AMJ, Amis AA (1998) The pivot-shift phenomenon: a clinical and biomechanical perspective. Knee 5(5):141–158

7. Bylski-Austrow DI, Grood ES, Hefzy MS et al (1990) Anterior cruciate ligament replacements: a mechanical study of femoral attachment location, flexion angle at tensioning, and initial tension. J Orthop Res 8(4):522–531

8. Campos JC, Chung CB, Lektrakul N et al (2001) Pathogenesis of the Segond fracture: anatomic and MR imaging evidence of an iliotibial tract or anterior oblique band avulsion. Radiology 219(2):381–386

9. Christel P, Djian P (2002) Anterio-lateral extra-articular tenodesis of the knee using a short strip of fascia lata. Rev Chir Orthop Reparatrice Appar Mot 88(5):508–513

10. Colombet PD (2011) Navigated intra-articular ACL reconstruction with additional extra-articular tenodesis using the same hamstring graft. Knee Surg Sports Traumatol Arthrosc 19(3):384–389

11. Delzell PB, Schils JP, Recht MP (1996) Subtle fractures about the knee: innocuous-appearing yet indicative of significant internal derangement. AJR Am J Roentgenol 167(3):699–703

12. Dejour H, Walch G, Neyret P et al (1988) Results of surgically treated chronic anterior laxities. Apropos of 251 cases reviewed with a minimum follow-up of 3 years. Rev Chir Orthop Reparatrice Appar Mot 74(7): 622–636

13. Dejour H, Dejour D, Ait Si Selmi T (1999) Chronic anterior laxity of the knee treated with free patellar graft and extra-articular lateral plasty: 10-year follow-up of 148 cases. Rev Chir Orthop Reparatrice Appar Mot 85(8):777–789

14. Dejour D, Vasconcelos W, Bonin N et al (2013) Comparative study between mono-bundle bone-patellar tendon-bone, double-bundle hamstring and mono-bundle bone-patellar tendon-bone combined with a modified Lemaire extra-articular procedure in anterior cruciate ligament reconstruction. Int Orthop 37:193–199

15. Dodds AL, Gupte CM, Neyret P et al (2011) Extra-articular techniques in anterior cruciate ligament reconstruction: a literature review. J Bone Joint Surg Br 93(11):1440–1448

16. Draganich LF, Hsieh YF, Reider B (1995) Iliotibial band tenodesis: a new strategy for attachment. Am J Sports Med 23(2):186–195

17. Duthon VB, Magnussen RA, Servien E et al (2013) ACL reconstruction and extra-articular tenodesis. Clin Sports Med 32(1):141–153

18. Ellison AE (1979) Distal iliotibial-band transfer for anterolateral rotatory instability of the knee. J Bone Joint Surg Am 61(3):330–337

19. Engebretsen L, Lew WD, Lewis JL et al (1990) The effect of an iliotibial tenodesis on intraarticular graft forces and knee joint motion. Am J Sports Med 18(2):169–176

20. Ferretti A, Conteduca F, Monaco E et al (2006) Revision anterior cruciate ligament reconstruction with doubled semitendinosus and gracilis tendons and lateral extra-articular reconstruction. J Bone Joint Surg Am 88(11):2373–2379

21. Giraud B, Besse JL, Cladiere F et al (2006) Intra-articular reconstruction of the anterior cruciate ligament with and without extra-articular supplementation by quadricipital tendon plasty: seven-year follow-up. Rev Chir Orthop Reparatrice Appar Mot 92(8):788–797

22. Jensen JE, Slocum DB, Larson RL et al (1983) Reconstruction procedures for anterior cruciate ligament insufficiency: a computer analysis of clinical results. Am J Sports Med 11(4):240–248

23. Krackow KA, Brooks RL (1983) Optimization of knee ligament position for lateral extraarticular reconstruction. Am J Sports Med 11(5):293–302

24. Lemaire M (1975) Chronic knee instability. Technics and results of ligament plasty in sports injuries. J Chir (Paris) 110(4):281–294

25. Lerat JL, Chotel F, Besse JL et al (1998) The results after 10-16 years of the treatment of chronic anterior laxity of the knee using reconstruction of the anterior cruciate ligament with a patellar tendon graft combined with an external extra-articular reconstruction. Rev Chir Orthop Reparatrice Appar Mot 84(8): 712–727

26. Losee RE, Johnson TR, Southwick WO (1978) Anterior subluxation of the lateral tibial plateau. A diagnostic test and operative repair. J Bone Joint Surg Am 60(8):1015–1030

27. Macintosh DL, Darby JA (1976) Lateral substitution reconstruction. Proceedings of the Canadian Orthopaedic Association. J Bone Joint Surg Br 58:142

28. Marcacci M, Zaffagnini S, Iacono F et al (1998) Arthroscopic intra- and extra-articular anterior cruciate ligament reconstruction with gracilis and semitendinosus tendons. Knee Surg Sports Traumatol Arthrosc 6(2):68–75

29. Marcacci M, Zaffagnini S, Giordano G et al (2009) Anterior cruciate ligament reconstruction associated with extra-articular tenodesis: a prospective clinical and radiographic evaluation with 10- to 13-year follow-up. Am J Sports Med 37(4):707–714

30. Marcacci M, Zaffagnini S, Marcheggiani Muccioli GM et al (2011) Arthroscopic intra- and extra-articular anterior cruciate ligament reconstruction with gracilis and semitendinosus tendons: a review. Curr Rev Musculoskelet Med 4(2):73–77

31. Monaco E, Labianca L, Conteduca F et al (2007) Double bundle or single bundle plus extraarticular tenodesis in ACL reconstruction? A CAOS study. Knee Surg Sports Traumatol Arthrosc 15(10): 1168–1174

32. Norwood LA Jr, Andrews JR, Meisterling RC et al (1979) Acute anterolateral rotatory instability of the knee. J Bone Joint Surg Am 61(5):704–709

33. Noyes FR, Barber SD (1991) The effect of an extra-articular procedure on allograft reconstructions for chronic ruptures of the anterior cruciate ligament. J Bone Joint Surg Am 73(6):882–892

34. O'Brien SJ, Warren RF, Pavlov H et al (1991) Reconstruction of the chronically insufficient anterior cruciate ligament with the central third of the patellar ligament. J Bone Joint Surg Am 73(2):278–286

35. Roth JH, Kennedy JC, Lockstadt H et al (1987) Intra-articular reconstruction of the anterior cruciate ligament with and without extra-articular supplementation by transfer of the biceps femoris tendon. J Bone Joint Surg Am 69(2):275–278

36. Strum GM, Fox JM, Ferkel RD et al (1989) Intraarticular versus intraarticular and extraarticular reconstruction for chronic anterior cruciate ligament instability. Clin Orthop Relat Res 245:188–198

37. Tashiro Y, Okazaki K, Miura H et al (2009) Quantitative assessment of rotatory instability after anterior cruciate ligament reconstruction. Am J Sports Med 37(5):909–916

38. Tashman S, Collon D, Anderson K et al (2004) Abnormal rotational knee motion during running after anterior cruciate ligament reconstruction. Am J Sports Med 32(4):975–983

39. Trojani C, Beaufils P, Burdin G (2012) Revision ACL reconstruction: influence of a lateral tenodesis. Knee Surg Sports Traumatol Arthrosc 20(8):1565–1570

40. Zaffagnini S, Marcacci M, Lo Presti M et al (2006) Prospective and randomized evaluation of ACL reconstruction with three techniques: a clinical and radiographic evaluation at 5 years follow-up. Knee Surg Sports Traumatol Arthrosc 14(11):1060–1069

41. Zaffagnini S, Signorelli C, Lopomo N et al (2012) Anatomic double-bundle and over-the-top single-bundle with additional extra-articular tenodesis: an in vivo quantitative assessment of knee laxity in two different ACL reconstructions. Knee Surg Sports Traumatol Arthrosc 20(1):153–159

Extra-articular Augmentation of Anterior Cruciate Ligament Reconstruction: The Monoloop Procedure

31

Cathal J. Moran, Peter C. Verdonk, Koen Lagae, and Geert DeClercq

Contents

C.J. Moran, MD, FRCS (Tr&Orth)
P.C. Verdonk, MD, PhD • K. Lagae, MD
G. DeClercq, MD (✉)
Orthopedisch Centrum SPM, AC Monica Hospitals,
Stevenslei 20, Deurne 2100, Belgium
e-mail: geert.declercq@azmonica.be

31.1 Introduction

Anterior cruciate ligament (ACL) injury is associated with symptomatic instability and increased risk of injury to the menisci and articular cartilage of the knee [1]. The aim of surgical intervention is to improve clinical symptoms, restore knee kinematics as best possible, and reduce the risk of further injury to the menisci and articular cartilage [2, 3]. Our ability to alter the natural history of the ACL-injured knee, in terms of the later degenerative change seen typically, remains unproven.

The techniques utilized to "normalize" excess translation and rotation/pivot in the ACL-injured knee have evolved over time, and there is ongoing debate as to the optimal technique to apply. This is due, in part, to the difficulty in replacing the unique anatomical structure and function of the native ACL, alongside limitations in our understanding of the role of potential concomitant injury to knee joint structures other than the ACL in pathological translational and pivot-shift phenomena [3–5]. However, an appropriately placed central graft appears effective in limiting translation in the sagittal plane, and it is generally accepted that placement of such a graft in an oblique plane provides a significant moment of resistance against the rotatory torque that occurs during the pivot shift. Whether the introduction of this single oblique central graft alone is sufficient to prevent instability in all patients is a matter of continued concern however. As many patients appear to have ongoing rotational instability

R. Siebold et al. (eds.), *Anterior Cruciate Ligament Reconstruction,*
DOI 10.1007/978-3-642-45349-6_31, © ESSKA 2014

following all-inside ACL surgery, it appears reasonable to consider historical literature that suggests optimal surgical restoration of knee stability in some cases needs simultaneous consideration of potentially unrecognized concomitant injury to structures at the periphery of the knee joint. Of specific concern is the role of capsular or ligamentous structures on the lateral side of the knee [6–10]. It has been repeatedly postulated that a combined intra-articular ACL reconstruction with extra-articular augmentation on the lateral side may be of benefit for some patients. Furthermore, Fu and others have extensively investigated the structure and function of the individual bundles of the ACL and the role that they play in both translational and rotational control of the knee [11]. The internal double-bundle concept has been very helpful in focusing our attention on anatomical factors in ACL reconstruction that may impact on outcomes following ACL surgery. It also highlights the limitations of traditional arthroscopic-alone-based techniques using an isolated central graft as the universal construct for all patients diagnosed with an ACL injury. We believe that, given the biomechanically short lever arm of centrally placed grafts, certain high-risk patients may warrant additional intervention to limit pathological rotation following what we recognize as an ACL injury.While we apply both single and double-bundle ACL reconstruction techniques in our practice, surgeons at our institution have also applied extra-articular augmentation in select cases for over 30 years [7]. We continue to believe it has a role to play in optimizing the outcome in many patients presenting with the primary finding of a ruptured ACL. In particular, we use this extra-articular augmentation in patients participating in activities with a high level of cutting or pivoting, patients with hyperlaxity or a pronounced pivot shift, and all cases of revision ACL reconstruction. Herein we describe our technique for a combined intra-articular ACL reconstruction with an extra-articular procedure we refer to as the monoloop technique. This technique is based on previously described forms of utilization of a section of the iliotibial band for extra-articular augmentation but in a refined procedure with limited potential for morbidity.

31.2 Surgical Technique

31.2.1 Setup, Examination Under Anesthesia, and Intra-articular Procedure

Regional anesthesia is used in all patients. Patients are set up on the operating table in a supine position with the table flat. Knee stability (translation and pivot) and range of motion are evaluated under anesthesia and recorded prior to arthroscopy. The knee is prepared and draped in a standard sterile fashion, and an Ioban dressing is applied to the entire surgical site. A tourniquet is used and inflated prior to surgery commencing. Routine knee arthroscopy is first performed and a note made of any intra-articular pathology. Management of any meniscal or cartilage lesions is performed before preparation and placement of an intra-articular ACL graft. We use an antero-medial approach with the knee in hyperflexion when creating our femoral tunnel (drilling from the standard anteromedial portal and viewing from the standard anterolateral portal). We typically use hamstring autografts with endobutton fixation on the femoral side. The intra-articular graft is passed and fixed on the femoral side prior to performing any extra-articular surgery on the lateral aspect of the knee. Fixation on the tibial side is performed with the use of both a post and an interference screw (BioRCI-HA, Smith & Nephew, Zaventem, Belgium) or soft tissue fixation staple (Smith & Nephew, Zaventem, Belgium) depending on surgeon preference. This tibial fixation is performed after completion of the extra-articular augmentation (Fig. 31.1).

31.2.2 Extra-articular Skin Incision and Preparation of the Graft

For the extra-articular augmentation procedure, the knee is flexed at 60° (Fig. 31.2a). Gerdy's tubercle and the iliotibial band (ITB) are palpated and marked. An incision of approximately 6 cm in length is made. This starts just proximal to Gerdy's tubercle and continues along the posterior 1/3 of the palpable ITB proximally (Fig. 31.2b). The subcutaneous tissues are then divided and elevated off the ITB from Gerdy's tubercle to approximately 14 cm proximally (Fig. 31.3a). This is possible through retraction and elevation of the incision edges. The posterior edge of the ITB is palpated, and a posterior line is incised in the ITB along the tensed portion in the posterior 1/3. This tensed portion of the ITB is readily palpated with the

Fig. 31.1 Key steps of monoloop procedure

1.	Routine arthroscopy + management of any meniscal/chondral lesions
2.	Intra-articular ACL reco nstruction - fixation femoral side only
3.	Preparation of monoloop extra-articular graft from ITB
4.	Routing of graft under LCL & under lateral intermuscular septum
5.	Fixation of monoloop graft with tibia in external rotation
6.	Fixation of intra-articular graft on tibial side

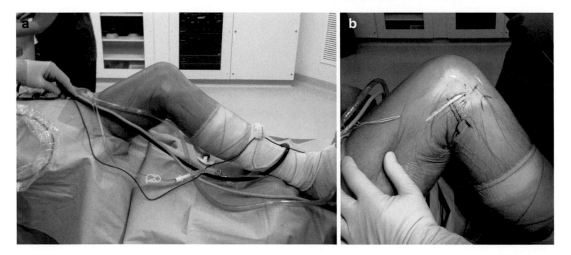

Fig. 31.2 (a) Setup and leg position. (b) Skin markings of major bony and soft tissue landmarks in addition to skin incision

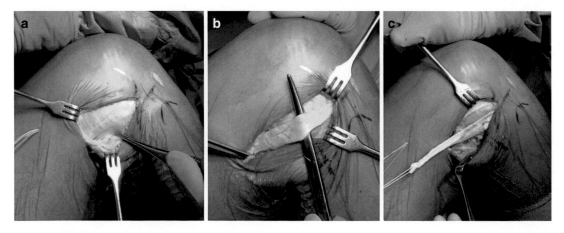

Fig. 31.3 (a) Iliotibial band (ITB) exposed and posterior aspect identified. (b) Strip of ITB, 1 cm wide and 12 cm in length (extending proximally from Gerdy's tubercle), is prepared. (c) Strip of ITB is released proximally and elevated. Leading suture placed in free end to aid passage of graft

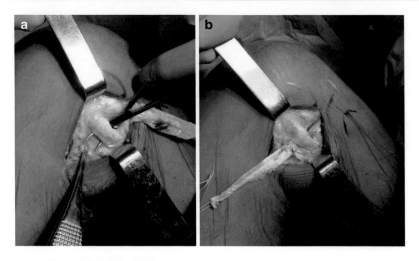

Fig. 31.4 (**a**) Lateral collateral ligament (LCL) is identified and a route to pass graft underneath is prepared. (**b**) ITB graft is passed under the LCL as shown

knee in 60° of flexion. With the addition of a second more anterior incision in the ITB, a strip of ITB of approximately 1 cm in width and 12 cm in length is elevated from the ITB (Fig. 31.3b). It is allowed to remain attached to Gerdy's tubercle but is freed up proximally (Fig. 31.3c).

31.2.3 Routing and Fixation of the Graft

The lateral collateral ligament is next identified. A 1 cm vertical incision is made on front and behind the LCL and the graft is routed under it (Fig. 31.4). The vastus lateralis muscle is then retracted, and the lateral intermuscular septum is identified on the distal femur (Fig. 31.5a). The fixation site is identified and cleared with the use of sharp dissection and electrocautery. Care must be taken not to disrupt the previously placed endobutton attached to the intra-articular graft as it should also lie in this area. The graft is then routed up under the lateral intermuscular septum, staying close to bone at the level of the septum (Fig. 31.5b, c). Depending on surgeon's preference, the monoloop graft is then laid down at a site of elevated cortical bone (sandwiched into the groove created) or simply laid against the native femur. In either event it is fixed in place with a soft tissue fixation staple (Fig. 31.6). It is important to keep the foot/tibia in external

rotation at the time of tensioning and fixation of the graft. The intra-articular graft must also be kept under tension distally to prevent subluxation of the tibia and/or fixation of the extra-articular graft in a subluxed position. The leading end of the extra-articular graft (emerging from the staple) is then sutured back to the first part of the graft, which is ascending and passing under the staple. If the leading sutures from the previously placed endobutton are still in place, these may be tied over the graft.

31.2.4 Completion of Procedure

A drain is placed in the lateral wound, and the proximal half of the incision in the ITB is then closed depending on surgeon preference. The intra-articular graft is then fixed distally on the tibia. Rehabilitation follows routine ACL reconstruction guidelines, with the additional component of 2 weeks in a brace to keep the knee flexed to a minimum of 20° to protect the extra-articular graft.

31.3 Discussion

The optimal technique for soft tissue reconstruction in patients presenting with a ruptured ACL is unclear. The earliest efforts at ACL reconstruction focused on open extra-articular techniques

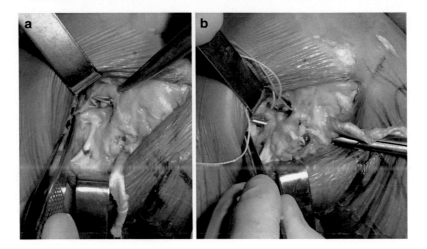

Fig. 31.5 (**a**) The vastus lateralis muscle is elevated, and the lateral intermuscular septum is identified and exposed. The previously placed cortical button should also be identified and protected. (**b**) A route for graft passage, first between capsule and lateral gastrocnemius, and then under the distal intermuscular septum while staying adjacent to bone, is prepared

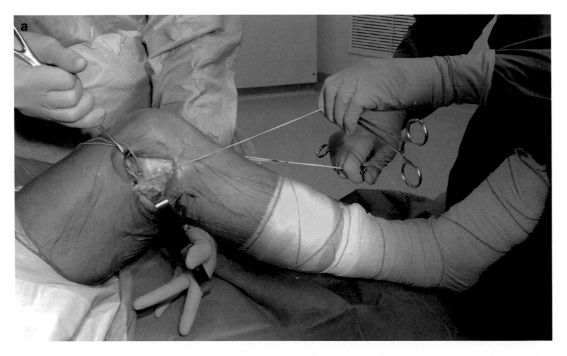

Fig. 31.6 (**a**) The graft is passed through the route prepared. The knee is then placed at 60° with the tibia in external rotation with tension placed on both intra- and extra-articular grafts for extra-articular fixation. (**b**) Soft tissue staple applied over graft which is held under tension. (**c**) Leading strand from cortical endobutton of intra-articular graft tied over extra-articular graft (optional). (**d**) Final appearance of extra-articular component prior to closure of wound

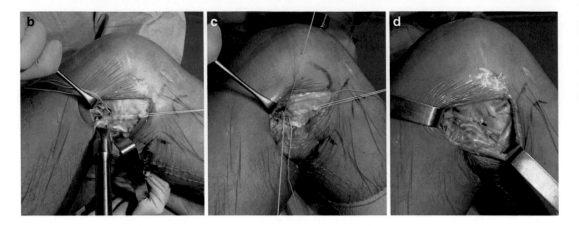

Fig. 31.6 (continued)

[6]. With arthroscopic advances came a movement in ACL surgery toward all-inside techniques. Most surgeons now apply a solely intra-articular technique, using either hamstring or patellar tendon grafts. Despite giving relatively consistent results, there is good evidence that current surgery does not restore normal kinematics and biomechanics, and in some cases does not prevent rotational instability. Although intra-articular techniques continue to be refined in an effort to prevent this, including the development of the double-bundle technique, it appears that there exists a subset of patients for whom an intra-articular procedure alone may be insufficient [6–10, 12].

The concept of the "slipping knee" has been recognized for nearly 100 years, and the term pivot shift has been in existence in the literature since 1972 [6]. Many investigators have linked this ACL injury phenomenon to concomitant injury to structures at the lateral aspect of the knee. The "pivot lesion" comprises characteristic bone bruising on the posterolateral tibial plateau and anterolateral femoral condyle that can be present on MRI scans of patients with acute ACL ruptures. Ségond has described an eponymous cortical tibial avulsion fracture which is seen on radiological imaging in many cases of ACL injury, noting that it occurs at the site of insertion of the middle third of the lateral capsular ligament [13]. Terry et al. demonstrated that during an injury that resulted in a clinically deficient

ACL, 93 % of IT bands were also torn [9]. More recently, Neyret and others have revisited the anatomy of the lateral aspect of the knee and have helped to refine our understanding of what is now known as the anterolateral ligament of the knee [14–16]. It is possible to speculate that lateral structures may act as secondary restraints to the pivot-shift phenomenon, supplementing the primary restraint role of the ACL. Reconstruction of the ALL (and/or related structures) may have a clinical role to play in those patients in whom its structure or function is disrupted.

A number of techniques for extra-articular reconstruction of the ruptured ACL have been described previously. These include the Macintosh procedure, Losee's "sling and reef" operation, Ellison's distal ITT transfer, Andrews operation, and the Lemaire procedure [6]. While space limits the ability to detail the precise components of all techniques here, these procedures tend to also have in common the use of long strips of isolated ITT band with various forms of extended soft tissue routing. Femoral tunnels are also required in many of these procedures. The shortcomings of these techniques, where used in the isolated setting, have been highlighted previously, including their failure to restore stability [6]. Secondary degenerative changes in the lateral compartment were also seen, possibly because without concomitant intra-articular ACL reconstruction, the joint may be secured in a subluxed position with altered mechanics. Extended periods of immobilization, with associated complications, in addition to donor site morbidity and concerns about cosmesis have also been described. It should also be noted that some studies have reported limited benefit to extra-articular augmentation of intra-articular reconstruction where universally applied [6, 10]. Dodds et al recently provided an excellent review of combined intra- and extra-articular ACL reconstruction techniques [6]. While they note that some reports do demonstrate efficacy of the combined approach, it is difficult to draw any definite conclusions regarding superiority to isolated intra-articular reconstruction at the present time. Ultimately we remain limited in our knowledge due to a lack of understanding of concomitant lateral sided injury, small study sizes, heterogeneous groups of patients, and absence of randomization common in reported literature.

We reserve the application of monoloop extra-articular augmentation to what we consider are high-risk groups for recurrent instability following ACL injury. These primarily include those patients involved in a significant level of pivoting activity (e.g., soccer players, martial arts participants, etc.), patients with hyperlaxity or a very pronounced pivot shift, and those patients undergoing revision ACL surgery. As revision ACL surgery, and any subsequent revisions, have been demonstrated to be associated with increasing levels of cartilage pathology and also inferior outcomes, we believe that this subset of patients always warrant maximal support for the intra-articular reconstruction. Many of these patients do not have a clinically or radiologically demonstrable injury to the lateral structures, but it is possible that we do not yet have enough understanding of these structures, or of their examination and imaging, to define a threshold level of injury that warrants extra-articular reconstruction. For now, we believe the addition of an extra-articular augmentation remains warranted in the "high-risk" cases noted. The reconstruction of lateral structures should not be associated with excess lateral compartment chondral stress when used alongside intra-articular reconstruction. Furthermore, application of the minimally invasive technique described in this paper should limit concerns with cosmesis and morbidity.

Regarding the future, it has been proposed that if the anatomy and biomechanics of ACL injury and reconstruction can be fully established, it may be possible to devise a more scientific approach to ACL reconstruction, taking into account the specific structures which have been damaged, and to allow repair of these tissues in acute cases or their reconstruction at later time points [6]. Good quality clinical data will also be of benefit. We look forward to both contributing to and seeing such information in the literature.

References

1. Sutherland AG, Cooper K, Alexander LA et al (2010) The long-term functional and radiological outcome after open reconstruction of the anterior cruciate ligament. J Bone Joint Surg [Br] 92-B:1096–1099
2. Kennedy J, Jackson MP, O'Kelly P, Moran R (2010) Timing of reconstruction of the anterior cruciate ligament in athletes and the incidence of secondary pathology within the knee. J Bone Joint Surg [Br] 92-B:363–366
3. Bull AMJ, Amis AA (1998) The pivot-shift phenomenon: a clinical and biomechanical perspective. Knee 5:141–158
4. Lane CG, Warren R, Pearle AD (2008) The pivot shift. J Am Acad Orthop Surg 16:679–688
5. Tashiro Y, Okazaki K, Miura H et al (2009) Quantitative assessment of rotator instability after anterior cruciate ligament reconstruction. Am J Sports Med 37:909–916
6. Dodds AL, Gupte CM, Neyret P, Williams AM, Amis AA (2011) Extra-articular techniques in anterior cruciate ligament reconstruction: a literature review. J Bone Joint Surg Br 93(11):1440–1448
7. Claes T, Declercq G, Martens M, Lefevre J (1986) Extra-articular ligamentoplasty for chronic ACL insufficiency. Acta Orthop Belg 52(4):515–525
8. Ristanis S, Stergiou N, Patras K et al (2005) Excessive tibial rotation during high- demand activities is not restored by anterior-cruciate ligament reconstruction. Arthroscopy 21:1323–1329
9. Terry GC, Norwood LA, Hughston JC, Caldwell KM (1993) How iliotibial tract injuries of the knee combine with acute anterior cruciate ligament tears to influence abnormal anterior tibial displacement. Am J Sports Med 21(1):55–60
10. O'Brien SJ, Warren RF, Wickiewicz TL et al (1991) The iliotibial band lateral sling procedure and its effect on the results of anterior cruciate ligament reconstruction. Am J Sports Med 19(1):21–24, discussion 24–5
11. Zelle BA, Vidal AF, Brucker PU, Fu FH (2007) Double-bundle reconstruction of the anterior cruciate

ligament: anatomic and biomechanical rationale. J Am Acad Orthop Surg 15:87–96

12. Marcacci M, Zaffagnini S, Giordano G, Iacono F, Lo PM (2009) Anterior cruciate ligament reconstruction associated with extra-articular tenodesis: a prospective clinical and radiographic evaluation with 10- to 13-year follow-up. Am J Sports Med 37:707–714

13. Ségond P (1879) Recherches cliniques et experimentales sur les épanchements sanguins du genou par entorse. Progres Med 7:297–341

14. Vincent JP, Magnussen RA, Gezmez F, Uguen A, Jacobi M, Weppe F, Al-Saati MF, Lustig S, Demey G, Servien E, Neyret P (2012) The anterolateral ligament of the human knee: an anatomic and histologic study. Knee Surg Sports Traumatol Arthrosc 20(1): 147–152

15. Pernin J, Verdonk P, Si Selmi TA, Massin P, Neyret P (2010) Long-term follow-up of 24.5 years after intra-articular anterior cruciate ligament reconstruction with lateral extra-articular augmentation. Am J Sports Med 38:1094–1102

16. Claes S, Vereecke E, Maes M, Victor J, Verdonk P, Bellemans J (2013) Anatomy of the anterolateral ligament of the knee. J Anat 223(4):321–328

ACL Rupture with Open Physis

32

Karl-Heinz Frosch, Romain Seil, Rainer Siebold,
Franck Chotel, Shinya Oka, and Achim Preiss

Contents

K-H. Frosch, MD (✉) • A. Preiss, MD
Department of Trauma and Reconstructive Surgery,
Asklepios Klinik St. Georg,
Lohmühlenstr. 5, 20099 Hamburg, Germany
e-mail: k.frosch@asklepios.com

R. Seil, MD, PhD (✉)
Department of Orthopaedic Surgery, Centre
Hospitalier de Luxembourg-Clinique d'Eich, and
Sports Medicine Research Laboratory,
Public Research Centre for Health,
76, rue d'Eich, L-1460 Luxembourg, Luxembourg
e-mail: rseil@yahoo.com

R. Siebold, MD (✉)
Institute for Anatomy and Cell Biology, Ruprecht-Karls
University Heidelberg, Im Neuenheimer Feld 307,
69120 Heidelberg, Germany

HKF: Center for Specialised Hip-Knee-Foot Surgery,
ATOS Hospital Heidelberg,
Bismarckstr. 9-15, 69115 Heidelberg, Germany
e-mail: rainer.siebold@atos.de

F. Chotel, MD, PhD
Department of Pediatric Orthopaedic Surgery,
Lyon University Hospital for Mother and Children,
Université Claude Bernard Lyon I,
59 Boulevard Pinel, F-69677 Bron, France

S. Oka, MD
Department of Orthopaedic Surgery,
Kobe University Graduate School of Medicine,
Hyōgo, Japan

HKF: Center for Specialised Hip-Knee-Foot Surgery,
ATOS Hospital Heidelberg,
Bismarckstr. 9-15, 69115 Heidelberg, Germany

R. Siebold et al. (eds.), *Anterior Cruciate Ligament Reconstruction*,
DOI 10.1007/978-3-642-45349-6_32, © ESSKA 2014

32.1 Clinical Findings with ACL Rupture in Kids and Adolescents

Shinya Oka and Rainer Siebold

32.1.1 Introduction

In recent years, the incidence of anterior cruciate ligament (ACL) injuries in skeletally immature patients increased significantly [26, 50]. Although available epidemiological information on ACL tears in skeletal immature patients is limited, the number of ≤10 age patients accounts for 0.4 % of all ACL injuries in Sweden [67]. Most of sports-related ACL injuries are noncontact in nature, that is, cutting or pivoting motion on a fixed foot during change of direction, sudden stopping or landing from a jump, or a hyperextension trauma [9]. The diagnostic accuracy of this young population is lower than in adults due to a lack of ability to state the circumstance of the injury or symptoms encountered since the injury [58]. For the physician it may be of help to assess the injury mechanism together with the patients. In any case it is very important to include the parents in the decision making of the treatment. A close cooperation and compliance of the young patients is essential, too.

32.1.2 Clinical Symptoms

Children presenting with ACL injury often report audible "pop" or "snap." This is followed by severe pain, a feeling of instability (often described as "giving way"), and an inability to continue their activity or sometimes to even bear weight. A hemarthrosis appears within hours of injury and continues few weeks. A limitation of knee range of motion due to hemarthrosis or some structural disturbance occurs at the same time. After a few weeks from injury, the young patients will be almost fully released from pain and inconvenience of limited knee motion in daily activities. However, feeling of instability or slight pain leads to inability of their sports activities and any other cutting, jumping, or pivoting activities.

Recurrent instability episodes with ACL rupture may cause subsequent intra-articular injuries like meniscal or cartilage damage with a high risk of early osteoarthritis [27, 47].

32.1.3 Physical Examination

The clinical examination should start with a close look on the gait pattern and alignment of the lower extremities and should check any atrophy of the lower limb, e.g., m. quadriceps femoris. The general documentation also includes articular effusion and swelling, range of motion, palpating for tenderness over the joint line and ligament insertion, valgus and varus instability, patellar tracking and instability, as well as concomitant musculoskeletal injuries. Clinicians should be aware that children and adolescents have increased ligamentous laxity than adults [31]. Therefore, the ligamentous status of the contralateral leg should be used for comparison and reference. Measuring heel height difference is also beneficial to check an extension contracture [54].

The inspection should also include assessment for acute hemarthrosis, which is helpful in determining the significance of the knee injury, e.g., ACL rupture, tibial spine avulsion, meniscal injury, osteochondral fracture, or patellar dislocation. An acute traumatic hemarthrosis after ACL rupture can be present in up to 47 % of children aged 7–12 and in up to 65 % of adolescents [80].

The Lachman, anterior drawer, and pivot shift tests are reliable in detecting an ACL insufficiency. However, assessment of knee kinematics are significantly affected by patients' conscious state [53] and may be difficult to be performed due to pain or fear in children. The pivot shift test is positive in 98 % of anesthetized patients with ACL insufficiency compared with only 35 % of patients who are awake during the examination [80].

32.1.4 Radiography

The routine standard radiographic evaluation of the knee includes an anteroposterior view a lateral view and a skyline view for the assessment of the patella. The bony age of the patients (status of the growth plates), bony injuries such as tibial spine avulsion, Segond fracture, epiphyseal injury, osteochondral fracture, and loose bodies have to be ruled out.

A Rosenberg view (anteroposterior "tunnel view" in 45° of flexion, weight bearing) might also be helpful to assess the intercondylar notch and the width of the medial and lateral joint lines.

Especially in kids and adolescents, a long leg standing radiograph (hip to ankle) gives important information on preoperative limb-length discrepancy or an angular deformity.

Anatomic risk factors for ACL injury such as increased anterior pelvic tilt, increased femoral anteversion, increased quadriceps angle, decreased intercondylar notch width, and increased posterior tibial slope should also be checked [2]. Radiographic changes of intercondylar notch and tibial eminences may indicate an ACL agenesis [52].

32.1.5 MRI

In kids and adolescents it is recommended to perform magnetic resonance imaging (MRI) to ensure the diagnosis. This is especially important when the clinical examination is difficult, to exclude additional injuries to the meniscus, the collateral ligaments including posterior cruciate ligament (PCL), or the cartilage and to assess the bony age of the growth plates (open or not).

MRI is an important tool to reconfirm the diagnosis for the parents and to establish a clear and confidential environment for the treatment.

The primary signs of an ACL tear are an abnormal ligament course referred to the Blumensaat line, an abnormal sign intensity defined as focally or diffusely increased signal intensity on intermediate- or T2-weighted images, and a ligament discontinuity such as a focal gap. Indirect signs of an ACL rupture are the presence of a bone bruise in the anterior part of the femoral lateral condyle and in the medial to posterior part of the tibial lateral condyle, an

abnormal PCL angle, and the presence of an anterior tibial displacement [49]. Additional oblique sagittal or coronal imaging may improve the specificity to detect a ligament discontinuity or abnormal signs [45].

32.2 Conservative or Operative Treatment?

Karl-Heinz Frosch and Achim Preiss

32.2.1 Introduction

Up into the 1990s conservative treatment of anterior cruciate ligament ruptures was seen as the favored treatment method in children and adolescents out of concern for not yet closed physes or for damaging the same, which then could result in potential growth disorders. More recently, publications favoring operative therapies in case of such injuries become more frequent as conservative therapies produce unsatisfactory clinical outcomes resulting in secondary damages. Barrack et al., for example, report on poor results after 38 months of conservative therapy [7]. Instabilities occur in up to 91 % of all cases after conservative therapy [72]. In 50–75 % of cases, secondary meniscal lesions can occur after an ACL rupture [7, 35, 62]. In case of persistent instability, the articular cartilage can progressively be damaged posteromedially over time [82]. In 11 of 18 patients, radiologically verified degenerative changes were detected after follow-up of 51 months [63]. Insufficiencies can also occur in peripheral ligament structures because secondary stabilizers counteract to anterior subluxation and are overstrained due to the missing anterior cruciate ligament. The rate of regaining high levels of sports activities after conservative therapy is low [5–41 %] [73].

32.2.2 Conservative Versus Operative Treatment

Due to unsatisfactory results of conservatively treated ACL ruptures in children and adolescents, we carried out a meta-analysis [69]. The aim of this meta-analysis was to evaluate the clinical outcome of the respective therapy as well as their specific complications regarding instability, insufficiency of the graft, axis deviation, and length differences. Therefore, an electronic search for publications on the subject of ACL rupture treatment in adolescents was performed in Medline, the Cochrane Controlled Trial Register, Embase, and Medpilot. Ten studies including 154 patients were analyzed regarding conservative treatment, 55 studies including 935 patients with regard to operative treatment.

Six of those ten studies compared operative with conservative therapy or a delayed reconstruction after initial conservative treatment [1, 6, 34, 55, 56, 64]. Four of those ten studies nearly only detail conservative treatments [27, 35, 63, 84]. For the analysis of operatively treated patients, a total of 57 studies were included [69]. Nine hundred and thirty-five patients with 941 operated knees were included in these studies.

On average the patients were aged 12.3 years (10.0–14.4 years). The duration of the patients' follow-up examinations resulted in a median of 29 months [24–72 months] [69].

In case of conservatively treated patients, there was no occurrence of leg-length discrepancies or axis deviations during the follow-up examinations.

In comparison to the aforementioned, the following data was detected in surgically treated patients.

32.2.3 Lysholm Score

The Lysholm score's mean for patients with surgery came to 95.5 ± 3.1 (median 96.5) and hence was significantly better than the score for conservatively treated patients, which came to 73.2 ± 17.8 (median 76.1) (Fig. 32.1).

32.2.4 Giving Way Phenomenon

In case of surgically treated ACL ruptures, the probability of the occurrence of a giving way phenomenon came to 2.8 (±6.9) %. In case of conservatively treated patients that probability

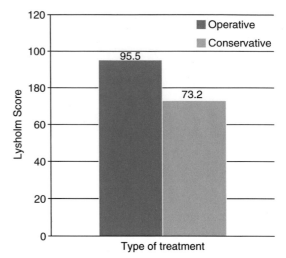

Fig. 32.1 Average Lysholm score grouped by type of treatment (Reprinted with permission of Springer Science and Business Media: Preiss et al. [69])

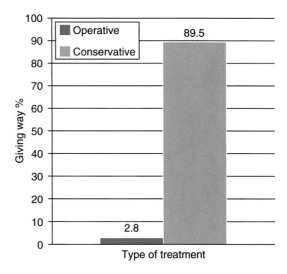

Fig. 32.2 Occurrence of a giving way phenomenon grouped by type of treatment (Reprinted with permission of Springer Science and Business Media: Preiss et al. [69])

came to an averaging 89.5 (±15.2) % and hence was significantly higher (Fig. 32.2).

32.2.5 Level of Sports Activity

The mean of surgically treated patients, who could regain their initial sports activity level,

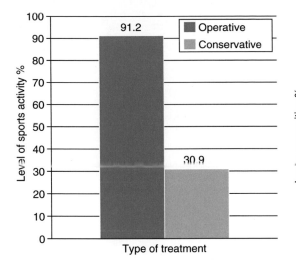

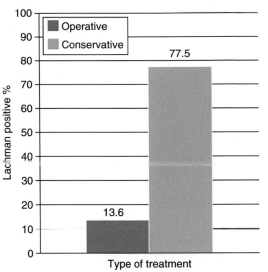

Fig. 32.3 Regain of initial level of sports activity grouped by type of treatment (Reprinted with permission of Springer Science and Business Media: Preiss et al. [69])

Fig. 32.4 Occurrence of a positive Lachman test grouped by type of treatment (Reprinted with permission of Springer Science and Business Media: Preiss et al. [69])

came to 91.2 ($\pm$ 3.1) % (median 96.5 %), and the mean of conservatively treated patients came to 30.9 ($\pm$ 33.8) % (median 24.7 %) (Fig. 32.3). Thus, significantly more patients with surgery regained their initial sports activity level than patients without surgery.

The duration from the accident (conservatively treated patients) or from the surgery to the follow-up examination had, in both operative and conservative studies, no significant influence on the probability of regaining one's initial level of sports activity.

32.2.6 Lachman Test

The mean of patients with surgery having a positive Lachman test grade of 2 or 3 during the follow-up examination came to 13.6 ($\pm$ 2.4) %; for patients treated conservatively, the mean was 77.5 ($\pm$ 43.7) % (Fig. 32.4). The group treated with surgery was significantly better, too.

> **Memory**
> The data presented here prove that operative therapy for ACL ruptures in children and adolescents has a significant advantage

over conservative treatment. Approximately 89 % of all children and adolescents with conservatively treated anterior cruciate ligament ruptures suffer from a giving way phenomenon. This is twice the rate as compared to adults. As, with regard to children and adolescents with ACL rupture, the risk of secondary meniscal injuries significantly increases already after 12 weeks of conservative therapy, one should decide rather early in favor of an operative therapy. Considering the data currently available, conservative therapy is the exception rather than the rule for ACL ruptures in children and adolescents.

32.3   Risk for Growth Plate and Timing of Surgery

Romain Seil and Franck Chotel

32.3.1 Introduction

There is a lack of current international guidelines with respect to the treatment of ACL-injured children, leaving the treating physicians in a therapeutic

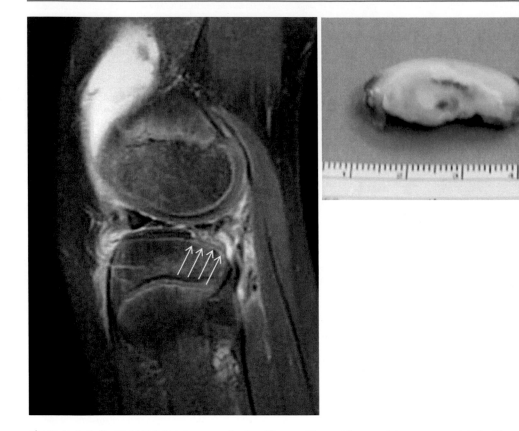

Fig. 32.5 *Left*: Sagittal MRI showing an avulsed cartilage fragment (*white arrows*, fragment *right* image) from the posterolateral tibia plateau in a 12-year-old boy who had sustained a severe knee sprain 6 months before surgery. The cartilage avulsion was associated with an ACL tear and a complex tear of the posterior horn of the lateral meniscus. It was missed at initial presentation

dilemma [65]. On the one hand, nonoperative treatment has shown to be successful in some patients, but the reasons for this are poorly understood [64, 81]. Furthermore, a strong association between the delay of surgery and the occurrence of meniscus and cartilage lesions strongly suggests that a nonoperative treatment may be detrimental to the intraarticular soft tissues [18, 30, 47, 48, 62]. On the other hand, surgery is difficult and highly specialized, due to the specific anatomy of children's knees and its serious complication potential [32, 38, 73, 74]. Surgical results are good [11, 12, 16, 41], but due to the remaining growth and knee maturation, they seem to be less predictable than in adults. Furthermore, there is a lack of high-quality outcome studies after surgical treatment [65]. ACL injuries have both short- and long-term consequences, affecting future knee structure and function with subsequent

meniscus and cartilage injuries, early development of osteoarthritis, and a serious economic burden, due to potentially shortened professional careers and later surgeries [70].

32.3.2 Indication and Timing for Surgery

Timing for surgery in the presence of a ligamentous ACL tear in a child is more difficult than in adults. There is no need for surgery in an acute setting, except if a dislocated meniscus bucket handle or a large cartilaginous avulsion is associated to the ACL injury (Fig. 32.5). In these cases, we recommend early cartilage and/or meniscus surgery. Simultaneous pediatric ACL reconstruction should only be considered if there is minor swelling and synovitis, if the surgical

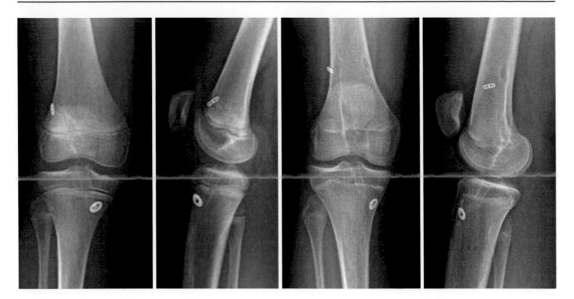

Fig. 32.6 Radiographic follow-up of two boys with images performed post surgery (*left*) and at the final follow-up (*right*). The boy sustained an ACL injury while playing football at the age of 11 (skeletal age=chronological age). A transphyseal fourfold semitendinosus-gracilis replacement with extracortical fixation was performed. At the age of 16, the boy was 20 cm taller. The graft showed some lengthening and relative thinning. Despite relative graft thinning and its vertical femoral position, the boy had negative Lachman and pivot shift testing. He returned successfully to a level II sport

environment is experienced with this type of surgery and if the parents are fully aware of the complication potential and the need for a close follow-up until the end of the growth period. Treating only the meniscus or the cartilage and leaving the ACL untreated in the long term cannot be recommended.

After the acute period, the timing and indication for surgery is becoming more complex and should take into consideration the child's individual needs and maturation process. This is especially true in a sportive environment, when it comes to the child's potential athletic career. A return to the same level of sports (and even a higher level in later years) should not be the primary motivation for surgery. Currently, we are not aware of a single child with a prepubertal ACL reconstruction who returned to a very high level or even a professional level I sport. For these reasons the child and the parents need to adhere to the long-term follow-up and should be fully informed on the possible outcome including surgery-specific complications. Functional instability is an indication for

surgery. However, instability symptoms with clearly identified giving way episodes are rarely spontaneously described by children, although they may report them if they are questioned specifically. For some authors, the sensation given during the pivot shift test can be recognized by the children and may be assimilated to functional instability [14]. Finally, ACL surgery should be indicated in the presence of a secondary meniscus tear.

Although significant evidence has been brought to the orthopedic literature over the last decade showing that pediatric ACL reconstructions are safe procedures and provide good results, surgery cannot yet be recommended on a systematic basis. There are two reasons for this: (a) Due to the nonanatomic graft placement in some techniques, the limited evidence on the fate of the ACL graft after implantation as well as the remaining knee growth and maturation, surgical results are less predictable than in adults (Fig. 32.6). It is known that children have very lax knees [8, 31] with sometimes physiologic grade C pivot shifts. Our own clinical experience

Fig. 32.7 The knee growth and maturation chart, which is based on the growth speed of the growth plates at the knee and the skeletal age, allows differentiating between three different periods of ligamentous ACL injuries in children and adolescents: (a) the prepubertal phase with a high remaining growth potential, (b) the pubertal phase, during which physeal growth potential decreases, and (c) the adult phase, when growth plate closure has occurred

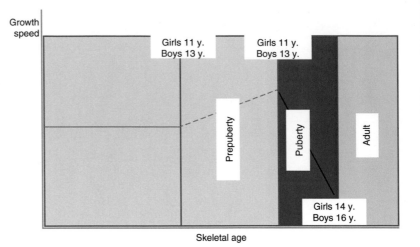

has shown that many of the ACL-injured and ACL-operated children remain hyperlax in the operated and nonoperated knee after the end of their growth period. This proportion seems to be much higher than in an adult ACL-injured population where hypermobile knees can be found in 5–10 % of ACL-injured individuals. It has been shown that the outcome of ACL surgery in these patients is inferior to normolax patients [38]. Although these data need further confirmation, they may suggest that children with ligamentous ACL injuries do not represent the same population as their adult counterparts. Currently, we are not able to predict which degree of knee stiffness a child reaches at the end of its growth period. Future studies will need to address this question specifically. (b) Several studies have reported a good outcome after nonoperative treatment of pediatric ACL injuries in approximately 50 % of the patients with little amount of subsequent meniscus and cartilage lesions [64, 80]. Some of them used functional tests to evaluate the child's ability to cope with the ACL tear. Two conditions seem to be mandatory for this outcome: a very close and individualized follow-up of this pediatric population and their parents and a frequent change from level I to level II sports. Future studies will have to address if creating an environment of systematic and regular functional testing and close follow-up will be as successful as the surgical treatment in a specific patient population.

Our knee growth and maturation chart (Fig. 32.7), which represents the growth speed of the growth plates at the knee and the skeletal age, allows us to differentiate between three different periods of ligamentous ACL injuries in children and adolescents[11]: (a) The prepubertal phase with a high remaining growth potential of the distal femoral and the proximal tibial physis. This phase ends at the skeletal age of 13 years in girls and 15 years in boys. During this phase, pediatric surgical techniques are mandatory. (b) The pubertal phase, during which physeal growth potential decreases. It lasts for approximately 1 year (13–14 in girls and 15–16 in boys). Pediatric surgical techniques are still mandatory at this stage, because growth plate injuries still can cause significant growth abnormalities. A second option, during this phase, is to delay surgery until skeletal maturity. (c) The adult phase, starting at 14 in girls and 16 in boys. At this moment, growth plate closure has occurred at the distal femur and the proximal tibia and adult procedures can be used.

It has been shown that defining the degree of maturation by relying on the Tanner stages alone is insufficient [77]. Moreover, the skeletal age [5] should be rather used than chronological age. Some authors modulate the reconstruction technique according to the patient's maturity: they recommend extraphyseal reconstruction for younger patients, transphyseal reconstruction for older patients and partial transphyseal procedures

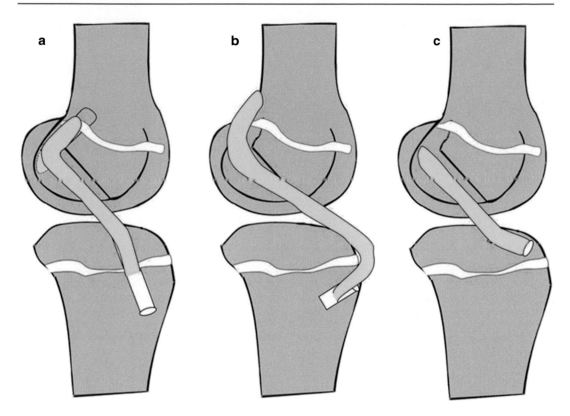

Fig. 32.8 According to the localization of the tibial and femoral tunnels, the surgical techniques can be divided into three categories: (**a**, *left*) transphyseal techniques, where the tunnels are drilled through the growth plates; (**b**, *middle*) extraepiphyseal techniques, where the graft is placed around the growth plate; and (**c**, *right*) epiphyseal techniques, where the tunnels are located in the tibial and femoral epiphysis, not injuring the growth plate. Finally, there are mixed techniques, where different types of graft placement are used on the tibial and the femoral side. Every surgical technique bears its own, specific complication potential

in between [28, 41, 57, 61]. The background for this strategy is based on the theoretical age-related risk of growth arrest. These authors claim that the extent of the deformity after a potential growth arrest is inversely proportional to the patient's age. However, we noticed in a recent survey [14] that growth changes occurred mainly in adolescents during the last year before knee physeal closure. The capacity of the growth plate to break small epiphyso-metaphyseal bone bridges spontaneously is important in young children, but it slows down with the maturation process[Yoo]. In others words, the amount of potential growth deformity is minor in older children, but the risk of growth arrest could be much higher. For this reason, we believe that there is a place for a delayed reconstruction in adolescents close to skeletal maturity.

32.3.3 Risk of a Growth Plate Injury

Many surgical techniques have been described in order to perform the best possible ACL replacement in children and at the same time to reduce the surgically induced complication potential to a minimum. Depending on the localization of the tibial and femoral tunnels, they can be divided into three categories (Fig. 32.8): (a) transphyseal techniques, where the tunnels are drilled through the growth plates, (b) epiphyseal techniques, where the tunnels are located in the tibial and femoral epiphysis, not injuring the growth plate and (c) extraepiphyseal techniques, where the graft is placed around the growth plate. Finally, there are mixed techniques, where different types of graft placement are used on the tibial and the femoral side. Every surgical technique bears its own, specific complication potential.

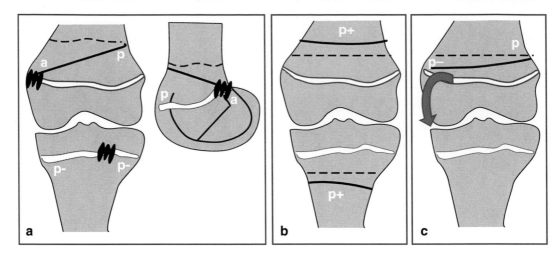

Fig. 32.9 The figure shows the main modes of potential growth abnormalities after pediatric ACL surgery (Fig. 32.9a): the process of growth type A: *a*rrest (**a**) is caused by a localized growth plate (*p*) injury which generates the formation of a transphyseal bone bridge. Bone bridge formation can be prevented with a soft tissue graft at the height of the injured growth plate. A transphyseal bone block, i.e., with a quadriceps or a bone-patellar tendon-bone graft, or a transphyseal hardware placement can cause such a sudden growth arrest as well. The second type (Fig. 32.9b) of growth abnormality is an overgrowth process (type B: *b*oost). It may be caused by a local hypervascularization which stimulates the physeal growth process. This growth disturbance is temporary and it usually becomes apparent in a limited period of 2 years following surgery. The third type (Fig. 32.9c) of growth disturbance (type C: de*c*elerate) may be caused by a so-called tenoepiphysiodesis effect. In this case, an excessive graft tension across the physis causes a deceleration of the remaining growth and a secondary growth abnormality

Growth disturbances after ACL replacements were classified into three categories [15] (Fig. 32.9): growth arrest, overgrowth, and decelerated growth.

The process of growth *a*rrest (A) is caused by a localized growth plate injury which generates the formation of a transphyseal bone bridge. Spontaneous breakage of the bone bridge may occur in very young children whose growth plate can create large distraction forces. Bone bridge formation can be prevented with a soft tissue graft at the height of the injured growth plate. A transphyseal bone block, i.e., with a quadriceps or a bone-patellar tendon-bone graft, or a transphyseal hardware placement can cause such a sudden growth arrest as well. A growth disturbance evolves throughout the remaining growth process. The amount of deformity is proportional to the localization and the size of the initial growth plate injury. A growth arrest can lead to axial deformities if it is located at the periphery of the physis or to symmetrical leg length discrepancies if it is located in the center of the growth plate. On the distal femur, peripheral growth plate injuries can be caused either by a tunnel with a too large diameter or a posterior blowout with an injury of the perichondral structures of the growth plate (Ranvier zone and perichondral ring of Lacroix) if a transphyseal technique is employed. If an epiphyseal tunnel is drilled (which should always be performed under fluoroscopy), the femoral tunnel is located distally to the growth plate. If a growth plate injury occurs with this technique, it will be much larger in comparison to the transphyseal technique, and asymmetric growth may be much more severe in comparison to an arrest which is caused by transphyseal drilling. Finally, if the surgeon chooses an extraepiphyseal technique (over the top technique), caution must be paid to avoid an excessive rasping of the over the top position for a better graft adherence. This surgical maneuver may injure the perichondral structures and lead to axial malalignment as well. Due to its posterolateral position, a growth arrest at the femoral tunnel will lead to a deformity in valgus and flexion. In such cases, anticipating the remaining growth allows to predict the amount of deformity.

On the tibial side, peripheral injuries may be caused by damaging the tibial tuberosity apophysis, either during harvesting of the hamstring tendons or through a too anterior positioning of the tibial tunnel entrance. In this case, the growth arrest will cause a recurvatum of the proximal tibia.

Yoo et al. reported MRI analysis of transphyseal ACL reconstruction in adolescents with open physis. Focal physeal disruptions developed in 5 of 43 adolescent patients without any clinical consequences [85]. The authors concluded that transphyseal techniques are not harmless and should not be used in young children. Unlike this conclusion, we believe that those focal bone bridges will break easier in younger children [13] and that these young children bear a lower risk of epiphysiodesis in comparison to adolescents. Hence, risks and consequences cannot be assimilated: in fact, adolescents are at a higher risk of epiphysiodesis but with low clinical consequences in terms of growth disturbances, while young children are at a lower risk of epiphysiodesis but with sometimes dramatic clinical consequences if the physeal bridge persists and continues to develop until the end of growth.

The second type of growth abnormality is an overgrowth process (type B: boost). It may be caused by a local hypervascularization which stimulates the physeal growth process. This phenomenon occurs mainly in very young children. The growth disturbance is temporary and it usually becomes apparent in a limited period of 2 years following surgery. It is usually symmetric and may lead to a moderate leg length discrepancy. In the study by McIntosh et al., 15 out of 16 patients had a leg length discrepancy of less than 10 mm, and 1 patient had the operated limb 15 mm longer than the healthy limb [59]. In Nakhostine's series, the youngest patient (12-year-old boy) had a leg length discrepancy of 15 mm [66]. The clinical impact of such a complication is usually low compared to a full growth arrest. Nevertheless, the need of a percutaneous epiphysiodesis has been reported because of a provisional leg discrepancy around 2 cm in an 8-years-old child at the time of ACL reconstruction [15].

Sometimes, a tibial valgus deformity can also occur, due to asymmetrical overgrowth. This is similar to the valgus deformities observed after metaphyseal pediatric proximal tibial fractures (so-called posttraumatic genu valgum). After an initial progressive increase of the deformity, a spontaneous correction has been documented and a close follow-up with nonoperative treatment of the deformity is recommended [15].

The third type of growth disturbance (type C: decelerate) may be caused by a so-called tenoepiphysiodesis effect. In this case, an excessive graft tension across the physis causes a deceleration of the remaining growth and a secondary growth abnormality. The exact amount of graft tension being able to cause such an abnormality in humans has not been defined yet. Kocher et al. reported two cases of genu valgum without physeal arrest which may have been caused by a lateral extraarticular tenodesis [38]. Experimental animal studies have shown that it should not exceed 80 N [20, 21]. Similarly, the use of a nonbiological, synthetic graft would cause the same effect. The mechanism behind this growth abnormality is called the Hueter-Volkmann principle [33, 83], according to early experimental studies which showed that an excessive pressure on the growth plate reduced longitudinal growth and vice versa. Many of the currently used ACL reconstruction techniques (even pediculated grafts and physeal-sparing techniques) could expose the young patient to this specific risk.

As a consequence of these possible growth abnormalities, children must undergo a much stricter postoperative follow-up as adults. Clinical and radiological controls should be mandatory until the end of the growth period. In case of a permanent growth abnormality, immediate surgical revision can be recommended if the cause of the complication has been clearly identified (i.e., transphyseal hardware or bone block placement). In such cases, a Langenskiöld procedure (soft tissue interposition) or an additional epiphysiodesis may be considered. If surgical revision is not considered immediately, a correction osteotomy with specific osteotomy plates or even Ilizarov fixators may be mandatory at the end of the growth period. Fortunately, these complications are extremely rare, especially if the surgical technique has been properly performed. Nevertheless, the children and their parents must be informed preoperatively that they may occur even in experienced hands.

32.4   Surgical Technique: Graft Choice, Drilling, and Fixation

Rainer Siebold and Shinya Oka

32.4.1   Introduction

An ACL reconstruction in kids and adolescents is challenging. The knee joint including tendons and bone might be tiny. Tendon harvest, bone tunnel drilling, and extracortical fixation require a high amount of concentration and experience even for experienced surgeons. Additional injuries have to be seen on MRI preoperatively, and a clear operative treatment plan has to be established before surgery. It is very important that the surgeon feels comfortable with operating and with the high level of responsibility. If not, it is much better to send the patient to a specialized center for treatment instead of risking a failure.

32.4.2   Graft Choice

The hamstring tendon graft (semitendinosus and gracilis tendons) is the favored graft in the younger patient. It has been used in many surgical ways to reconstruct the ACL [1, 4, 10, 16, 17, 29, 41, 43, 44, 71]. The most common technique is a transphyseal approach with a fourfold semitendinosus and gracilis tendon graft and extracortical fixation.

As a pure tendon graft, a hamstring graft avoids physeal issues associated with bone blocks, e.g., bone bridge formation. Empty bone tunnels demonstrated to form bony bridges in animal studies [74, 78]. The hamstring tendon graft is long enough to fill the perforated growth plates by soft tissue. Fixation can be accomplished well

away from the physis in an extracortical fashion, e.g., with buttons or posts.

Some authors also reported favorable clinical outcomes using a patella tendon (BTB or BT) graft in transphyseal or physeal-sparing technique [6, 12, 19, 56, 62, 76]. However, damaging the anterior tibial tubercle apophysis during harvest of the patellar tendon may result in a tibial recurvatum deformity with premature arrest of the apophysis [22]. In addition, care has to be taken not to position bone plugs across the physis to avoid local growth arrest [38]. Frosch et al. presented from a meta-analysis of 55 original studies that the relative risk of the occurrence of leg length difference or axis deviations was reduced to 45 % when a hamstring tendon graft was used rather than a patellar tendon graft [26].

Kocher et al. reported good results with physeal sparing, intra and extra-articular reconstruction of the ACL combined with the use of an iliotibial band (ITB) graft for skeletal immature patients at Tanner stage I or II [39]. This procedure is known as a modification of MacIntosh procedure. The iliotibial band graft is detached proximally and left attached distally at Gerdy's tubercle. The graft is brought through the knee in the over-the-top position and passed underneath the intermeniscal ligament. The proximal part of the graft is sutured to the intermuscular septum and periosteum of the lateral femoral condyle through a lateral knee incision, and the distal part is sutured to the periosteum of the proximal medial tibial metaphysis.

32.4.3   Drilling

The current options for ACL reconstruction are divided into physeal-sparing procedures, partial transphyseal procedures, and transphyseal procedure.

The most commonly performed approach in skeletally immature patients is a transphyseal ACL reconstruction. The surgical technique is similar to adults and familiar to most surgeons. Many authors reported excellent clinical results using a transphyseal technique with essentially no growth plate complications.

However, there is still concern about the incidence of growth plate disturbance using that technique. Yoo et al. reported on 5 out of 43 adolescent patients which had a focal physeal disruption revealed on MRI without a perceived clinical disturbance [85].

Kercher et al. calculated volumetric measurements using MRI simulation and concluded that the graft radius may be the most important variable affecting the volume of physeal injury and potential arrest [36]. Volumetric injury of 7 % has been shown to create a high risk of partial physeal closure in animal models [51]. Less than 3 % injury occurred to the growth plate when an 8-mm tunnel is drilled across the physis. Shea et al. also reported using an MRI model that double-bundle ACL reconstruction substantially increases the volume of physeal injury in skeletally immature patients who undergo ACL reconstruction [75]. Finally peripheral drill-holes may have a greater probability of causing physeal arrest than more central drill-holes [23].

Bone tunnel drilling in physeal-sparing procedures is usually more challenging compared to the common transphyseal bone tunnel approach. They were developed to allow more anatomical ACL reconstructions in skeletally immature patients with less risk to the physis. Anderson et al. reported a physeal-sparing ACL reconstruction where the tibial and femoral bone tunnels were drilled with fluoroscopic aid [3, 4]. Lawrence et al. also reported a physeal-sparing procedure where they used intraoperative CT scanning with three-dimensional (3D) reconstruction to reconfirm the precise localization of the all-epiphyseal femoral and tibial tunnels [46]. Both studies reported no growth disturbance and good clinical outcomes.

Physeal-sparing bone tunnel drilling may also be achieved by femoral anterograde outside-in drilling and tibial and femoral retrograde inside-out drilling to the level of the growth plates. However, these procedures are technically challenging and the surgeon should be very experienced when using them in adults and children. Frosch et al. argue that the position of drilling near the growth plate may cause the heat damage to the epiphysis which may also risk growth arrest [26].

32.4.4 Fixation

Most surgeons favor an extracortical suspensory fixation using buttons, discs, posts, or staples when operating on kids. An intraosseous fixation technique such as interference screws or a press-fit fixation with bone plugs is very critical to cause growth disturbancy and may better be avoided. A survey of the Herodicus Society and the ACL Study Group reported 15 cases of growth disturbances. The most common reported causes were fixation across the lateral distal physis of the femur with an interference screw, a staple, a transfixation pin, or a bone block [38].

Tensioning of the soft-tissue graft may also have an influence on the growth plate, as excessive tensioning may induce premature physeal closure. Edwards et al. reported that significant growth disturbance occurred with an excessively tensioned fascia lata autograft and a transphyseal ACL reconstruction using a canine model [20, 21].

32.5 Literature Results

Karl-Heinz Frosch

Surgical care of anterior cruciate ligament ruptures in children and adolescents produces significantly better results than conservative therapy. Literature, however, describes a wide range of various surgical techniques, which are – to some extent – quite differently evaluated and also lead to different clinical results.

32.5.1 Cruciate Ligament Suture

On the assumption that the risk of inducing a growth disorder can be minimized and also because of its principally high healing potential in children and adolescents, various authors favored the method of suturing the ruptured anterior cruciate ligament. In 67 patients, who were treated with a cruciate ligament suture and were included in the meta-analysis of Frosch et al.

[26], no growth disorder was detected. With regard to the IKDC score, however, just 40 % of the patients showed good or very good results. This implies that the majority of patients, which underwent a cruciate ligament suture, suffer from persistent instability; this is also reflected in a moderate averaging Lysholm score of 79.6 points [26]. Hence, the suture of ACL ruptures in children and adolescents cannot be recommended as a standard therapy.

32.5.2 Cruciate Ligament Reconstruction

In principle, cruciate ligament reconstruction in children and adolescents produces good clinical results [24, 26, 69]. In a meta-analysis Preiss et al. determined an averaging Lysholm score of 95.5 points. Applying conservative therapy, however, only 73.2 points was accomplished on average [69]. The return to the initial level of sports activity after anterior cruciate ligament reconstruction in children and adolescents came to 91.2 %. In that regard only 2.8 % of patients suffered from a postoperative persistent giving way phenomenon [69]. 86.4 % of patients in growing age with anterior cruciate ligament reconstruction had a negative Lachman test after surgery [69]. Therefore, these results are comparable with those of adults. To our knowledge there are no articles about anterior cruciate ligament reconstruction in children and adolescents, which would predominately report on moderate or poor clinical results. Good to very good clinical results after anterior cruciate ligament reconstruction are even reported on children less than 12 years of age, while there was no considerable increase of the rate of postoperative growth disorders [40].

32.5.3 Risks of Surgical Therapy

In a meta-analysis including 935 patients with an average age of 13 years, the relative risk of suffering from a growth disorder after anterior cruciate ligament reconstruction was approximately 2 %

[26]. On average the period of time for a follow-up came to 40 months. Only 59 children aged 12 years or less were identified in this study [26]. Additionally, one has to keep in mind that the risk of suffering from a growth disorder is dependent on the surgical technique. The rate of postoperatively monitored axis deviations or leg-length discrepancies came to 5.8 % using growth plate-saving techniques and to 1.9 % applying transphyseal techniques [26]. The risk of the occurrence of a postoperative leg-length discrepancy or axis deviation came to 3.2 % in case of a transplant fixation close to the joint line and to 1.4 % when fixation was carried out far from the joint line [26]. The risk of suffering from a postoperative growth disorder is 3.6 % in case of using a patellar tendon transplant, and it is 1.9 % when hamstring transplants are used.

In case of the 941 knee joints, which were included in the study, in 23 cases an axis deviation of more than 3° or a leg-length discrepancy of more than 1 cm was postoperatively detected [26]. In those 23 patients a leg-length discrepancy was diagnosed in 48 % of cases; 31 % showed a genu recurvatum, 17 % a genu valgum, and 4 % a genu varum [26]. From a total of 55 articles, however, only 9 authors carried out postoperative full-leg radiographs, and, in case of 7, growth disorders were diagnosed. This suggests that the number of unreported cases of growth disorders after anterior cruciate ligament reconstruction in children and adolescents is likely to be considerably higher than stated in the literature. In this context a study from McIntosh et al. [59] is of interest as they determined an averaging leg elongation of the operated leg of 6.2 mm by means of precise pre- and postoperative measuring, whereby 15 of 16 examined patients showed leg-length differences.

The ACL Study Group obtained somewhat different growth disorder ratios. From a total of 15 cases with growth disorders after anterior cruciate ligament reconstruction, they diagnosed 10 genua valga, 3 genua recurvata, and 2 cases of postoperative leg-length discrepancies [38].

32.5.4   Classification of Growth Disorders After Anterior Cruciate Ligament Reconstruction

Chotel et al. [15] classified growth disorders after anterior cruciate ligament reconstruction in children and adolescents and categorized them into three types [13]. In Type A localized growth plate damages occur along with the formation of a focal bone bridge. Due to the remaining growth of undamaged growth plate areas, a genu valgum, varum, or recurvatum will develop depending on the damage's localization.

Type B [15] is associated with excessive growth of the damaged limb. This is probably induced by an irritation of the physis caused by the surgical trauma, which possibly leads to hyper-vascularization of the physis and its stimulation. A consequence of this is leg elongation.

Type C [15] is associated with decrease in leg length. The likeliest cause is supposed to be a "teno-epiphysiodesis effect": the transplant tension decreases the length growth of the limb resulting in a leg-length decrease of the affected leg.

In addition complex malpositions can be generated by using implants intersecting the growth plate or by using bone blocks for fixation purposes.

32.5.5   Genu Valgum

The development of genu valgum can be evoked by the implant material when perforating a physis laterally on the femur [42]. In three cases within the current literature, no statements were given with regard to the development of a genu valgum [26]. However, it is known from animal experiments [60, 74] that peripheral, dorsal, and transphyseal drilling of the femoral canal can involve injury of the Ranvier's groove, which then can lead to an early closure of the lateral femur's growth plate and, hence, to a genu valgum [60, 74]. Therefore, one must keep in mind that a sufficiently broad bone bridge should dorsally remain during the femoral placement of the tunnel. Principally one has to ensure that a soft tissue transplant in the

tunnel lies at growth plates' level as empty tunnels can also evoke growth disturbances including early closure of the growth plates [60, 74].

The ACL Study Group [38] described the following scenarios for the incurrence of genu valgum: caused by implant material, by bone blocks at growth plate's level, by oversized tunnel diameter (12 mm) and also by lateral extra-articular tenodesis and by peripheral injury of the femoral growth plate caused by "over the top" technique.

From animal experiments studies as well as from our own clinical experiences, a genu valgum can be prevented by the avoidance of a too dorsal and peripheral tunnel placement, by using hamstring transplants unharmfully crossing the growth plate, and also by a fixation far from the joint line [60, 74].

32.5.6   Genu Varum

According to current literature a genu varum occurs on rather rare occasions. The ACL Study Group did not record a genu varum [38]. In the current meta-analysis, which included 941 patients, only one case of a postoperative genu varum was described [26]. A reason for this was not specified by the authors. Discussed to be causes for the development of a genu varum are either peripheral growth plate damages of the tibial canal or an epiphysiodesis effect of the growth plate caused by fixation materials or bone blocks at growth plate's level.

32.5.7   Genu Recurvatum

With regard to the development of a genu recurvatum, a number of causes need to be discussed. Particularly the apophysis of the proximal tibia or the ventral part of the proximal physis of the tibia can be peripherally damaged during the placement of the tibial tunnel, which, as a result, could lead to an early closure of the growth plate [38, 60]. In principle one also has to consider in this context that tangential drilling near the growth plate could cause heat damage which then may lead to an early closure [78]. A further possibility for the development of a genu recurvatum – particularly in case of growth plate-protecting techniques – could be evoked by ventrally pulling out a transplant from the knee joint proximal to the tibial physis and by fixation distal to the growth plate; the foregoing could make the transplant block the growth of the growth plate in the sense of a "teno-epiphysiodesis effect" [15].

32.5.8 Leg-Length Discrepancy

Whether or not leg-length discrepancies in connection with anterior cruciate ligament reconstruction in children and adolescents can also be prevented by optimized surgical techniques remains currently uncertain. It is admittedly described by animal experiments that the incurrence of growth disturbances, leg-length discrepancies in particular, can be prevented with the help of adequate surgical methods [60, 74]; however, in that case, the observation period of 24 weeks must be regarded as rather short. With a 2 % statistical risk of postoperatively suffering from a 1-cm leg-length discrepancy, it principally is a debatable point whether this can be of any evidence at all considering the small numbers of animals used for the experiments. In individual cases it may be difficult to prevent a stimulation of the physis with subsequent stimulation of the length growth [59] as a response of the epiphyseal plate is histologically verifiable in the tunnel area even without subsequent growth disturbance [60].

Further analysis of the development of a growth disturbance after anterior cruciate ligament reconstruction in children and adolescents shows that a decrease in leg length described there was caused by staples used for the fixation of the tibial and femoral growth plate [50]. In addition a decrease in leg length in case of congenital anisomelia with accompanying cruciate ligament insufficiency was observed [61] and also another one after contralateral femur fracture [66]. However, when evaluating the leg length, most studies' problem is that the leg length was not measured accurately before surgery [26]. Therefore, the leg-length discrepancy

cannot always be ascribed to the cruciate ligament surgery with absolute certainty [26].

32.5.9 Arthrofibrosis and Restricted Mobility

In case of children less than 10 years of age, a brace will be used for aftercare purposes. Forearm crutches are not appropriate in this age group because of low body weight and, in most cases, lack of compliance. For children 10 years or older, we recommend the placement of an orthesis with restricted range of motion (0–0–90°) and also forearm crutches with partial weight-bearing of 10–20 kg for a 4-week period. In our view mobilization of the knee joint should be worked on in all age groups and in a controlled manner by means of physiotherapy two to three times per week in the first 6 weeks. From week 6 onwards, aftercare activities can be intensified depending on age in the form of, for instance, extended ambulatory physiotherapy [EAP] [25].

Attention should be paid to the fact that arthrofibrosis is one of the most common complications (8.3 % of all cases) after anterior cruciate ligament reconstruction – even in children and adolescents [68]. Risk factors, which may lead to a development of arthrofibrosis after anterior cruciate ligament reconstruction, are the female gender, the age group between 16 and 18 years, and the usage of BTB transplants [68]. However, an early surgery within the first 4 weeks after trauma has no influence on the development of an arthrofibrosis.

Because of the current data situation, we consider it necessary to also treat children postoperatively with physiotherapy after anterior cruciate ligament reconstruction.

References

1. Aichroth PM, Patel DV, Zorrilla P (2002) The natural history and treatment of rupture of the anterior cruciate ligament in children and adolescents. A prospective review. J Bone Joint Surg Br 84(1):38–41
2. Alentorn-Geli E, Myer GD, Silvers HJ, Samitier G, Romero D, Lazaro-Haro C, Cugat R (2009) Prevention

of non-contact anterior cruciate ligament injuries in soccer players. Part 2: a review of prevention programs aimed to modify risk factors and to reduce injury rates. Knee Surg Sports Traumatol Arthrosc 17(8):859–879. doi:10.1007/s00167-009-0823-z

3. Anderson AF (2003) Transepiphyseal replacement of the anterior cruciate ligament in skeletally immature patients. A preliminary report. J Bone Joint Surg Am 85-A(7):1255–1263

4. Anderson AF (2004) Transepiphyseal replacement of the anterior cruciate ligament using quadruple hamstring grafts in skeletally immature patients. J Bone Joint Surg Am 86-A(Suppl 1 (Pt. 2)):201–209

5. Anderson M, Green WT, Messner MB (1963) Growth and predictions of growth in the lower extremities. J Bone Joint Surg Am 45:1–14

6. Arbes S, Resinger C, Vecsei V, Nau T (2007) The functional outcome of total tears of the anterior cruciate ligament (ACL) in the skeletally immature patient. Int Orthop 31(4):471–475. doi:10.1007/s00264-006-0225-5

7. Barrack RL, Bruckner JD, Kneisl J et al (1990) The outcome of nonoperatively treated complete tears of the anterior cruciate ligament in active young adults. Clin Orthop Relat Res 259:192–199

8. Baxter MP (1988) Assessment of normal pediatric knee ligament laxity using the genucom. J Pediatr Orthop 8(5):546–550

9. Boden BP, Dean GS, Feagin JA Jr, Garrett WE Jr (2000) Mechanisms of anterior cruciate ligament injury. Orthopedics 23(6):573–578

10. Bollen S, Pease F, Ehrenraich A, Church S, Skinner J, Williams A (2008) Changes in the four-strand hamstring graft in anterior cruciate ligament reconstruction in the skeletally-immature knee. J Bone Joint Surg Br 90(4):455–459. doi:10.1302/0301-620X.90B4.19416

11. Bonnard C, Chotel F (2007) Knee ligament and meniscal injury in children and adolescents. [Article in French]. Rev Chir Orthop Reparatrice Appar Mot 93(6 Suppl):95–139

12. Bonnard C, Fournier J, Babusiaux D, Planchenault M, Bergerault F, de Courtivron B (2011) Physeal-sparing reconstruction of anterior cruciate ligament tears in children: results of 57 cases using patellar tendon. J Bone Joint Surg Br 93(4):542–547. doi:10.1302/0301-620X.93B4.25801

13. Chotel F, Seil R (2013) Growth disturbances after transphyseal ACL reconstruction in skeletally immature patients: Who is more at risk? Young child or adolescent? J Pediatr Orthop 33(5):585–586

14. Chotel F, Bonnard C, Accadbled F et al (2007) Résultats et facteurs pronostiques de la reconstruction du LCA sur genou en croissance. A propos d'une série multicentrique de 102 cas. Rev Chir Orthop Reparatrice Appar Mot 93:3S131–3S138

15. Chotel F, Henry J, Seil R, Chouteau J, Moyen B, Bérard J (2010) Growth disturbances without growth arrest after ACL reconstruction in children. Knee Surg Sports Traumatol Arthrosc 18:1496–1500

16. Cohen M, Ferretti M, Quarteiro M, Marcondes FB, de Hollanda JP, Amaro JT, Abdalla RJ (2009) Transphyseal anterior cruciate ligament reconstruction in patients with open physes. Arthroscopy 25(8):831–838. doi:10.1016/j.arthro.2009.01.015

17. Courvoisier A, Grimaldi M, Plaweski S (2011) Good surgical outcome of transphyseal ACL reconstruction in skeletally immature patients using four-strand hamstring graft. Knee Surg Sports Traumatol Arthrosc 19(4):588–591. doi:10.1007/s00167-010-1282-2

18. Dumont GD, Hogue GD, Padalecki JR, Okoro N, Wilson PL (2012) Meniscal and chondral injuries associated with pediatric anterior cruciate ligament tears: relationship of treatment time and patient-specific factors. Am J Sports Med 40(9):2128–2133

19. Edwards PH, Grana WA (2001) Anterior cruciate ligament reconstruction in the immature athlete: long-term results of intra-articular reconstruction. Am J Knee Surg 14(4):232–237

20. Edwards TB, Greene CC, Baratta RV et al (2001) The effect of placing a tensioned graft across open growth plates. A gross and histologic analysis. J Bone Joint Surg Am 83:725–734

21. Edwards TB, Greene CC, Baratta RV, Zieske A, Willis RB (2001) The effect of placing a tensioned graft across open growth plates. A gross and histologic analysis. J Bone Joint Surg Am 83-A(5):725–734

22. Fabricant PD, Jones KJ, Delos D, Cordasco FA, Marx RG, Pearle AD, Warren RF, Green DW (2013) Reconstruction of the anterior cruciate ligament in the skeletally immature athlete: a review of current concepts: AAOS exhibit selection. J Bone Joint Surg Am 95(5):e28. doi:10.2106/JBJS.L.00772

23. Ford LT, Key JA (1956) A study of experimental trauma to the distal femoral epiphysis in rabbits. J Bone Joint Surg Am 38-A(1):84–92

24. Frosch KH, Preiss A, Giannakos A (2012) Probleme und Komplikationen nach vorderer. Kreuzbandplastik im Wachstumsalter Arthroskopie 25:260–265

25. Frosch KH, Habermann F, Fuchs M, Michel A, Junge R, Schmidtmann U, Stürmer KM (2001) Is prolonged ambulatory physical therapy after anterior cruciate ligament-plasty indicated? Comparison of costs and benefits. Unfallchirurg 104(6):513–518

26. Frosch KH, Stengel D, Brodhun T, Stietencron I, Holsten D, Jung C, Reister D, Voigt C, Niemeyer P, Maier M, Hertel P, Jagodzinski M, Lill H (2010) Outcomes and risks of operative treatment of rupture of the anterior cruciate ligament in children and adolescents. Arthroscopy 26(11):1539–1550. doi:10.1016/j.arthro.2010.04.077

27. Graf BK, Lange RH, Fujisaki CK, Landry GL, Saluja RK (1992) Anterior cruciate ligament tears in skeletally immature patients: meniscal pathology at presentation and after attempted conservative treatment. Arthroscopy 8(2):229–233

28. Guzzanti V (2003) The natural history and treatment of rupture of the anterior cruciate ligament in children and adolescents. J Bone Joint Surg Br 85(4):618–619; author reply 619

29. Guzzanti V, Falciglia F, Stanitski CL (2003) Preoperative evaluation and anterior cruciate ligament reconstruction technique for skeletally immature patients in Tanner stages 2 and 3. Am J Sports Med 31(6):941–948

30. Henry J, Chotel F, Chouteau J, Fessy MH, Bérard J, Moyen B (2009) Rupture of the anterior cruciate ligament in children: early reconstruction with open physes or delayed reconstruction to skeletal maturity? Knee Surg Sports Traumatol Arthrosc 17(7): 748–755

31. Hinton RY, Rivera VR, Pautz MJ, Sponseller PD (2008) Ligamentous laxity of the knee during childhood and adolescence. J Pediatr Orthop 28(2):184–187. doi:10.1097/BPO.0b013e3181652120

32. Hudgens JL, Dahm DL (2012) Treatment of anterior cruciate ligament injury in skeletally immature patients. Int J Pediatr 2012:932702

33. Hueter C (1862) Anatomische Studien an den Extremitätengelenken Neugeborener und Erwachsener. Virchow Arch 25:575–599

34. Janarv PM, Nystrom A, Werner S et al (1996) Anterior cruciate ligament injuries in skeletally immature patients. J Pediatr Orthop 16:673–677

35. Kannus P, Jarvinen M (1988) Knee ligament injuries in adolescents. Eight year follow-up of conservative management. J Bone Joint Surg Br 70:772–776

36. Kercher J, Xerogeanes J, Tannenbaum A, Al-Hakim R, Black JC, Zhao J (2009) Anterior cruciate ligament reconstruction in the skeletally immature: an anatomical study utilizing 3-dimensional magnetic resonance imaging reconstructions. J Pediatr Orthop 29(2):124–129. doi:10.1097/BPO.0b013e3181982228

37. Kim SJ, Chang JH, Kim TW, Jo SB, Oh KS (2009) Anterior Cruciate Ligament Reconstruction with Use of a Single or Double-Bundle Technique in Patients with Generalized Ligamentous Laxity. J Bone Joint Surg Am 91:257–262

38. Kocher MS, Saxon HS, Hovis WD, Hawkins RJ (2002) Management and complications of anterior cruciate ligament injuries in skeletally immature patients: survey of the Herodicus Society and the ACL Study Group. J Pediatr Orthop 22(4):452–457

39. Kocher MS, Garg S, Micheli LJ (2005) Physeal sparing reconstruction of the anterior cruciate ligament in skeletally immature prepubescent children and adolescents. J Bone Joint Surg Am 87(11):2371–2379. doi:10.2106/JBJS.D.02802

40. Kocher MS, Garg S, Micheli LJ (2006) Physeal sparing reconstruction of the anterior cruciate ligament in skeletally immature prepubescent children and adolescents. Surgical technique. J Bone Joint Surg Am 88(Suppl 1):283–293

41. Kocher MS, Smith JT, Zoric BJ, Lee B, Micheli LJ (2007) Transphyseal anterior cruciate ligament reconstruction in skeletally immature pubescent adolescents. J Bone Joint Surg Am 89(12):2632–2639. doi:10.2106/JBJS.F.01560

42. Koman JD, Sanders JO (1999) Valgus deformity after reconstruction of the anterior cruciate ligament in a skeletally immature patient. A case report. Bone Joint Surg Am 81:711–715

43. Kopf S, Schenkengel JP, Wieners G, Starke C, Becker R (2010) No bone tunnel enlargement in patients with open growth plates after transphyseal ACL reconstruction. Knee Surg Sports Traumatol Arthrosc 18(11):1445–1451. doi:10.1007/s00167-009-1041-4

44. Kumar S, Ahearne D, Hunt DM (2013) Transphyseal anterior cruciate ligament reconstruction in the skeletally immature: follow-up to a minimum of sixteen years of age. J Bone Joint Surg Am 95(1):e1. doi:10.2106/JBJS.K.01707

45. Kwon JW, Yoon YC, Kim YN, Ahn JH, Choe BK (2009) Which oblique plane is more helpful in diagnosing an anterior cruciate ligament tear? Clin Radiol 64(3):291–297. doi:10.1016/j.crad.2008.10.007

46. Lawrence JT, Bowers AL, Belding J, Cody SR, Ganley TJ (2010) All-epiphyseal anterior cruciate ligament reconstruction in skeletally immature patients. Clin Orthop Relat Res 468(7):1971–1977. doi:10.1007/s11999-010-1255-2

47. Lawrence JT, Argawal N, Ganley TJ (2011) Degeneration of the knee joint in skeletally immature patients with a diagnosis of an anterior cruciate ligament tear: is there harm in delay of treatment? Am J Sports Med 39(12):2582–2587. doi:10.1177/0363546511420818

48. Lawrence JT, Argawal N, Ganley TJ (2011) Degeneration of the knee joint in skeletally immature patients with a diagnosis of an anterior cruciate ligament tear: is there harm in delay of treatment? Am J Sports Med 39(12):2582–2587

49. Lee K, Siegel MJ, Lau DM, Hildebolt CF, Matava MJ (1999) Anterior cruciate ligament tears: MR imaging-based diagnosis in a pediatric population. Radiology 213(3):697–704. doi:10.1148/radiology.213.3.r99dc26697

50. Lipscomb AB, Anderson AF (1986) Tears of the anterior cruciate ligament in adolescents. J Bone Joint Surg Am 68(1):19–28

51. Makela EA, Vainionpaa S, Vihtonen K, Mero M, Rokkanen P (1988) The effect of trauma to the lower femoral epiphyseal plate. An experimental study in rabbits. J Bone Joint Surg Br 70(2):187–191

52. Manner HM, Radler C, Ganger R, Grill F (2006) Dysplasia of the cruciate ligaments: radiographic assessment and classification. J Bone Joint Surg Am 88(1):130–137. doi:10.2106/JBJS.E.00146

53. Matsushita T, Oka S, Nagamune K, Matsumoto T, Nishizawa Y, Hoshino Y, Kubo S, Kurosaka M, Kuroda R (2013) Differences in knee kinematics between wake and anesthetized patients during the Lachman and Pivot-Shift tests for anterior cruciate ligament deficiency. Orthop J Sports Med 1 (1). doi:10.1177/2325967113487855

54. Mauro CS, Irrgang JJ, Williams BA, Harner CD (2008) Loss of extension following anterior cruciate ligament reconstruction: analysis of incidence and etiology using IKDC criteria. Arthroscopy 24(2):146–153. doi:10.1016/j.arthro.2007.08.026

55. Mccarroll JR, Rettig AC, Shelbourne KD (1988) Anterior cruciate ligament injuries in the young

athlete with open physes. Am J Sports Med 16: 44–47

56. McCarroll JR, Shelbourne KD, Porter DA, Rettig AC, Murray S (1994) Patellar tendon graft reconstruction for midsubstance anterior cruciate ligament rupture in junior high school athletes. An algorithm for management. Am J Sports Med 22(4):478–484

57. McCarroll JR, Shelbourne KD, Patel DV (1995) Anterior cruciate ligament injuries in young athletes. Recommendations for treatment and rehabilitation. Sports Med 20(2):117–127

58. McConkey MO, Bonasia DE, Amendola A (2011) Pediatric anterior cruciate ligament reconstruction. Curr Rev Musculoskelet Med 4(2):37–44. doi:10.1007/s12178-011-9076-9

59. McIntosh AL, Dahm DL, Stuart MJ (2006) Anterior cruciate ligament reconstruction in the skeletally immature patient. Arthroscopy 22:1325–1330

60. Meller R et al (2008) Hindlimb growth after a transphyseal reconstruction of the anterior cruciate ligament: a study in skeletally immature sheep with wide-open physes. Am J Sports Med 36(12): 2437–2443

61. Micheli LJ, Rask B, Gerberg L (1999) Anterior cruciate ligament reconstruction in patients who are prepubescent. Clin Orthop Relat Res 364:40–47

62. Millett PJ, Willis AA, Warren RF (2002) Associated injuries in pediatric and adolescent anterior cruciate ligament tears: does a delay in treatment increase the risk of meniscal tear? Arthroscopy 18(9):955–959

63. Mizuta H, Kubota K, Shiraishi M et al (1995) The conservative treatment of complete tears of the anterior cruciate ligament in skeletally immature patients. J Bone Joint Surg Br 77:890–894

64. Moksnes H, Engebretsen L, Risberg MA (2008) Performance-based functional outcome for children 12 years or younger following anterior cruciate ligament injury: a two to nine-year follow-up study. Knee Surg Sports Traumatol Arthrosc 16(3):214–223

65. Moksnes H, Engebretsen L, Risberg MA (2012) The current evidence for treatment of ACL injuries in children is low: a systematic review. J Bone Joint Surg Am 94(12):1112–1119

66. Nakhostine M, Bollen SR, Cross MJ (1995) Reconstruction of mid-substance anterior cruciate rupture in adolescents with open physes. J Pediatr Orthop 15(3):286–287

67. Nordenvall R, Bahmanyar S, Adami J, Stenros C, Wredmark T, Fellander-Tsai L (2012) A population-based nationwide study of cruciate ligament injury in Sweden, 2001–2009: incidence, treatment, and sex differences. Am J Sports Med 40(8):1808–1813. doi:10.1177/0363546512449306

68. Nwachukwu BU, McFeely ED, Nasreddine A, Udall JH, Finlayson C, Shearer DW, Micheli LJ, Kocher MS (2011) Arthrofibrosis after anterior cruciate ligament reconstruction in children and adolescents. J Pediatr Orthop 31(8):811–817

69. Preiss A, Brodhun T, Stietencron I, Frosch KH (2012) Rupture of the anterior cruciate ligament

in growing children: surgical or conservative treatment? A systematic review. Unfallchirurg 115(9): 848–854

70. Renström PA (2013) Eight clinical conundrums relating to anterior cruciate ligament (ACL) injury in sport: recent evidence and a personal reflection. Br J Sports Med 47(6):367–372

71. Salzmann GM, Spang JT, Imhoff AB (2009) Double-bundle anterior cruciate ligament reconstruction in a skeletally immature adolescent athlete. Arthroscopy 25(3):321–324. doi:10.1016/j.arthro.2008.11.008

72. Seil R, Kohn D (2000) Ruptures of the anterior cruciate ligament (ACL) during growth. Bull Soc Sci Med Grand Duche Luxemb 1:39–53

73. Seil R, Robert H (2004) Complete anterior cruciate ligament tears in children. Rev Chir Orthop Reparatrice Appar Mot 90(8 Suppl):3S11–3S20. Review. French

74. Seil R, Pape D, Kohn D (2008) The risk of growth changes during transphyseal drilling in sheep with open physes. Arthroscopy 24(7):824–833. doi:10.1016/j.arthro.2008.02.007

75. Shea KG, Grimm NL, Belzer JS (2011) Volumetric injury of the distal femoral physis during double-bundle ACL reconstruction in children: a three-dimensional study with use of magnetic resonance imaging. J Bone Joint Surg Am 93(11):1033–1038. doi:10.2106/JBJS.J.01047

76. Shelbourne KD, Gray T, Wiley BV (2004) Results of transphyseal anterior cruciate ligament reconstruction using patellar tendon autograft in tanner stage 3 or 4 adolescents with clearly open growth plates. Am J Sports Med 32(5):1218–1222. doi:10.1177/0363546503262169

77. Slough JM, Hennrikus W, Chang Y (2013) The reliability of tanner staging performed by orthopaedic sports medicine surgeons. Med Sci Sports Exerc 45(7):1229–1234

78. Sobau C, Ellermann A (2004) Anterior cruciate ligament reconstruction with hamstring tendons in the young. Unfallchirurg 107:676–679

79. Stadelmaier DM, Arnoczky SP, Dodds J, Ross H (1995) The effect of drilling and soft tissue grafting across open growth plates. A histologic study. Am J Sports Med 23(4):431–435

80. Stanitski CL, Harvell JC, Fu F (1993) Observations on acute knee hemarthrosis in children and adolescents. J Pediatr Orthop 13(4):506–510

81. Streich NA, Barié A, Gotterbarm T, Keil M, Schmitt H (2010) Transphyseal reconstruction of the anterior cruciate ligament in prepubescent athletes. Knee Surg Sports Traumatol Arthrosc 18(11): 1481–1486

82. Strobel MW (2005) Vordere Kreuzbandinsuffizienz. In: Wirth CJ, Zichner L, Kohn D (eds) Orthopädie und orthopädische Chirurgie, Germany:Georg Thieme Verlag, Stuttgart, pp 263–288

83. Volkmann R (1862) Chirurgische Erfahrungen über Knochenverbiegungen und Knochenwachstum. Arch Pathol Anat 24:512–540

84. Woods GW, O'connor DP (2004) Delayed anterior cruciate ligament reconstruction in adolescents with open physes. Am J Sports Med 32:201–210

85. Yoo WJ, Kocher MS, Micheli LJ (2011) Growth plate disturbance after transphyseal reconstruction of the anterior cruciate ligament in skeletally immature adolescent patients: an MR imaging study. J Pediatr Orthop 31(6):691–696. doi:10.1097/BPO.0b013e3182210952

Bony Avulsion with Open Physis

33

Elisabeth Abermann, Peter Gföller, Christian Hoser, and Christian Fink

Contents

E. Abermann, MD
LKH Feldkirch, OSM Research Foundation,
Carinagasse 47, 6800 Feldkirch, Austria

P. Gföller • C. Hoser, MD
OSM Research Foundation, Sportsclinic Austria,
Olympiastr. 39, 6020 Innsbruck, Austria

C. Fink, MD (✉)
Research Knee – Sports Medicine, OSM Research
Foundation, Sportsclinic Austria,
Olympiastr. 39, 6020 Innsbruck, Austria
e-mail: christian.fink@sportsclinicaustria.com

The avulsion fracture of the tibial attachment is also commonly known as fracture of the anterior tibial spine or the intercondylar eminence. Both these terms are misnomers as this avulsion fracture usually involves only the intercondylar depression anterior to the spine where the ACL attaches [1]. Less frequently, a large fractured piece may involve the tibial spine and may also extend medially and laterally to lift up wings of articular cartilage [2]. However, most authors do not really make this differentiation. The epiphyseal ossification process does not reach the tibial eminence until late childhood or early adolescence [3], which seems to be the most common time frame for this type of fracture [3, 4]. Intercondylar fractures of the tibia are relatively common in children and adolescents compared to adults (annual incidence of 3/100,000 children) [4] as incomplete ossification in this area may render it more vulnerable to tensile forces than the ACL itself [5–7]. It has also been proposed that the injury occurs in consequence to greater elasticity of the ligaments in children [8]. The fragment is mostly oval, bigger than the cross section of the ACL according to the anchorage zone of the ACL, and consists of bone and cartilage.

R. Siebold et al. (eds.), *Anterior Cruciate Ligament Reconstruction*,
DOI 10.1007/978-3-642-45349-6_33, © ESSKA 2014

However, avulsions without bony portions are possible and are tricky because they can hardly be detected on plain radiographs. The anterior part can reach under the anterior horn of the medial/lateral meniscus or intermeniscal ligament [9]. The mechanism of injury for tibial eminence fractures is similar to an ACL tear [10]; however, it involves a chondroepiphyseal avulsion of the ACL insertion on the anteromedial tibial eminence [8, 11]. Common injury mechanisms are hyperextension of the knee, a direct blow on the distal end of the femur with the knee flexed [4], or forced flexion with rotation [12].

33.1 Clinical Symptoms and Findings: X-Ray, CT, and MRI

33.1.1 Clinical Examination

Clinical symptoms are different in acute and chronic avulsions. Patients with acute avulsion fractures typically hold the injured knee in a slightly flexed position and show pain and effusion around the knee from associated hemarthrosis similar to patients with a ligamentous ACL injury. Reluctance of weight bearing, limitation in range of motion, and positive Lachman and Pivot shift test are often present, too. Restriction of motion can occur due to mechanical impingement of the bony fragment [13]. Initial examination is sometimes difficult due to severe pain and the evaluation of the ligamentous laxity may be limited. Even under anesthesia some patients may have only IKDC grade B laxity (nearly normal) – pivot shift more than Lachman and still have an ACL avulsion [14]. Chronic cases show knee extension limitation and grade II or more instability due to non- or malunion.

33.1.2 X-Ray

Standard radiographs, involving anteroposterior, lateral, and oblique views, are usually diagnostic. The appearance of a tiny bone fragment in the intercondylar notch with cortical irregularity of the adjacent tibial eminence suggesting a donor site for the fragment is the usual finding in this

entity [15]. Because the avulsed fragment may be mostly nonossified cartilage with only a small, thin ossified portion, the fracture can be difficult to recognize and is best seen on the lateral radiograph (Figs. 33.1 and 33.2) [3]. However, these injuries can easily be missed by untrained eyes if not suspected [2].

33.1.3 CT

Computed tomographic scanning allows precise definition of the fracture anatomy [5] and bony architecture (Fig. 33.1) [10]. Apart from that a CT scan cannot bring any further information and has the disadvantage of additional radiation exposure.

33.1.4 MRI

As we see the avulsion fracture as a ligamentous injury with bony involvement, and not primarily as a fracture of the tibial head, we recommend MRI as the additional investigation of first choice after conventional radiograph for every suspected avulsion fracture (Fig. 33.2). It is as useful to understand the fracture anatomy and determine the amount of dislocation as a CT scan and can beyond that confirm that the entire substance of ACL is intact (Fig. 33.3). Furthermore, it provides the benefit of diagnostic imaging of associated meniscal, ligamentous, or chondral pathology (Fig. 33.4) [5].

33.1.5 Classification

The classification of Meyers and McKeever, described in 1959, is still today the most common (Fig. 33.5). Their classification divides the fractures into three groups based on the degree of fragment dislocation: type I represents a nondisplaced to minimally displaced fracture at the anterior margin. Type II fractures involve the anterior third of the avulsed bone displaced proximally, with an intact posterior hinge resembling a bird's beak. Type III fractures are characterized by completely displaced fragments. In addition, completely displaced type III was subdivided into types IIIA and IIIB, the former being merely displaced and the

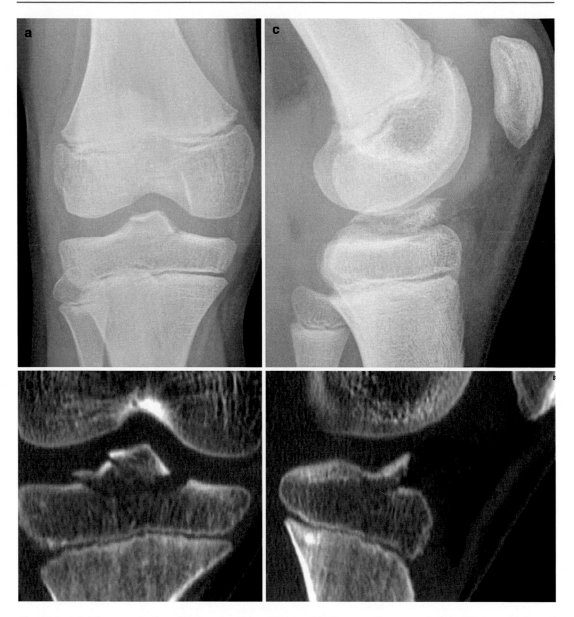

Fig. 33.1 (**a**) AP x-ray of a large fragment avulsion fracture. (**b**) Corresponding coronal plain CT scan. (**c**) Lateral x-ray of the same knee. (**d**) Corresponding sagittal plain CT scan

latter being displaced and rotated [16]. Zarycznyj added type IV in which the fragment is comminuted (Fig. 33.5) [10]. However, this classification takes no account of the size of the fragment [17]. Therefore, Zifko and Gaudernak introduced another classification on the basis of the anatomy of the anterior intercondylar eminence to distinguish between type A, isolated avulsion of the ACL, and type B, fractures including the intercondylar eminence [18].

33.1.6 Associated Pathologies

Historically, tibial eminence fractures were rarely associated with additional injuries, suggesting a rate of meniscal injuries of less than 5 % [16, 19, 20]. However, most of these studies were based on conventional radiographic findings and did not address injuries to the subchondral bone and soft tissues of the knee. Nonetheless, McLennan et al. already stated in 1982 that

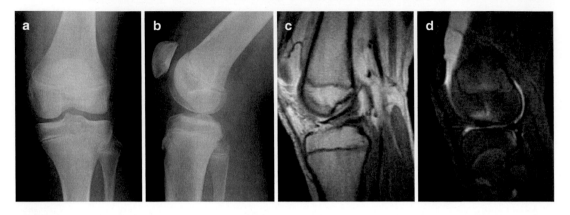

Fig. 33.2 (**a, b**) AP and lateral x-ray of a very small bony fracture fragment, which can hardly be seen on the conventional radiography. (**c**) Sagittal plain of the corresponding MRI. (**d**) Typical bone bruises on the lateral femoral condyle and the posterior tibial edge

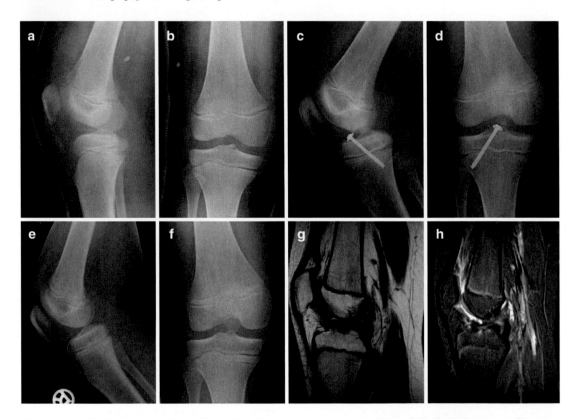

Fig. 33.3 (**a, b**) Radiographs of an ACL avulsion in an 11-year-old boy with cast immobilization. (**c, d**) Postoperative radiographs after screw fixation, dislocation of the fragment can be seen already. (**e, f**) Radiographs 1 year after screw fixation with still displaced fragment. (**g, h**) Corresponding sagittal plain MRI pictures showing an absorbed ACL

meniscal tears were the most commonly associated injuries with fractures of the tibial intercondylar eminence [21]. Shea et al. found a high incidence of concomitant bone contusions (90 %) in children who sustained a tibial eminence fracture. The patterns and location of bone contusions seen in these injuries were similar to those seen with ACL tears in adults (Fig. 33.2).

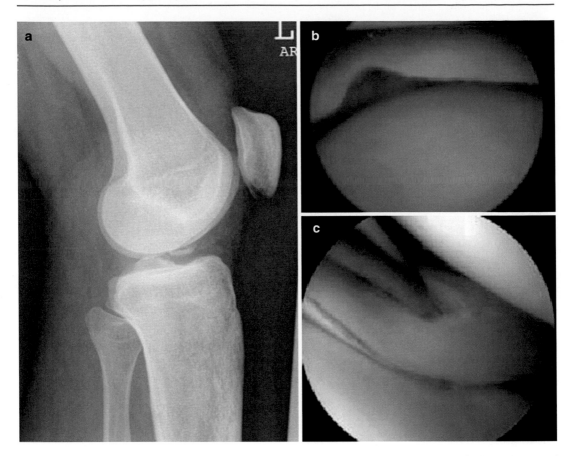

Fig. 33.4 Type III ACL avulsion fracture with lateral meniscal tear: (**a**) lateral x-ray, arthroscopic findings with (**c**) and without probe (**b**)

Meniscal tears were present in 40 % of the children (Fig. 33.4) [22].

33.2 Conservative or Operative Treatment and Timing of Surgery

As with other injuries about the knee joint, treatment was historically limited to immobilization and developed, in the course of time, to include open surgical repair [5]. Nonetheless, the appropriate management of tibial eminence fractures in children is still controversial, with techniques advocating cast immobilization (Fig. 33.3a, b) with [23, 24] or without [20, 25] closed reduction, open reduction with internal fixation [23, 26], arthroscopic reduction with suture (Figs. 33.6 and 33.7) [5, 27–30] or suture anchor fixation (Figs. 33.3c, d, 33.8 and 33.9) [31], and arthroscopic reduction with wire [32], absorbable pin [33], or screw fixation (Figs. 33.10 and 33.11) [21, 28, 34, 35].

Like in ACL reconstructions, isometry and tension are essential in the treatment of tibial intercondylar eminence avulsions to restore normal knee kinematics and must be obtained with the initial treatment [36]. Furthermore, anatomic reduction and rigid fixation that allow for early range of motion should be achieved [10]. Theoretically, over-reduction should be avoided to prevent excessive tightening of the ACL resulting in a limitation of knee motion [34]. On the other hand, some believe that permanent intersubstance stretching of the ACL occurs prior to the fracture and therefore recommend

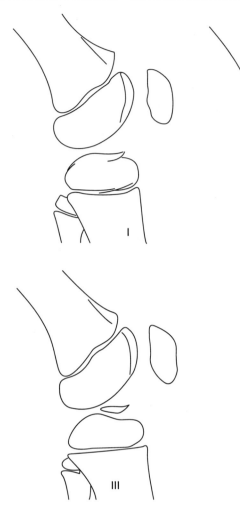
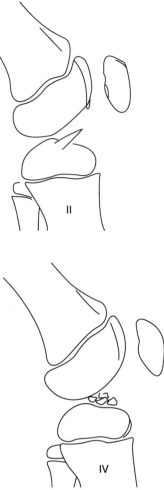

Fig. 33.5 Schematic drawing of the types of fractures of the intercondylar eminence of the tibia which occur in the child. Type *I* – minimum displacement, Type *II* – dis-placement of the anterior third to half of the avulsed fragment, Type *III* – fragment is completely lifted from its bone bed [16], Type *IV* – comminuted fragment [10]

over-reduction [8]. Other authors suggest regaining a normal ACL tension by pulling the inferior portion of ACL fibers with pullout suturing [27, 29]. And finally, Wilfinger et al. conclude that some dislocation resulting in slight laxity can be tolerated without any handicap in daily life and sports [25]. However, most current authors consent that any displacement requires at least anatomic reduction.

Concerning the timing of surgery, Patel et al. described an earlier return to full preinjury activity level for acute definitive treatment [37]. We share this impression and recommend an early surgical approach in case of any upcoming doubts concerning a successful outcome with conservative treatment. The idea is not to injure the knee joint for a second time when the healing process has already started.

In general, treatment is based on the Meyers and McKeever classification. For type I fractures immobilization in extension is generally recommended. However, some controversy exists regarding the degree of knee extension. Ligament isometry of the ACL in vivo and in cadavers

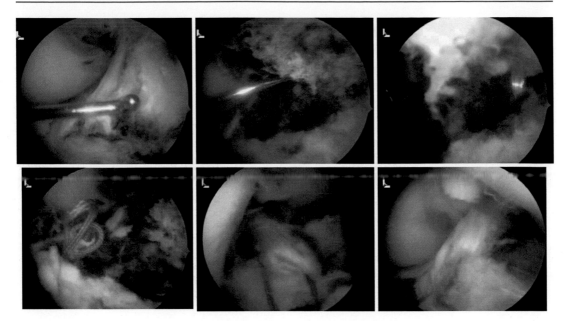

Fig. 33.6 Suture fixation: the fragment is cleaned until it can be reduced. Two 2.4 mm K-wires are placed at the medial and lateral border of the crater. Two No. 2 (absorbable or non-absorbable) sutures are placed through the ACL and close to the bone. The two sutures are then retrieved through the two bone tunnels and pulled tight

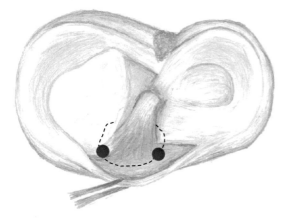

Fig. 33.7 Axial view of the tibia with a schematic drawing of an ACL avulsion crater, a released intermeniscal ligament, and proper position of the drill holes (*red dots*)

showed maximum tensioning at 0 and 45° and the least tensioning at 30° [36]. Therefore, from a biomechanical point of view, immobilization in 20–30° of flexion appears to be the best position for fracture healing and maintenance of reduction.

Several authors recommended immobilization in slight flexion from 10° to 30° [3, 16, 19]. However, other authors prefer immobilization in full extension to avoid extension deficits [10]. Full weight bearing is allowed if tolerated. No matter which position is preferred, close follow-up radiographs should be performed in the first weeks to detect displacement of the fragment as soon as possible.

The treatment of type II fractures is still seen controversial in the literature. In all cases, closed reduction may be attempted by aspiration of the hemarthrosis and knee extension or hyperextension (concepting the femoral condyles to reduce the fracture) [5, 25]. However, McLennan et al. found that the fracture pattern was not congruous with the femoral condyle footprint at any point of flexion as evident in the computerized reconstructions and cadaveric studies at 0°, 20°, 30°, and 45°. It was documented during arthroscopy, too, that the femoral condyles at no point of knee motion had any

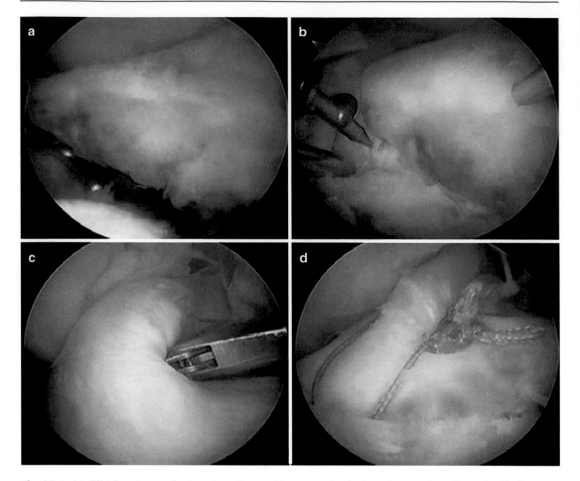

Fig. 33.8 (**a**) Tibial eminence fracture in a 7-year-old boy. (**b**) Transitory fixation with a K-wire and anchor location. (**c**) Piercing of inferomedial part of ACL with suture hook through anterolateral portal. (**d**) Suture in place (Reprinted with permission from Vega [31])

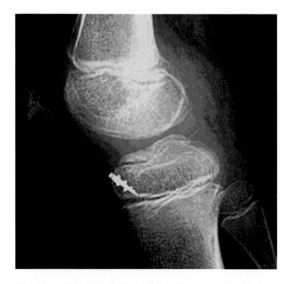

Fig. 33.9 Lateral postoperative radiograph of knee with a metallic anchor in adequate position avoiding open physis (Reprinted with permission from Vega [31])

bony contact with the cartilaginous wings of the fracture, and reduction was maintained by lack of ligament tension [36]. Kocher et al. stated that according to the previous biomechanical remarks they often experienced closed reduction at 30° flextion. Anyway, anteroposterior and lateral radiographs should be taken to verify reduction, and, with difficult visualization, CT or MRI should be performed [10]. Often, anatomic reduction cannot be achieved due to meniscal entrapment or interposition of the intermeniscal ligament (Fig. 33.7) [14]. For these cases, Wiley and Baxter found a correlation between fracture displacement at healing and knee laxity and functional outcome [38]. Therefore, nowadays, arthroscopic reduction and internal fixation of tibial intercondylar eminence fractures is the emerging treatment of

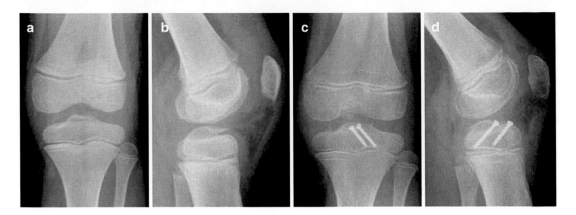

Fig. 33.10 Radiographs of the left knee of an 8-year-old boy with an ACL avulsion before (**a, b**) and after (**c, d**) screw fixation

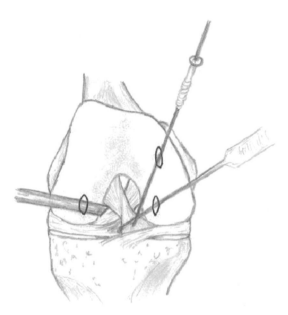

Fig. 33.11 Example of a screw fixation: the arthroscope is introduced through the inferior anterolateral portal. A hook probe is used from the inferior anteromedial portal to reduce the fragment. A guide wire is introduced through a superior anteromedial portal and drilled in the antegrade inferoposterior direction to fix the fragment. The hole is drilled with a cannulated drill bit and the screw is placed intra-articularly over the guide wire

choice and should be considered for all cases of displaced type II fractures [5].

Type III fractures are nowadays widely approached surgically because closed reduction is even more difficult in these fractures. The fact that the displaced osseous fragment is attached simultaneously to the anterior cruciate ligament and to the anterior horn of the lateral meniscus, both pulling in different directions, may explain why type III tibial eminence fractures are commonly irreducible by manipulation [39]. Arthroscopic reduction and internal fixation have become the standard procedure and additionally allow treating concomitant pathology like meniscal or osteochondral lesions. However, all techniques involving transphyseal drilling may be associated with growth disturbances. Although up to date fixation methods using cannulated screws (Fig. 33.10) or pullout sutures (Fig. 33.6) – currently the most common techniques – have equally excellent results, not every treatment can be applied to all fracture types. Screw fixation has the advantage of stronger fixation strength, but should only be applied to a large fracture fragment, otherwise risking comminution of the fragment (Fig. 33.3) [27]. Nevertheless, the potential for posterior malreduction is higher with screw fixation compared to transosseous sutures, because the screw is applied obliquely from anterior to posterior [40]. Furthermore screw heads may cause impingement and/or cartilage damage, necessitating removal. Additionally, neurovascular injuries due to protruding screws at the back of the tibia have been described [10]. Therefore, intraoperative use of fluoroscopy is mandatory with screw fixation. Suture fixation also has its shortcomings, such as a longer operation time, suture knot slippage, and being technically more demanding [41]. Alternatively, suture anchors, which avoid the risks of transphyseal drilling, may become an interesting solution for the future (Figs. 33.8 and 33.9) [31].

33.3 Surgical Technique

The patient is placed supine. A leg holder may be used. In case of screw fixation, it is important to allow at least for 120° of knee flexion. A tourniquet facilitates visualization. In all cases the calf compartments must be continually palpated to assure that fluid extravasation does not result in compartment syndrome. While intercondylar eminence avulsion fractures are contained injuries, they may be associated with capsular disruption. Standard anterolateral and anteromedial portals are used for visualization, but additional portals for instrumentation are commonly needed. Thorough lavage is required to remove hemarthrosis or loose chondral or osteochondral fragments. Depending on the situation, additional pathology like meniscal injuries may be treated before or after fixation of the avulsed fragment. The fragment and the fracture bed must be cleaned from fibrous tissue or clots [5]. Once the fracture site has been debrided, a tibial ACL guide or a probe is used to attempt a reduction [10]. If there is an entrapped anterior horn of the medial/lateral meniscus or intermeniscal ligament, it can be released by using an arthroscopic probe. In some cases, entrapment may recur unless the fracture is simultaneously reduced. In this case it might be helpful to place a temporary suture around the anterior horn of the medial meniscus from the anteromedial portal to retract it during reduction and fixation [14]. If the intermeniscal ligament prevents reduction and cannot be mobilized, resection is performed. Following reduction of the tibial fragment, temporal fixation may be obtained with a K-wire. This step is performed through a transpatellar tendon or medial parapatellar tendon approach under direct arthroscopic visualization (Fig. 33.11) [31].

At this point one should have decided upon the definitive fixation technique. Commonly, there are three possible pathways.

33.3.1 Screw Fixation

The fracture fragment should be at least three times the diameter of the fixation screw to pre-

vent comminution [35]. Several authors describe screw fixation with one transphyseal screw with or without a washer [26, 28, 34, 35, 42]. The screw can be introduced through a superior anteromedial portal [42] or an anterior transpatellar tendon portal (Fig. 33.11) [35]. Preferably a cannulated 3.5 or 4 mm screw is used. In this case an appropriate guide wire is introduced first to hold the fragment in place [42]. For the guide wires to be vertically oriented in the tibial spine, they must be passed near the inferior pole of the patella [35] and the knee has to be flexed to about 100–120°. Screw length is determined with a measuring device and the hole is drilled with a cannulated drill bit and threaded with a cannulated tap over the guide wire. In case of a thin or comminuted fracture, a washer is added. Eventual impingement of the screw has to be checked throughout full range of motion [42].

However, we prefer the technique of Kocher et al. who described a modified technique using two 3.5 mm AO cannulated screws within the epiphysis. A more horizontal placement, from anterior to posterior, is used to avoid crossing the proximal tibial physis (Fig. 33.10). Fluoroscopic assistance is mandatory in order to avoid screw protrusion across the proximal tibial physis [40].

Arthroscopic screw removal is recommended between 8 and 12 weeks postoperatively [40].

33.3.2 Pullout Suture Technique

The technique may be performed using only two portals; however, accessory portals may facilitate the technique [5].

A 90° suture lasso (Arthrex) is placed percutaneously (or via an accessory portal) through the fibers of the ACL in its midcoronal plane and as close to the bony fragment (distal) as possible [5]. Instead of the lasso a bended 80 mm cannula loaded with a loop of Seralon 3/0 (Serag Wiessner) can be used. The wire loop within the lasso is secured with an arthroscopic grasper and pulled through either of the portals and loaded with a No. 2 PDS (Ethicon) or Fiberwire (Arthrex) suture. With one end of the suture secured, the lasso is then retrieved, pulling the other end of the suture back through the ligament fibers and out through the skin (or accessory portal) [5]. The two ends are gathered with a hemostat for future identification. An additional two or more sutures are passed through the ACL fibers parallel to the previous sutures (Fig. 33.6) [27].

The drill holes one each side of the fracture bed must be established next. A short longitudinal incision is made approximately 3 cm distal to the joint line and midportion from the tibial tuberosity and the medial edge of the tibia. A standard ACL tibial aimer is used to place two 2.4 mm guide wires. The position of the drilled holes is essential for the stability of the reduced fragment. It should be attempted to place the guide wires more anterior than the mid-transverse axis of the crater. Anterior positioning helps to reduce the risk of fragment tilting after tightening the sutures (Fig. 33.7). In case of attachment of the lateral meniscus to the fragment, Ahn et al. stress the importance of anchoring the meniscus to the tibia. This can be achieved by creating a lateral hole piercing the anterior horn of the lateral meniscus and anchoring the meniscus together with the fragment [27].

An arthroscopic suture retriever or a wire loop is passed up through each drill hole to pull down the respective ends of the reduction suture. A standard arthroscopic grasper must be placed through one of the portals in order to "hand" the respective ends of the suture to the narrow-shafted grasper or pull them through the wire loop. Once the respective ends of the suture have been passed through the tunnels, the fragment is reduced by pulling down the suture ends while removing any entrapped soft tissue. When the fragment is in correct position, the sutures are tied over a bony bridge at approximately 30° of knee flexion. The reduced fragment is reexamined under arthroscopic vision with a probe testing its fixation during a full range of motion [27].

33.3.3 Suture Anchor Fixation

For the definitive fixation, a titanium or bioabsorbable anchor (Corkscrew or Bio-Corkscrew; Arthrex, Naples, FL) is used loaded with two strands of No. 2 braided polyester suture (Ethibond; Ethicon, Somerville, NJ or FiberWire; Arthrex). After introduction of a clear cannula through the anteromedial portal, the anchor is placed 2–3 mm in front of the fracture rim, not through the bony fragment (Fig. 33.8). The best alignment of the anchor is 45° in the frontal plane, avoiding a too vertical introduction of the implant. Angulation of the anchor reduces the risk of suture pullout and growth plate damage. The anchor does not penetrate the physes when this angulation is used (Fig. 33.9) [31].

A straight or curved suture hook or suture retriever is loaded with one of the suture strands. The instrument is pushed through the more anterior part of the ACL just above its tibial insertion, from the medial direction, leaving the suture on the lateral surface of the ACL (Fig. 33.8). With a suture grasper, the suture is retrieved through the cannula. At this point, the knee is flexed between 20° and 45° to relax the more anterior fibers of the ACL, and a sliding knot is made externally and slid inside with a knot pusher. Additionally, two or three half-hitch knots with alternating posts on reverse throws are made (Fig. 33.8). Because the most anterior fibers of the ACL are anterior to the axis of knee flexion, they do tighten with increased knee flexion. Provided that the sutures pass through these anterior fibers, there may be a tension band effect. The same procedure is repeated with the second strand, passing through the base of the ACL more posteriorly. Finally, the reduction of the fracture is reexamined, and the quality of the suture and the bony reduction is checked during knee flexion and extension. If bone reduction is not maintained during flexion and extension, the placement of an additional anchor is advised [31].

33.4 Pitfalls and Complications (e.g., Stability, Extension Deficit)

Fractures with displacement after attempting closed reduction (Fig. 33.3) require careful evaluation to rule out meniscal entrapment [5]. This may prevent anatomic reduction of the tibial eminence fragment, which may result in increased

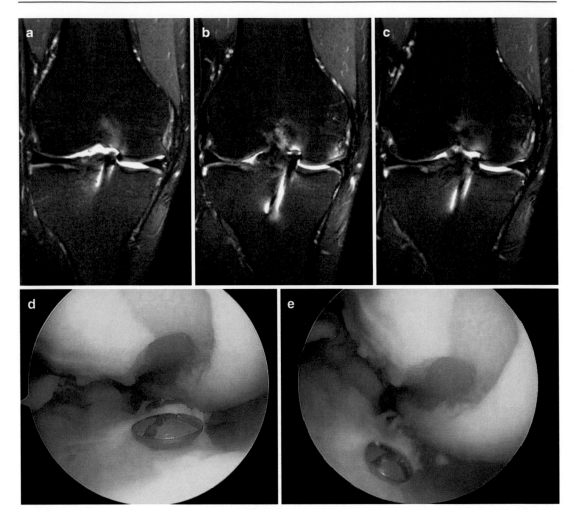

Fig. 33.12 Impingement of the screw head on the medial femoral condyle. (**a–c**) Coronal plain MRI pictures with obvious osteochondral destruction. (**d, e**) Arthroscopic view

anterior laxity or a block to extension [23, 36, 38, 43, 44]. Furthermore, meniscal entrapment itself may cause knee pain after fracture healing [45]. Kocher et al. found that approximately half (47 %) of type II tibial eminence fractures that they treated did not reduce adequately with knee extension [14]. Several authors have reported meniscal entrapment under the displaced tibial eminence fragment blocking anatomic closed reduction. Its presence may be a rationale for considering arthroscopic or open reduction in cases of type II and type III tibial eminence fractures [30, 45–47]. Kocher et al. observed an incarcerated anterior horn of the medial or lateral meniscus or intermeniscal ligament in 54 % of patients with irreducible fractures. Meniscal

entrapment occurred in up to 26 % of type II fractures and 65 % of type III fractures that did not reduce in extension [14].

Concomitant injury of the ACL substance may result in persistent ACL laxity, even if anatomic reduction of the avulsed fragment has been achieved [48].

Possible impingement of the screw heads has to be checked throughout full range of motion. Due to different configurations of the notch and the lateral edge of the medial femoral condyle, there may be a lot of space in flexion but still impingement with increasing extension (Fig. 33.12). An approach to avoid this complication in noncomminuted displaced tibial eminence fractures is the use of physeal-sparing headless compression screws [2,

49]. However, Sharma et al. observed migration of Herbert screws deep into the tibial plateau albeit without any clinical consequences in two out of five cases [2].

The most common complications following treatment of bony ACL avulsions in children include loss of motion due to arthrofibrosis [37, 50], persistent anterior laxity [40], quadriceps weakness, retropatellar knee pain [38], and growth disturbances [51]. Quadriceps weakness and retro patellar pain are commonly associated with an extension deficit. Persistent anterior knee laxity despite anatomic surgical reduction, fixation, and fracture healing has been frequently reported [20, 21, 24, 26, 30, 35, 36, 38, 52]. A positive Lachman test has been reported in up to 87 % of patients following anatomic reduction and internal fixation of type III fractures [53]. Interstitial injury of the ACL with elongation is likely associated with tibial spine fracture. At the time of tibial spine fixation, the ACL often appears hemorrhagic within its sheath, but grossly intact and in continuity [40]. Noyes et al. frequently found an elongation and disruption of the ligament architecture despite gross ligament continuity in experimentally produced tibial spine fractures at both slow and fast loading rates [8]. However, laxity is rarely severe enough to limit activity, and objective laxity may not necessarily manifest as subjective instability [28, 38, 52]. Some authors indicate that residual anterior knee laxity, due to elongation of the femur-ACL-tibia complex after fracture healing in a preadolescent child, may diminish during growth [25, 28, 43, 54]. A possible mechanism for such a reduction could be that the ACL only grows properly in response to tensile forces, which are reduced if the ligament is slack. Since growth enlarges the skeletal parts of the knee joint, the tensile forces are gradually restored and growth of the ACL will resume [54]. Van Laer et al. believe that the peri- and postpubertal ligament tightening should bring back sufficient ACL tension and recommend a wait-and-see strategy, if subjective symptoms are absent [55].

In contrast arthrofibrosis and decreased range of motion are well-defined sequelae that limit functional capability and often necessitate additional surgeries. Arthrofibrosis, being a consequence of both knee injury and reconstruction, represents a wide spectrum of pathologic changes resulting in loss of knee motion [50]. Arthrofibrosis is defined as a 10° extension deficit and/or 25° of flexion loss 3 months after treatment that persists despite aggressive physical therapy and is not caused by nonunion, malunion, new injury, ligamentous or meniscal pathology, or bony deformity [56, 57]. Van der Have et al. found a prevalence of 10 % after operative treatment of displaced tibial eminence fractures, however, with postoperative immobilization of 4–6 weeks. In case of knee stiffness, mobilization under anesthesia is recommended, but only in conjunction with arthroscopic lysis of adhesions because of an otherwise high incidence of distal femoral physeal fractures [50].

Growth disorders are rare but have been described as a consequence of iatrogenic injury of the epi- or apophysis [51]. Most severe cases with coronal or sagittal plane deformities are reported following transepiphyseal compression screw fixation (Figs. 33.13 and 33.14) [17, 51, 55]. Once this injury is recognized, restoration of limb alignment becomes the objective. First, the offending screw must be removed. Afterwards growth plate modulation with temporary hemiepiphysiodesis and guided growth [51, 58] or osteotomies [55] may become necessary to compensate for angular deformities. In order to avoid this complication, early removal of the metalwork – within 8 weeks postoperatively – is recommended [59]. Furthermore, growth plate-sparing methods with suture anchors [31] and direct [40, 49] or indirect [17] intraepiphyseal screw fixation may be preferable. Using transphyseal suture fixation, no difference of growth disturbance could be found with respect to absorbable or non-absorbable suture materials. Ahn et al. described one case of a genu recurvatum of more than 10° in a series of 14 patients after absorbable suture fixation [27].

33.5 Rehabilitation

Postoperative rehabilitation protocols are controversial in literature. However, there is a general trend towards earlier functional treatment. Nonetheless, some authors still recommend cast

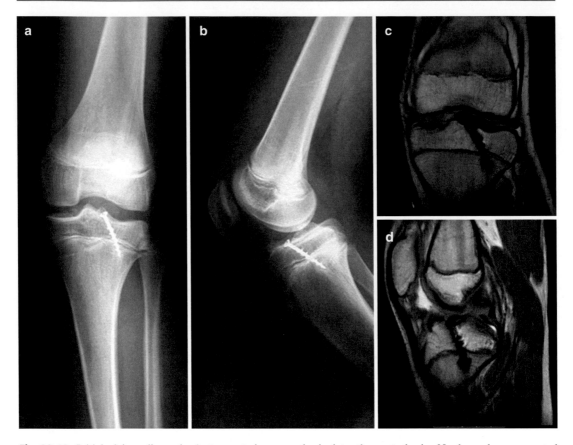

Fig. 33.13 Initial plain radiographs (anteroposterior **a**; lateral **b**) and T1-weighted MRI (coronal **c**; sagittal **d**) show screw fixation extending through the proximal tibial physis into the metaphysis. No bony bar was noted on MRI (Reprinted with permission from Fabricant et al. [51])

immobilization for 3–6 weeks following surgery [28, 33, 41, 49, 60]. As mentioned previously, immobilization after knee ligament injury and reconstruction remains a risk factor for arthrofibrosis. An intra-articular fracture and hematoma, combined with immobilization, undoubtedly contribute to stiffness. Accelerated rehabilitation to reduce stiffness after tibial spine fractures must be weighed against the possibility of fracture displacement and malunion [50]. Patel et al. found a 12 times higher likelihood to develop arthrofibrosis if range-of-motion (ROM) therapy was started later than 4 weeks after treatment and that earlier commencement of ROM therapy is associated with earlier physician clearance for full activity. Patients started ROM exercises between 4 and 11 days postoperatively, and no nonunion or malunion was seen in the follow-up radiographs [37]. For arthroscopically fixed tibial eminence fractures, several

authors report ROM exercises during the first 2 weeks postoperatively, if stable fixation is achieved during surgery [5, 12, 28, 30, 37, 42, 50]. Rehabilitation exercise starts with cycling as soon as the range of motion is sufficient, followed by slow jogging. Patients are allowed to return to athletic activity after the fracture has completely healed and they have achieved normal range of motion and quadriceps strength, which is commonly achieved about 3–4 months postoperative.

33.6 Literature Results

33.6.1 Different Types of Surgical Fixation

Sharma et al. found no statistically significant difference in joint laxity in children fixed with

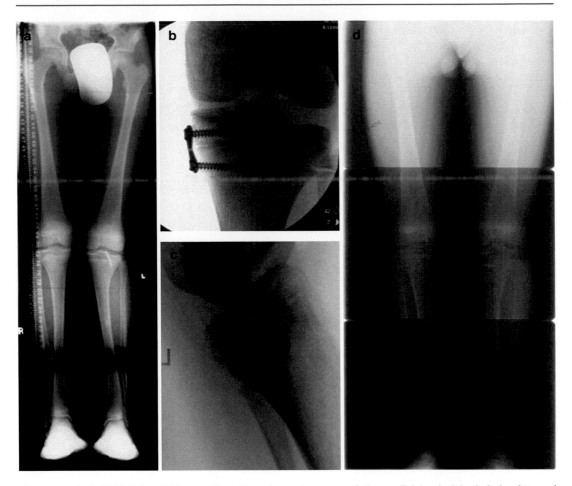

Fig. 33.14 (**a**) Initial full-length hip-to-ankle radiographs show 19° of genu valgum in the left lower extremity as a result of cessation of growth of the lateral proximal tibial physis. (**b, c**) Anteroposterior and lateral intraoperative fluoroscopic imaging confirming correct extraphyseal placement of the medial hemiepiphysiodesis plate and screws. (**d**) Eleven months after open medial hemiepiphysiodesis, full-length hip-to-ankle radiographs demonstrated correction of the anatomic and mechanical axis of the left knee (Reprinted with permission from Fabricant et al. [51])

absorbable sutures compared to non-absorbable materials (screw, wire loop). Clinical results were slightly better for absorbable fixation but did not reach statistical significance [2]. Seon et al. found similar results in Lachman testing after 2 years of follow-up for screw and suture fixation and comparable Lysholm scores for both techniques [41].

A biomechanical human cadaver study showed a significantly higher anterior tibial translation after 500 cycles of loading in pullout suture fixation than in antegrade screw fixation. Concerning the loss of graft fixation after cyclic loading, no significant difference occurred between the two groups. Antegrade screw fixation with a washer was the most effective technique to obtain initial rigid fixation [48]. However, Bong et al. showed in a cadaveric study that Fiberwire sutures (Arthrex) had a statistically significant higher failure load than cannulated screws with washer. Furthermore, there was a difference in failure modes with cutting through the anterior tibial cortex or the fracture fragment with suture fixation and screw pullout from the fracture bed on the other side [61]. The limitation in these two studies is the average age of the tested specimen, which is relatively high and far from childhood. Mahar et al. concluded that mechanically, the two devices are similar and that both means of fixation could withstand tensile forces before failure of a magnitude unlikely reached during the early rehabilitation period [62]. Eggers et al. observed in a skeletally immature porcine cadaver model that an additional screw does not increase but further decrease pullout strength significantly [63].

Hapa et al. found no difference in total displacement after cyclic loading between pullout suture fixation with non-absorbable sutures and suture anchor fixation in skeletally mature intact ovine knees. They reported lower maximal failure loads for suture anchors than suture fixation, which could be clinically relevant, but might be overcome by using a double-loaded anchor [64].

33.6.2 Long-Term Results in Literature

Subjective outcome, measured by IKDC, Tegner and Lysholm scores are predominantly excellent and good regardless of the treatment pathway [27, 31, 42, 60, 65–67]. As shown by Noyes et al. in a biomechanical cadaver study, it is very hard to adequately restore the pretraumatic stability, due to the occurrence of an elongation of more than 50 % of the original length of the fibers of the ACL prior to the avulsion fracture [8]. Several authors, reporting residual laxity in both conservatively and surgically treated patients, support these experimental findings [6, 24, 38, 44, 52–54]. However, this may be partially compensated by continued growth. It has been observed that younger children achieve greater stability [28, 43, 54]. Furthermore, it has been widely shown how the residual laxity differs depending on the type of the fracture with type I fractures resulting in less laxity than type II and III fractures [25, 52, 60]. However, there are authors [27, 31, 42, 67] who report normal laxity (tested by an instrumented Lachman test) especially following arthroscopic reduction and internal fixation. Functional outcome according to the one-leg-hop test was good following conservative and surgical approach with nearly equal or better results on the injured leg in 68 and 78 %, respectively [25, 65]. The findings of Janarv et al. indicate that an anterior tibial spine fracture may cause changes in the mechanical properties of the ACL with an obviously reduced ultimate load to failure in adulthood [54].

Memory

Bony ACL avulsions are relatively common in children and adolescents. Today, this injury should be seen as a ligamentous ACL injury with bony involvement rather than a fracture. This implicates the use of MRI to search for additional pathology (e.g., meniscal lesions) rather than a CT scan, which is primarily focused on the bony structure of the fragment, in addition to plain radiographs.

Arthroscopically assisted fixation of displaced fragments (Type II, III) is the treatment of choice. If the size of the attached bone is appropriate, screw fixation is recommended. For smaller or fragmented bony avulsions, suture fixation or bone anchors appear superior. Early operative treatment results in better outcome and a lower complication rate than delayed surgery. The fixation strength of the operative techniques used should allow for an early functional treatment.

Conservative treatment with immobilization should be reserved for non-displaced avulsions (type I) only if additional pathology can be excluded (MRI!).

References

1. Fyfe IS, Jackson JP (1981) Tibial intercondylar fractures in children: a review of the classification and the treatment of mal-union. Injury 13(2):165–169
2. Sharma A et al (2008) An analysis of different types of surgical fixation for avulsion fractures of the anterior tibial spine. Acta Orthop Belg 74(1):90–97
3. Beaty JH, Kumar A (1994) Fractures about the knee in children. J Bone Joint Surg Am 76(12):1870–1880
4. Skak SV et al (1987) Epidemiology of knee injuries in children. Acta Orthop Scand 58(1):78–81
5. Lubowitz JH, Elson WS, Guttmann D (2005) Part II: arthroscopic treatment of tibial plateau fractures: intercondylar eminence avulsion fractures. Arthroscopy 21(1):86–92
6. Accousti WK, Willis RB (2003) Tibial eminence fractures. Orthop Clin North Am 34(3):365–375
7. Parikh SN et al (2010) Management of fractures in adolescents. J Bone Joint Surg Am 92(18): 2947–2958
8. Noyes FR, DeLucas JL, Torvik PJ (1974) Biomechanics of anterior cruciate ligament failure: an analysis of strain-rate sensitivity and mechanisms of

failure in primates. J Bone Joint Surg Am 56(2): 236–253

9. Weinberg AM et al (2006) Der tibiale Anteil des Kniegelenkes (proximale Tibiaepiphyse). In: Weinberg AM, Tscherne H (eds) Unfallchirurgie im Kindesalter Band 2. Springer, Berlin

10. Mortimer SL, Hunter RE (2010) Arthroscopic treatment of tibial eminence fractures. In: Hunter RE, Sgaglione NA (eds) AANA advanced arthroscopy the knee. Elsevier Inc., Philadelphia

11. Woo SL et al (1991) Tensile properties of the human femur-anterior cruciate ligament-tibia complex. The effects of specimen age and orientation. Am J Sports Med 19(3):217–225

12. Kieser DC, Gwynne-Jones D, Dreyer S (2011) Displaced tibial intercondylar eminence fractures. J Orthop Surg (Hong Kong) 19(3):292–296

13. Merkel DL, Molony JT Jr (2012) Recognition and management of traumatic sports injuries in the skeletally immature athlete. Int J Sports Phys Ther 7(6):691–704

14. Kocher MS et al (2003) Tibial eminence fractures in children: prevalence of meniscal entrapment. Am J Sports Med 31(3):404–407

15. Gottsegen CJ et al (2008) Avulsion fractures of the knee: imaging findings and clinical significance. Radiographics 28(6):1755–1770

16. Meyers MH, McKeever FM (1970) Fracture of the intercondylar eminence of the tibia. J Bone Joint Surg Am 52(8):1677–1684

17. Mylle J, Reynders P, Broos P (1993) Transepiphyseal fixation of anterior cruciate avulsion in a child. Report of a complication and review of the literature. Arch Orthop Trauma Surg 112(2):101–103

18. Zifko B, Gaudernak T (1984) Problems in the therapy of avulsions of the intercondylar eminence in children and adolescents. Treatment results based on a new classification. Unfallheilkunde 87(6):267–272

19. Meyers MH, Mc KF (1959) Fracture of the intercondylar eminence of the tibia. J Bone Joint Surg Am 41-A(2):209–220; discussion 220–222

20. Molander ML, Wallin G, Wikstad I (1981) Fracture of the intercondylar eminence of the tibia: a review of 35 patients. J Bone Joint Surg Br 63-B(1):89–91

21. McLennan JG (1982) The role of arthroscopic surgery in the treatment of fractures of the intercondylar eminence of the tibia. J Bone Joint Surg Br 64(4): 477–480

22. Shea KG et al (2011) Bone bruises and meniscal tears on MRI in skeletally immature children with tibial eminence fractures. J Pediatr Orthop 31(2):150–152

23. Oostvogel HJ, Klasen HJ, Reddingius RE (1988) Fractures of the intercondylar eminence in children and adolescents. Arch Orthop Trauma Surg 107(4): 242–247

24. Willis RB et al (1993) Long-term follow-up of anterior tibial eminence fractures. J Pediatr Orthop 13(3):361–364

25. Wilfinger C et al (2009) Nonoperative treatment of tibial spine fractures in children-38 patients with a minimum follow-up of 1 year. J Orthop Trauma 23(7):519–524

26. Mulhall KJ et al (1999) Tibial spine fractures: an analysis of outcome in surgically treated type III injuries. Injury 30(4):289–292

27. Ahn JH, Yoo JC (2005) Clinical outcome of arthroscopic reduction and suture for displaced acute and chronic tibial spine fractures. Knee Surg Sports Traumatol Arthrosc 13(2):116–121

28. Hunter RE, Willis JA (2004) Arthroscopic fixation of avulsion fractures of the tibial eminence: technique and outcome. Arthroscopy 20(2):113–121

29. Kogan MG, Marks P, Amendola A (1997) Technique for arthroscopic suture fixation of displaced tibial intercondylar eminence fractures. Arthroscopy 13(3): 301–306

30. Mah JY et al (1998) Follow-up study of arthroscopic reduction and fixation of type III tibial-eminence fractures. J Pediatr Orthop 18(4):475–477

31. Vega JR et al (2008) Arthroscopic fixation of displaced tibial eminence fractures: a new growth plate-sparing method. Arthroscopy 24(11):1239–1243

32. Zaricznyj B (1977) Avulsion fracture of the tibial eminence: treatment by open reduction and pinning. J Bone Joint Surg Am 59(8):1111–1114

33. Shepley RW (2004) Arthroscopic treatment of type III tibial spine fractures using absorbable fixation. Orthopedics 27(7):767–769

34. Lubowitz JH, Grauer JD (1993) Arthroscopic treatment of anterior cruciate ligament avulsion. Clin Orthop Relat Res 294:242–246

35. Berg EE (1995) Pediatric tibial eminence fractures: arthroscopic cannulated screw fixation. Arthroscopy 11(3):328–331

36. McLennan JG (1995) Lessons learned after second-look arthroscopy in type III fractures of the tibial spine. J Pediatr Orthop 15(1):59–62

37. Patel NM et al (2012) Tibial eminence fractures in children: earlier posttreatment mobilization results in improved outcomes. J Pediatr Orthop 32(2):139–144

38. Wiley JJ, Baxter MP (1990) Tibial spine fractures in children. Clin Orthop Relat Res 255:54–60

39. Lowe J et al (2002) The anatomy of tibial eminence fractures: arthroscopic observations following failed closed reduction. J Bone Joint Surg Am 84-A(11): 1933–1938

40. Kocher MS, Foreman ES, Micheli LJ (2003) Laxity and functional outcome after arthroscopic reduction and internal fixation of displaced tibial spine fractures in children. Arthroscopy 19(10):1085–1090

41. Seon JK et al (2009) A clinical comparison of screw and suture fixation of anterior cruciate ligament tibial avulsion fractures. Am J Sports Med 37(12):2334–2339

42. Senekovic V, Veselko M (2003) Anterograde arthroscopic fixation of avulsion fractures of the tibial eminence with a cannulated screw: five-year results. Arthroscopy 19(1):54–61

43. Gronkvist H, Hirsch G, Johansson L (1984) Fracture of the anterior tibial spine in children. J Pediatr Orthop 4(4):465–468

44. Janarv PM et al (1995) Long-term follow-up of anterior tibial spine fractures in children. J Pediatr Orthop 15(1):63–68

45. Chandler JT, Miller TK (1995) Tibial eminence fracture with meniscal entrapment. Arthroscopy 11(4): 499–502

46. Burstein DB, Viola A, Fulkerson JP (1988) Entrapment of the medial meniscus in a fracture of the tibial eminence. Arthroscopy 4(1):47–50

47. Falstie-Jensen S, Sondergard Petersen PE (1984) Incarceration of the meniscus in fractures of the intercondylar eminence of the tibia in children. Injury 15(4):236–238

48. Tsukada H et al (2005) A biomechanical comparison of repair techniques for anterior cruciate ligament tibial avulsion fracture under cyclic loading. Arthroscopy 21(10):1197–1201

49. Johnson DL, Durbin TC (2012) Physeal-sparing tibial eminence fracture fixation with a headless compression screw. Orthopedics 35(7):604–608

50. Vander Have KL et al (2010) Arthrofibrosis after surgical fixation of tibial eminence fractures in children and adolescents. Am J Sports Med 38(2):298–301

51. Fabricant PD, Osbahr DC, Green DW (2011) Management of a rare complication after screw fixation of a pediatric tibial spine avulsion fracture: a case report with follow-up to skeletal maturity. J Orthop Trauma 25(12):e115–e119

52. Baxter MP, Wiley JJ (1988) Fractures of the tibial spine in children. An evaluation of knee stability. J Bone Joint Surg Br 70(2):228–230

53. Smith JB (1984) Knee instability after fractures of the intercondylar eminence of the tibia. J Pediatr Orthop 4(4):462–464

54. Janarv PM, Hirsch G (2001) Growth influences knee laxity after anterior tibial spine fracture: a study on rabbits. Acta Orthop Scand 72(2):173–180

55. von Laer L, Kraus R, Linhart WE (eds) (2013) Eminentiafrakturen. Frakturen und Luxationen im Wachstumsalter1986. Georg Thieme Verlag, Stuttgart

56. Freeman MA, Pinskerova V (2005) The movement of the normal tibio-femoral joint. J Biomech 38(2): 197–208

57. Shelbourne KD, Patel DV, Martini DJ (1996) Classification and management of arthrofibrosis of the knee after anterior cruciate ligament reconstruction. Am J Sports Med 24(6):857–862

58. Wiemann JM 4th, Tryon C, Szalay EA (2009) Physeal stapling versus 8-plate hemiepiphysiodesis for guided correction of angular deformity about the knee. J Pediatr Orthop 29(5):481–485

59. Goudarzi YM (1985) Operative treatment of avulsion fractures of the intercondylar eminence in childhood. Aktuelle Traumatol 15(2):66–70

60. Perugia D et al (2009) Clinical and radiological results of arthroscopically treated tibial spine fractures in childhood. Int Orthop 33(1):243–248

61. Bong MR et al (2005) Suture versus screw fixation of displaced tibial eminence fractures: a biomechanical comparison. Arthroscopy 21(10):1172–1176

62. Mahar AT et al (2008) Biomechanical comparison of four different fixation techniques for pediatric tibial eminence avulsion fractures. J Pediatr Orthop 28(2): 159–162

63. Eggers AK et al (2007) Biomechanical evaluation of different fixation methods for tibial eminence fractures. Am J Sports Med 35(3):404–410

64. Hapa O et al (2012) Biomechanical comparison of tibial eminence fracture fixation with high-strength suture, EndoButton, and suture anchor. Arthroscopy 28(5):681–687

65. Huang TW et al (2008) Arthroscopic suture fixation of tibial eminence avulsion fractures. Arthroscopy 24(11):1232–1238

66. Casalonga A et al (2010) Tibial intercondylar eminence fractures in children: the long-term perspective. Orthop Traumatol Surg Res 96(5):525–530

67. Park HJ et al (2007) Arthroscopic evaluation after surgical repair of intercondylar eminence fractures. Arch Orthop Trauma Surg 127(9):753–757

Part VIII

One-Stage Revision

Systematic Approach from Porto School

34

Hélder Pereira, Nuno Sevivas, Rogério Pereira,
Alberto Monteiro, Ricardo Sampaio,
Joaquim Miguel Oliveira, Rui Luís Reis,
and João Espregueira-Mendes

Contents

H. Pereira, MD (✉)
Clínica Espregueira-Mendes F.C. Porto Stadium –
FIFA Medical Centre of Excellence,
3B's Research Group – Biomaterials, Biodegradables
and Biomimetics, Univ. Minho, Headquarters of the
European Institute of Excellence on Tissue
Engineering and Regenerative Medicine,
Ave Park, S. Cláudio de Barco,
4806–909, Taipas, Guimarães, Portugal

ICVS/3B's – PT Government Associated Laboratory,
Braga, Guimarães, Portugal

Clínica Espregueira-Mendes F.C. Porto Stadium –
FIFA Medical Centre of Excellence, Porto, Portugal

Orthopedic Department, Centro Hospitalar Póvoa de
Varzim – Vila do Conde, Vila do Conde, Portugal
e-mail: heldermdpereira@gmail.com

N. Sevivas
Clínica Espregueira-Mendes F.C. Porto Stadium –
FIFA Medical Centre of Excellence,
ICVS/3B's – PT Government Associated Laboratory,
Braga, Guimarães, Portugal

Clínica Espregueira-Mendes F.C. Porto Stadium –
FIFA Medical Centre of Excellence, Porto, Portugal

R. Pereira • A. Monteiro
Clínica Espregueira-Mendes F.C. Porto Stadium –
FIFA Medical Centre of Excellence, Porto, Portugal

R. Sampaio
Imaging Department, Hospital da Boavista,
Porto, Portugal

J.M. Oliveira, BSc, PhD
R.L. Reis, CEng, MSc, PhD, DSc
Clínica Espregueira-Mendes F.C. Porto Stadium –
FIFA Medical Centre of Excellence,
3B's Research Group – Biomaterials, Biodegradables
and Biomimetics, Univ. Minho, Headquarters of the
European Institute of Excellence on Tissue
Engineering and Regenerative Medicine,
Ave Park, S. Cláudio de Barco,
4806–909, Taipas, Guimarães, Portugal

ICVS/3B's – PT Government Associated Laboratory,
Braga, Guimarães, Portugal

J. Espregueira-Mendes, MD, PhD
Clínica Espregueira-Mendes F.C. Porto Stadium –
FIFA Medical Centre of Excellence, 3B's Research
Group – Biomaterials,
Biodegradables and Biomimetics, Univ. Minho,
Headquarters of the European Institute of Excellence
on Tissue Engineering and Regenerative Medicine,
Ave Park, S. Cláudio de Barco,
4806–909, Taipas, Guimarães, Portugal

ICVS/3B's – PT Government Associated Laboratory,
Braga, Guimarães, Portugal

Clínica Espregueira-Mendes F.C. Porto Stadium –
FIFA Medical Centre of Excellence, Porto, Portugal

R. Siebold et al. (eds.), *Anterior Cruciate Ligament Reconstruction*,
DOI 10.1007/978-3-642-45349-6_34, © ESSKA 2014

34.1   Introduction

The high prevalence of anterior cruciate ligament (ACL) reconstruction [1–3] reinforces the importance of developing strategies aiming at prevention, diagnosis, and treatment of possible complications and/or failure of such procedures. Revision of ACL reconstruction always presents a challenge in orthopedic practice. However, in present time it must enter in the "routine" of any knee reconstruction surgeon [4–19]. Revision of ACL repair, regardless of the inherent cause, must be considered a demanding and delicate clinical procedure. Its results have been considered as predictably less satisfactory than those of the primary operation [20]. Somewhat inferior patient-reported outcome scores comparing to previously published results of primary ACL reconstruction have been shown, but clinical relevance of these findings remains to be clarified [21]. Furthermore, higher remaining laxity, higher graft failure rate, and meniscal or cartilage degeneration have also been described [1, 22]. Despite several reports of favorable results and return to sports at the same level after AC revision, clinical failure rates up to 25 % have been reported [17].

Confinement of revision to motivated patients has been associated to higher success rate [20]. Besides the previous, dramatically elevated failure rate after revision ACL repair, nearly three to four times the failure rate in prospective series of primary ACL reconstructions [21] have also been reported. Patients are more and more demanding and frequently expect full restore of joint kinematics and function and do not satisfy with mere symptomatic control and adapting way of life to limit the risk of arthritis [23].

Herein we described the systematic approach for complications or failure after primary ACL repair and/or re-rupture. This aims to summarize our systematic approach in a practical sense developed through years dedicated to this problem. In our sense it is mandatory to organize clinical knowledge in order to develop an efficient approach. We strongly believe that a systematic and organized approach is mandatory in

order to diminish errors and pitfalls considering such a multifactorial and complex issue. There is no foolproof strategy concerning revision of ACL repair; however, "a reasonable strategy is surely more prone to good results than no strategy at all."

34.2   What Have We Learned from Primary ACL Repair

Recent insights from basic sciences dedicated to ACL research (anatomy, biology, physiopathology, or biomechanics) have influenced current clinical practice [24]. Clinical progresses related to graft selection, tunnel placement, graft fixation, and rehabilitation protocols have been developed [25]. The biology of graft incorporation and "ligamentization" process continues to require intense investigation; however, increased awareness has assisted in prevention on complications such as excessive graft elongation, pullout, or slippage [14].

Technical improvements have also increased our options permitting different and more effective graft fixation systems [26].

The currently accepted "double-bundle concept" considers two functional bundles – anteromedial (AM) and posterolateral (PL) – according to the relative location of the tibial insertion site [27].

In the 1990s, single-bundle ACL reconstruction intended to reconstruct the AM portion of the ACL aiming isometric graft placement, and the reported outcomes were generally good [28, 29]. The need to improve rotational stability led to the actual leading concept of anatomical graft placement (lower and more distal comparing to over-the-top position on the femur in a flexed knee). Probably this change in concepts (from "isometric" to further anatomical graft positioning) aroused from the recognition that some patients treated in the past kept referring limited return to the same level activity after ACL surgery particularly during pivoting activities [30].

Some defend that the rotational control demands anatomical double-bundle ACL reconstruction [31, 32], at least in selected cases [30].

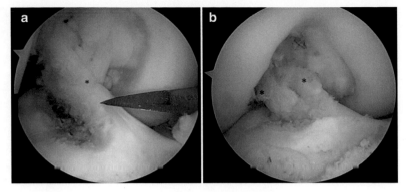

Fig. 34.1 Augmentation procedure with reconstruction of PL bundle (*). Notice on (**a, b**) (*) the macroscopic aspect of AM bundle remnant

Other authors defend advantages of augmentation/partial repair [33, 34] (Fig. 34.1).

Young, active, skeletally mature patients have higher failure rates after various surgical procedures, including stabilization for primary ACL reconstruction [35]. Despite being successful in restoring knee stability, only up to 50 % of young, active, skeletally mature patients have returned to their prior level of activity or sport [35] after revision ACL repair. Young patients have been considered a particularly demanding population in this field [35].

However, results have been improving through time, and outcome close to those achieved by primary reconstructions with a little less satisfactory results has been achieved [20].

Research dedicated to ACL ruptures in females is also evolving. It has been recognized that the risk of a primary ACL injury is up to three times higher in women athletes when compared to men [36]. When performing primary ACL repair (particularly in youngsters and female), maximal preservation of bone stock and minimal surgical aggression should be kept in mind considering the possibility for ACL revision through lifetime [37].

We know there are intrinsic risk factors, such as anatomy (e.g., morphology, notch width, lower extremity valgus), hormonal factors, and biomechanical factors (e.g., hamstring weakness, jump-land pattern) besides genetic, cognitive function, previous injury, and extrinsic risk factors [38, 39]. Equally, all these should be taken into account when facing a failed ACL repair or planning revision.

34.3 Possible Causes for Failure of ACL Repair

Revision ACL reconstruction obliges surgeons to deal with a panoply of problems such as tunnel malposition, tunnel widening, preexisting hardware, and concomitant injuries to other structures in the knee joint [40].

In a recent report from MARS Group, causes of failure as deemed by the revising surgeons included subsequent trauma (32 %), technical error (24 %), biologic failure (7 %), combination (37 %), infection (<1 %), and unclear (<1 %) [41].

Our definition of failure of ACL repair is patient-reported subjective unsatisfactory result of any source. In this sense, patient's complaints are more meaningful than any imaging study or further associated report. The first step is to recognize, understand, classify, and stratify the implicated cause of failure in any particular case. A careful preoperative evaluation is mandatory given the multifactorial aspect of this condition. The compliance and motivation of the patient must be considered within realistic expectations. It has been established that outcome is associated to the cause of failure [4, 13, 19, 42].

The treatment strategy depends on the cause, patient features, and surgeon's experience. Several techniques, grafts, and methods of fixation might be considered.

For practical purposes, we divide causes for failure in three major groups: (1) instability, (2) diminished range of motion, and (3) persistent pain. It must be kept in mind that the same case

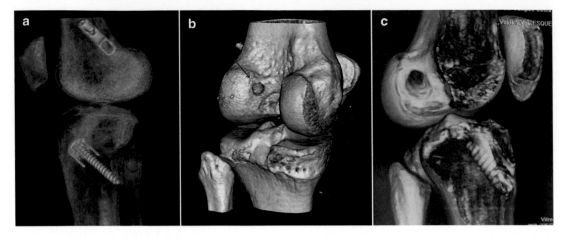

Fig. 34.2 Red arrow indicates position of previous femoral tunel on 3D CT reconstruction. On the left, we notice a fixation system which, despite providing strong fixation, creates some problems when there is a need for revision. On the other hand, it might be a user-friendly solution in revision after loop systems (**a**). (**b, c**) Confirm position of femoral tunnels for preoperative planning. *Red arrow* indicates position of previous femoral tunel on 3D CT reconstruction

might combine several aspects from any of the former groups.

The most frequent while preventable etiology for failure of ACL repair continues to be surgical errors [4, 5, 17, 19, 42, 43]. However, a new traumatic event [7, 22], biological factors [11, 44], or infection might be implicated [21, 35, 41, 43].

A multicenter study enrolling 10 French orthopedic centers concluded that the main cause for failure of ACL reconstruction was femoral tunnel malposition (36 % of the cases) [45]. Furthermore, authors observed better functional result and knee stability in the non-meniscectomized group comparing to patients submitted to meniscectomy [45]. Failures might correlate with fixation systems (e.g., screw migration [46] or malposition [47], graft pullout or slippage [48], foreign body or similar reactions [46, 49, 50]), malpositioning of the tunnels [47, 51], and aggressive rehabilitation neglecting integration and "ligamentization" periods [14, 21]. The trend for double-bundle repair has created a new set of challenges, mainly due to increased bone stock damage and more fragile hold ground during revision as consequence of the additional tunnels. One must consider their orientation and distance between tunnels as well as the implicated fixation methods (Fig. 34.2). Several options might

be valid including the use of the same tunnels (e.g., re-ruptures), reconstructing only one (ruptured) bundle, or option for two-step revision [17]. Tunnel widening is rarely the "cause" of revision surgery even if it might pose determinant problems to repair [51, 52]. Patients complaining of instability during high-demand activities with otherwise faultless ACL reconstructions require specific approach both in diagnosis and treatment [53].

Below it is summarized the basic clinical approach for patients presenting complaints after ACL repair [54].

1. *Instability*
   (a) *Always present after surgery*
      - *Major instability* – insufficient graft fixation (pullou*t or slippage), graft plastic deformation, or tunnel* malpositioning.
      - *Asymptomatic for daily living and instability during high-demand sports or pivoting* – vertical graft (Fig. 34.3); evaluation by MRI with PKTD (Fig. 34.4); discuss patient's expectations and options for revision surgery (including augmentation, single-bundle revision – Fig. 34.1).
   (b) *Full recovery after primary procedure and secondary onset of new instability (after new traumatic event)* – re-rupture.

Fig. 34.3 Notice orientation of vertical and anterior femoral tunnel (*green line*). *Yellow line* represents the aimed orientation for revision. Hardware was not removed to avoid creating additional fragility to bone stock. *Blue lines* demonstrate the limits of femoral tunel (**a**). *Red circle* represents the planed position for femoral tunnel (**b**)

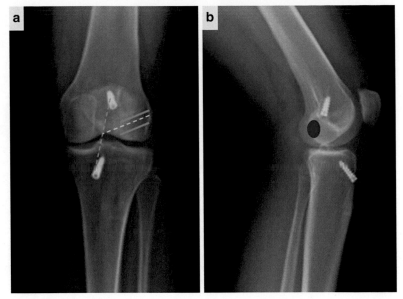

(c) *Initial rigidity* – tunnel malposition; patient denotes limited range of motion after surgery that might improve when excessive graft elongation, migration, or rupture occurs. Subsequent secondary instability might develop.

(d) *Not-diagnosed/"neglected" correlated injuries* [55] – posterior cruciate ligament, medial collateral ligament, and posterolateral or posteromedial corner injuries.

2. *Reduced knee mobility*
   (a) *Extension deficit*
      • *Cyclops* [56]
      • *Intercondylar notch scarring* (Fig. 34.5)
      • *Tibial tunnel too anterior (graft impingement)*
      • *Femoral tunnel too posterior* – usually well tolerated; risks of posterior wall breakage (perioperative or on long-term follow-up)
   (b) *Flexion deficit*
      • *Femoral tunnel too anterior* – one of the most frequent errors
      • *Tibial tunnel too posterior*
   (c) *Extension and flexion deficit (capsulitis/arthrofibrosis)* [57–59]– characterized by constant pain and stiffness, inflamed and swollen knee, quadriceps lag, and limited patella mobility; infrapatellar

contracture syndrome [60]; incorrect tunnel placement might be implicated.

3. *Persistent pain*
   • *Associated synovitis, chondral or meniscal lesions* [45], *MCL strains* [55], *and neural lesions (infrapatellar branch of saphenous nerve or medial femoral cutaneous nerve)* [61, 62] – Proper treatment for specific pathologies.
   • *Anterior knee pain* – Patellofemoral (PF) joint is a frequent source of pain after almost any knee surgery. We indicate ACL repair only if/when full range of motion (ROM) is accomplished. Muscle weakness and altered ROM cause abnormal PF kinematics. Meticulous graft harvesting technique is mandatory to minimize retropatellar fat fibrosis, patellar tendon shortening, or medial displacement of patella. Rehabilitation protocol, when adapted to individual characteristics and not dictated by calendar, is mandatory.
   • *Infection* – Rare (under 1 %) but potentially devastating complication [6, 63–65]. Staphylococcal species are among the most common. Elevation of C-reactive protein after ACL reconstruction is an indicator of postoperative septic complication, more sensitive than erythrocyte sedimentation rate or white blood cell (WBC) count [63]. Effusion

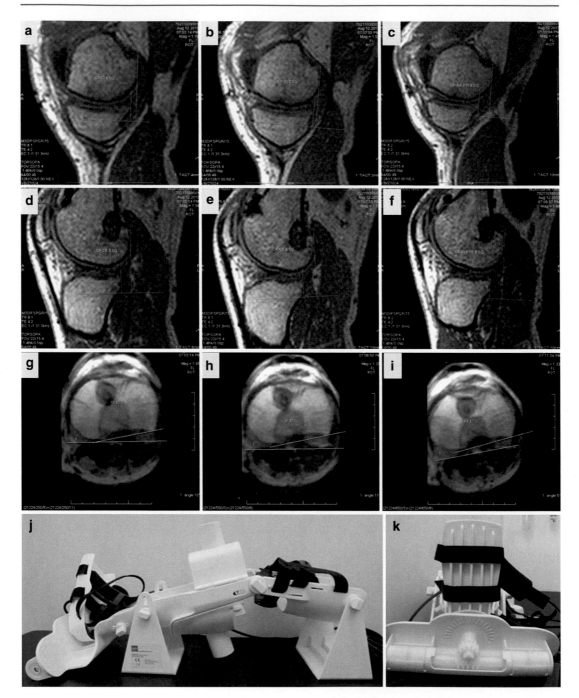

Fig. 34.4 Standard protocol evaluation of postoperative ACL revision at 9 months follow-up. Sagittal view with foot in neutral position without load application correspondent to medial (**a**) and lateral compartments (**c**). Result after load applications correspondent to medial (**b**) and lateral compartments (**d**). In this case, the differential would be, respectively, of 1 and 2 mm. Image correspondent to load after maximum internal foot rotation in lateral compartment (**e**) and after maximum external foot rotation in medial compartment (**f**). Evaluation of angular and linear tibial dislocation from axial views: without load (**g**) and with load after internal (**h**) and external foot rotation (**i**). Evaluation confirmed successful ACL revision, concordant to subjective scores and satisfaction degree from the patient. Photography of PKTD device (**j**) which enables knee rotation from the footplate (**k**)

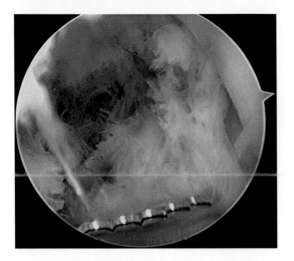

Fig. 34.5 Intercondylar notch scarring subsequent to ACL primary reconstruction with vertical and anterior femoral tunnel

companies, the so-called biomaterials, "biodegradable" screws, and/or cross-pins have been implicated in complications such as screw breakage, tunnel enlargement, allergic or foreign body reactions, cyst or abscess formation, and delayed migration.

- *Complex regional pain syndrome* – Defined as an exaggerated response to "aggression" producing intense prolonged pain, vasomo tor disturbance, delayed functional recovery, and trophic changes [67]. This rare condition often requires management by a multidisciplinary team, including chronic pain management specialists, physical therapists, and orthopedic surgeons [68].

34.4 Study Protocol for "Failed/Problematic ACL Repair"

Clinical history and evaluation are critical when dealing with ACL injuries. In our days, higher demands from patients and clinicians dictate that knee evaluation can no longer rely in surgeon's hands alone. Objective anteroposterior and rotation laxity quantification is required. Study of bone morphology is mandatory to detect possible risk factors and prepare treatment [39, 69–71]. The International Knee Documentation Committee Subjective Knee Form is a responsive measure of symptoms, function, and sports activity for patients with a variety of knee conditions [72]. We follow IKDC form in assessment of all cases.

is nearly always present, and aspiration analyzed for WBC differential and count, Gram stain, and culture will help in diagnosis and treatment orientation. MRI and bone scan assist in understanding the extent of infection. It is highly advised a prompt intervention in acute postoperative cases with antibiotic therapy combined with arthroscopic irrigation and debridement. Graft removal shall be done whenever it becomes nonfunctional, in ongoing infections after few days of treatment or late onset.

- *Symptomatic varus or initial femorotibial arthritis* – Consider selection for high tibial valgization osteotomy (HTO). Although technically more demanding, it has shown good results over the years [66]. Risk of stiffness must be considered. Sequence of procedures, above or below tubercle high tibial osteotomy (HTO), simultaneous or independent procedures, fixation method, patient selection criteria, and surgeon's experience are key factors in defining treatment options. If an opening wedge technique is considered, keep in mind to avoid increasing tibial slope. This is usually caused when a plate is used and placed in an anterior position.
- *Pain related to foreign material* [46, 49] – Despite the information provided by selling

Radiological evaluation is always performed and includes full-leg standing anteroposterior view (mechanical axes), standing anteroposterior and schuss view (evaluate arthritic changes besides previous tunnel placement in frontal plane), standing lateral view in full extension and 30° of flexion (need to evaluate tibial slope [70] and previous tunnel placement based on Bernard's quadrant method) [73], and skyline view (30° or 45° of flexion) to evaluate patellofemoral articulation. This radiological protocol is a valuable, low-cost, accessible tool which helps gathering varied and fundamental information concerning

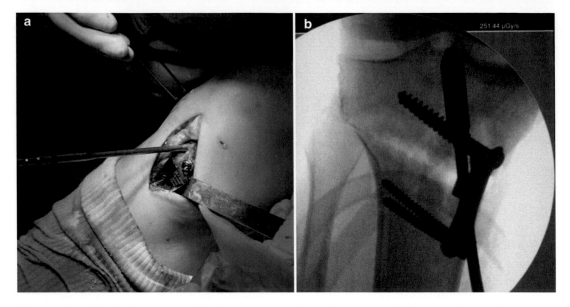

Fig. 34.6 Combined ACL revision and HTO procedure (**a**) with radioscopic control of tunnel placement (**b**)

limb alignment, original tunnel placement, fixation methods used, tunnel widening, tunnel angles [74] (orientation), osteolysis, and articular degenerative changes (Fig. 34.3).

Excessive varus alignment with pre-arthritic changes might cause excessive strains on the ACL plasty and persistent complains. In such cases, high valgus tibial osteotomy must be considered [75] (Fig. 34.6). Likewise, tibial slope higher than 15° might need a bony procedure, and previous patellofemoral joint problems can be implicated and even aggravated by ACL repair surgery.

CT scan is useful to study tunnel placement as well as the extent of the existent bony defect (Fig. 34.7).

MRI evaluation is important to evaluate the state of the previous ACL graft (integrity and incorporation) and possible associated lesions (e.g., chondral, menisci, and ligaments) [48]. The ideal tool to evaluate the knee should be a mean to assess both the "anatomy" and the "function" in the same examination. In order to improve the diagnostic capacity of both CT and MRI, the Porto-knee testing device (PKTD) was developed permitting assessment of the amount of anteroposterior and rotation laxities between bony landmarks in response to a stress load [53, 76] (Fig. 34.4).

In those cases in which we were previously unable to detect any "major" problem despite describing subjective sensation of instability during sports or pivoting activities, it is now possible to objectively quantify rotational laxity and discuss with patient's further possibilities [53].

All cases undergo analytic evaluation with complete hemogram (including white blood cell count), erythrocyte sedimentation rate, and C-reactive protein to exclude infection. In cases with higher suspicion for infection, labeled leukocyte scintigraphy, intra-articular fluid analysis, and several synovial biopsies should be performed. Inflammatory disease must also be ruled out.

34.5 Options for Treatment

34.5.1 Goals and Prognosis for ACL Revision

In a recent meta-analysis considering more than 1,000 cases, worse IKDC and/or Lysholm scores derived from ACL revision procedure when compared to primary surgery [21]. Furthermore, a significantly higher failure rate was found [21]. The MARS Group aimed to study the predictor factors for worse outcomes after ACL revision as compared to primary. Despite traumatic reinjury is supposed by several surgeons to be the most

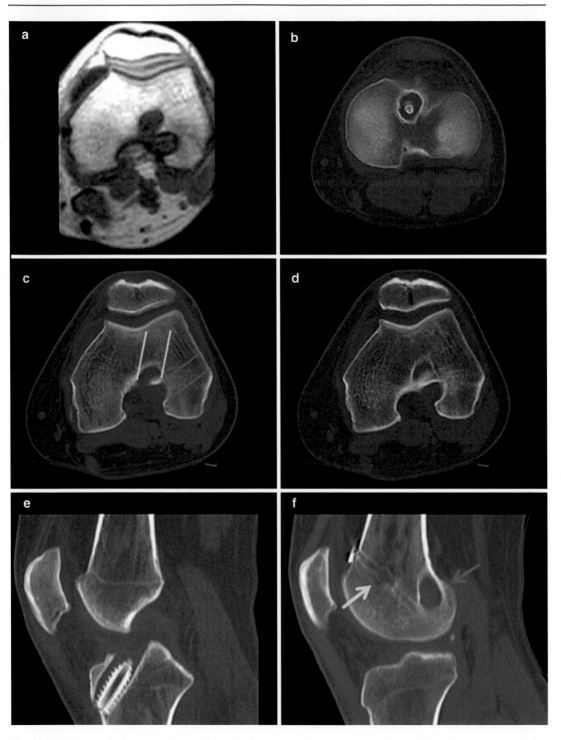

Fig. 34.7 Notice vertical and anterior positions of primary tunnel on MRI (**a**) and CT (**c, d, f** – *yellow arrow* and *line*). CT protocol also assessed the tibial tunnel (**b, e**). Final femoral tunnel position is represented by *blue lines* and *blue arrow*

common single mode of failure, the problem seems to be multifactorial, and a combination of several factors represents the most common mode of failure [41]. Concomitant knee injury is extremely common in patients undergoing ACL revision, and the use of allograft graft (in the

USA) has been more common than autograft in the revision setting [41].

At 2 years follow-up, the ACL ligament from contralateral normal knee is at a similar risk of ACL tear as the graft after primary anterior cruciate ligament reconstruction [77]. The MOON cohort group studied predictors of activity level 2 years after ACL and concluded that preoperative activity is a strong predictor of posttreatment activity [78]. However, no definite association of gender and revision surgery on activity level following ACL repair could definitely be established [78]. At minimum 6 years,

ACL revision surgery, allograft choice, lateral meniscus status, BMI, and smoking status were found to be predictors of sports activity and function after ACL repair. Suggestions derived to avoid allograft include leaving "stable" partial and complete lateral meniscal tears alone, not smoking, and lowering BMI in order to improve outcomes [79].

Return to sports at the same level has been reached; however, the multiplicity of factors involved advises extreme care in assuming this as the objective in all cases [17]. Given the multifactorial character of this issue, expectations should be addressed in an individual basis, considering the specificity of each case but also keeping in mind realistic goals.

Identification of the milestone, the "key problem" around each patient/case, is mandatory to define a strategy prone to success. The patient must be involved in this decision. To do so he must receive adequate information in order to be able to assume informed consent. We believe that the use of the aphorism – "It is too complex" – often hides the inability of surgical team to provide suitable information for the "nonexpert."

Sometimes a lower activity level might suit for a patient's demand [80, 81], and in other situations even a high functional score might be considered not good enough and motive for dissatisfaction.

Based in literature and in our department's experience, we conclude that the patient must realize that the results of ACL revision surgery are usually good but are not as reliable as in primary procedures [4, 18, 82, 83].

34.5.2 Revision Surgery Setting

Standard equipment should globally be considered as insufficient for an ACL revision. Difficulties must be anticipated and a complete set of hardware must be available. This includes equipment for removing previous implants (e.g., trephines, screwdrivers), drills of several sizes (for overdrilling or augmentation), material for bone grafting (autologous, allografts, tissue engineering, biologic enhancement therapy [84, 85]), several fixation devices (complementary between them), and radioscopy device and technician [15].

Tip and Pearl

We advise the removal of previous fixation material only if it presents an obstacle to our surgery (Fig. 34.8). An empty tunnel after removal of a screw represents an area of increased bone fragility with higher risk of wall breakage of the new tunnel, thus compromising graft fixation and creating a tough new difficulty to solve.

Removal of staples or plates from the medial tibial metaphyseal cortex must be carefully considered under the same consideration as it may result in damage to the cortical bone.

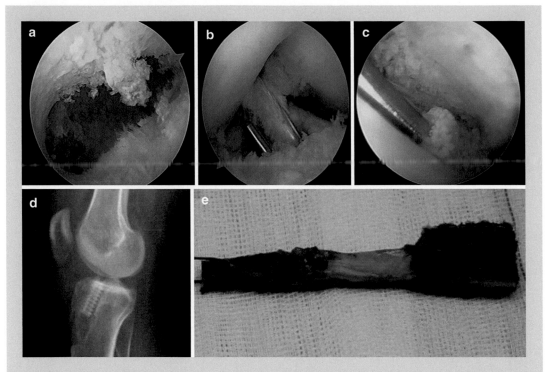

Fig. 34.8 Asymmetric, ovoid tibial tunnel after removal of graft remnants and implant (**a**). A custom-fit bone block of BPTB autograft (**e**) was used and interference screw provided fixation close to articular surface as desired (**b, c, d**)

Two main situations advise for a two-step reconstruction: severe bone loss (requiring a first surgery to fill the void and a second-time reconstruction) and important stiffness (initial surgery to allow recovery of full range of motion prior to new ligament repair). Two-step reconstruction will be addressed separately.

Because the landmarks are often less distinct comparing to primary reconstruction, the tibial tunnel sometimes might be referenced by imaging control. We do not consider the posterior cruciate ligament or the intercondylar spines alone to be reliable references, and our goal is the nearest anatomical reconstruction [80]. A revision notchplasty is sometimes needed to improve the view of the posterior cortical border, avoid lateral impingement with the graft, and permit full ROM particularly in chronic patients with osteophytes.

It must be noticed that "roofplasty" is not a harmless procedure. When one "finds" the need to do it, is advisable to make a stop and think it over. Try to assume that something might be wrong with your reconstruction, and thoroughly revise everything step by step before continuing.

The correct positioning of the tunnels is the key point. The most common error is to place them too anterior either on femoral or tibial side. Regarding the femoral tunnel, an outside-in technique might be appropriate if the previous approach was inside-out and vice versa [75, 80]. Besides correct position in articular surface of lateral condyle, it might be important to achieve divergent tunnels ensuring lower risk of bone fracture. Correct tunnel position can be accomplished by either outside-in or inside-out techniques (by anteromedial or accessory anteromedial portal).

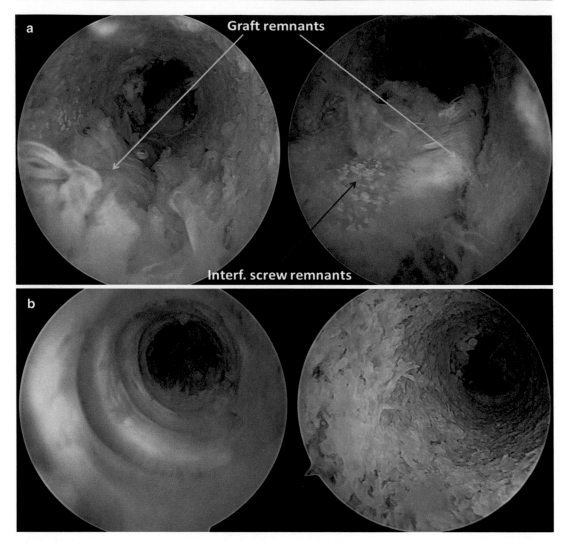

Fig. 34.9 Introducing the scope within tibial tunnel, we can evaluate graft and screw remnants (**a**). Notice the macroscopic aspect (suggesting different biologic conditions) after removal of a so-called bioabsorbable screw (*left*) and after slight overdrilling (*right*) (**b**)

If the previous tunnels are in good position, they can be redrilled in the same place, but care must be taken given the significant risk of creating large bone defects by convergence between your drill and previous tunnel. In such cases, sometimes it is possible to overcome this problem by harvesting a patellar tendon graft with a larger amount of bone from the tibia (Fig. 34.8).

Similarly for tibial tunnels one can achieve asymmetric tunnels after overdrilling (Fig. 34.8) or removal of hardware and graft remnants (Fig. 34.9). Besides adapting bone block to the defect, complementary fixation (double fixation) by staples or post-screws might be considered while warranting stable graft close to articular surface (Fig. 34.10).

When previous tunnels are incorrectly placed, it may be possible to create a new one without significant implications (Fig. 34.11). Obviously, the most difficult cases are those in which you find the initial tunnels in a slightly nonanatomical position because the resultant bony defect can be excessively large. In the presence of large bone defects, sometimes it is possible to solve situation by bone grafting, but if you come upon high risk, we advise a two-stage procedure [17, 80].

If you find a properly reconstructed AM bundle in a patient with rotatory instability, you can choose an augmentation procedure (Fig. 34.1) and reconstruct only the PL bundle similarly with an augmentation primary procedure. Probably for historical reasons we never had to deal with the opposite situation in the setting of revision.

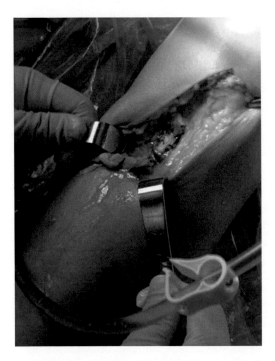

Fig. 34.10 Complementary fixation with a staple after interference screw after revision using hamstrings autograft

After formerly exposed one should conclude that in revision surgery, graft harvesting must be done only after definitive tunnels are created and characterized, once needed graft properties might depend and vary accordingly.

Associated knee ligamentous instability must be treated to avoid failure of the ACL revision surgery. Acute lateral collateral or posterolateral ligamentous injury should be repaired with or without augmentation. High-grade medial collateral sprains with posteromedial corner injuries should be repaired or allowed to heal before reconstruction. Complete posterior cruciate ligament (PCL) ruptures should undergo simultaneous or staged reconstruction [19].

Anatomical femoral tunnel position (Fig. 34.12) is important in reproducing function of the anterior cruciate ligament [86, 87] (Table 34.1).

34.5.3 Choosing the Graft for ACL Revision

The choice of graft for any ACL repair procedure (primary or revision) is still controversial [88, 89]. The debate concerning selection of autograft (and which type) or an allograft in ACL revision also remains to clarify and mainly depends on experience and local conditions [90]. Given the considerable difficulty in assessing allografts in our country, our choice is mainly for autograft. An allograft avoids donor site morbidity and can proportionate a big bone block useful to fill bone gaps. Besides

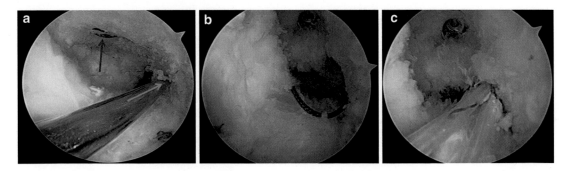

Fig. 34.11 *Red arrow* shows metallic screw on an anterior and vertical tunnel (**a**). *Green arrow* indicates correct position of tunnel during revision. A new tunnel and revision of the plasty derived without further implications with previous tunnel (**b, c**)

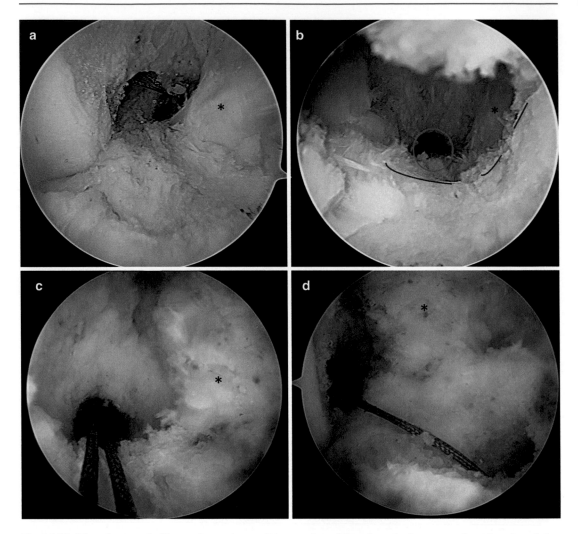

Fig. 34.12 There is no such thing as "excessive care" in anatomical tunnel positioning, besides careful intra-articular evaluation (**a, d**). In order to establish dynamic evaluation of relation between both tunnels, we often complementarily investigate by introducing the scope inside the tibial tunnel and studying through the range of motion the relation between both tunnels, with or without graft passing sutures (**b, c**). *Blue circle* indicates femoral tunnel, while *red lines* demonstrate the bony limit of tibial tunnel looked from inside. PCL is also used as complementary landmark (*)

Table 34.1 Summary of consequences derived from tunnel positioning [86, 87]

Femoral tunnel displacement	Predictable effect
Anterior	Tightens in flexion/loosens in extension
Posterior	Loosens in flexion/tightens in extension
Tibial tunnel displacement	Predictable effect
Anterior	Tightens in flexion/notch impingement with extension
Posterior	Tightens in extension/impingement with posterior cruciate ligament
Medial/lateral	Impingement at ipsilateral femoral condyle

some concerns with infection, disease transmission risk, late re-cellularization, and some tendency toward late failure [91], the increased costs with this option also have to be considered.

Our rule is to prefer autograft, and only in selected cases we use allografts, namely, when we have to repair multiligament lesions involving PCL, ACL, and/or posterolateral corner.

Our most frequent graft choice in primary or revisions is patellar tendon. In selected cases hamstrings or even quadriceps tendons might be considered, and several techniques must be possible by any ACL revision surgeon.

We agree that ACL revision surgery requires "à la carte" treatment [92], and the surgical team must control many surgical options to solve quite different challenges. Without further considerations, our preference for patellar bone graft relies in results, team experience, and possibility of harvesting a larger bone block to overcome big bone defects if that is the case. Like other authors, in some circumstances, we prefer to harvest the graft in the contralateral limb [16] specially if the revision surgery is done less than 18 months after the primary surgery and the initial graft is well positioned; when more than 18 months pass by, we re-harvest the graft from the same location [9].

> **Tip and Pearl**
> When it is not expected the need for bigger bone blocks (bad position on tibia and femur of previous graft) and cortical suspensory fixation seems a good option, we choose for four-strand hamstring graft and also avoid a second aggression to the extensor apparatus.
>
> Quadriceps tendon is also a reliable graft which we use mainly for re-revisions but represents a valid option for any ACL reconstruction [89].

Table 34.2 summarizes our algorithm for autograft management in ACL revision.

To date, there is no tissue-engineered ACL construct that has been successfully implanted in humans [93]; however, promising ongoing research envisions positive perspectives for future [94].

34.5.4 Choice of Fixation Method

A variety of devices for bone and soft tissue fixation must be available aiming to not restrict the

Table 34.2 Algorithm for autograft-based choice in ACL revision surgery

Primary graft		Revision graft
Bone-patellar tendon-bone (BPTB) in bad position (both femur and tibia)		Four-strand hamstring; cortical suspensory fixation
Bone-patellar tendon-bone (BPTB) well positioned	<18 months after primary ACL repair	Contralateral BPTB
	≥18 months after primary ACL repair	Ipsilateral BPTB
Four-strand hamstring		BPTB
Re-revisions/limitations for BPTB or hamstrings harvest		Quadriceps tendon

choice of the graft and use the best bone support [95].

Whatever the chosen method, it has to withstand the early postoperative rehabilitation forces until the graft integration has occurred.

Different fixation methods might be considered for femur or tibia and sometimes combined for increase fixation (suspensory cortical, cross-pins, staples, washers, posts, or apertural intra-tunnel) [95]. The analysis of characteristics of each type of fixation is not the issue of this work but must be recognized.

Generally, fixation devices distant to the joint line (i.e., buttons, staples, washers or post-screws) fail to reconstruct the complex nature of the native tibial or femoral ACL insertion close to the joint surface [25]. As a consequence, the strain that is induced in a substitute during cyclic loading is significantly larger when compared to the intact ACL [96]. This allows for longitudinal ("bungee effect") and transverse ("windshield-wiper effect") graft motion within the bone tunnel, which in turn may lead to bone tunnel dilation, may impair healing of the graft to the bone tunnel, and may complicate revision surgery due to loss of bone material [25]. Furthermore, it should be considered that the linear stiffness of grafts fixated distant to the joint line is less than placing the graft close to the entrance of the bone tunnel [25] (Fig. 34.8). Considering the previous we tend to opt for fixation close to joint line even if this requires a double fixation. Moreover, when using suspensory cortical methods, we tend to opt for a device that enables to fill the entire tunnel with the graft. Besides a shorter system, adjustable-length loop devices warrant more preservation of bone stock comparing to fixed-loop systems requiring space to turn and disarm the holding button [97]. However, all these systems have provided adequate fixation [97].

We must understand that any given fixation method must provide: sufficient resistance to pullout or slippage; avoid graft damage; minimal obstacle to integration process; diminished risk of bony wall damage; low long-term complications rate; be amenable to extract when something goes wrong; the surgeon must be skilled and confident in its application.

34.6   Rehabilitation

The initial goals for rehabilitation protocol after revision ACL repair are similar to primary procedure. An "early" rehabilitation program must be individually suited and guided by the specific objectives and demands of each patient (not by calendar). It must respect and consider the limb alignment, bone quality, patient compliance, and the preoperative variables that might interfere with the rehabilitation progression (bone grafting, quality of graft fixation, combined surgical procedures).

It is admissible that usually the process requires longer time, with slower progression in weight-bearing and functional exercises. This rehabilitation program must be tailored for the individual patient.

As general rule, active knee flexion and full passive extension start 24 h after surgery. Ice therapy is regularly used to reduce the inflammatory response and swelling. Patients are instructed to use crutches to walk until a nearly normal gait pattern has been recovered. Weight bearing depends mainly of achieved fixation. The patients are discharged 48 h after surgery, and rehabilitation continues in an outpatient form.

Ninety degrees of flexion with full extension should be reached in the first 2 weeks postoperative. The first stage includes gradual mobilization,

strengthening (isometric, closed chain, and some open chain), and dynamic stability exercises. Running is permitted when minimal swelling and pain-free knee have been achieved [80].

At a later stage of the program, the patient will get sports-specific training aiming proprioceptive performance until full return to sports.

It should always be kept in mind the processes of intraosseous incorporation and "ligamentization" of the graft [14]. This is a long continuous sequence of events leading to graft transformation in a tissue that resembles, but does not completely matches, the native ligament. It is commonly divided in an early phase dominated by graft necrosis and hypocellularity, followed by the proliferation phase (higher biomechanical fragility), and finally the ligamentization phase culminating in graft remodeling until the maximum of resistance with closest similarity to native ACL. We can predict that generally the patient can return to contact sports 9 months after surgery, but all factors (patient related and surgery related) must be considered, and in some cases a longer period might be required.

Our main objective must not be jeopardized by disrespecting some "golden rules" dictated by biology.

> **Memory**
> Revision of a "failed" reconstruction of the ACL is multifactorial, requires meticulous investigation, and often demands individualized surgery.
>
> It is mandatory to correctly identify the main cause of failure starting from patient's complaints.
>
> Several cases require revision after secondary trauma following successful primary repair (re-rupture).
>
> However, in many others the cause will be an error attributable to initial surgery, neglected correlated lesions, infection, cyclops, arthritis, chondral or meniscal lesions, and patellofemoral pathology among others.

This represents a highly demanding issue whose successful repair requires an experienced surgical team skillful in primary ACL repair and dedicated to knee surgery. Besides proper preoperative planning, some decisions can only be taken preoperatively. Only if you have previously safeguarded all options, you might find the best among several possibilities for each case. There are many variables and obstacles to withstand, and the surgeon must be familiar with several different techniques to be able to choose the most suited to every individual patient.

Globally good results are to be expected but not as consistently as in primary procedures.

References

1. Mohtadi NG, Chan DS, Dainty KN, Whelan DB (2011) Patellar tendon versus hamstring tendon autograft for anterior cruciate ligament rupture in adults. Cochrane Database Syst Rev (9):CD005960.
2. Griffin LY, Agel J, Albohm MJ et al (2000) Noncontact anterior cruciate ligament injuries: risk factors and prevention strategies. J Am Acad Orthop Surg 8:141–150
3. Prodromos C, Rogowski J, Joyce BT (2008) The economics of anterior cruciate ligament reconstruction. In: Prodromos C, Brown C, Fu FH, Georgoulis AD, Gobbi A, Howell SM et al (eds) The anterior cruciate ligament: reconstruction and basic science. Saunders Elsevier, Philadelphia, pp 79–83
4. Uribe JW, Hechtman KS, Zvijac JE, Tjin ATEW (1996) Revision anterior cruciate ligament surgery: experience from Miami. Clin Orthop Relat Res 325:91–99
5. Carson EW, Anisko EM, Restrepo C, Panariello RA, O'Brien SJ, Warren RF (2004) Revision anterior cruciate ligament reconstruction: etiology of failures and clinical results. J Knee Surg 17:127–132
6. Burks RT, Friederichs MG, Fink B, Luker MG, West HS, Greis PE (2003) Treatment of postoperative anterior cruciate ligament infections with graft removal and early reimplantation. Am J Sports Med 31:414–418
7. Harner CD, Giffin JR, Dunteman RC, Annunziata CC, Friedman MJ (2001) Evaluation and treatment of recurrent instability after anterior cruciate ligament reconstruction. Instr Course Lect 50:463–474
8. DeFranco MJ, Bach BR Jr (2009) A comprehensive review of partial anterior cruciate ligament tears. J Bone Joint Surg Am 91:198–208
9. Colosimo AJ, Heidt RS Jr, Traub JA, Carlonas RL (2001) Revision anterior cruciate ligament reconstruction with a reharvested ipsilateral patellar tendon. A J Sports Med 29:746–750
10. Carson EW, Brown CJ (2003) Revision anterior cruciate ligament surgery. Lippincott, Williams & Wilkins, Philadelphia
11. Greis PE, Johnson DL, Fu FH (1993) Revision anterior cruciate ligament surgery: causes of graft failure and technical considerations of revision surgery. Clin Sports Med 12:839–852
12. Espregueira-Mendes J (2005) Revision of failures after reconstruction of the anterior cruciate ligament. In: Lemaire JS, Horan F, Villar R (eds) EFORT – European instructional course lectures, 7th edn. The British Editorial Society of Bone and Joint Surgery, London, pp 184–189
13. Johnson DL, Swenson TM, Irrgang JJ, Fu FH, Harner CD (1996) Revision anterior cruciate ligament surgery: experience from Pittsburgh. Clin Orthop Relat Res 325:100–109
14. Menetrey J, Duthon VB, Laumonier T, Fritschy D (2008) "Biological failure" of the anterior cruciate ligament graft. Knee Surg Sports Traumatol Arthrosc 16:224–231
15. Thomas NP, Pandit HG (2008) Revision anterior cruciate ligament. In: Prodromos C, Brown C, Fu FH, Georgoulis AD, Gobbi A, Howell SM, et al (eds) The anterior cruciate ligament: reconstruction and basic science. Saunders Elsevier, Philadelphia, p 443–457
16. Shelbourne KD, O'Shea JJ (2002) Revision anterior cruciate ligament reconstruction using the contralateral bone-patellar tendon-bone graft. Instr Course Lect 51:343–346
17. Thomas NP, Kankate R, Wandless F, Pandit H (2005) Revision anterior cruciate ligament reconstruction using a 2-stage technique with bone grafting of the tibial tunnel. Am J Sports Med 33:1701–1709
18. Wirth CJ, Kohn D (1996) Revision anterior cruciate ligament surgery: experience from Germany. Clin Orthop Relat Res 325:110–115
19. Wolf RS, Lemak LJ (2002) Revision anterior cruciate ligament reconstruction surgery. J South Orthop Assoc 11:25–32
20. Denti M, Lo Vetere D, Bait C, Schonhuber H, Melegati G, Volpi P (2008) Revision anterior cruciate ligament reconstruction: causes of failure, surgical technique, and clinical results. Am J Sports Med 36:1896–1902
21. Wright RW, Gill CS, Chen L et al (2012) Outcome of revision anterior cruciate ligament reconstruction: a systematic review. J Bone Joint Surg Am 94:531–536
22. Getelman MH, Friedman MJ (1999) Revision anterior cruciate ligament reconstruction surgery. J Am Acad Orthop Surg 7:189–198
23. Friel NA, Chu CR (2013) The role of ACL injury in the development of posttraumatic knee osteoarthritis. Clin Sports Med 32:1–12
24. Musahl V, Becker R, Fu FH, Karlsson J (2011) New trends in ACL research. Knee Surg Sports Traumatol Arthrosc 19(Suppl 1):S1–S3

25. Dargel J, Gotter M, Mader K, Pennig D, Koebke J, Schmidt-Wiethoff R (2007) Biomechanics of the anterior cruciate ligament and implications for surgical reconstruction. Strateg Trauma Limb Reconstr 2:1–12

26. Dargel J, Schmidt-Wiethoff R, Heck M, Bruggemann GP, Koebke J (2008) Comparison of initial fixation properties of sutured and nonsutured soft tissue anterior cruciate ligament grafts with femoral cross-pin fixation. Arthroscopy 24:96–105

27. Girgis FG, Marshall JL, Monajem A (1975) The cruciate ligaments of the knee joint. Anatomical, functional and experimental analysis. Clinl Orthop Relat Res 106:216–231

28. Yunes M, Richmond JC, Engels EA, Pinczewski LA (2001) Patellar versus hamstring tendons in anterior cruciate ligament reconstruction: a meta-analysis. Arthroscopy 17:248–257

29. Freedman KB, D'Amato MJ, Nedeff DD, Kaz A, Bach BR Jr (2003) Arthroscopic anterior cruciate ligament reconstruction: a metaanalysis comparing patellar tendon and hamstring tendon autografts. Am J Sports Med 31:2–11

30. Muller B, Hofbauer M, Wongcharoenwatana J, Fu FH (2013) Indications and contraindications for double-bundle ACL reconstruction. Int Orthop 37:239–246

31. Yagi M, Wong EK, Kanamori A, Debski RE, Fu FH, Woo SL (2002) Biomechanical analysis of an anatomic anterior cruciate ligament reconstruction. Am J Sports Med 30:660–666

32. Yamamoto Y, Hsu WH, Woo SL, Van Scyoc AH, Takakura Y, Debski RE (2004) Knee stability and graft function after anterior cruciate ligament reconstruction: a comparison of a lateral and an anatomical femoral tunnel placement. Am J Sports Med 32:1825–1832

33. Pujol N, Colombet P, Cucurulo T et al (2012) Natural history of partial anterior cruciate ligament tears: a systematic literature review. OrthopTraumatol, Surg Res 98:S160–S164

34. Sonnery-Cottet B, Lavoie F, Ogassawara R, Scussiato RG, Kidder JF, Chambat P (2010) Selective anteromedial bundle reconstruction in partial ACL tears: a series of 36 patients with mean 24 months follow-up. Knee Surg Sports Traumatol Arthrosc 18:47–51

35. Reinhardt KR, Hammoud S, Bowers AL, Umunna BP, Cordasco FA (2012) Revision ACL reconstruction in skeletally mature athletes younger than 18 years. Clin Orthop Relat Res 470:835–842

36. Sutton KM, Bullock JM (2013) Anterior cruciate ligament rupture: differences between males and females. J Am Acad Orthop Surg 21:41–50

37. Lubowitz JH, Schwartzberg R, Smith P (2013) Randomized controlled trial comparing all-inside anterior cruciate ligament reconstruction technique with anterior cruciate ligament reconstruction with a full tibial tunnel. Arthroscopy 29:1195–1200

38. Smith HC, Vacek P, Johnson RJ et al (2012) Risk factors for anterior cruciate ligament injury: a review of the literature-part 2: hormonal, genetic, cognitive

function, previous injury, and extrinsic risk factors. Sports Health 4:155–161

39. Smith HC, Vacek P, Johnson RJ et al (2012) Risk factors for anterior cruciate ligament injury: a review of the literature – part 1: neuromuscular and anatomic risk. Sports Health 4:69–78

40. Cheatham SA, Johnson DL (2013) Anticipating problems unique to revision ACL surgery. Sports Med Arthrosc Rev 21:129–134

41. Wright RW, Huston LJ, Spindler KP et al (2010) Descriptive epidemiology of the Multicenter ACL Revision Study (MARS) cohort. Am J Sports Med 38:1979–1986

42. Noyes FR, Barber-Westin SD, Roberts CS (1994) Use of allografts after failed treatment of rupture of the anterior cruciate ligament. J Bone Joint Surg Am 76:1019–1031

43. Wright R, Spindler K, Huston L et al (2011) Revision ACL reconstruction outcomes: MOON cohort. J Knee Surg 24:289–294

44. Corsetti JR, Jackson DW (1996) Failure of anterior cruciate ligament reconstruction: the biologic basis. Clin Orthop Relat Res 325:42–49

45. Trojani C, Sbihi A, Djian P et al (2011) Causes for failure of ACL reconstruction and influence of meniscectomies after revision. Knee Surg Sports Traumatol Arthrosc 19:196–201

46. Pereira HM, Correlo VM, Silva-Correia J, Oliveira JM, Reis Ceng RL, Espregueira-Mendes J (2013) Migration of "bioabsorbable" screws in ACL repair. how much do we know? A systematic review. Knee Surg Sports Traumatol Arthrosc 21:986–994

47. Sanchis-Alfonso V, Tinto-Pedrerol M (2004) Femoral interference screw divergence after anterior cruciate ligament reconstruction provoking severe anterior knee pain. Arthroscopy 20:528–531

48. Bencardino JT, Beltran J, Feldman MI, Rose DJ (2009) MR imaging of complications of anterior cruciate ligament graft reconstruction. Radiographics 29:2115–2126

49. Konan S, Haddad FS (2009) A clinical review of bioabsorbable interference screws and their adverse effects in anterior cruciate ligament reconstruction surgery. Knee 16:6–13

50. Konan S, Haddad FS (2009) The unpredictable material properties of bioabsorbable PLC interference screws and their adverse effects in ACL reconstruction surgery. Knee Surg Sports Traumatol Arthrosc 17:293–297

51. Gomoll AH, Bach BRJ (2006) Managing tunnel malposition and widening in revision anterior cruciate ligament surgery. Oper Tech Sports Med 14:36–44

52. Maak TG, Voos JE, Wickiewicz TL, Warren RF (2010) Tunnel widening in revision anterior cruciate ligament reconstruction. J Am Acad Orthop Surg 18:695–706

53. Espregueira-Mendes J, Pereira H, Sevivas N et al (2012) Assessment of rotatory laxity in anterior cruciate ligament-deficient knees using magnetic resonance imaging with Porto-knee testing device. Knee Surg Sports Traumatol Arthrosc 20:671–678

54. Pereira H, Sevivas N, Varanda P, Monteiro A, Monllau JC, Espregueira-Mendes J (2013) Failed anterior cruciate ligament repair. In: Pre-Pub, G. Bentley (ed.), Surgical Orthopaedics and Traumatology, Springer, Berlin/Heidelberg

55. Jarvela T, Kannus P, Jarvinen M (2001) Anterior cruciate ligament reconstruction in patients with or without accompanying injuries: a re-examination of subjects 5 to 9 years after reconstruction. Arthroscopy 17:818–825

56. Sonnery-Cottet B, Lavoie F, Ogassawara R et al (2010) Clinical and operative characteristics of cyclops syndrome after double-bundle anterior cruciate ligament reconstruction. Arthroscopy 26:1483–1488

57. Magit D, Wolff A, Sutton K, Medvecky MJ (2007) Arthrofibrosis of the knee. J Am Acad Orthop Surg 15:682–694

58. Shelbourne KD, Johnson GE (1994) Outpatient surgical management of arthrofibrosis after anterior cruciate ligament surgery. Am J Sports Med 22:192–197

59. Skutek M, Elsner HA, Slateva K et al (2004) Screening for arthrofibrosis after anterior cruciate ligament reconstruction: analysis of association with human leukocyte antigen. Arthroscopy 20:469–473

60. Paulos LE, Wnorowski DC, Greenwald AE (1994) Infrapatellar contracture syndrome. Diagnosis, treatment, and long-term followup. Am J Sports Med 22:440–449

61. Sanders B, Rolf R, McClelland W, Xerogeanes J (2007) Prevalence of saphenous nerve injury after autogenous hamstring harvest: an anatomic and clinical study of sartorial branch injury. Arthroscopy 23:956–963

62. Vardi G (2004) Sciatic nerve injury following hamstring harvest. Knee 11:37–39

63. Sechriest VF 2nd, Carney JR, Kuskowski MA, Haffner JL, Mullen MJ, Covey DC (2013) Incidence of knee sepsis after ACL reconstruction at one institution: the impact of a clinical pathway. J Bone Joint Surg Am 95(843–9):S1–S6

64. Indelli PF, Dillingham M, Fanton G, Schurman DJ (2002) Septic arthritis in postoperative anterior cruciate ligament reconstruction. Clin Orthop Relat Res 398:182–188

65. Zalavras CG, Patzakis MJ, Tibone J, Weisman N, Holtom P (2005) Treatment of persistent infection after anterior cruciate ligament surgery. Clin Orthop Relat Res 439:52–55

66. Zaffagnini S, Bonanzinga T, Grassi A et al (2013) Combined ACL reconstruction and closing-wedge HTO for varus angulated ACL-deficient knees. Knee Surg Sports Traumatol Arthrosc 21:934–941

67. Dowd GS, Hussein R, Khanduja V, Ordman AJ (2007) Complex regional pain syndrome with special emphasis on the knee. J Bone Joint Surg Br 89:285–290

68. Hogan CJ, Hurwitz SR (2002) Treatment of complex regional pain syndrome of the lower extremity. J Am Acad Orthop Surg 10:281–289

69. Wahl CJ, Westermann RW, Blaisdell GY, Cizik AM (2012) An association of lateral knee sagittal anatomic factors with non-contact ACL injury: sex or geometry? J Bone Joint Surg Am 94:217–226

70. Sonnery-Cottet B, Archbold P, Cucurulo T et al (2011) The influence of the tibial slope and the size of the intercondylar notch on rupture of the anterior cruciate ligament. J Bone Joint Surg Br 93:1475–1478

71. Hashemi J, Mansouri H, Chandrashekar N, Slauterbeck JR, Hardy DM, Beynnon BD (2011) Age, sex, body anthropometry, and ACL size predict the structural properties of the human anterior cruciate ligament. J Orthop Res 29:993–1001

72. Irrgang JJ, Anderson AF, Boland AL et al (2006) Responsiveness of the International Knee Documentation Committee Subjective Knee Form. Am J Sports Med 34:1567–1573

73. Bernard M, Hertel P, Hornung H, Cierpinski T (1997) Femoral insertion of the ACL. Radiographic quadrant method. Am J Knee Surg 10:14–21; discussion 22

74. Koga H, Muneta T, Yagishita K, Ju YJ, Sekiya I (2012) The effect of graft fixation angles on anteroposterior and rotational knee laxity in double-bundle anterior cruciate ligament reconstruction: evaluation using computerized navigation. Am J Sports Med 40:615–623

75. Carson EW, Brown CJ et al (2003) Revision anterior cruciate ligament surgery. In: Callaghan JJ (ed) The adult knee. Lippincott, Williams & Wilkins, Philadelphia

76. Pereira H, Sevivas N, Pereira R et al (2012) New tools for diagnosis, assessment of surgical outcome and follow-up. In: Hernández J, Monllau JC (eds) Lesiones Ligamentosas de La Rodilla. Marge Books, Barcelona, pp 185–194

77. Wright RW, Dunn WR, Amendola A et al (2007) Risk of tearing the intact anterior cruciate ligament in the contralateral knee and rupturing the anterior cruciate ligament graft during the first 2 years after anterior cruciate ligament reconstruction: a prospective MOON cohort study. Am J Sports Med 35:1131–1134

78. Dunn WR, Spindler KP (2010) Predictors of activity level 2 years after anterior cruciate ligament reconstruction (ACLR): a Multicenter Orthopaedic Outcomes Network (MOON) ACLR cohort study. Am J Sports Med 38:2040–2050

79. Spindler KP, Huston LJ, Wright RW et al (2011) The prognosis and predictors of sports function and activity at minimum 6 years after anterior cruciate ligament reconstruction: a population cohort study. Am J Sports Med 39:348–359

80. Thomas NP, Pandit HG (2008) Revision anterior cruciate ligament. In: Prodromos C, Brown C, Fu FH et al (eds) The anterior cruciate ligament: reconstruction and basic science. Saunders Elsevier, Philadelphia, pp 443–457

81. Safran MR, Harner CD (1996) Technical considerations of revision anterior cruciate ligament surgery. Clin Orthop Relat Res 325:50–64

82. Noyes FR, Barber-Westin SD (2001) Revision anterior cruciate surgery with use of bone-patellar

tendon-bone autogenous grafts. J Bone Joint Surg Am 83-A:1131–1143

83. Espregueira-Mendes J (2005) Revision of failures after reconstruction of the anterior cruciate ligament. In: Lemaire JS, Horan F, Villar R (eds) EFORT – European instructional course lectures, 7 edn. The British Editorial Society of Bone and Joint Surgery, London, p, 184–189

84. Yan LP, Silva-Correia J, Correia C et al (2013) Bioactive macro/micro porous silk fibroin/nano-sized calcium phosphate scaffolds with potential for bone-tissue-engineering applications. Nanomedicine (Lond) 8:359–378

85. Oliveira JM, Sousa RA, Malafaya PB et al (2011) In vivo study of dendronlike nanoparticles for stem cells "tune-up": from nano to tissues. Nanomedicine 7:914–924

86. Musahl V, Plakseychuk A, VanScyoc A et al (2005) Varying femoral tunnels between the anatomical footprint and isometric positions: effect on kinematics of the anterior cruciate ligament-reconstructed knee. Am J Sports Med 33:712–718

87. Csizy M, Friederich NF (2002) Bore canal site in surgical reconstruction of the anterior cruciate ligament. Position – placement errors – anatomic measurement. Orthopade 31:741–750

88. Samuelsson K, Andersson D, Karlsson J (2009) Treatment of anterior cruciate ligament injuries with special reference to graft type and surgical technique: an assessment of randomized controlled trials. Arthroscopy 25:1139–1174

89. Gorschewsky O, Klakow A, Putz A, Mahn H, Neumann W (2007) Clinical comparison of the autologous quadriceps tendon (BQT) and the autologous patella tendon (BPTB) for the reconstruction of the anterior cruciate ligament. Knee Surg Sports Traumatol Arthrosc 15:1284–1292

90. Mariscalco MW, Magnussen RA, Mehta D, Hewett TE, Flanigan DC, Kaeding CC (2013) Autograft versus nonirradiated allograft tissue for anterior cruciate ligament reconstruction: a systematic review. Am J Sports Med doi:10.1177/0363546513497566. [Epub ahead of print]

91. Prodromos CC, Joyce BT (2008) Allograft complications and risk factors. In: Prodromos C, Brown C, Fu FH et al (eds) The anterior cruciate ligament: reconstruction and basic science. Saunders-Elsevier, Philadelphia, pp 561–564

92. Karlsson J (2010) Anatomy is the key. Knee Surg Sports Traumatol Arthrosc 18:1

93. Leong NL, Petrigliano FA, McAllister DR (2013) Current tissue engineering strategies in anterior cruciate ligament reconstruction. J Biomed Mater Res A. doi:10.1002/jbm.a.34820. [Epub ahead of print]

94. Fare S, Torricelli P, Giavaresi G et al (2013) In vitro study on silk fibroin textile structure for anterior cruciate ligament regeneration. Mater Sci Eng C 33:3601–3608

95. Harvey A, Thomas NP, Amis AA (2005) Fixation of the graft in reconstruction of the anterior cruciate ligament. J Bone Joint Surg Br 87:593–603

96. Fu FH, Bennett CH, Lattermann C, Ma CB (1999) Current trends in anterior cruciate ligament reconstruction. Part 1: biology and biomechanics of reconstruction. Am J Sports Med 27:821–830

97. Petre BM, Smith SD, Jansson KS et al (2013) Femoral cortical suspension devices for soft tissue anterior cruciate ligament reconstruction: a comparative biomechanical study. Am J Sports Med 41:416–422

One-Stage Revision: Danish Approach

35

Martin Lind

Contents

M. Lind, MD, PhD
Division of Sports Trauma,
University Hospital of Aarhus, Tage Hansens Gade 2,
DK 8000 Aarhus, Denmark
e-mail: martinlind@dadlnet.dk

35.1 Causes for ACL Reconstruction Failure

35.1.1 Incidence of Failure

The incidence of failure after anterior cruciate ligament reconstruction (ACLR) is highly dependent on the failure definition. Failure after ACL reconstruction can be defined as need for revision ACLR, unsatisfactory outcome scores in objective or subjective clinical outcome instruments like the Lysholm and International Knee Documentation Score, excessive knee laxity above a specific level (typically 5 mm side-to-side increased objective laxity), or continuous subjective knee instability. Since revision ACLR is not performed on all patients with insufficient knee stability or poor subjective outcome after ACLR, then the revision rates after ACLR underestimate the true failure rate. Recent ACL revision rates based on data from national registries have found a revision rate of 4 % after 5 years [31] (Fig. 35.1). Even though the revision rate after ACL reconstruction appears to be relatively low in the range of 4–5 % after 5 years, a higher proportion of ACL reconstruction procedures are presently revision procedures. Data from national registries have shown that approximately 10 % of all ACL procedures are revision procedures [20, 30].

35.1.2 Failure Mechanisms

The main causes for ACL reconstruction failure are new trauma, technical failure, concomitant

R. Siebold et al. (eds.), *Anterior Cruciate Ligament Reconstruction*,
DOI 10.1007/978-3-642-45349-6_35, © ESSKA 2014

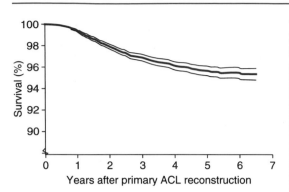

Fig. 35.1 Survival of ACL graft after primary ACL reconstruction. Kaplan-Meier survival profile for 14,878 patients from a national cohort followed for up to 6 years

Table 35.1 Causes for ACL reconstruction failure leading to revision ACL reconstruction as described in the literature

Cause for revision in %	Lind et al. (2012) [29]	MARS Group (2010) [57]	Trojani et al. (2011) [51]
New trauma	38	32	30
Femoral tunnel position	24	19	36
Tibial tunnel position	6	9	11
Tunnel widening	2		
Unknown cause	24	24 (biologic)	15
Fixation failure		5	5

ligament instability, and biological failure. The term biological failure is poorly defined and covers mainly unknown causes for failure (Table 35.1). A recent French multicenter study investigating descriptive data of ACL revision in 293 patients demonstrated that the main causes for ACL graft failure were femoral tunnel position (36 %), new trauma (30 %), and unknown cause (15 %) [52].

35.1.2.1 New Trauma

The main reason for failure of ACL reconstruction is a new trauma. New trauma has been estimated to be the cause for ACL graft failure in approximately 35 % of cases. [31, 59]

In 80 % of cases, the new trauma occurs during sports activities. In some pivoting sports like team handball, the risk for reinjury after ACL reconstruction is very high in the range of 25 % [37].

35.1.2.2 Technical Failure

Recent focus on the anatomy of the ACL insertions and the possibility to perform more anatomical correct ACL reconstructions have revealed that previous techniques resulted in suboptimal tunnel placement especially in the femur, where a tendency to a vertical tunnel placement was a standard until a decade ago (Fig. 35.2). Both too vertical and anterior placement of the tunnels in femur will result in impingement against the posterior cruciate ligament, which will over time result in graft tissue stretching and fretting, which

can lead to new instability. In the tibia a too anteriorly placed tunnel will result in impingement against the roof of the intercondylar notch, and this is another possible failure mechanism caused by graft impingement. Excessive graft tension exerted during surgery has been demonstrated to result in poor graft ligamentation and subsequent increased graft laxity [60]. The implants used for graft fixation in the bone tunnels can also be a cause for failure. Ligamentation and anchorage of the graft to the tunnel wall near the joint normally result in graft incorporation within 3–6 months, so insufficient implant fixation will normally result in early failure. Normal graft loading during rehabilitation can result in forces up to 500 N, so a fixation method needs to withstand forces of this magnitude [50].

35.1.2.3 Biological Failure

Biological failure is often defined as an exclusion diagnosis. If no obvious new trauma or surgical errors exist, a biological failure of some kind must be the reason for failure. However, the biological response of the grafted tissue is related to the mechanical and biochemical environment into which the graft is placed. Thus, the "biological failure" of the ACL graft is a complex pathological entity, and its nature is not insufficiently understood. Biological failure mechanisms can be early extensive graft necrosis, disturbances in

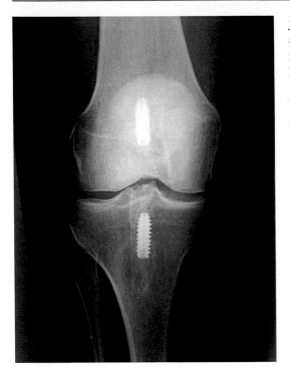

Fig. 35.2 Anterior-posterior radiograph of a patient with a vertical un-anatomical placement of the femoral tunnel. The metal interference screw is seen positioned at the 12 o'clock position

joint-near fixation methods [11]. Suspensory fixation methods in which there is excessive elasticity of the graft fixation implants can result in poor ligamentization in the bone tunnels. Continued adverse mechanical loading between graft and bone tunnel can subsequently lead to tunnel widening. Also resorbable implants can cause cystic bone resorption around the implants due to acidic degradation products that are released during implant degradation [9, 10, 36]

There is however no direction correlation between increased laxity after ACLR and tunnel widening.

35.1.2.4 Concomitant Lesions

Failure to identify and treat injuries to collateral ligaments and PCL can cause increased loads on the ACL graft after reconstruction. Posterolateral instability is the most commonly unrecognized concurrent ligament insufficiency and is seen in 10–15 % of chronically ACL-deficient knees [12].

35.2   Management of Patients with ACLR Failure: History, Clinical Symptoms, X-Ray, MRI, and CT

35.2.1   History

Careful patient evaluation is very important for proper planning and treatment of failed ACL reconstruction. Probably the most important step in the revision surgery is the preoperative planning. This is to avoid repetition of the failures related to the primary ACL reconstruction. Patient activity level and symptom characteristics after primary ACLR should be determined. Subjective complaints of failed ACLR may include instability sensation, pain, swelling, giving way, locking, noise, stiffness, or a limp. It is important to distinguish between pain and instability symptoms. All past operative records should be carefully reviewed for information about the previous intra-articular injuries and treatments. Regarding the previous ACLR it is important to know the type of graft, placement of graft, and graft fixation techniques and the

revascularization, and poor cell repopulation and proliferation that lead to late or insufficient ligamentization process [34]. When using allograft tendons for ACLR, an adverse immune reaction can play a role for graft disruption especially for irradiated graft that seems to be able to induce a more extensive immune response than nonirradiated allografts [9].

Tunnel widening following anterior cruciate ligament (ACL) reconstruction is a well-described phenomenon [6, 9, 55]. The basis of tunnel widening is multifactorial with several possible mechanical and biological contributing factors [22]. Suspensory graft fixation results in a more elastic graft construct and may contribute to the so-called bungee effect, which has been suggested to contribute to tunnel widening [11, 22, 38]. Tunnel widening is more frequent when using cortical fixation techniques, such as button fixations or fixation posts, compared to implants used. Physical examination should include assessment of knee effusion, range of motion, and detailed ligamentous laxity examination. Gait and alignment should be noted. Any valgus or varus deformity should be noted and possibly further evaluated by full extremity radiography. A varus or valgus thrust can indicate concomitant laxity of the medial or posterolateral corner. Such instabilities can be evaluated by valgus and varus stress tests and rotatory tests such as the dial test. Clinical finding of collateral instabilities can further be evaluated by stress radiographs where a side-to-side difference in joint space opening can indicate a significant collateral ligament insufficiency which should be addressed in a revision procedure [27]. Objective tests of ACL laxity include the anterior drawer and pivot-shift tests. Instrumented laxity examination is beneficial, and results can be compared with previous examinations. A side-to-side laxity difference of more than 5 mm has been defined as failure of ACLR [54].

35.2.2 Imaging

The primary investigation is radiographs in two or three planes. These are used to determine the presence and location of hardware. Secondly the radiographs reveal tunnel placements and tunnel widening. Tunnel widening can be measured as the diameter between the sclerotic margins of the bone tunnel [26] (Fig. 35.3). On lateral radiographs sagittal tibial tunnel position at the tibial plateau can be divided from anterior to posterior in four equal quadrants as described by Amis and Jakob [1]. The tibial tunnel should enter the joint in the posterior third of quadrant 2. For the femoral tunnel, Blumensaat line can be divided into four equal quadrants, and the tunnel should be in the most posterior quadrant [2]. On frontal radiographs the tibial tunnel should be in the center of the tibial plateau, and the femoral tunnel should be between 40° and 70° from central vertical axis.

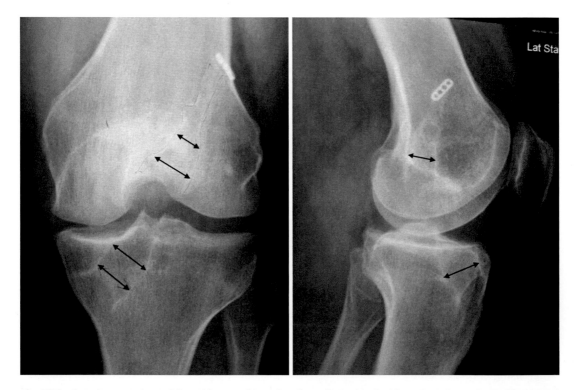

Fig. 35.3 Anterior-posterior and lateral knee radiographs of a patient with significant both femoral and tibial tunnel widening after hamstring ACL reconstruction. *Arrows* indicate the tunnel walls

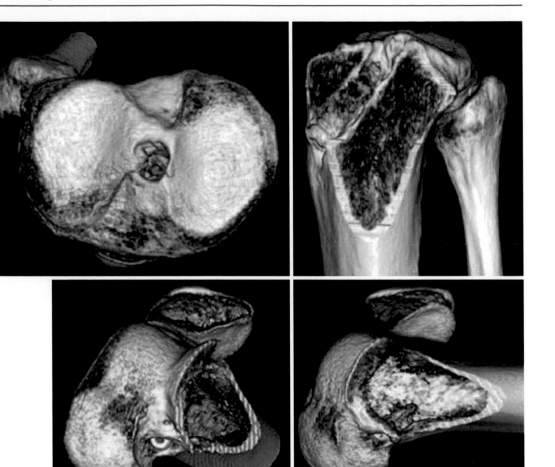

Fig. 35.4 3D reconstruction CT scanning is ideal to identify tunnel position and tunnel configurations prior to revision ACL reconstruction

Magnetic resonance imaging (MRI) is a useful adjunct to the radiological evaluation. MRI scanning can determine the integrity of the reconstructed ACL and evaluate the status of cartilage and menisci.

A CT scanning can supplement evaluation of bone tunnels and tunnel widening and gives more detailed information than the standard radiographs. It is recommended to use supplementary CT scanning if radiographs demonstrate potentially problematic tunnel positions or tunnel widening. 3D reconstructions may further add to the information retrieved from CT scannings especially to identify the tunnel entrances to the joint and to identify possible new tunnel placement (Fig. 35.4).

35.3   Surgical Tactics for Revision: Removal of Implants and Assessment of Bone Tunnels

When planning revision ACL reconstruction, the surgeon should have access to a variety of techniques to deal with malpositioned tunnels, bone loss, tunnel expansion, and implants needing removal. When all informations are available, decisions can be made with respect to timing, removal of old fixation devices (special removal instruments must be available), graft choice, tunnel placement, graft fixation, single- or two-stage technique. To avoid failure of the ACL revision, the patient must be carefully "educated" to prevent early return to sport or pivoting activities.

Thus, it is important that the operation is planned in a period where postoperative rehabilitation period suits the patient's social life and sports activities.

35.3.1 Timing

Before surgery it is mandatory that problems with lack of extension and flexion have been cleared. In some cases this is due to arthrofibrosis or infrapatellar contracture syndrome. In these cases arthroscopic release procedures and intensive rehabilitation must be done prior to revision ACLR.

35.3.2 Implant Removal

If the index tunnels and implants are correctly or nearly correctly placed, the screws have to be removed. Size and mark of screws used in previous surgery must be determined, and the appropriate screwdriver must be available for the surgeon. Care must be taken to remove any bone ingrowth from the inside and around the top of the screw, before the correct-sized screwdriver is engaged with the screw. The screwdriver has to be as parallel to the screw as possible. Stripping or damaging the threads of the screw during either insertion or removal may require a more extensive bone removal and subsequently a staged operation. In case of metallic screws placed in the proximal tibial or when there is complete bony overgrowth, fluoroscopy can be very helpful for identification of hidden screw position. A trick for screw identification is to use a K-wire and to drill the K-wire to the end of the screw using fluoroscopy. Subsequently it is possible to drill with standard reamers to expose the end of the screw, which then can be removed with minimal bone loss.

Changing the angle of drilling and thereby avoiding removal of the originally inserted screw can often facilitate tibial tunnel preparation when a new tibial tunnel is created [16]. Special attention should be given to the "absorbable interference screws," which, although radiolucent, may require removal even several years postoperatively. Poor quality bone tissue might exist around bone tunnels in which resorbable implants have

been placed due to inflammatory possesses occurring during implant resorption. Cystic bone resorption has been documented as caused by resorbable implants [9, 10, 36]. Therefore, it is advisable always to remove such implants during revision ACLR procedures.

35.3.3 Tunnel Placement

Probably the most common technical failure of ACL reconstructions is nonanatomical femoral and tibial tunnel placement. Previous standard operative technique for ACLR has been to place the ACL graft in a near upright position in the femur to accommodate the use of femoral offset guides during transtibial ACLR techniques (Fig. 35.2). Only recently rediscovery of anatomical ACLR principles has changed tunnel placement to more correct anatomical positions especially in the femur. Regarding tunnel placement at primary ACLR, there are principally three situations to be considered.

35.3.3.1 Primary ACLR with Well-Placed Tunnels

Well-positioned tunnels with no enlargement can be reused, and routine fixation methods can normally be applied. In case of mild tunnel widening or osteolysis, a graft with a large bone plug may be used, which typically will be an allograft. For femoral tunnel widening a technique using a conical bone plug placed from outside-in has been described. With this technique only press-fit fixation is necessary. Another option in the femur is to use double interference screw fixation to fill up an oversized tunnel [39, 44]. On the tibia side, a large interference screw can be used to fill the tunnel or an allograft can be used with the bone plug sized to the enlarged tunnel diameter. If there is any doubt of the bone quality in the tibia, backup fixation with bicortical screw and washer is recommended. In cases with acceptable tunnel placement, old hardware is removed, and the drill hole is debrided and redrilled by stepwise increasing reamer diameter until a clean bone tunnel is achieved. Straight reamers may be preferred relative to acorn reamers to avoid possible drill migration or drifting. One method for insurance

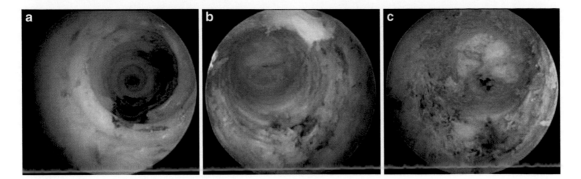

Fig. 35.5 Sequential drilling is essential for tunnel preparation in revision ACL reconstruction. In the (**a**) panel a metallic interference screw has been removed. In panel (**b**) reaming has been performed with an 8 mm reamer. In panel (**c**) reaming has been performed with a 10 mm reamer. The bone tunnel is now clean with fresh cancellous bone in tunnel wall. In the lower deep part of the tunnel, cortical remnants of the bone block from the patella bone autograft used at index surgery are visible

of drill direction is to drill the K-wire into the femoral notch roof during the sequential drilling. Another is to stabilize the tip of the K-wire with an instrument during drilling. Use the arthroscope to look up in the drill hole to make sure that old graft tissue, sutures, and implant remnant are removed and that sclerotic bone is removed from the tunnel walls (Fig. 35.5). In these cases it is normally necessary to increase the graft size from the first to the second operation.

35.3.3.2 Primary ACLR Operation with Malpositioned Tunnels

If a tunnel is clearly malpositioned, a new drill hole can be made through a different approach to obtain a tunnel with more correct anatomical position. In these cases old hardware can be left in situ to optimize the compactiveness of the surrounding bone for the revision fixation procedure. If new tunnels can be placed without confluence of malpositioned index tunnels, routine fixation can be used depending on graft choice and surgeon's experience. However, if the surgeon suspects weakened cancellous bone and thereby reduced fixation strength, extra cortical fixation may be considered. This extra fixation can in the femur be a hybrid fixation principle with cortical button and an interference screw if soft tissue graft is used. Combining a metal interference screw with a bicortical fixation post in the distal femur can enhance femoral fixation of grafts with a bone plug. In the tibia a backup fixation with a bicortical screw and washer can be combined with any intraosseous fixation implant.

35.3.3.3 Primary ACLR with Partly Malpositioned Tunnels

It is important to emphasize that a correct tunnel placement has little to do with the intraosseous placement or angulations. More important is the entry point of the tunnel in the joint. In cases of partially malpositioned tunnel placement, there are options to avoid staged procedures. It is however important to understand that increased tunnel obliquity results in increased tunnel ovularity and opening area.

In case of a partially posterior tibial tunnel, it is possible to correct this by shifting the tibial tunnel 2–3 mm anterior during the reaming and debridement of the primary tunnel. During graft fixation an interference screw is placed posterior to the graft and close to joint entry to ensure that the graft heals to the anterior aspects of the new tunnel. A similar principle can be used for partially anterior tibial tunnel, where the tunnel instead is shifted posteriorly and the screw is placed anterior to the graft. Care should be taken during screw placement in these cases since the anterior screw position can cause fracture to the anterior cortex. Also the tunnel length is short in the anterior aspects of an anteriorized tunnel so that the tip of the screw might enter the joint space causing graft impingement or cartilage damage to femur joint surface. In the femur the typical problem with a partially malplaced tunnel is a tunnel that is moderately high in the notch but where preparation of a new tunnel might result in communication to the old tunnel during drilling. In such cases hardware in the old can be replaced by a composite bioresorbable screw or a PEEK screw. These screws can accept minimal damage during drilling of the new tunnel. It is advisable to use a composite resorbable screw containing hydroxyapatite calcium phosphate since these screws resorb very slowly and integrate well with surrounding bone, which will maintain bony integrity around the revision femoral bone tunnel [42].

Fluoroscopic imaging can be a valuable tool during revision ACLR procedures both for hardware removal and for optimization of tunnel positioning.

35.3.4 Revision After Double-Bundle ACLR

The recent focus on double-bundle ACLR will in the coming years lead to an increasing number of patients that need revision of failed double-bundle reconstructions. Revision in these cases exerts special challenges since we lack experience with the problems created of having four tunnels that need revision. The issue of having two tunnels in both the tibia and femur will make single-stage revisions more difficult. The safest option will be to choose a staged procedure with initial bone grafting of all four tunnels. An option for single-stage approach will be to perform a single-bundle revision of the anteromedial ACL bundle after filling the posterolateral tunnels with cortico-cancellous allograft plugs or allograft screws.

35.3.5 Concomitant Ligament Lesions

As previously mentioned, several cases of graft failures are caused by overload of the graft due to concomitant ligament lesion not detected at the time of the primary reconstruction. Isolated revision of the torn ACL graft without restoration of other ligament insufficiencies might lead to a new graft failure due to overtensioning, which can cause lack of graft incorporation in the bone tunnel and poor intra-articular tissue ingrowth and revascularization. Also concomitant ligament insufficiency can result in graft rupture due to new episodes of giving away when the patient returns to sports. Thus, it is advisable that concomitant ligament lesions with laxity of more than IKDC grade 3 and 4 should be reconstructed at the time of the ACL revision procedure. Standard collateral ligament reconstruction techniques should be used [28, 61]. Especially if rotatory instability is present in combination collateral ligament instability. Rotatory instability can be detected clinically by dial test and external and internal rotatory tests [32].

35.3.6 Rehabilitation

The postoperative rehabilitation protocol depends on a variety of factors. Important surgical factors to consider include the type of graft used, fixation stability, concomitant reconstruction of secondary stabilizers, and any meniscal or cartilage pathology. Patient considerations include age, activity level, size, compliance, and expectations of the patient. The rehabilitation can in most cases follow the principles for primary ACL reconstruction. However, if the graft fixation strength is not optimal, a more restrictive rehabilitation regimen must be used. The use of braces in ACL surgery is controversial and is still under debate with respect to primary ACL reconstruction [58]. Risberg et al. found in a randomized controlled trial (RCT) no difference between use and nonuse of braces in primary ACL reconstructions [3]. No RCT has been described in revision ACL surgery. However, biomechanical investigations indicate that braces can reduce load on the reconstructed ACL graft in both weight-bearing and non-weight-bearing situations. In the noncomplicated revision situations, brace usage is probably not indicated. In cases of poor bone quality and suboptimal graft fixation, a brace and reduced range of motion for 4–6 weeks can be used to ensure reduced graft loading during the initial phases of graft healing. In cases where valgus or varus instability has been treated with collateral ligament reconstruction, the use of brace is needed in the period where the graft undergoes revascularization and incorporation to bone tunnel (6–10 weeks) [4, 53].

35.4 Indication for One- or Two-Stage Revision

The primary indication for considering revision ACLR is recurrent knee instability after previous ACLR. If the patient complains of reoccurrence of sudden knee failure and sensation of subluxation, then these symptoms are signs of graft failure, which potentially can be managed with a revision ACLR. Pain and problems with range of motions after ACLR are not necessarily corrected by a revision ACLR and should therefore be evaluated and treated independently. There is good evidence in the literature that a revision ACLR can restore knee stability to almost the same level as a primary reconstruction [29, 31]. However, symptoms and function and patient's subjective perception of knee functions are poorer than after primary ACLR [29, 31]. Indications for staged surgery should be reserved to cases where the quality of bone either at the joint entry points or in the fixation zones in the tibia or in the lateral femoral condyle is too poor to perform a one-stage revision ACLR with proper tunnel placement and secure graft fixation. Another indication is in cases with partly incorrectly placed bone tunnels, where the new graft position cannot be corrected by redrilling combined with graft bone block position or fixation implant positioning. In the first situation, insufficient graft fixation and potential poorer graft incorporation can lead to new mechanical failure. In the latter situations, a one-stage procedure probably would result in a repetition of the failure due to the same poor graft position that resulted in failure after the primary procedure. To avoid the above-mentioned problems, a staged procedure is necessary.

Staged revision ACLR involves in the first stage procedure removal of all hardware, debridement, and redrilling of the old tunnels with oversized drill diameter to remove sclerotic bone in the tunnel wall and subsequently autologous or allogenic bone transplantation in both femoral and tibial drill holes. Normally bone allograft is used as either milled bone chips or bone plugs drilled out from a femoral head. The bone graft tissue is subsequently compressed into the debrided tunnels. Autologous bone graft is normally harvested from the iliac crest. The second stage operation is performed 4–6 months later when the bone graft has been incorporated in the bone tunnel. A CT scanning is performed prior to the second stage procedure to ensure proper incorporation of the allograft bone in the tunnels (Fig. 35.6). A significant advantage at the second stage procedure of revision ACLR is that the construction typically can be performed like a primary reconstruction.

However, since studies have indicated that increased time to revision correlates with development of radiographic arthritis and meniscal and chondral lesions, the surgeon must use caution when deciding for a 2-stage procedure when a 1-stage procedure may be sufficient [40]. A 2-stage revision normally requires a 4- to 6-month window between procedures. This will subject patients to a prolonged period of continued knee instability, which may result in further cartilage and meniscal injury to the involved knee. Two-stage protocols also require a second anesthetic and further periods of activity modification. When possible, preference should be given to a 1-stage procedure in all situations in which adequate placement and fixation of the graft can be achieved.

35.5 Graft Choice and Surgical Technique (Table 35.2)

A major surgical strategy issue is which graft to choose for revision ACLR. In the literature there is very sparse evidence for which graft type provides the best outcome. The choice primarily stands between autografts and allograft. The choice of graft depends on which grafts have been used at the index surgery and on the placement of tunnels and tunnel size after debridement. Also the previous fixation method has to be taken into consideration during the planning along with the

Fig. 35.6 Standard radiographs of a patient with tibial (**a**) and femoral (**b**) tunnel widening. The patient was treated with a staged revision ACL reconstruction. After bone grafting a CT scanning was performed 5 months later to confirm proper bone tunnel filling and incorporation of the bone graft in the tibia (**c**) and femur (**d**)

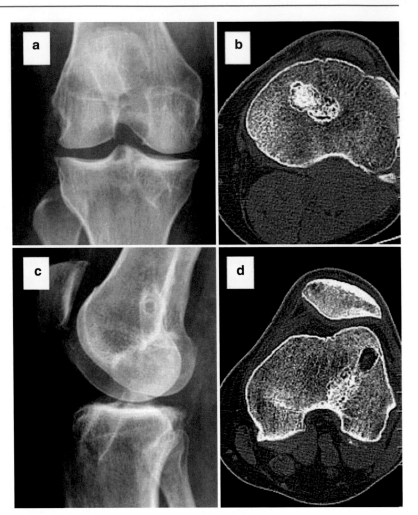

Table 35.2 Technical tricks and pearls

Removal of screws hidden in bone	Blindly drill K-wire to identify screw location. Then sequentially drill hole for removal of screw
Graft translation in partially malpositioned bone tunnels	Position graft fixation implant so that the graft is translated in the needed direction
Tunnel widening	Healthy bone tissue is typically found 1–2 mm earlier than the sclerotic bone margins seen on radiographs. Await staging decision until after bone debridement
Partially malpositioned tunnels	Reuse of partially malpositioned tunnel induces a risk for poor graft positioning and graft impingement. A low threshold for staged procedure is a good strategy in these cases

suspected reason for failure of the previous graft. Other factors of importance are patient's age, general health, activities of daily living, and specific sports demands postoperatively [44]. In the literature there is a tendency to favor autografts over allograft. This strategy is supported by a recent study based on a national cohort of revision ACLR patients demonstrating a twofold increase in failure rate for revisions performed with allografts compared to autografts [31].

If the primary surgery was performed with a hamstring graft and the tunnels are placed acceptable, the preferable graft choice would be to use ipsilateral patella-tendon-bone or a quadriceps tendon graft with dimensions of the bone plugs cut to match the size of the bone tunnels. After hamstring graft primary surgery, the typical tunnel issues are moderate tibial tunnel widening (up to 12 mm) and posterior tibial tunnel placement due to transtibial technique at primary surgery. A graft with bone plugs can be fitted into tunnels with moderate tunnel widening or misplacement. A moderately posteriorly placed tibial tunnel can be corrected by ensuring that the tunnel is redrilled 2–3 mm anteriorly. With a bone plug in the new tibial tunnel, the graft can be shifted anteriorly by placing the tibial interference screw posterior to the bone plug. In cases where the index surgery was with patella tendon bone graft and the tunnels are placed acceptable, the use of hamstring grafts from either the ipsilateral or contralateral side depends on the diameter of the tunnels and/or the position of the tunnels. In cases of previous patella-tendon-bone graft usage, there is typically no tunnel widening as the patella-tendon graft bone plugs have been integrated into the tunnels. If tunnel widening has developed, a 7–9 mm hamstring graft can be too small for proper filling of the debrided tunnels. In these cases an allograft or a staged procedure with initial bone grafting is advocated. After bone grafting a problem-free usage of hamstring autograft for the second stage procedure can be performed. Another typical tunnel placement problem due to transtibial technique is a too vertical femoral tunnel placement. Often it is possible to drill a new femoral tunnel at the correct anatomical femoral ACL attachment position using drilling through the anteromedial portal.

Thus, it might be difficult to go from patella tendon graft to hamstring graft at revision procedures due to smaller graft diameter of the hamstring tendons, but more feasible to go from hamstring graft to patella-tendon-bone graft.

When an autologous tendon graft is planned for revision ACLR, the graft must be harvested as the last surgical step after determining if all the technical steps of the revision can be implemented [7].

When using allografts for revision ACL surgery, donor site morbidity issues are eliminated, but allograft usage adds concerns for bacterial or viral contamination from the graft, even though these risks are very minimal [35]. Allografts should be used as fresh frozen, because grafts treated with irradiation have shown significant worse results in recent studies [41, 45]. Allografts should not be obtained from too old donors as the tendon-to-bone interface weakens with increasing patient's age [56]. The preferred allografts for revision ACL surgery are patella tendon bone grafts, quadriceps tendon grafts, and Achilles tendon grafts, but also soft tissue graft such as tibialis tendon grafts can be used. Both deep frozen and cryopreserved allografts have been shown to repopulate with host cells and to reinnervate with nerve fibers (A fibers, afferent, and efferent C fibers) [19, 48]. Both allografts and autografts provide a fibrous framework for new ligamentous healing. Maximal tensile strength of allografts is less than that of autografts, but stronger than the native ACL if the diameter of allograft is sufficient [46, 47]. Due to these biomechanical issues, it is advisable to use allografts with a diameter of 10–11 mm. When using allografts, it is imperative that the surgeon is knowledgeable with graft processing techniques and the Tissue Banks certification. In the setting of multi-ligament reconstructions, in which also revision ACLR is performed, allograft tissue can diminish surgical time and associated surgical site morbidity. Also allografts might be the only options since potential autografts might have been used at the primary ACLR.

Use of the contralateral knee graft is an option, especially in situations where allograft tissue is unavailable. In some European countries, legal issues prevent the use of allograft tissue. A major issue with contralateral graft usage is the potential introduction of donor site morbidity to a healthy knee. Patella tendon harvest is associated with more donor site morbidity than hamstring harvest with a higher incidence of anterior knee pain and kneeling problems [24, 25]. If contralateral graft harvest is necessary, it is advocated to harvest hamstring grafts instead of patella tendon graft.

Presently there is no documentation for a place for synthetic grafts in revision ACLR [17]. Recently a new synthetic graft type, the Ligament Advanced Reinforcement System (LARS), has gained some popularity in selected countries. This synthetic graft has advantageous mechanical properties and could therefore be an option for revision ACLR for athletes with high demands for knee function. However, the literature is still limited regarding outcome and complications [33]. The poor history of previous synthetic ACL grafts should lead to caution about usage of synthetic grafts for revision ACLR.

Graft choice in revision ACLR surgery is therefore based on detailed knowledge of the history of the previous surgery, tunnel placement, bone quality, and the availability of grafts and on the surgeon's experience and preferences. An algorithm for management strategy can be seen in Fig. 35.7.

35.6   Pitfalls and Complications

35.6.1 Technical Pitfalls (Table 35.3)

Numerous potential technical pitfalls exist when performing revision ACLR.

In cases of anteriorly placed tibial tunnels where revision is performed without staging, there is a potential risk for fracture of the anterior tibial cortex if the new tibial fixation screw is placed between the graft and the anterior tibial cortex wall. This technique can be used to correct the graft position into a more posterior direction, but care must be taken when placing the fixation implant to avoid cortical fracture which can result in long-term pain problems and fixation failure. In the similar situation where a screw is used to correct graft position in an anteriorly positioned tunnel, there is a risk for screw protrusion into the joint since the anterior aspects of the tibial tunnel are shorter than the average tunnel length. Thereby a screw length and tunnel length mismatch can occur. Recently there has been a trend to drill more horizontal tibial tunnels for transtibial single-bundle ACL reconstruction in order to be able to reach the anatomical insertion area when drilling the femur tunnel. Care should be taken to

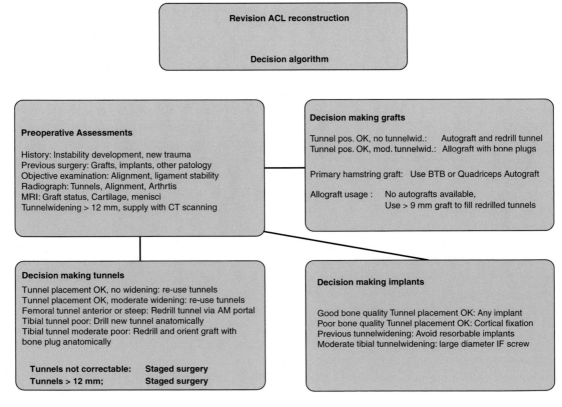

Fig. 35.7 Algorithm for revision ACL surgery

Table 35.3 Technical pitfalls

Implant protrusion	Reusage of partially misplaced bone tunnels increases the risk of implant protrusions
Tibial plateau collapse	Horizontal tibial tunnels established when trying to attempt anatomical femoral drill hole position can undermine tibial plateau when debrided further for revision reconstruction. Consider staged procedure
Anterior tibial cortex fracture	Insert implants with care when placed anteriorly to the graft in the tibia
Associated ligament insufficiency	Be prepared to reconstruct collateral ligament if found to be insufficient during the procedure

reuse such tunnels during ACL revision procedures. Redrilling of a tunnel just below the medial tibial plateau might result in too extensive removal of subchondral bone with subsequent medial tibial cartilage collapse as a complication.

When performing tunnel bone transplantation in staged procedures, an easy solution is just to remove the screw and then only transplant the screw cavity. This typically results in poor bone quality in the proximal and joint-near part of the tibial tunnel. It is therefore advisable to debride and transplant the entire tunnel during staged procedures.

35.6.2 Complications and Failure After Revision ACLR

Only two studies have studied large enough cohorts of revision ACL patients to determine reliable failure rates. In a national cohort re-revision occurred in 5.4 % of cases within 5 years. In a case series of 126 patients, 6 % were re-revised after average 6 years [29]. Lack of improvement of knee stability was seen in 15 % of patients, and this failure definition was not different from after primary ACLR where 12 % demonstrated lack of stability improvement. Another important type of failure after revision ACLR is chronic pain problems, which can result in significant disability. As chronic pain normally does not result in re-revision ACLR, the incidence

of this complication is poorly described in the literature. It is thought that the most likely cause for chronic pain is the accumulated injuries to cartilage and menisci combined with scar tissue formation due to multiple surgeries [52, 57].

35.7 Literature Results

35.7.1 Results After Anterior Cruciate Ligament Revision Surgery

Most of the literature on revision ACL reconstruction is related to technical aspects of performing revision procedures such as different fixation methods and graft types. The studies evaluating the outcome of revision ACL reconstruction have typically involved small case series and therefore have low level of evidence. Recently national registries and multicenter study collaborations like the Multi-center ACL Revision Study group (MARS group) have generated study populations that more reliably present epidemiology and outcome in relation to revision ACLR [30, 59] (Table 35.4). Weiler et al. compared the subjective and objective results after revision ACL minimum of 2 years postoperatively to a matched group of patients who had primary hamstring ACL reconstruction. They demonstrated 6.5 % in the revision group who experienced graft failure, compared to 5.6 % in the primary reconstruction group. The manual maximum KT-1000 arthrometer side-to-side difference was 2.1 ± 1.6 mm for the revision group and 2.2 ± 1.1 mm for the primary reconstruction group. The Lysholm score was significantly better in the primary reconstruction group. The incidence of postoperative positive pivot-shift test results was not significantly different [54].

Recent data from the Danish register for ACL reconstruction have demonstrated results after revision ACLR for a national prospective cohort. Tegner and KOOS scores increased significantly from preoperatively to postoperatively (Tegner score from 3 to 4, KOOS symptoms 50–57, KOOS pain 66–77, activity of daily living 73–83, KOOS sports 32–51, KOOS

Table 35.4 Clinical outcome after revision anterior cruciate ligament reconstruction in different previous studies

Author, year, reference	Study design	Number of patients	Follow-up (years)	Outcome measure	Results at follow-up
Noyes et al. (2001) [39]	Cohort	54	2.7	Cincinnati	87
Taggart et al. (2004) [49]	Case series	26	1–5	Lysholm	85
				Tegner	4.8
Fules et al. (2003) [14]	Case series	26	4.2	Lysholm	87
				Obj. IKDC	B 22/26
Grossman et al. (2005) [21]	Case series	27	3–9	Lysholm	87
				Tegner	5.2
Lind et al. (2012) [29]	Case series	128	2–9	KOOS	Symp 72
				Tegner	Pain 76
					ADL 82
					Sports 50
					QoL 52
					Tegner 4
Wright et al. (2011) [59]	MOON cohort	39	2		IKDC score 76
					Re-revision 4 %
Lind et al. (2009) [30]	National registry	222	2	KOOS	Symp 75
				Tegner	Pain 77
					ADL 83
					Sports 51
					QoL 47
					Tegner 3.9
Lind et al. (2012) [31]	National registry	1,099	1–6	KOOS (1 year)	Symp 73
				Tegner	Pain 78
					ADL 84
					Sports 52
					QoL 48
					Tegner 4

quality of life 32–47) [30]. The 1-year follow-up outcome after RACLR was poorer than after primary ACLR by 5–13 points for the different KOOS subscales with the quality of life subscore being the most different compared to primary ACLR.

In cases of new instability due to failure of the primary ACL reconstruction, revision surgery can result in regained stability to a level similar to after primary ACLR [23, 29, 31]. No high-evidence studies have been published, but several case–control studies demonstrate improved stability and function after revision surgery [5, 8, 21]. Eberhardt et al. showed that 67 % were able to return to sports activity, but 63 % had pain at activity, and 63 % showed signs of osteoarthritis 37 months after revision surgery compared to pre-op radiographs [8]. The risk of osteoarthritis

was significantly higher if the athlete continued sports activity [8].

Comparing revision surgery to primary ACLR, Carson et al. found significantly lower Hospital for Special Surgery knee ligament evaluation score 2 years after surgery (case–control study design) [5]. In a similar retrospective study, Grossmann et al. reported follow-up Lysholm score and subjective IKDC score minimum of 6 years after revision to be 87 and 86, respectively [21]. Furthermore the authors reported marked higher side-to-side knee laxity difference based on KT-1000 measurements when using allograft compared to autograft [21]. Similar findings of inferior outcome after revision ACL reconstruction were found in two national cohort studies with lower scores in knee-specific outcome score and function scores [18, 31]. One of the two national cohort studies also demonstrated more osteoarthritis development in revision patients compared to primary ACLR patients. The 2- to 11-year follow-up results after revision ACL utilizing a nonirradiated patellar tendon allograft were less favorable than in patients who had a primary anterior cruciate ligament reconstruction, with a lower subjective satisfaction level and a higher percentage of patients with grade 1+ or higher pivot-shift results [13]. Similar finding was done in a national cohort of 1,099 patient, with a doubled re-revision rate for allograft revisions [31].

Using the quadriceps tendon for revision surgery, good results were reported mean 26 months after surgery with 97 % showing max-manual KT-1000 side-to-side translation <5 mm [15].

Any concomitant injuries to the knee will affect the results after revision surgery. Rollier et al. demonstrated inferior functional outcome if initial ACLR was done with a synthetic ligament and the knee presented meniscal or cartilage damage [43].

A recent study demonstrated a cumulative meniscus lesion incidence of 70 % after 2.5 years follow-up after ACL revision. They demonstrated that meniscectomy negatively influenced both functional outcome and knee stability. This accumulated incidence of meniscus and cartilage injuries in ACL revision patients is a likely contributing cause for case of chronic pain after ACL revision [51].

Data from the American MARS cohort demonstrated current or previously treated meniscal injury in 74 % of patients. Articular cartilage damage grade 2 or worse was noted in 73 %. Both meniscal and articular cartilage damage was seen in 57 % [57].

In conclusion, secondary instability after primary ACL surgery can be treated with revision surgery, resulting in improved stability and function. However, the results are poorer after revision ACLR than after primary ACLR. Use of allograft results in similar knee function compared to autograft but inferior stability and a higher risk of failure due to re-revision. Concomitant lesion will negatively influence the pain and knee scores. Return to sports activity can be expected in approximately 60 %, but with significantly higher risk of osteoarthritis.

> **Memory**
> Failure mechanisms of ACLR are numerous, and new trauma and poor anatomical placement of the tunnels for ACL graft fixation seem to be the most important failure mechanisms. The surgical technique for ACL revision reconstruction needs to correct failure causes and address concomitant ligament lesions. It is often necessary to use allograft tendons as the new ACL graft and fixation methods should be suited for the graft choices and bone quality. The outcome of ACL revision surgery has previously been poorly described in small case series, but recent data from national registries and larger cohort studies provide more reliable results. Outcome after revision ACLR is poorer than after primary ACLR, and patients need to be informed about these results in order to have realistic expectations to the clinical outcome after revision ACLR.

References

1. Amis AA, Jakob RP (1998) Anterior cruciate ligament graft positioning, tensioning and twisting. Knee Surg Sports Traumatol Arthrosc 6(Suppl 1):S2–S12
2. Bernard M, Hertel P, Hornung H, Cierpinski T (1997) Femoral insertion of the ACL. Radiographic quadrant method. Am J Knee Surg 10(1):14–21; discussion 21–12
3. Beynnon BD, Good L, Risberg MA (2002) The effect of bracing on proprioception of knees with anterior cruciate ligament injury. J Orthop Sports Phys Ther 32(1):11–15
4. Beynnon BD, Uh BS, Johnson RJ, Fleming BC, Renstrom PA, Nichols CE (2001) The elongation behavior of the anterior cruciate ligament graft in vivo. A long-term follow-up study. Am J Sports Med 29(2):161–166
5. Carson EW, Anisko EM, Restrepo C, Panariello RA, O'Brien SJ, Warren RF (2004) Revision anterior

cruciate ligament reconstruction: etiology of failures and clinical results. J Knee Surg 17(3):127–132

6. Clatworthy MG, Annear P, Bulow JU, Bartlett RJ (1999) Tunnel widening in anterior cruciate ligament reconstruction: a prospective evaluation of hamstring and patella tendon grafts. Knee Surg Sports Traumatol Arthrosc 7(3):138–145

7. Denti M, Lo Vetere D, Bait C, Schonhuber H, Melegati G, Volpi P (2008) Revision anterior cruciate ligament reconstruction: causes of failure, surgical technique, and clinical results. Am J Sports Med 36(10):1896–1902

8. Eberhardt C, Kurth AH, Hailer N, Jager A (2000) Revision ACL reconstruction using autogenous patellar tendon graft. Knee Surg Sports Traumatol Arthrosc 8(5):290–295

9. Fahey M, Indelicato PA (1994) Bone tunnel enlargement after anterior cruciate ligament replacement. Am J Sports Med 22(3):410–414

10. Fauno P, Christiansen SE, Lund B, Lind M (2010) Cyst formation 4 years after ACL reconstruction caused by biodegradable femoral transfixation: a case report. Knee Surg Sports Traumatol Arthrosc 18(11):1573–1575

11. Fauno P, Kaalund S (2005) Tunnel widening after hamstring anterior cruciate ligament reconstruction is influenced by the type of graft fixation used: a prospective randomized study. Arthroscopy 21(11):1337–1341

12. Ferretti A, Monaco E, Labianca L, De Carli A, Conteduca F (2008) Double bundle or single bundle plus extra-articular tenodesis in ACL reconstruction? A CAOS study. Knee Surg Sports Traumatol Arthrosc 16(1):98

13. Fox JA, Pierce M, Bojchuk J, Hayden J, Bush-Joseph CA, Bach BR Jr (2004) Revision anterior cruciate ligament reconstruction with nonirradiated fresh-frozen patellar tendon allograft. Arthroscopy 20(8):787–794

14. Fules PJ, Madhav RT, Goddard RK, Mowbray MA (2003) Revision anterior cruciate ligament reconstruction using autografts with a polyester fixation device. Knee 10(4):335–340

15. Garofalo R, Djahangiri A, Siegrist O (2006) Revision anterior cruciate ligament reconstruction with quadriceps tendon-patellar bone autograft. Arthroscopy 22(2):205–214

16. George MS, Dunn WR, Spindler KP (2006) Current concepts review: revision anterior cruciate ligament reconstruction. Am J Sports Med 34(12):2026–2037

17. Getelman MH, Friedman MJ (1999) Revision anterior cruciate ligament reconstruction surgery. J Am Acad Orthop Surg 7(3):189–198

18. Gifstad T, Drogset JO, Viset A, Grontvedt T, Hortemo GS (2013) Inferior results after revision ACL reconstructions: a comparison with primary ACL reconstructions. Knee Surg Sports Traumatol Arthrosc 21(9):2011–2018

19. Goertzen MJ, Buitkamp J, Clahsen H, Mollmann M (1998) Cell survival following bone-anterior cruciate ligament-bone allograft transplantation: DNA fingerprints, segregation, and collagen morphological

analysis of multiple markers in the canine model. Arch Orthop Trauma Surg 117(4–5):208–214

20. Granan LP, Forssblad M, Lind M, Engebretsen L (2009) The Scandinavian ACL registries 2004–2007: baseline epidemiology. Acta Orthop 80(5):563–567

21. Grossman MG, ElAttrache NS, Shields CL, Glousman RE (2005) Revision anterior cruciate ligament reconstruction: three- to nine-year follow-up. Arthroscopy 21(4):418–423

22. Hoher J, Moller HD, Fu FH (1998) Bone tunnel enlargement after anterior cruciate ligament reconstruction: fact or fiction? Knee Surg Sports Traumatol Arthrosc 6(4):231–240

23. Johnson DL, Swenson TM, Irrgang JJ, Fu FH, Harner CD (1996) Revision anterior cruciate ligament surgery: experience from Pittsburgh. Clin Orthop Relat Res 325:100–109

24. Kartus J, Movin T, Karlsson J (2001) Donor-site morbidity and anterior knee problems after anterior cruciate ligament reconstruction using autografts. Arthroscopy 17(9):971–980

25. Kjaergaard J, Fauno LZ, Fauno P (2008) Sensibility loss after ACL reconstruction with hamstring graft. Int J Sports Med 29(6):507–511

26. L'Insalata JC, Klatt B, Fu FH, Harner CD (1997) Tunnel expansion following anterior cruciate ligament reconstruction: a comparison of hamstring and patellar tendon autografts. Knee Surg Sports Traumatol Arthrosc 5(4):234–238

27. Laprade RF, Bernhardson AS, Griffith CJ, Macalena JA, Wijdicks CA (2010) Correlation of valgus stress radiographs with medial knee ligament injuries: an in vitro biomechanical study. Am J Sports Med 38(2):330–338

28. Lind M, Lund B, Fauno P, Christiansen S (2009) Revision anterior cruciate ligament reconstruction. Challenges and approaches. Min Orthop Traumatol 60:341–351

29. Lind M, Lund B, Fauno P, Said S, Miller LL, Christiansen SE (2012) Medium to long-term follow-up after ACL revision. Knee Surg Sports Traumatol Arthrosc 20(1):166–172

30. Lind M, Menhert F, Pedersen AB (2009) The first results from the Danish ACL reconstruction registry: epidemiologic and 2 year follow-up results from 5,818 knee ligament reconstructions. Knee Surg Sports Traumatol Arthrosc 17(2):117–124

31. Lind M, Menhert F, Pedersen AB (2012) Incidence and outcome after revision anterior cruciate ligament reconstruction: results from the Danish registry for knee ligament reconstructions. Am J Sports Med 40(7):1551–1557

32. Lubowitz JH, Bernardini BJ, Reid JB 3rd (2008) Current concepts review: comprehensive physical examination for instability of the knee. Am J Sports Med 36(3):577–594

33. Machotka Z, Scarborough I, Duncan W, Kumar S, Perraton L (2010) Anterior cruciate ligament repair with LARS (ligament advanced reinforcement system): a systematic review. Sports Med Arthrosc Rehabil Ther Technol 2:29

34. Malinin TI, Levitt RL, Bashore C, Temple HT, Mnaymneh W (2002) A study of retrieved allografts used to replace anterior cruciate ligaments. Arthroscopy 18(2):163–170

35. Marrale J, Morrissey MC, Haddad FS (2007) A literature review of autograft and allograft anterior cruciate ligament reconstruction. Knee Surg Sports Traumatol Arthrosc 15(6):690–704

36. Martinek V, Friederich NF (1999) Tibial and pretibial cyst formation after anterior cruciate ligament reconstruction with bioabsorbable interference screw fixation. Arthroscopy 15(3):317–320

37. Myklebust G, Steffen K (2009) Prevention of ACL injuries: how, when and who? Knee Surg Sports Traumatol Arthrosc 17(8):857–858

38. Nebelung W, Becker R, Merkel M, Ropke M (1998) Bone tunnel enlargement after anterior cruciate ligament reconstruction with semitendinosus tendon using Endobutton fixation on the femoral side. Arthroscopy 14(8):810–815

39. Noyes FR, Barber-Westin SD, Roberts CS (1994) Use of allografts after failed treatment of rupture of the anterior cruciate ligament. J Bone Joint Surg Am 76(7):1019–1031

40. Ohly NE, Murray IR, Keating JF (2007) Revision anterior cruciate ligament reconstruction: timing of surgery and the incidence of meniscal tears and degenerative change. J Bone Joint Surg Br 89(8):1051–1054

41. Rappe M, Horodyski M, Meister K, Indelicato PA (2007) Nonirradiated versus irradiated Achilles allograft: in vivo failure comparison. Am J Sports Med 35(10):1653–1658

42. Robinson J, Huber C, Jaraj P, Colombet P, Allard M, Meyer P (2006) Reduced bone tunnel enlargement post hamstring ACL reconstruction with poly-L-lactic acid/hydroxyapatite bioabsorbable screws. Knee 13(2):127–131

43. Rollier JC, Besse JL, Lerat JL, Moyen B (2007) Anterior cruciate ligament revision: analysis and results from a series of 74 cases. Rev Chir Orthop Reparatrice Appar Mot 93(4):344–350

44. Safran MR, Harner CD (1996) Technical considerations of revision anterior cruciate ligament surgery. Clin Orthop Relat Res 325:50–64

45. Schwartz HE, Matava MJ, Proch FS et al (2006) The effect of gamma irradiation on anterior cruciate ligament allograft biomechanical and biochemical properties in the caprine model at time zero and at 6 months after surgery. Am J Sports Med 34(11):1747–1755

46. Shino K, Inoue M, Horibe S, Nagano J, Ono K (1988) Maturation of allograft tendons transplanted into the knee. An arthroscopic and histological study. J Bone Joint Surg Br 70(4):556–560

47. Shino K, Kawasaki T, Hirose H, Gotoh I, Inoue M, Ono K (1984) Replacement of the anterior cruciate ligament by an allogeneic tendon graft. An experimental study in the dog. J Bone Joint Surg Br 66(5):672–681

48. Shino K, Oakes BW, Horibe S, Nakata K, Nakamura N (1995) Collagen fibril populations in human anterior cruciate ligament allografts. Electron microscopic analysis. Am J Sports Med 23(2):203–208; discussion 209

49. Taggart TF, Kumar A, Bickerstaff DR (2004) Revision anterior cruciate ligament reconstruction: a midterm patient assessment. Knee 11(1):29–36

50. Tohyama H, Beynnon BD, Johnson RJ, Renstrom PA, Arms SW (1996) The effect of anterior cruciate ligament graft elongation at the time of implantation on the biomechanical behavior of the graft and knee. Am J Sports Med 24(5):608–614

51. Trojani C, Beaufils P, Burdin G et al (2012) Revision ACL reconstruction: influence of a lateral tenodesis. Knee Surg Sports Traumatol Arthrosc 20(8):1565–1570

52. Trojani C, Sbihi A, Djian P et al (2011) Causes for failure of ACL reconstruction and influence of meniscectomies after revision. Knee Surg Sports Traumatol Arthrosc 19(2):196–201

53. Uchio Y, Ochi M, Adachi N, Kawasaki K, Kuriwaka M (2003) Determination of time of biologic fixation after anterior cruciate ligament reconstruction with hamstring tendons. Am J Sports Med 31(3):345–352

54. Weiler A, Schmeling A, Stohr I, Kaab MJ, Wagner M (2007) Primary versus single-stage revision anterior cruciate ligament reconstruction using autologous hamstring tendon grafts: a prospective matched-group analysis. Am J Sports Med 35(10):1643–1652

55. Wilson TC, Kantaras A, Atay A, Johnson DL (2004) Tunnel enlargement after anterior cruciate ligament surgery. Am J Sports Med 32(2):543–549

56. Woo SL, Hollis JM, Adams DJ, Lyon RM, Takai S (1991) Tensile properties of the human femur-anterior cruciate ligament-tibia complex. The effects of specimen age and orientation. Am J Sports Med 19(3):217–225

57. Wright RW, Huston LJ, Spindler KP et al (2010) Descriptive epidemiology of the Multicenter ACL Revision Study (MARS) cohort. Am J Sports Med 38(10):1979–1986

58. Wright RW, Preston E, Fleming BC et al (2008) A systematic review of anterior cruciate ligament reconstruction rehabilitation: part II: open versus closed kinetic chain exercises, neuromuscular electrical stimulation, accelerated rehabilitation, and miscellaneous topics. J Knee Surg 21(3):225–234

59. Wright R, Spindler K, Huston L et al (2011) Revision ACL reconstruction outcomes: MOON cohort. J Knee Surg 24(4):289–294

60. Yoshiya S, Kurosaka M, Ouchi K, Kuroda R, Mizuno K (2002) Graft tension and knee stability after anterior cruciate ligament reconstruction. Clin Orthop Relat Res 394:154–160

61. Zantop T, Schumacher T, Diermann N, Schanz S, Raschke MJ, Petersen W (2007) Anterolateral rotational knee instability: role of posterolateral structures. Winner of the AGA-DonJoy Award 2006. Arch Orthop Trauma Surg 127(9):743–752

ACL Two-Stage Revision Surgery: Practical Guide

36

João Espregueira-Mendes,
Hélder Pereira, Alberto Monteiro,
Joaquim Miguel Oliveira, Rui Luís Reis,
Pedro Luís Ripóll, and Neil Thomas

Contents

J. Espregueira-Mendes, MD, PhD
3B's Research Group – Biomaterials, Biodegradables
and Biomimetics, Univ. Minho, Headquarters of the
European Institute of Excellence on Tissue
Engineering and Regenerative Medicine,
Ave Park, S. Cláudio de Barco,
4806–909, Taipas, Guimarães, Portugal

ICVS/3B's – PT Government Associated Laboratory,
Braga, Guimarães, Portugal

Clínica Espregueira-Mendes F.C. Porto Stadium –
FIFA Medical Centre of Excellence, Porto, Portugal

H. Pereira, MD (✉)
3B's Research Group – Biomaterials, Biodegradables
and Biomimetics, Univ. Minho, Headquarters of the
European Institute of Excellence on Tissue
Engineering and Regenerative Medicine,
Ave Park, S. Cláudio de Barco,
4806–909, Taipas, Guimarães, Portugal

ICVS/3B's – PT Government Associated Laboratory,
Braga, Guimarães, Portugal

Clínica Espregueira-Mendes F.C. Porto Stadium –
FIFA Medical Centre of Excellence, Porto, Portugal

Orthopedic Department, Centro Hospitalar Póvoa de
Varzim – Vila do Conde, Vila do Conde, Portugal
e-mail: heldermdpereira@gmail.com

A. Monteiro, MD
Clínica Espregueira-Mendes F.C. Porto Stadium –
FIFA Medical Centre of Excellence, Porto, Portugal

J.M. Oliveira, BSc, PhD
R.L. Reis, CEng, MSc, PhD, DSc
3B's Research Group – Biomaterials, Biodegradables
and Biomimetics, Univ. Minho, Headquarters of the
European Institute of Excellence on Tissue
Engineering and Regenerative Medicine,
Ave Park, S. Cláudio de Barco,
4806–909, Taipas, Guimarães, Portugal

ICVS/3B's – PT Government Associated Laboratory,
Braga, Guimarães, Portugal

P.L. Ripóll, MD
Ripoll y De Prado Sport Clinic, Ripoll, Spain

N. Thomas, MD
North Hampshire Hospital and the Hampshire Clinic,
Basingstoke, UK

R. Siebold et al. (eds.), *Anterior Cruciate Ligament Reconstruction*,
DOI 10.1007/978-3-642-45349-6_36, © ESSKA 2014

36.1   Introduction

Reconstruction of the anterior cruciate ligament (ACL) has become an increasingly common orthopedic procedure. Around 200,000 ACL ruptures per year occur in the United States [16, 17]. The overall incidence has been reported between 36.9 and 60.9 per 100,000 persons per year [12, 34]. Considering surgical treatment, it is estimated that more than 100,000 ACL repairs are performed annually in the United States [5], 34,000 ACL repairs are performed in France [46], and approximately 50,000 ACL reconstructions have been reported in the United Kingdom [41]. This condition thus represents a heavy economic burden with major societal impact. With a success rate for primary reconstruction ranging from 75 to around 90 % [47], one must consider that surgery for revision of ACL repair has become a frequent procedure for a knee-dedicated surgeon. Nevertheless, it should not be forgotten that this procedure presents a continuous challenge to knee surgeons in most cases. This is mainly due to a multiplicity of problems that might arise, thus dictating failure of ACL repair [36] and leading to patient- and problem-related treatment options [48].

This chapter will focus only in the subgroup of patients who might be selected for two-stage revision procedure. A review from literature is provided complemented by institutional and personal experience aiming to provide a useful and practical tool.

36.2   Patient Selection for Two-Stage ACL Revision

The radiologist is a strong ally in the diagnosis process. This member of the diagnostic health-care team should be able to recognize the types of primary repair. It must be able to assess for the complications of primary surgery, such as tunnel malpositioning, tunnel widening, and fixation device failure [18]. Nevertheless, when correct bone tunnel position implicates conflict with previous tunnels and/or hardware, consequently all materials should be carefully removed to recreate biologic and biomechanical conditions for adequate graft placement and further graft integration.

By its turn, bone tunnel enlargement has been reported after ACL reconstruction surgery [13]. Although the long-term outcome of this phenomenon is not yet well known, tunnel lysis or expansion may be clinically significant in revision surgery. This is mainly due to the fact that the enlarged tunnels may complicate graft placement and fixation [13, 41]. Thus, two-stage revision surgery ensures adequate restoration of bone stock. By this mean, it is possible to ensure the biologic conditions for healing of the bone tunnels, which will then provide a good bed for fixation of the ACL graft [41].

Anatomic (posterior and proximal) placement of the intra-articular exit (apertural) of the femoral tunnel is required since it can provide minimal lengthening of the ACL substitute during range of motion, including when full extension is achieved [29]. A more anterior and distal position of the femoral tunnel within the roof of the notch is a recognized cause of failure, leading to the increase in length of the graft with flexion [6]. Similarly, it has also been stated the need for correct positioning of the tibial tunnel [6, 13]. A tibial tunnel in the anterior half of the anatomic tibial footprint may cause roof graft impingement in extension. In addition, repeated impingements can induce weakening of the graft with subsequent increased risk of failure [1].

Bearing in mind the aforementioned, if a significant void bony defect arises after a primary ACL reconstruction (Fig. 36.1), it will jeopardize the necessary biologic conditions for graft integration. In addition, it will also impair the correct apertural placement of the graft. Even if suspensory fixation could provide pullout stability, it would not be possible to recreate joint kinematics [13]. When this is the case, i.e., if insufficient bone stock impairs adequate apertural fixation of the plasty, primary bone grafting and a two-stage reconstruction are advised.

> **Tricks and Pearls**
> Moreover, if widening of the tunnel is higher than 100 % of the original one, or its width measures from 16 to 20 mm on preoperative X-ray or CT, the option for two-stage repair is also suggested [2].

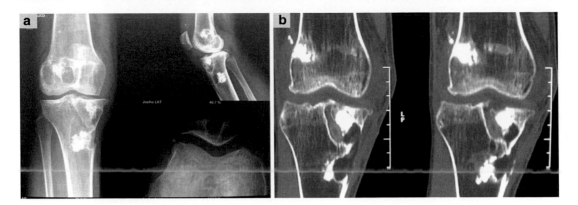

Fig. 36.1 Anteroposterior, lateral, and Merchant's X-ray views (**a**) from a clinical case presenting severe osteolysis in both femur and tibia following ACL reconstruction with BPTB. Complementary CT images aiming the study of bone stock (**b**)

Considering anatomic and technical issues, we have found more frequently such indications involving the tibial than femoral tunnel [41, 42].

36.3 Graft Choice and Surgical Technique of Two-Stage Revision

Several graft options exist for ACL reconstruction (primary or revision), and, up to date, surgeons are far from reaching consensus concerning which represents the best option [14, 40].

Choice between autograft and allograft is a matter of continuous debate [27]. Several issues remain, but personal/institutional experience and legal issues play a decisive role. Allograft helps to overcome morbidity of graft harvesting and enables availability of large amount of tissue when it is available (Fig. 36.2). As recently reported, when ACL autografts fail traumatically, they frequently fail near their femoral origin. However, allograft reconstructions are more likely to fail in other locations or stretch [26]. Despite some issues that still remain to be overcome, namely, those related to biologic conditions on allografts, it keeps being a valuable option particularly in re-revision cases or associated to severe tissue damage [35, 42, 44].

Some allograft inherent risks and considerable costs should be considered prior its application [22, 28, 37, 38, 45].

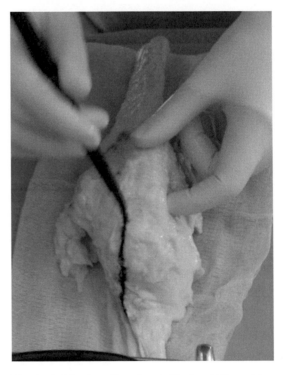

Fig. 36.2 Massive allograft suitable for ACL revision surgery. Large grafts might be tailored according to the needs from each particular case

Novel regenerative possibilities include tissue engineering and regenerative medicine principles. These are under intense research and promise to overcome the need for cadaver allografts for future for either bone or ligament replacement [8, 20, 33, 50]. Figure 36.3 shows an example of

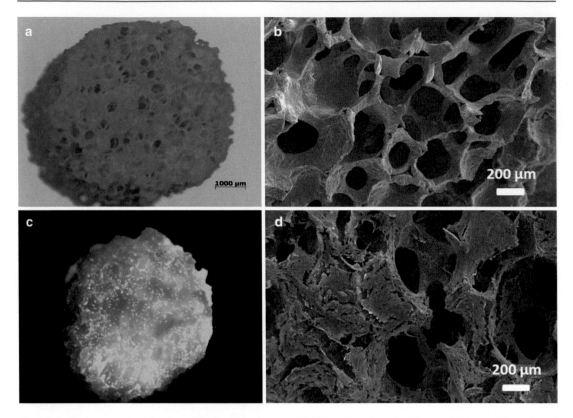

Fig. 36.3 Hydroxyapatite (HAp) scaffold for bone tissue engineering: stereomicroscopy image (**a**), SEM image of HAp scaffolds (**b**), fluorescence microscopy image of HAp scaffolds seeded with rat bone marrow stromal cells (BMSCs) cultured for 21 days (LIVE/DEAD assay; *green color* shows live cells) (**c**) and SEM image of hydroxyapatite scaffold seeded with bone marrow stromal cells, after 21 days of culturing (**d**). It is possible to observe that BMSCs adhered to the HAp scaffolds, proliferated, and were viable after 21 days of culturing (in vitro). It has been demonstrated that these HAp scaffolds present a good biocompatibility, and when seeded with BMSCs, it supported de novo bone formation in vivo, thus being a promising future alternative to autografts in bone regeneration procedures [43]

the scaffolds that have been developed in the context of bone tissue engineering.

Despite the previously exposed, there are several viable options for ligament autograft [36] in any form of ACL repair (primary or revision). Likewise, autologous bone grafting from iliac crest [41] or other sources (e.g. proximal tibia) [10] can be used. This is also the case when a two-stage revision is to be considered.

Surgeons still lean toward the use of autografts due to technical, biologic, and legal issues. Generally, clinicians lean toward favoring a graft source different from that used in primary reconstruction. That is, if hamstrings were used as primary choice, then bone-patellar tendon-bone (BPTB) is the choice for the revision procedure. Conversely, if BPTB was firstly used, hamstrings are selected in the revision. This issue is further discussed elsewhere.

Tissue engineering also presents promising new options for future concerning ligament replacement [8]. However, in current practice, prosthetic ligaments as primary grafts lead to some of the most difficult cases with increased intra-articular scarring and more pronounced tunnel widening. Therefore, we do not encourage their use for the time being [41].

36.3.1 Graft Fixation

The techniques for graft fixation that have been used during the revision procedure are mainly dependent on the remaining bone stock and the chosen graft [19, 42].

Initial fixation is critical for the outcome, but it is particularly important until adequate graft integration takes place.

> **Tricks and Pearls**
> In order to increase primary resistance and obtain stability close to the articular surface, "double fixation" combining complementary devices might be an appropriate option during several "difficult ACL revision" cases [19].

Either suspensory cortical fixation (fixed or adjustable loop) or interference screws might be complemented with interference screws, staples, or post with sutures. Such double fixation might provide additional strength or increase stability close to joint line.

Fixation devices distant from the joint line (e.g., buttons, staples, washers, or post-screws) will provide a less stable reconstruction [7, 11]. This will permit abnormal graft motion within the bone tunnel causing the so-called bungee effect (longitudinal) and/or windshield-wiper effect (transverse). Ultimately, these phenomena might contribute to the enlargement of bone tunnels, and it can jeopardize integration of the graft. Ultimately, it can increase risk for failure, thus posing higher difficulty in subsequent surgeries if that might be the case [7].

Whatever is the chosen technique, it will be mandatory to achieve sufficient bone stock for further primary fixation and integration of the transplant. This is the rationale behind the two-stage revision option in cases of major defects around primary tunnels.

36.3.2 Two-Stage Revision Technique

36.3.2.1 Stage I
All patients should be submitted to careful clinical examination under anesthesia and observations

recorded. Arthroscopic thorough examination follows using standard arthroscopic portals. Possibility of ongoing infection must be definitely ruled out. Assessment and appropriate treatment of meniscal and chondral injuries should take place. Then, the graft remnant must be removed as well as unwanted osteophytes. Notch assessment and notchplasty when strictly necessary should also occur. Usually one should expect more macroscopic cartilage damage changes than previously suggested by preoperative assessment.

After the soft tissues are debrided and the entrances of the tunnels exposed, the surgeon will have a definitive picture of the defect and hardware-related issues. Hardware is removed only when it is required.

> **Tricks and Pearls**
> If the original tunnel interferes with the placement of the new tunnel, it should be inspected with the arthroscope in air medium (osteoscopy) (Fig. 36.4).

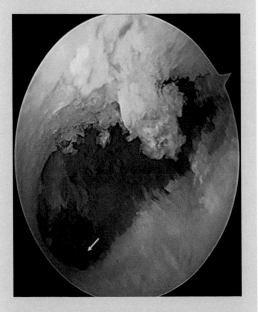

Fig. 36.4 Osteoscopy image with the arthroscope inside the tibial tunnel. This enables inspection of macroscopic aspects of the bone of tunnel walls. Notice the oval aspect of the tunnel in the articular surface. *Yellow arrow* represents the location of femoral tunnel

The sclerotic walls of the tunnel should be drilled with a fine 2 mm drill, and the tunnel curetted and rasped until the tunnel walls had been taken back to clean bone. Bone in the form of dowel grafts must be then harvested from the iliac crest, placed into the tunnel, and carefully impacted. Bone graft from the ipsilateral iliac crest can be used.

Compression is a critical point once extreme care is required to avoid additional damage. For tibial tunnel, we must avoid to breach the exit point within the joint, which is achieved by viewing the relevant articular surface of the tibial plateau with the arthroscope during bone graft compression.

Arthroscopic bone grafting of femoral tunnel is a demanding procedure. Several options have been proposed either sliding graft through a guidewire [30] or using a tube harvester similar to osteochondral autograft transfer system (OATS) procedure and a press-fit technique [10].

It should be highlighted that additional difficulties are to be expected if the primary ligament used is a synthetic one. In our experience, the first-stage revision surgery is more demanding and time-consuming given the higher synovitis. Besides, it can increase intra-articular scarring associated to the synthetic graft. Tunnel widening also tends to be higher after the foreign body reaction. Extra care is often required to identify the posterior cruciate ligament (PCL) before clearing the intercondylar notch.

36.3.2.2 Stage II

The second stage procedure might be summarized in five steps: (1) examination under anesthesia, (2) macroscopic arthroscopic assessment, (3) relevant meniscal and chondral surgery, (4) graft harvesting, and (5) revision ACL reconstruction.

After minimizing bone voids in stage I, the revision procedure itself becomes "similar" to a primary procedure. The main focus is now given for achieving the correct anatomic placement of the tunnels.

Because the landmarks were often less distinct than those in a primary procedure, the tibial tunnel was referenced off the PCL on the medial side of the midintercondylar point. Moreover, the femoral tunnel was referenced from the over-the-top position using appropriate tools. Perioperative radioscopic imaging using an image intensifier is occasionally required to ensure optimal placement (see also Chap. 34).

36.4   Timing for Revision ACL Reconstruction After Spongiosaplasty

After stage I procedure, one might predict a period of 4–6 months until stage II might take place.

Many approaches are used to repair skeletal defects in reconstructive orthopedic surgery.

Autogenous cancellous bone graft, with its osteogenic, osteoinductive, and osteoconductive properties, remains the gold standard [23]. Neovascularization takes place within the bone graft as early as 2 days after implantation. With time, there is a repopulation of the marrow spaces with primitive MSCs.

Despite autogenous cancellous bone grafts lack mechanical strength, their favorable biologic activity (osteoinduction, osteoconduction, and new bone formation) provides early stability at the recipient site [23]. The biology of the graft and the mechanical environment of the host-graft interface are critical for the successful graft integration. Besides graft integration, minimal biomechanical features must be achieved prior to final ACL reconstruction. Bone maturation will continue up to several years after surgery [4, 23].

Compared with autograft cancellous bone, allograft bone of any source is a poorer promoter of bone healing [23]. Cancellous chips are the most common type of allogeneic cancellous graft used.

When revision requires a two-stage procedure with bone grafting of the tunnels prior to the definitive ligament repair, radiologists might play an important role in order to assess for adequate bone graft incorporation [18]. X-ray analysis and more relevantly computed tomography (CT) have proven to be powerful tools in this subject (Figs. 36.5 and 36.6).

Fig. 36.5 3D CT reconstructions from a case of re-revision after BPTP ACL repair. Notice the placement of two separate tibial tunnels (*red* and *yellow arrows*) and bone loss due to graft harvesting (*)

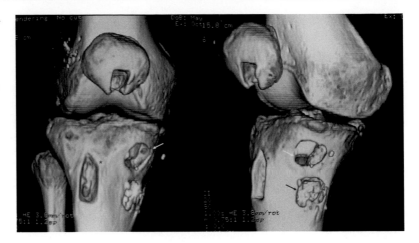

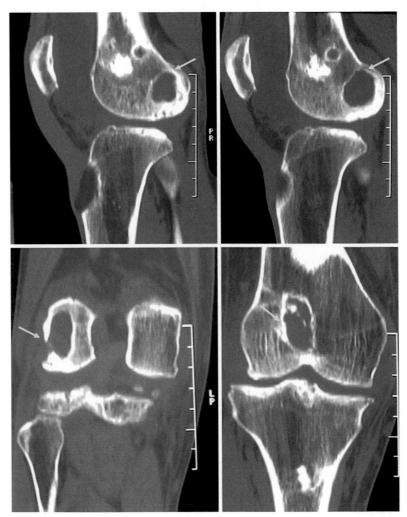

Fig. 36.6 CT images representing severe bone loss around femoral tunnel (*yellow arrows*)

A CT scan obtained at 4 months should be used to assess healing of the bone graft. Blurring of the tunnel margins, reactive sclerosis, and the presence of bone within the tunnel are signs of adequate healing.

In upcoming future, we envision that tissue engineering and regenerative medicine strategies can provide an adequate grafting material mimicking bone tissue. The main challenge for scientists in manufacturing bone graft substitutes is to obtain a scaffold that has sufficient mechanical strength and bioactive properties and can be vascularized in order to promote a viable new tissue [24, 39]. Such approach would overcome the morbidity of autologous bone harvesting and possibly achieving a faster maturation of implanted material. Our study group has been working thoroughly on development of several possibilities for bone replacement on orthopedic application combining scaffolds, cells, and nanotechnologies [31–33] (Fig. 36.3). One additional feature would be to provide a more user-friendly method for arthroscopic implantation [25] and furthermore combining bioactive molecules (e.g., growth factors) or medications [49, 50] to enhance and/or fasten tissue maturation.

36.5   Pitfalls and Complications of Two-Stage Revision

As aforementioned, the complications and pitfalls of two-stage revision must consider the additional morbidity of bone harvesting. Anterior iliac crest should be regarded as a good site for bone harvesting, i.e., considering its relatively low morbidity rate, early ambulation, and hospital discharge [9]. However, up to 28 % postoperative pain and nearly 5 % sensory disturbances have been reported [9]. The safe zone on the proximal tibia (anterior tibial metaphysis) has recently been described [43] for this propose with minimal complications noticed: 1.7 % transitory sensory disturbances and one case over thirty with hypoesthesia at a five-year follow-up causing no particular limitation [10]. Allografts constitute a valid option but present lower biologic activity and inherent risks [45], while

tissue-engineered implants are giving the first steps toward clinical application [33].

Preservation of tunnel's bone walls is sometimes difficult to achieve, and it requires extreme care during bone impaction with appropriate arthroscopic control of apertural limits of tibial tunnel. Given the risk of wall breakage during surgery, surgeons should "expect the unexpected" and must be prepared for the worst-case scenario. Ultimately, it is required a complete surgical set with several distinct and complementary fixation options, i.e., besides surgical tools to prepare "bone beds" or additional fixation strategies.

Surgical time might be on the upper limit of the globally expected for ACL surgery which might predispose to vascular issues despite no evidence has been provided in this matter [15].

Complications inherent to any elective knee arthroscopy should also be considered [3].

Further possible complications are parallel to any ACL revision procedure which is described in detail on a specific chapter (see also Chap.34).

However, it must be bear in mind that most cases selected for two-stage revision are among the most difficult patients requiring ACL repair. So being, expectations for outcome must be realistic, adequate to the specific condition, and previously discussed with the patient.

36.6   Literature Results of Two-Stage Revision

There are limited reports from literature focused on patient selection, technical issues, or outcome from two-stage ACL revision procedures.

Patients having revision ACL reconstruction after a failed repair had improvement in their functional status as compared with pre-revision status. However, they did not achieve the same level of satisfactory results as primary ACL reconstruction [21, 48]. Outcome of repeat revision has been reported as excellent or good in 70 % of the cases, although decreased after the second revision [46]. The main causes of failure have been recurrent trauma and surgical technical errors [46, 48].

A case-control clinical study has reported technical aspects and results of two-stage ACL repair with bone grafting of the tibial tunnel and the use of a different femoral tunnel [41]. Comparing to primary ACL repair, ACL revision cases presented a higher incidence of chondral and meniscal lesions. At final follow-up, IKDC scores of 61.2 ± 19.6 were obtained in the two-stage revision group comparing to 72.8 ± 10.2 for primary ACL repair. No significant differences were found between laxity measurements using KT-2000 arthrometer [41].

Considering two-stage revision requiring bone grafting of femoral tunnel, a recent study considering autologous hamstring tendon graft by a single-bundle transtibial ACL reported very good results at mean 6.7-year follow-up [10]. At the last follow-up, IKDC scores significantly improved from 18 class C and 12 D to 27 patients A and B plus 3C. Mean Lysholm score improved from 65.4 (48–82; SD, 7.9) to 90.2 (72–100; SD, 7.9). Twenty-four of 30 patients (80 %) were able to hop 90–100 % (grade A) as compared to the uninjured side. Significantly improved outcome concerning KT-1000 side-to-side difference and Lachman and pivot-shift measures was also registered. At a 24-month follow-up, 20 of 30 patients (66.7 %) had returned to the preoperative sport activity level (9 elite athletes, 11 county levels); 9 patients had changed to lower nonimpact sports, and 3 had to quit sports activities. All patients were able to undertake the knee-walking test without significant complaints [10]. Minor complaints related to graft harvesting were reported.

A short clinical experience of four cases that required bone tunnel repositioning and two-stage technique by means of sliding the structural iliac crest bone graft through a guidewire reported no complications from either the intra-articular bone grafting procedure or the bone graft harvesting [30].

Prospective controlled studies would be desirable in order to increase evidence level concerning two-stage ACL revision. However, it must be assumed that this is a difficult task considering the somewhat low incidence and multifactorial aspect of this condition. However, it can be concluded that in properly selected cases, two-stage revision is an adequate and feasible option while enabling good results however generally lower than primary ACL reconstruction. Ongoing research and upcoming new options might provide improved outcome particularly by diminishing the morbidity associated to graft harvesting and fasten the process of bone formation.

> **Memory**
>
> Two-stage revision after failed ACL repair must be understood as a challenging multifactorial entity. Preoperative planning is mandatory, and one should be prepared even for the unexpected. Surgeons must be experienced in primary ACL procedures and be aware of multiple options and devices to enable choosing the best approach in each specific case. In properly selected cases, good/fair results might be achieved. However, poorer outcome comparing to primary repair should be expected.

References

1. Aglietti P, Buzzi R, Giron F, Simeone AJ, Zaccherotti G (1997) Arthroscopic-assisted anterior cruciate ligament reconstruction with the central third patellar tendon. A 5-8-year follow-up. Knee Surg Sports Traumatol Arthrosc 5:138–144
2. Bach BR Jr (2003) Revision anterior cruciate ligament surgery. Arthroscopy 19(Suppl 1):14–29
3. Bohensky MA, deSteiger R, Kondogiannis C, Sundararajan V, Andrianopoulos N, Bucknill A et al (2013) Adverse outcomes associated with elective knee arthroscopy: a population-based cohort study. Arthroscopy 29:716–725
4. Burchardt H (1987) Biology of bone transplantation. Orthop Clin North Am 18:187–196
5. Chadwick CC, Rogowski J, Joyce BT (2008) The economics of anterior cruciate ligament reconstruction. In: Prodromos C, Brown C, Fu FH, Georgoulis AD, Gobbi A, Howell SM et al (eds) The anterior cruciate ligament: reconstruction and basic science. Saunders Elsevier, Philadelphia, pp 79–83
6. Csizy M, Friederich NF (2002) Bore canal site in surgical reconstruction of the anterior cruciate ligament. Position–placement errors–anatomic measurement. Orthopade 31:741–750
7. Dargel J, Gotter M, Mader K, Pennig D, Koebke J, Schmidt-Wiethoff R (2007) Biomechanics of the

anterior cruciate ligament and implications for surgical reconstruction. Strategies Trauma Limb Reconstr 2:1–12

8. Fare S, Torricelli P, Giavaresi G, Bertoldi S, Alessandrino A, Villa T et al (2013) In vitro study on silk fibroin textile structure for anterior cruciate ligament regeneration. Mater Sci Eng C Mater Biol Appl 33:3601–3608

9. Fasolis M, Boffano P, Ramieri G (2012) Morbidity associated with anterior iliac crest bone graft. Oral Surg Oral Med Oral Pathol Oral Radiol 114:586–591

10. Franceschi F, Papalia R, Del Buono A, Zampogna B, Diaz Balzani L, Maffulli N et al (2013) Two-stage procedure in anterior cruciate ligament revision surgery: a five-year follow-up prospective study. Int Orthop 37:1369–1374

11. Fu FH, Bennett CH, Lattermann C, Ma CB (1999) Current trends in anterior cruciate ligament reconstruction. Part 1: biology and biomechanics of reconstruction. Am J Sports Med 27:821–830

12. Gianotti SM, Marshall SW, Hume PA, Bunt L (2009) Incidence of anterior cruciate ligament injury and other knee ligament injuries: a national population-based study. J Sci Med Sport 12:622–627

13. Gomoll AH, Bach BRJ (2006) Managing tunnel malposition and widening in revision anterior cruciate ligament surgery. Oper Tech Sports Med 14:36–44

14. Gorschewsky O, Klakow A, Putz A, Mahn H, Neumann W (2007) Clinical comparison of the autologous quadriceps tendon (BQT) and the autologous patella tendon (BPTB) for the reconstruction of the anterior cruciate ligament. Knee Surg Sports Traumatol Arthrosc 15:1284–1292

15. Greene JW, Deshmukh AJ, Cushner FD (2013) Thromboembolic complications in arthroscopic surgery. Sports Med Arthrosc 21:69–74

16. Griffin LY, Albohm MJ, Arendt EA, Bahr R, Beynnon BD, Demaio M et al (2006) Understanding and preventing noncontact anterior cruciate ligament injuries: a review of the Hunt Valley II meeting, January 2005. Am J Sports Med 34:1512–1532

17. Griffith TB, Allen BJ, Levy BA, Stuart MJ, Dahm DL (2013) Outcomes of repeat revision anterior cruciate ligament reconstruction. Am J Sports Med 41:1296–1301

18. Groves C, Chandramohan M, Chew C, Subedi N (2013) Use of CT in the management of anterior cruciate ligament revision surgery. Clin Radiol 68(10):e552–e559

19. Harvey A, Thomas NP, Amis AA (2005) Fixation of the graft in reconstruction of the anterior cruciate ligament. J Bone Joint Surg Br 87:593–603

20. Janicki P, Schmidmaier G (2011) What should be the characteristics of the ideal bone graft substitute? Combining scaffolds with growth factors and/or stem cells. Injury 42(Suppl 2):S77–81

21. Johnson DL, Swenson TM, Irrgang JJ, Fu FH, Harner CD (1996) Revision anterior cruciate ligament surgery: experience from Pittsburgh. Clin Orthop Relat Res 325:100–109

22. Joyce MJ (2005) Safety and FDA regulations for musculoskeletal allografts: perspective of an orthopaedic surgeon. Clin Orthop Relat Res 435:22–30

23. Khan SN, Cammisa FP Jr, Sandhu HS, Diwan AD, Girardi FP, Lane JM (2005) The biology of bone grafting. J Am Acad Orthop Surg 13:77–86

24. Killion JA, Kehoe S, Geever LM, Devine DM, Sheehan E, Boyd D et al (2013) Hydrogel/bioactive glass composites for bone regeneration applications: Synthesis and characterisation. Mater Sci Eng C Mater Biol Appl 33:4203–4212

25. Lin G, Cosimbescu L, Karin NJ, Tarasevich BJ (2012) Injectable and thermosensitive PLGA-g-PEG hydrogels containing hydroxyapatite: preparation, characterization and in vitro release behavior. Biomed Mater 7(2):024107

26. Magnussen RA, Taylor DC, Toth AP, Garrett WE (2012) ACL graft failure location differs between allografts and autografts. Sports Med Arthrosc Rehabil Ther Technol 4:22

27. Mariscalco MW, Magnussen RA, Mehta D, Hewett TE, Flanigan DC, Kaeding CC (2013) Autograft versus nonirradiated allograft tissue for anterior cruciate ligament reconstruction: a systematic review. Am J Sports Med. doi:10.1177/0363546513497566

28. MTF (2005) Allograft safety and ethical considerations. Proceedings of the fourth symposium sponsored by the Musculoskeletal Transplant Foundation. September 2003. Edinburgh, Scotland, United Kingdom. Clin Orthop Relat Res 435:2–117

29. Musahl V, Plakseychuk A, VanScyoc A, Sasaki T, Debski RE, McMahon PJ et al (2005) Varying femoral tunnels between the anatomical footprint and isometric positions: effect on kinematics of the anterior cruciate ligament-reconstructed knee. Am J Sports Med 33:712–718

30. Oetgen ME, Smart LR, Medvecky MJ (2008) A novel technique for arthroscopically assisted femoral bone tunnel grafting in two-stage ACL revision. Orthopedics 31:16–18

31. Oliveira JM, Kotobuki N, Tadokoro M, Hirose M, Mano JF, Reis RL et al (2010) Ex vivo culturing of stromal cells with dexamethasone-loaded carboxymethyl-chitosan/poly(amidoamine) dendrimer nanoparticles promotes ectopic bone formation. Bone 46:1424–1435

32. Oliveira JM, Sousa RA, Kotobuki N, Tadokoro M, Hirose M, Mano JF et al (2009) The osteogenic differentiation of rat bone marrow stromal cells cultured with dexamethasone-loaded carboxymethylchitosan/poly(amidoamine) dendrimer nanoparticles. Biomaterials 30:804–813

33. Oliveira JM, Sousa RA, Malafaya PB, Silva SS, Kotobuki N, Hirose M et al (2011) In vivo study of dendronlike nanoparticles for stem cells "tune-up": from nano to tissues. Nanomedicine 7:914–924

34. Parkkari J, Pasanen K, Mattila VM, Kannus P, Rimpela A (2008) The risk for a cruciate ligament injury of the knee in adolescents and young adults: a population-based cohort study of 46 500 people with a 9 year follow-up. Br J Sports Med 42:422–426

35. Pascual-Garrido C, Carbo L, Makino A (2013) Revision of anterior cruciate ligament reconstruction with allografts in patients younger than 40 years old: a 2 to 4 year results. Knee Surg Sports Traumatol Arthrosc [Epub ahead of print]

36. Pereira H, Sevivas N, Varanda P, Monteiro A, Monllau JC, Espregueira-Mendes J (2013) Failed Anterior Cruciate Ligament Repair. In: Surgical Orthopaedics and Traumatology, Bentley G (ed.), Springer-Verlag Berlin Heidelberg, pp. 1–16

37. Prodromos CC, Joyce BT (2008) Allograft complications and risk factors. In: Prodromos C, Brown C, Fu FH, Georgoulis AD, Gobbi A, Howell SM, Johnson DL, Paulos LE, Shelbourne KD (eds) The anterior cruciate ligament: reconstruction and basic science. Saunders-Elsevier, Philadelphia, pp 561–564

38. Robertson A, Nutton RW, Keating JF (2006) Current trends in the use of tendon allografts in orthopaedic surgery. J Bone Joint Surg Br 88:988–992

39. Salgado AJ, Coutinho OP, Reis RL (2004) Bone tissue engineering: state of the art and future trends. Macromol Biosci 4:743–765

40. Samuelsson K, Andersson D, Karlsson J (2009) Treatment of anterior cruciate ligament injuries with special reference to graft type and surgical technique: an assessment of randomized controlled trials. Arthroscopy 25:1139–1174

41. Thomas NP, Kankate R, Wandless F, Pandit H (2005) Revision anterior cruciate ligament reconstruction using a 2-stage technique with bone grafting of the tibial tunnel. Am J Sports Med 33:1701–1709

42. Thomas NP, Pandit HG (2008) Revision anterior cruciate ligament. In: Prodromos C, Brown C, Fu FH, Georgoulis AD, Gobbi A, Howell SM, Johnson DL, Paulos LE, Shelbourne KD (eds) The anterior cruciate ligament: reconstruction and basic science. Saunders Elsevier, Philadelphia, pp 443–457

43. Tornctta P 3rd, Riina J, Geller J, Purban W (1999) Intraarticular anatomic risks of tibial nailing. J Orthop Trauma 13:247–251

44. Vangsness CT Jr, Garcia IA, Mills CR, Kainer MA, Roberts MR, Moore TM (2003) Allograft transplantation in the knee: tissue regulation, procurement, processing, and sterilization. Am J Sports Med 31:474–481

45. Wang CJ, Chan YS, Weng LH, Yuan LJ, Chen HS (2004) Comparison of autogenous and allogenous posterior cruciate ligament reconstructions of the knee. Injury 35:1279–1285

46. Wegrzyn J, Chouteau J, Philippot R, Fessy MH, Moyen B (2009) Repeat revision of anterior cruciate ligament reconstruction: a retrospective review of management and outcome of 10 patients with an average 3-year follow-up. Am J Sports Med 37:776–785

47. Wright R, Spindler K, Huston L, Amendola A, Andrish J, Brophy R et al (2011) Revision ACL reconstruction outcomes: MOON cohort. J Knee Surg 24:289–294

48. Wright RW, Gill CS, Chen L, Brophy RH, Matava MJ, Smith MV et al (2012) Outcome of revision anterior cruciate ligament reconstruction: a systematic review. J Bone Joint Surg Am 94:531–536

49. Wu CC, Wang CC, Lu DH, Hsu LH, Yang KC, Lin FH (2012) Calcium phosphate cement delivering zoledronate decreases bone turnover rate and restores bone architecture in ovariectomized rats. Biomed Mater 7:035009

50. Yan LP, Silva-Correia J, Correia C, Caridade SG, Fernandes EM, Sousa RA et al (2013) Bioactive macro/micro porous silk fibroin/nano-sized calcium phosphate scaffolds with potential for bone-tissue-engineering applications. Nanomedicine (Lond) 8:359–378

Bone Harvest from Iliac Crest and Bone Tunnel Filling

37

Rainer Siebold and Hans H. Pässler

Contents

R. Siebold (✉)
Institute for Anatomy and Cell Biology,
Ruprecht-Karls University Heidelberg,
Im Neuenheimer Feld 307, 69120 Heidelberg, Germany

HKF: Center for Spezialised Hip-Knee-Foot Surgery,
ATOS Hospital Heidelberg, Bismarckstr. 9-15, 69115
Heidelberg, Germany
e-mail: rainer.siebold@atos.de

H.H. Pässler
HKF: Center for Spezialised Hip-Knee-Foot Surgery,
ATOS Hospital Heidelberg, Bismarckstr. 9-15,
69115 Heidelberg, Germany

37.1   Principle

Through a mini-incision one or more corticocancellous bone plugs are harvested with special harvesting tubes (Fig. 37.1). The tubes are also used to insert the bone plugs into the tibial and femoral bone tunnels.

37.2   Advantages

A small 2–3-cm incision provides adequate access for harvesting the cylindric bone plugs from the iliac crest. The morbidity at the donor site is small with little postoperative pain. The bone plugs are harvested according to the diameter of the tibial and femoral bone tunnels and are introduced press-fit into the bony defect.

37.3   Surgical Technique

In case of revision ACL surgery, an arthroscopy is performed first. The old bone tunnels are cleaned. Therefore bone tunnels are overdrilled, starting with smaller drills, until the required diameter is achieved.

Next, the iliac crest is exposed through a 2–3-cm incision in the skin lines 2–3 cm posterior to the spina iliaca anterior superior. Carefully expose the periost of the iliac crest and use electrocautery for haemostasis and longitudinal periosteal incision. With an elevator, move the periosteum aside medially and laterally. If the bone plugs are

R. Siebold et al. (eds.), *Anterior Cruciate Ligament Reconstruction*,
DOI 10.1007/978-3-642-45349-6_37, © ESSKA 2014

Fig. 37.1 Harvesting tubes with trocar, internal diameters 8–14 mm (Richard Wolf, Germany)

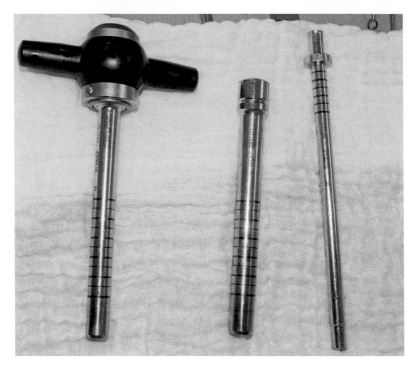

to be used for filling of old drill tunnels, we recommend not to remove the periosteum.

To mark the harvesting tube direction, insert one short 1.8-mm diameter K-wires each down the internal and the external aspect of the iliac crest. The harvesting tubes with trocar have internal diameters between 8 and 14 mm (Richard Wolf). The instruments are non-disposable.

Carefully harvest the required corticocancellous bone plug by using a mallet (Fig. 37.2). The depth (length) of the bone plug can be controlled by the scale on the harvesting tube. When the necessary length of the plug is achieved, remove the harvesting tube with the captured bone plug (Fig. 37.3).

The harvesting tube is also used for inserting the bone plugs into the tibial and femoral bone tunnels. The femoral bone plug is inserted through a low anteromedial portal or transtibial into the knee joint, depending on the femoral bone tunnel location. The tibial bone tunnel defect is filled from distal to proximal under arthroscopic visualisation (Fig. 37.4). The final result of press-fit bone tunnel filling with the plugs is displayed in Fig. 37.5, and the bone healing 6 months later in Fig. 37.6.

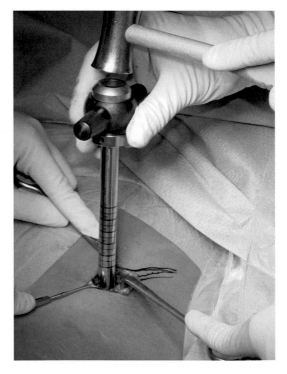

Fig. 37.2 Harvest of bone plug(s) from iliac crest

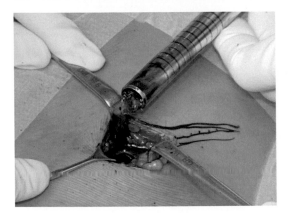

Fig. 37.3 Harvesting tube with captured bone plug

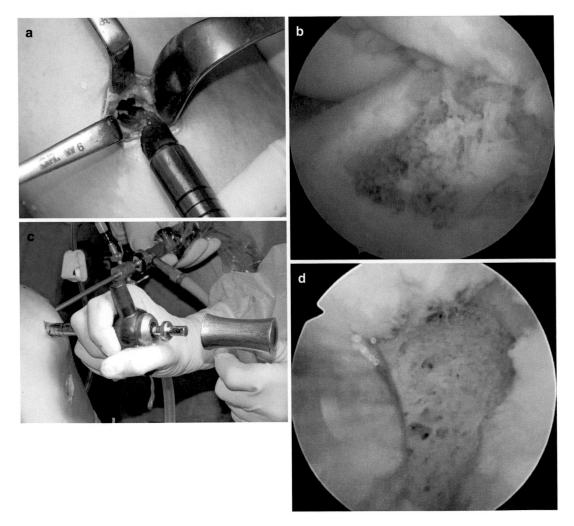

Fig. 37.4 Insertion of bone plugs into bone tunnels with harvesting tube: (**a**, **b**) tibial, (**c**, **d**) femoral

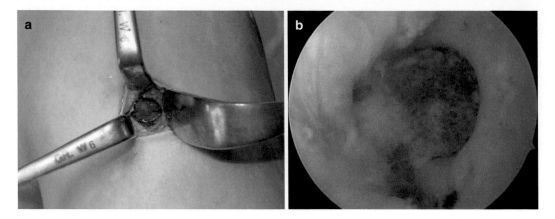

Fig. 37.5 Press-fit situation after insertion of plugs: (**a**) tibial, (**b**) femoral

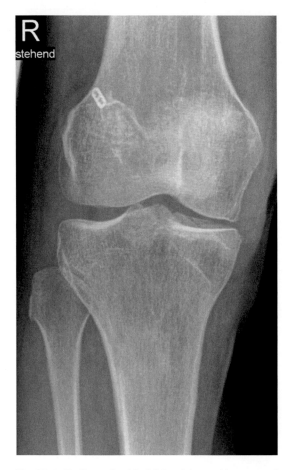

Fig. 37.6 Radiograph with tibial and femoral bone tunnel healing 5 months after spongiosaplasty

Surgical Technique

38

Pedro Pessoa

Contents

P. Pessoa, MD
Department of Knee, Orthopaedic Hospital
Santíago do Outão, Setúbal, Portugal
e-mail: ppessoa@sapo.pt

38.1   Introduction

The treatment of anterior instability is important for preventing meniscal and cartilage changes. The patient most often looks for an expert on the chronic phase as well as eventual advanced degenerative changes.

In *Arthroscopy* (2005), Nebelung verified that in a group of 19 athletes who underwent conservative treatment after ACL rupture, 79 % had meniscal injuries after 10 years. After 20 years, that number increased to 90 %, and 68 % of them had cartilage damage Outerbridge class IV. Also, 35 years later, 65 % had undergone a total knee replacement. So, it is clear that the conservative option remains a poor one [1, 2, 8, 9, 11].

The main goal of treatment is stabilizing the knee and preventing the degenerative changes. So, the assessment of cartilage and meniscal injuries and sagittal and coronal malalignment must be performed.

Clinical evaluation is most important. Instability is an early complaint; pain is a more delayed symptom.

Over time, stiffness increases and the patient complaints are mainly pain with a decrease of stability.

Surgical therapeutic options are reconstruction of the anterior cruciate ligament, alone or with other surgical procedures such as osteotomy, meniscal repair, or replacement. On sagittal or coronal malalignment, ACL repair alone can be insufficient to prevent the evolution of osteoarthritis.

R. Siebold et al. (eds.), *Anterior Cruciate Ligament Reconstruction*,
DOI 10.1007/978-3-642-45349-6_38, © ESSKA 2014

Unicompartmental replacement can be considered when there is isolated symptomatic osteoarthritis of either the medial or lateral compartment [4].

Indications
  Standing varus malalignment
  Symptomatic isolated medial compartment arthritis with instability
Contraindications
  Deformity over 15°
  Flexion contracture over 15°
  Knee flexion under 90°
  Excessive medial bone loss (over 3 mm)
  Inflammatory arthritis
  Patella baja

Anteroposterior radiographs on single leg stance and a profile view on weightbearing at 30° of flexion are important (Figs. 38.1, 38.2, and 38.3). The MRI allows us to access the cartilage, meniscal, and ligament status.

For a chronic anterior cruciate ligament deficiency with a mild arthrosis, a coronal malalignment, and a *varus* context, the most consistent solution would be to combine the ACL reconstruction with a high tibial osteotomy (HTO) for alignment correction [3, 5, 7, 10, 12–16].

Performing it at once or twice [5, 7], with intra-articular plasty or combined with an extra-articular

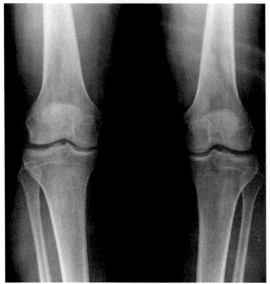

Fig. 38.2 The x-ray on weightbearing gives us information about the true degree of arthrosis

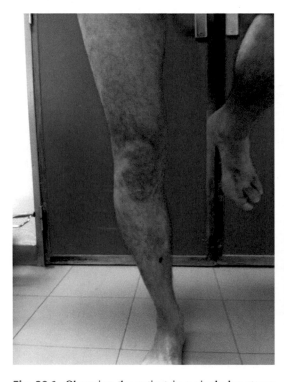

Fig. 38.1 Observing the patient in a single leg stance gives us information about the stability of the knee

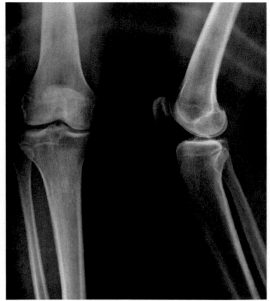

Fig. 38.3 The x-ray in profile with 30° flexion shows a more conclusive image of the articular line

plasty, using a single bundle or double bundle, are matters of personal choice.

Simultaneous high tibial *valgus* osteotomy and ACL reconstruction is most often indicated at chronic anterior knee instability for patients younger than 40 years. It is a surgical procedure with low morbidity and a high degree of satisfaction (80 %), and it is highly successful in limiting pain (60 %) and reducing instability (90 %). It is found that 40 % of patients regain sports activity [1, 2, 8, 9, 11, 13].

The loss of meniscal tissue worsens the prognosis; so whenever possible we try to repair the meniscus. If the patient has undergone a previous subtotal meniscectomy, we proceed to a meniscal replacement. If a remaining meniscal rim exists, we prefer the "synthetic scaffold"; if not, the option will be a meniscal allograft.

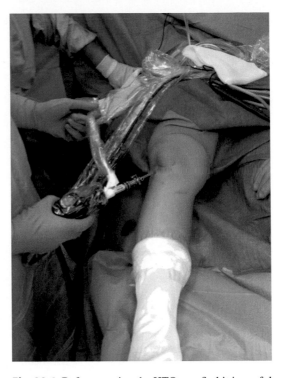

Fig. 38.4 Before starting the HTO, we find it is useful to arthroscopically inspect the knee. If there is involvement of more than 1 compartment, the technique is not indicated

38.2 Technique 1: Subtraction High Tibial Osteotomy

1. Start with an arthroscopic evaluation about meniscal and chondral status; if an evolved osteoarthritis process compromises the lateral compartment, the HTO must not be performed (Fig. 38.4).
2. Proceed with graft collection. Hamstrings are most often used (Fig. 38.5).
3. During the 1st arthroscopy, a femoral tunnel is performed in anatomical position, through the medial portal, getting a reference lead (Fig. 38.6a, b).

> **Pearls**
> • A lateral post is used instead of a leg holder to allow the surgeon to hyperflex the knee to 120° while performing the femoral tunnel.

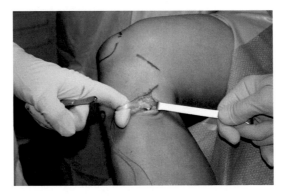

Fig. 38.5 Operative view of hamstrings harvesting

4. Begin the osteotomy. Fibula osteotomy is performed about the proximal half 1/3 fibular transition. The knee position—bent at 90°—allows muscle relaxation and facilitates the

bone access (Fig. 38.7). Feel the fibula and make a 2-cm longitudinal incision (Fig. 38.8a, b). The fibula osteotomy is performed with a saw and finished with laminar osteotome. Always use 2 (Holman) guards to engage the fibula segment, protecting the lateral popliteal sciatic nerve.

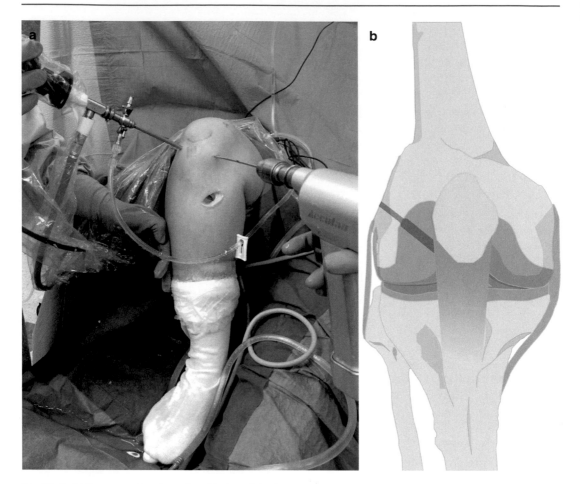

Fig. 38.6 (**a**) Intraoperative view of perforation of the femoral tunnel through the medial portal with the knee in hyperflexion. (**b**) Schematic view of the femoral tunnel

Pearls
- The fibula osteotomy at the proximal 1/3–half 1/3 transition is easily performed with reduced morbidity (Fig. 38.9). Alternatively, the dislocation of the fibula at a proximal level in most cases complicates the process of osteoclasia and the osteotomy closure and can lead to chronic instability in the same proximal tibiofibular articulation.

5. Next, the tibial osteotomy is performed. Skin incision in S lazy, launched at the interline level, extending distally between Gerdy's tubercle and the head of the fibula (Fig. 38.10).

6. Muscles are partly detached from the tibia anterolateral face. Mark up the osteotomy with 2 K-wires and the help of image intensifier (Fig. 38.11a, b).
7. The tibial osteotomy is performed with a saw and ends up with an osteotome drive. Cut up the wedge bone and make up the inner cortical osteoclasia (Fig. 38.12a–c). The fixation is usually performed with the use of a Coventry staple (Fig. 38.13a, b). If necessary, 2 staples or a plate and screws can be used.

Avoid Pitfalls
- When placing the staples, confirm with the arthroscope whether they are totally extra-articular. The fluoroscopic imaging can be misleading.

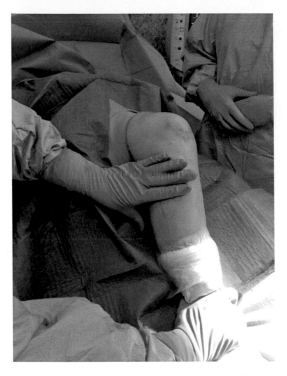

Fig. 38.7 Preparing for fibular osteotomy. Bending the knee to 90° facilitates the approach

> **Pearls**
> • The approach made for hamstring graft harvest at the medial side of the knee can be used to place a retractor and protect the posterior surface of leg vessels when the tibial osteotomy is performed.

8. After the osteotomy closure, the surgery is finished with the second intra-articular phase, performing the tibial tunnel with usual (55°) angle, passage of the graft, and its fixation with femoral button and screw or tibial knob (Figs. 38.14, 38.15, and 38.16a, b).

9. Use an intra-articular 12-mm drain tube and 2 silastic vascular drains at the osteotomy spot (Fig. 38.17).

> **Avoid Pitfalls**
> Be careful when placing the lateral retractor to avoid exaggerated pressure over the common peroneal nerve. Always use a drain over the osteotomy site to avoid postoperative hematoma and late compression of the common peroneal nerve.

> **Pearls**
> • After the tibia osteotomy fixation, the ACL ligament reconstruction, whatever the technique, is easily performed and does not require modification of the surgical procedure. When combining an ACL reconstruction with an osteotomy, it is essential that the fixation is reliable, allowing us to undertake the ACL rehabilitation with no mobility restriction.

> **Pearls**
> • Another possibility is the "all-inside" ligamentoplasty technique, making the harvest of the graft in the knee posterior face and the tunnels inside-out. Thus we avoid a second incision on the inner side of the knee (Fig. 38.18a–d).

> **Avoid Pitfalls**
> • If you choose to harvest the hamstring graft in the posterior aspect of the knee, use the closed tenotome and position the knee in 45° flexion with the leg in external rotation to avoid sectioning the graft.

38.3 Technique 2: Addition High Tibial Osteotomy

1. Start with the first arthroscopic inspection (Fig. 38.19), proceeding with evaluation and repair of meniscal and chondral lesions. Appreciate the lateral enclosure.

2. At this first arthroscopic inspection, the femoral tunnel should be performed in anatomical position, through the medial portal (Fig. 38.20). The tibial tunnel is also performed at the usual angle (55°).

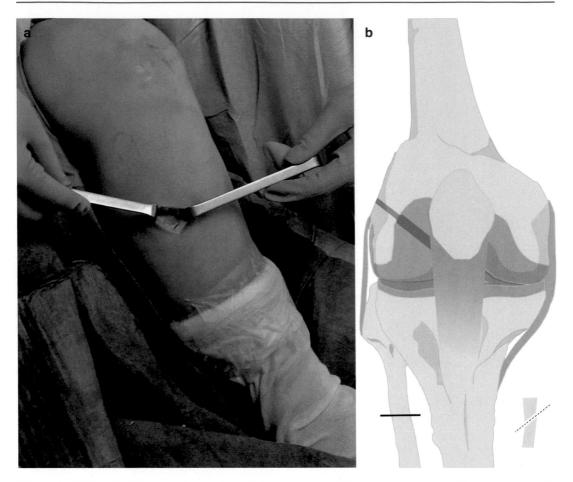

Fig. 38.8 (a) The fibula is exposed at the level of the osteotomy, taking care to protect the adjacent structures. (b) Schematic view of the level of the fibular osteotomy

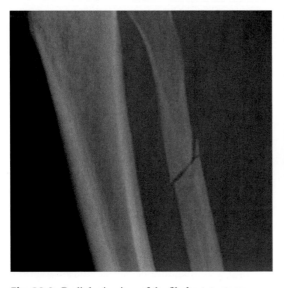

Fig. 38.9 Radiologic view of the fibular osteotomy

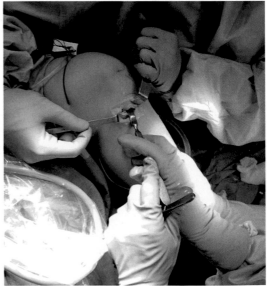

Fig. 38.10 Exposing the tibia for the proximal osteotomy

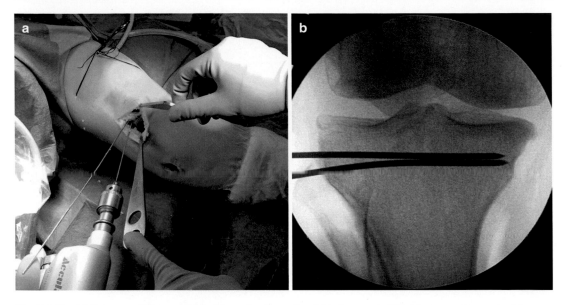

Fig. 38.11 (a) It is essential to mark the place for the osteotomy with 2 K-wires that will guide the saw. (b) Using the image intensifier is useful for confirmation of the right placement of the K-wires and to control the progression of the bone saw

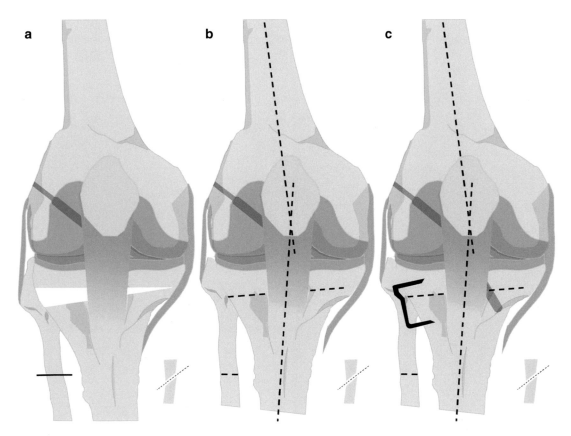

Fig. 38.12 (a) Schematic view of the tibial osteotomy. (b) Schematic view of the alignment correction after closing the osteotomy. (c) Schematic view of osteotomy fixation with a staple

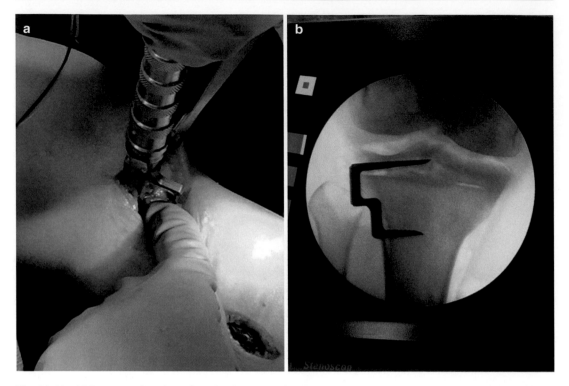

Fig. 38.13 (**a**) Intraoperative view of staple placement. (**b**) The position of the staple should be confirmed with the image intensifier

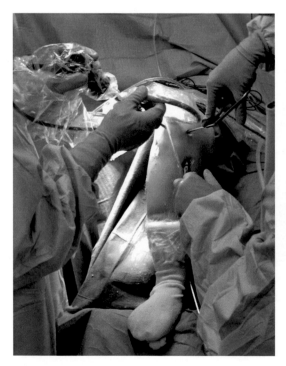

Fig. 38.14 Intraoperative view of the tibial tunnel in place

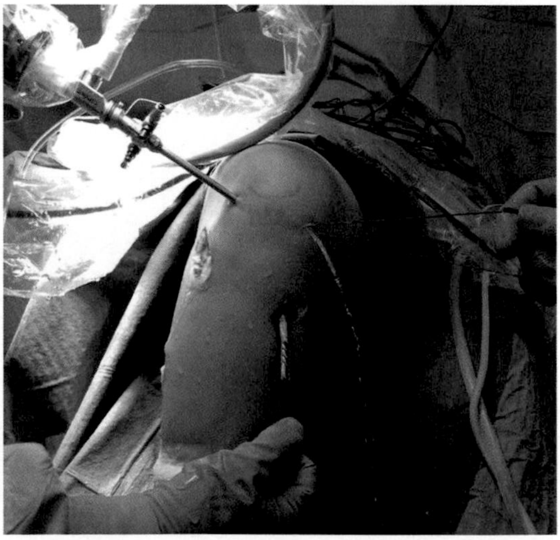

Fig. 38.15 The hamstrings graft is introduced through the tibial tunnel and carefully pulled under arthroscopic control

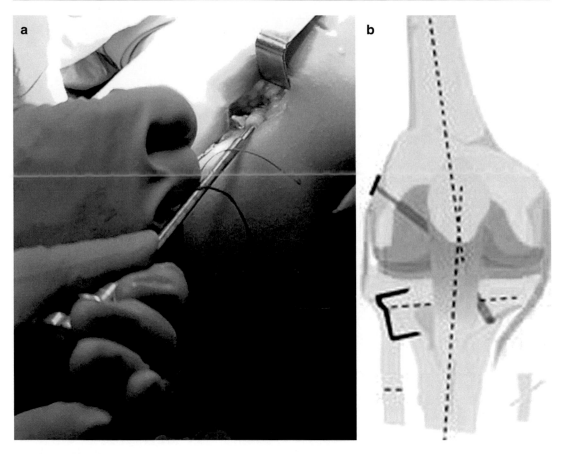

Fig. 38.16 (**a**) The graft is fixed proximally with a cortical suspension device and distally with an interferential screw. (**b**) Schematic view of alignment correction with the graft fixed in place

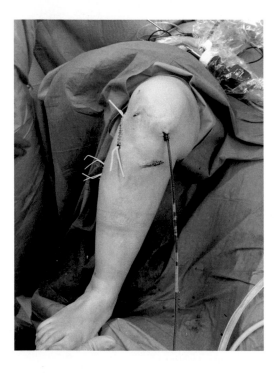

3. Make the graft collection. Feel the hamstrings at the medial face of tibial level, about 2 cm of the anterior tuberosity. The oblique incision extends proximally about 5 cm (Fig. 38.21).
4. Then begin the osteotomy. The surface beam should be protected from the medial collateral ligament; place a retractor in the tibial posterior face to protect the vessels (Fig. 38.22). The popliteal artery, even with the knee in flexion, is about 0.5 mm from the level at which the osteotomy is performed (Fig. 38.23a–c).

Fig. 38.17 Using a drain in every surgical approach avoids postoperative complications

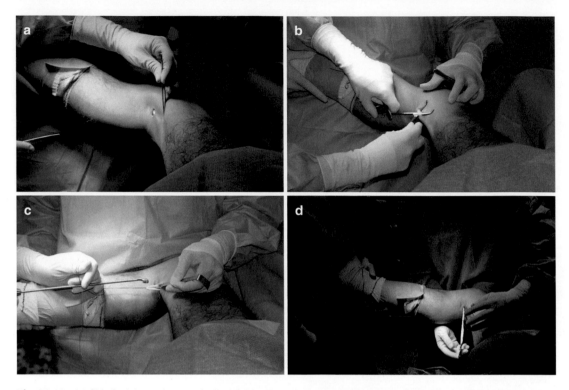

Fig. 38.18 (**a**) Skin incision to harvest the hamstrings through a posterior approach. (**b**) Using the all-inside technique, only 1 of the hamstrings is harvested. (**c**) An open tenotome is used. (**d**) The hamstring is safely harvested

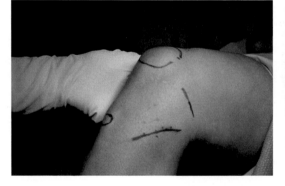 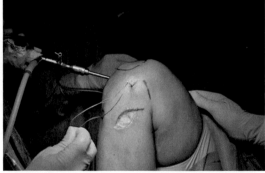

Fig. 38.19 The anatomical references are drawn prior to the start of the arthroscopic inspection of the knee

Fig. 38.20 The femoral tunnel is drilled through the medial portal with the knee in hyperflexion to obtain an anatomical placement

Fig. 38.23 (**a**) Schematic view of femoral and tibial tunnel position. (**b**) Schematic view of osteotomy placement and direction. (**c**) Schematic view highlighting the importance of the manual osteotome

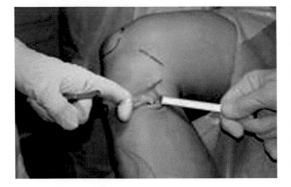

Fig. 38.21 The hamstrings are harvested

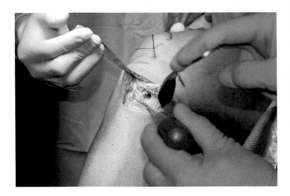

Fig. 38.22 The osteotomy is started with a bone saw and carefully finished with use of an osteotome

Prevent Complications

- During the osteotomy an image intensifier is used for control, so we can see if the saw/osteotome follows the intended route; confirm this before making the osteoclasia (Figs. 38.24 and 38.25).
- The risk of a fracture of the tibial plateau is not negligible, despite being a complication that usually does not require a modification of the surgical procedure; however, it requires some changes to the postoperative protocol.
- A postoperative hematoma at the incision for the osteotomy is another possible complication, though it can be partially resolved by replacing the vascular drains by aspirative tubular drains (with vacuum).

5. When you add this plate, it should be placed as posterior as possible, in order to intervene as little as possible with the tibial tunnel (Fig. 38.26). Screw drilling must be controlled by placing the arthroscope at the tibial tunnel

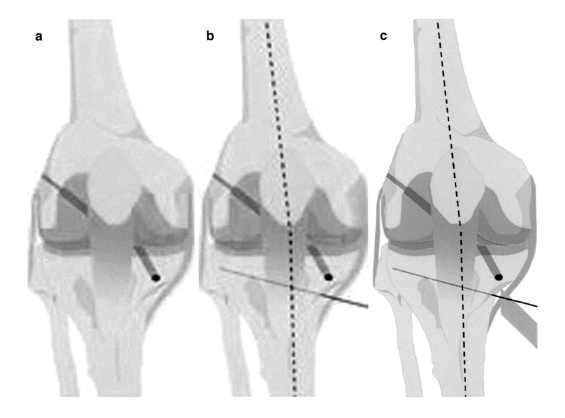

a   b   c

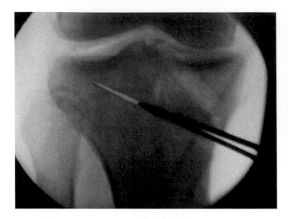

Fig. 38.24 Using the K-wire and image intensifier control to confirm the direction of the osteotomy

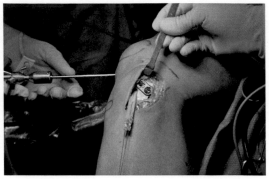

Fig. 38.27 The hamstring graft is introduced through the tibial tunnel after plate fixation

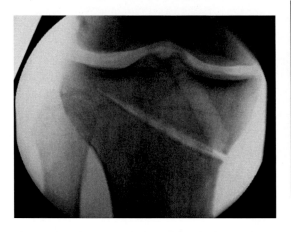

Fig. 38.25 The ostoclasia is performed after confirmation of adequate direction

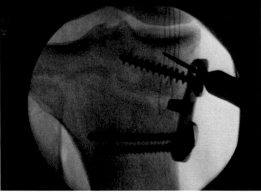

Fig. 38.28 The plate fixation is controlled with the use of image intensifier

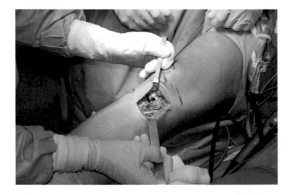

Fig. 38.26 The plate is placed as posterior as possible to avoid interference with the tibial tunnel

to prevent the screws from interfering with graft passage.

6. In a later surgical step, we pass a forceps through the tibial tunnel, under arthroscopic control; then the femoral tunnel/portal anatomical passage wire is retracted. Next, the graft is passed through the tibial tunnel, tensioned, and fixed with a screw (Figs. 38.27, 38.28, and 38.29a, b).

7. Whether the tibial tunnel should be performed prior or after the osteotomy closure and fixation is still controversial. We leave the choice to the surgeon (Figs. 38.30, 38.31, 38.32, 38.33, 38.34, and 38.35).

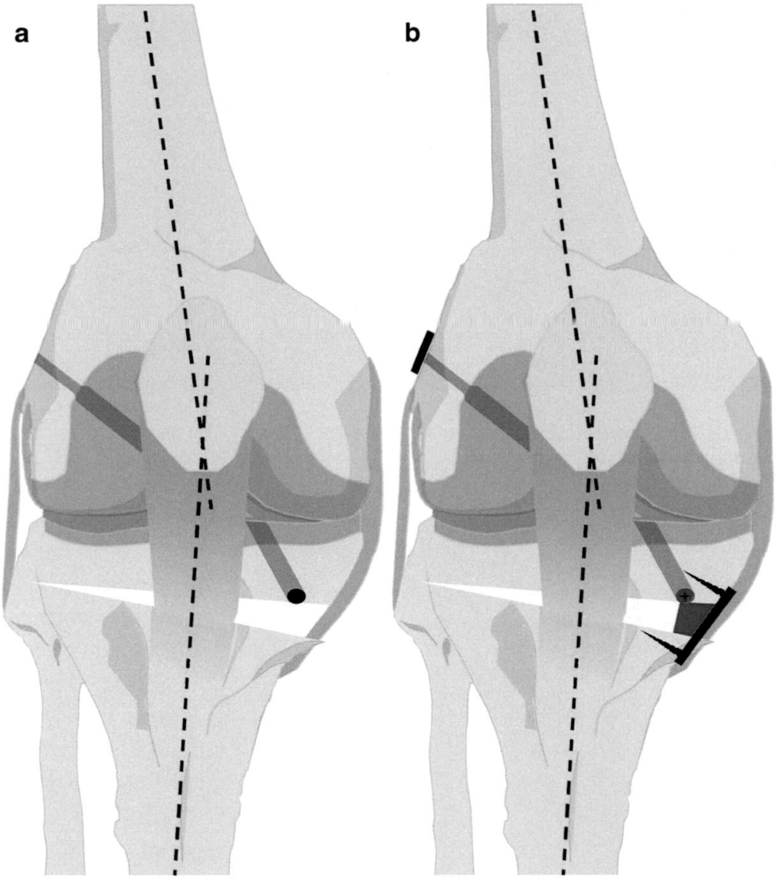

Fig. 38.29 (**a**) Schematic view of alignment correction after osteotomy opening. (**b**) Schematic view of fixation of the opening osteotomy with Puddu-like plate

a

b

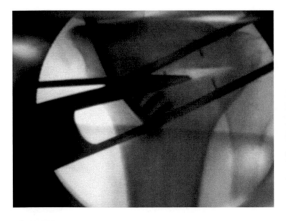

Fig. 38.30 Tibial osteotomy is performed prior to tibial tunnel drilling

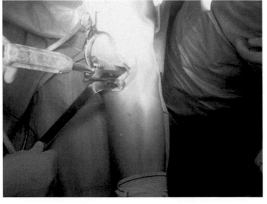

Fig. 38.31 The osteotomy is opened with help of a spacer

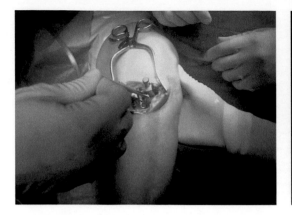

Fig. 38.32 The opening is maintained by the spacer during the plate selection and fixation

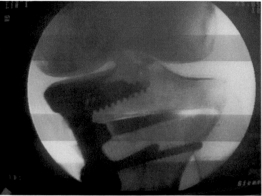

Fig. 38.34 Plate fixation with control of image intensifier

38.4 Recovery

Postoperatively the patient remains hospitalized for 2 days, starts mobilizing and strengthening. The ligament reconstruction rehabilitation protocol does not change.

There is no plastered immobilization. The patient is left with an intra-articular suction drain and a vascular silastic drain at the tibial incision. It is placed a simple bandage, reinforced by a layer of cotton and an elastic bandage, from the foot to the root of the thigh.

The patient starts continuous passive motion 24 h after surgery and rises on the first day.

Drains are removed at 24/48 h.

The patient should walk with crutches for 4 weeks, non-weightbearing for the first week and weightbearing afterward. Knee flexion by the second day after surgery should be 90° and 120° at sixth week.

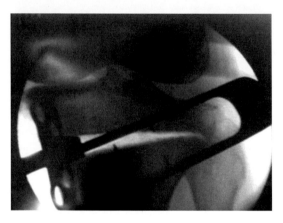

Fig. 38.33 Plate positioning with control of image intensifier

---

Pearls

- When the screws are placed on the osteotomy plate, put the optic in the tibial tunnel and prevent drilling through this tunnel (Fig. 38.36).
- The screw placement is not always easy. To obviate this difficulty, we first perform the femoral tunnel, then we place the tibial plate and screws and only after the tibial tunnel is performed, diverging more or less, and with a more open or closed angle (50°/70°).

Memory

Chronic ACL insufficiency and knee instability lead in the long term to the development of knee osteoarthritis. This degenerative process will be exacerbated if there is also limb malangulation. Performing ACL reconstruction and corrective tibial osteotomy at the same time

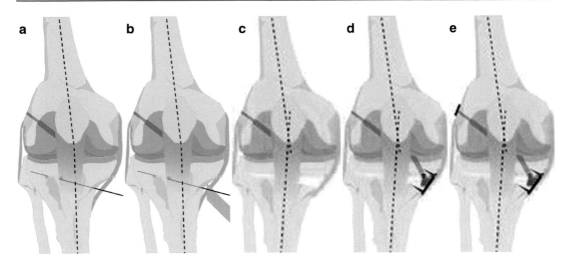

Fig. 38.35 (**a**) Schematic view of tibial osteotomy direction marked with a K-wire. (**b**) Schematic view of tibial osteotomy with saw and osteotome. (**c**) Schematic view of alignment correction after opening of the osteotomy. (**d**) Schematic view of tibial tunnel drilled after plate fixation. (**e**) Schematic view of graft positioned in placed

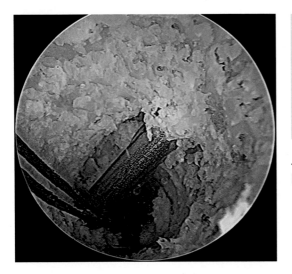

Fig. 38.36 When drilling the holes for placement of the screws, an arthroscopic view of the tibial tunnel is useful to confirm that the tunnel is not violated

The technique of simultaneous ACL reconstruction and corrective high tibial osteotomy shows excellent results and a relative low complication rate. However, it should be performed by a skilled surgeon with good experience in knee pathology.

is a technique increasingly used, but this requires proper preoperative planning. When planning this surgery, the surgeon may desire to include additional cartilage surgery or allograft meniscus replacement, and in this case the tourniquet time is an important aspect to consider.

References

1. Aqueskirchner JD, Bernau A, Burkart AC, Imhoff AB (2002) Knee instability and varus malangulation – simultaneous cruciate ligament reconstruction and osteotomy (indication, planning and operative technique, results). Z Orthop Ihre Grenzgeb 140(2):185–193
2. Bonin N, Ait Si Selmi T, Donell ST, Dejour H, Neyret P (2004) Anterior cruciate reconstruction combined with valgus upper tibial osteotomy: 12 years follow-up. Knee 11(6):431–437
3. Boss A, Stutz G, Oursin C, Gächter A (1995) Anterior cruciate ligament reconstruction combined with valgus tibial osteotomy (combined procedure). Knee Surg Sports Traumatol Arthrosc 3(3):187–191
4. Citak M, Bosscher F, Musali V, Pearle A, Suero E (2011) "Anterior cruciate ligament reconstruction after unicompartmental knee arthroplasty" – Knee Surgery Sport Traumatol. Arthroscopy 19:1683–1688
5. Imhoff AB, Linke RD, Agneskirchner J (2004) Corrective osteotomy in primary varus, double varus and triple varus knee instability with cruciate ligament replacement. Orthopade 33(2):201–207

6. Kim SJ, Moon HK, Chun YM, Chang WH, Kim SG (2011) Is correctional osteotomy crucial in primary varus knees undergoing anterior cruciate ligament reconstruction. Clin Orthop Relat Res 469(5):1421–1426, Epub 2010 Sep 25

7. Lattermann C, Jakob RP (1996) High tibial osteotomy alone or combined with ligament reconstruction in anterior cruciate ligament-deficient knees. Knee Surg Sports Traumatol Arthrosc 4(1):32–38

8. Lerat JL, Moyen B, Garin C, Mandrino A, Besse JL, Brunet-Guedj E (1993) Anterior laxity and internal arthritis of the knee. Results of the reconstruction of the anterior cruciate ligament associated with tibial osteotomy. Rev Chir Orthop Reparatrice Appar Mot 79(5):365–374

9. Nebelung W, Wuschech H (2005) Thirty five years follow-up of anterior cruciate ligament deficient knee in high level athletes. Arthroscopy 21:696–702

10. Neuschwander DC, Drez D Jr, Paine RM (1993) Simultaneous high tibial osteotomy and ACL reconstruction for combined genu varum and symptomatic ACL tear. Orthopedics 16(6):679–684

11. Noyes FR, Barber SD, Simon R (1993) High tibial osteotomy and ligament reconstruction in varus angulated, anterior cruciate ligament-deficient knees. A stwo- to seven-year follow-up study. Am J Sports Med 21(1):2–12

12. Noyes FR, Barber-Westin SD, Hewett TE (2000) High tibial osteotomy and ligament reconstruction for varus angulated anterior cruciate ligament-deficient knees. Am J Sports Med 28(3):282–296

13. O'Neill DF, James SL (1992) Valgus osteotomy with anterior cruciate ligament laxity. Clin Orthop Relat Res 278:153–159

14. Roscher E, Martinek V, Imhoff AB (1998) Anterior cruciate ligament-plasty and high valgus tibial osteotomy as a combined procedure in anterior instability and varus deviation. Zentralbl Chir 123(9):1019–1026

15. Stutz G, Boss A, Gächter A (1996) Comparison of augmented and non-augmented anterior cruciate ligament reconstruction combined with high tibial osteotomy. Knee Surg Sports Traumatol Arthrosc 4(3):143–148

16. Williams RJ 3rd, Kelly BT, Wickiewicz TL, Altchek DW, Warren RF (2003) The short-term outcome of surgical treatment for painful varus arthritis in association with chronic ACL deficiency. J Knee Surg 16(1):9–16

Results of Combined High Tibial Osteotomy (HTO) and ACL Reconstruction

39

Christophe Hulet, Aude Sebilo, and Sylvie Collon

Contents

39.1   Introduction

An ACL-deficient knee combined with medial meniscectomy and varus malalignment can be a risk factor precipitating the progression of arthritis. In these particular clinical conditions, combined surgery associated with ACL reconstruction and HTO represents an interesting salvage procedure for such complex patients who are usually young and willing to improve their function for both pain and instability. The purpose of the surgery is to keep participating in sports leisure activity.

39.2   Literature Results

According to the literature, from 1990 to 2013, over a 23-year period, we found only 18 publications associating HTO and ACL reconstruction, a staged concomitant procedure using a variety of PCL grafts or osteotomy technique. The main characteristics of the papers are summarized in Table 39.1.

In all these publications, the material of the study presents similar characteristics. The number of patients in each series is very low, from 5 to 51 cases, compared to the number of isolated ACL reconstruction during the same period. In most situations, these young patients (20–25 years old) were sportsmen, most often competitors. They have had an ACL injury in 80–90 % of cases with at least 10–15 years of evolution. Therefore, they had chronic anterior laxity with a former long delay between injury and surgery (more than 10

C. Hulet, MD, Pr (✉)
A. Sebilo, MD • S. Collon, MD
Orthopedic Department, Comete INSERM
U1075 – UCBN EA 3917, Caen University
Hospital, Avenue de la Côte de Nacre,
14033 Caen, France
e-mail: hulet-c@chu-caen.fr

R. Siebold et al. (eds.), *Anterior Cruciate Ligament Reconstruction*,
DOI 10.1007/978-3-642-45349-6_39, © ESSKA 2014

Table 39.1 Association of ACL reconstruction and high tibial osteotomy

Author	FU (years)	n	Age	% Medial meniscectomy	Delay for surgery	Open-wedge or closing osteotomy	Time table
Badhe et al. [1]	2.8	14	34	?	8.3 years	10 F/4 O	6 same time
Boileau and Neyret [2]	4	58	28	73	5 years	51C/7 O	52 same time 6 later
Bonin et al. [3, 4]	12	30	30	63	7 years	25C/5O	Same time
Boss et al. [5]	6.25	27	36	74	?	24C/3 O	Same time
Boussaton and Potel [6]	6.5	51	36	78	9 years	51C	Same time
Dejour et al. [7]	3.6	44	29	61	6 years	37C/7 O	Same time
Demange et al. [8]		8	39.1	?	?	O	Same time
Garin et al. [9]	3	18	36	77		13C/5 O	Same time
Imhoff et al. [10]	?	55	33				Same time
Lattermann and Jakob [11]	5.8	27	37	92.5	8.3 years	17C/10 O	8 same time 8 later
Lerat et al. [12]	4	51	37	86	9.5 years	39C/12 O	Same time
Neuschwander et al. [13]	2.5	5	27	100	7 years	7C	Same time
Noyes et al. [14]	4.5	41	29	73	6.5 years	41C	3 same time 38 later
Noyes et al. [15]	5	41	32	93	10 years	41C	16 later
O'Neill and James [16]	3	10	32.1	100		10C	7 same time 3 later
Zaffagnini et al. [17]	6.5	32	40.1	53	10 years	32C	Same time
Williyears III et al. [18]	3.5	25	35.5	96		25C	13 same time

years). They also present severe cartilage damage, and during this period a medial meniscectomy was very frequently observed from 56 to 100 % of medial meniscectomy. Zaffagnini et al. [17] also report a high frequency of previous ACL reconstruction (40 %). The mean age of this study (40.1 years) was older than in other previous studies, and the mean delay from injury to injury was longer (10.4±8.1 years).

At the time of surgery, patients were active but presented both knee pain and knee instability as objectives measured by instrumental laxity measurement. The main symptoms for indications were instability and pain in the medial compartment. Radiographically, there was pre-arthritic change in most of the patients with joint space narrowing less than 50 %. There was a varus deformity with a global hip knee angle in the varus (3.8±2.7° for Zaffagnini et al. [17] and 3° for Bonin et al. [3, 4]. The results are interesting with low morbidity and low failure rate at femoral follow-up. With a mean 6.5 years of follow-up, the failure rate was 6 % for Zaffagnini et al. [17] and two cases of stiffness for Bonin et al. [3, 4].

In the earliest series, it was a staged procedure [11, 14, 15], and there was an evolution with combined procedure using closing wedge or medial addition as an HTO technique. Special care was performed to avoid increasing tibial posterior slope. Increased slope causes a significant anterior and superior translation of the tibial plateau with respect to the femoral condyle [19], leading to an increase in anterior instability.

Actually, procedures were performed in combined concomitant surgery due to the low morbidity indicated in the initial studies. For the HTO, closing wedge, or medial addition, there was no superiority from one technique compared to the other one [20, 21]. In medial osteotomy addition, the internal precision angular correction is better (57–70 %). It is more readily reproducible and is associated with a deflection osteotomy [20, 22]. This osteotomy leaves intact the fibula. The risk of increasing tibial slope with decreased patellar height should be taken into account. A staple or a plate performs the fixation, which is sometimes a challenging issue in performing tibial tunnel and distal attachment. The stability of the transplant in such conditions requires a second tibial attachment.

The closing-wedge osteotomy is above the tuberosity with a less angular accuracy in the correction (26–78 % [21]). It requires an osteotomy of the fibula associated with risks to the common peroneal nerve and compartment syndrome. There is a risk of destabilization of the tibiofibular joint. The tibial slope is less modified, and Lerat [23] observed a better correction of the anterior tibial translation. It relaxes the patellar tendon with an increase in the patellar height. The stability of the graft is better because it is continuous in a bone tunnel; a single mode of attachment is sufficient [22, 24]. The osteosynthesis plate may cause a conflict with the anterior-posterior direction of the tibial tunnel. All these elements should be involved in choosing the type of osteotomy, but for Lerat [23], the experience of the operator is also crucial for the reliability of the techniques as osteotomy is one of the most uncertain. Regarding the mechanical axis, the goal is to achieve 3° valgus deformity [3, 4, 7, 14, 15], up to 6° in Lattermann's report [11]. The axial correction should be at least up to 6° of valgus deformity from the initial varus deformity to change the constraints of the knee to overload the lateral compartment and unload the medial compartment. Particular attention is required during the surgery to avoid increasing the posterior tibial slope. Lerat [23] and the Sofcot group [25] showed that the open-wedge HTO increases slope with a mean of 0.6° compared to closing wedge with tibial slope decrease of 0.7. During the procedure, whatever your option, great care should be addressed to avoid increase of PT slope. This objective could be achieved by using computer-assisted surgery as described by Demange et al. [8] with better accuracy.

For the ACL reconstruction, both the intra-articular graft and in some situation an extra-articular tenodesis were added to better control the ATT laxity. However, with the small number available, no statistical significant difference could be shown. An ACI procedure could be associated simultaneously as described by Elser [26].

Clinically, patients are satisfied or very satisfied in 80–90 % of cases. A significant number of active patients were able to resume moderate sports activity (44–47 %) [3, 4, 12, 17], but it does not seem reasonable to encourage them to return to sports competition. Age at surgery is not a limiting factor in the recovery of a recreational sport. The knee stability obtained is essential [3, 4, 7, 11, 14, 15], and it is closely related to the disappearance of knee pain. Factors that limit return to sports activities were as follows: long delay between initial injury and surgery, previous surgeries, cartilage lesion, and residual laxity greater than 10 mm [6]. Also, the changes of the global morphotype with valgus lead to change the balance in single leg stance with all proprioceptive sensations. This new situation needs at least 1 year of assimilation and good adaptation to the new position for the most active patients prior to return to sports activity.

The result on pain is good (55–64 % of cases). The instability is well controlled: 78–90 % of negative Lachman and 88–96 % of negative pivot shift tests. For Bonin et al. [3, 4], the overall results are significantly related to the importance of preoperative tibial translation and revision. At final revision some patients still had relevant anterior laxity (27 % grade C for Bonnin et al. [3, 4], 2 % for Zaffagnini et al. [17]). However, in such condition, with knee major instability, the anterior tibial translation remains greater than normal.

Radiographically, the midterm (4–5 years) evolution of OA medial femorotibial compartment was stabilized. At 8.5 years, Zaffagnini et al. [17] found only an increase of one case for grade C compared to the preop level (18 versus 17). This inhibitory effect on the evolution OA is sustainable beyond 10 years. Bonin et al. [3, 4] reviewed the patients 11 years later in the same group as Dejour et al. [7] and found only five cases of aggravation of class (17 %).

These results should be compared with the isolated ACL grafts with 10 years of follow-up, where the rate of change in OA varies between 15 and 25 % [24, 27]. In case of isolated ACL reconstruction without medial meniscectomy, the growth rate is 10 % in OA against more than 40 % when a medial meniscectomy pre- or intra-operatively was performed [24]. These highly significant differences confirm the prognostic role important to the medial meniscal preservation of the capital [28]. In all these studies, the percentage of medial meniscectomy was between 60 and 100 %.

Fig. 39.1 Evolution of symptoms and discomfort during natural history of ACL tear at the stage of chronic anterior laxity (5–10 years of natural history) with pre-arthritis or joint space narrowing less than 50 %

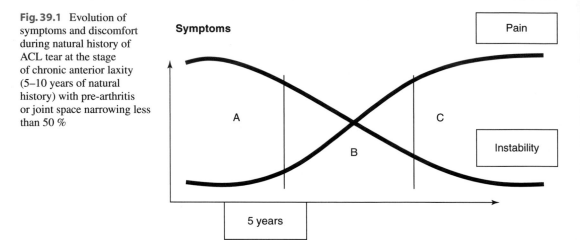

A Instability dominates, *B* Pain and instability coexist, *C* Pain dominates

A controversial topic regarding HTO is the relevance of posterior tibial slope and its effect on ACL-deficient knee with a chronic laxity. This is participating to the sagittal imbalance. Bonin et al. [29] showed the important role played by the genu varum and tibial slope. When the tibial slope exceeds 13°, it is considered excessive deflection, and an osteotomy may be associated with the ACL graft [22, 30]. There is a significant correlation between the correction of the posterior tibial slope and correction of the anterior tibial translation [29]. Deflection tibial osteotomy (i.e., to say a front closure) internally associated to an ACL graft is recommended [22, 31]. The slope should be standardized around 4°. The indication must be made in a patient with unstable little osteoarthritis, anterior tibial translation difference of more than 10 mm, and a posterior tibial slope of more than 13°.

Globally, patients are subjectively very happy after this double intervention. The improvement is clear on functional impairment, and there is a significant decrease in residual laxity. Osteoarthritis is not obviously worsened. However, patients with a decrease of 5 years have a net decrease in the level of sports, and the period of rehabilitation and recovery is long.

39.3 Conclusion

In patient with a history of chronic ACL deficiency with previous medial meniscectomy, the clinical evaluation should focus on these parameters for better indication [30].

The most important parameters were:

The determination of the main symptom (Fig. 39.1). During the natural history of ACL deficiency, pain and instability occurred in a different way. Instability is the most important parameter after the ACL tear but with time decreased progressively to the second level.

At the opposite, pain is not very relevant compared to ACL tear, but with time and previous surgery could be the first symptom after the untreated ACL tear.

- The evaluation of the laxity with instrumental measurement.
- The capital medial meniscus.
- The radiological analysis of the knee osteoarthritis with specific attention to the schuss view and the pre-arthritic changes described by Dejour et al. [7] (joint space narrowing less than 50 %).
- The functional objectives and patient's motivation and expectation.

Memory

The combined procedure of HTO and ACL reconstruction, in patients with medial OA, varus alignment and previous medial meniscectomy, allowed to restore correct alignment, knee laxity, and instability and resume to a recreational level of leisure activities or sports with midterm follow-up. It is a very interesting salvage procedure to improve function and relief pain. It may avoid a more aggressive surgical procedure such as knee arthroplasty in young patients.

References

1. Badhe NP, Forster IW (2002) High tibial osteotomy in knee instability: the rationale of treatment and early results. Knee Surg Sports Traumatol Arthrosc 10:38–43

2. Boileau P, Neyret PH (1991) Résultats des ostéotomies tibiales de valgisation associées aux plasties du ligament croisé antérieur dans le traitement des laxités antérieures chroniques évoluées. 7ème Journée du genou. Lyon, ALRM Edition p 232–238

3. Bonin N, Aït Si Selmi T, Neyret P (2004) Ostéotomies et laxité antérieure. Cahiers d'Enseignement SOFCOT, vol 86. Expansion scientifique française, Paris, p 96–103

4. Bonin N, Aït Si Selmi T, Donell ST, Dejour H, Neyret P (2004) Anterior cruciate reconstruction combined with valgus upper tibial osteotomy : 12 years follow-up. Knee 11:431–434

5. Boss A, Stutz G, Oursin C, Gächter A (1995) Anterior cruciate ligament reconstruction combined with valgus tibial osteotomy (combined procedure). Knee Surg Sports Traumatol Arthrosc 3:187–191

6. Boussaton M, Potel JF (2003) Ostéotomie tibiale de valgisation associée à une ligamentoplastie du ligament croisé antérieur utilisant le tendon rotulien: réflexions et indications. Perspectives en arthroscopie (SFA), vol 3. Springer, Paris, p 37–41

7. Dejour H, Neyret P, Boileau P, Donell ST (1994) Anterior cruciate reconstruction combined with valgus tibial osteotomy. Clin Orthop 299:220–228

8. Demange MK, Camanho GL, Pe´cora JR, Gobbi RG, Tirico LE, da Mota E, Albuquerque RF (2011) Simultaneous anterior cruciate ligament reconstruction and computer-assisted open-wedge high

9. Garin C, Lerat JL, Moyen B (1989) Laxité chronique antérieure et arthrose. Etude d'une série de 31 cas de ligamentoplastie associée à une ostéotomie de valgisation tibiale. Journées Lyonnaises de Chirurgie du Genou et de Traumatologie du Sport. SAURAMPS Ed 99–105

10. Imhoff AB, Linke RD, Agneskirchner J (2004) Korrekturosteotomie bei primary-varus-, double-varus-und triple-varus-knieistabilität mit kreuzbandersatz. Orthopäd 33:201–207

11. Lattermann C, Jakob RP (1996) High tibial osteotomy alone or combined with ligament reconstruction in anterior cruciate ligament-deficient knees. Knee Surg Traumatol Arthrosc 4:32–38

12. Lerat JL, Moyen B, Garin C, Mandrino A, Besse JL, Brunet-Guedj E (1993) Laxité antérieure et arthrose interne du genou. Résultats de la reconstruction du ligament croisé antérieur associée à une ostéotomie tibiale. Rev Chir Orthop 79:365–374

13. Neuschwander DC, Drez D, Praine RM (1993) Simultaneous high tibial osteotomy and ACL reconstruction for combined genu varum and symptomatic ACL tear. Orthopedics 16(6):679–684

14. Noyes FR, Barber SD, Simon R (1993) High tibial osteotomy and ligament reconstruction in varus angulated, anterior cruciate ligament-deficient knee. A two- to seven-year follow-up study. Am J Sports Med 21:2–12

15. Noyes FR, Barber-Westin SD, Hewett T (2000) High tibial osteotomy and ligament reconstruction for varus angulated anterior cruciate ligament deficient knees. Am J Sports Med 28:282–296

16. O'Neill DF, James SL (1992) Valgus osteotomy with anterior cruciate ligament laxity. Clin Orthop 278:153–159

17. Zaffagnini S, Bonanzinga T, Grassi A, Marcheggiani Muccioli GM, Musiani C, Raggi F, Iacono F, Vaccari V, Marcacci M (2013) Combined ACL reconstruction and closing-wedge HTO for varus angulated ACL-deficient knees. Knee Surg Sports Traumatol Arthrosc 21(4):934–941

18. Williams RJ III, Wickiewicz TL, Warren RF (2000) Management of unicompartmental arthritis in the anterior cruciate ligament-deficient knee. Am J Sports Med 28:749–760

19. Agneskirchner JD, Hurschler C, Stukenborg-Colsman C, Imhoff AB, Lobenhoffer P (2004) Effect of high tibial flexion osteotomy on cartilage pressure and joint kinematics: a biomechanical study in human cadaveric knees. Arch Orthop Trauma Surg 124:575–584

20. Lobenhoffer P, Agneskirchner JD (2003) Improvements in surgical technique of valgus high tibial osteotomy. Knee Surg Sports Traumatol Arthrosc 11:132–138

21. Hulet C (2005) Osteoarthritis and Knee laxity Cahiers d'Enseignement SOFCOT, vol 87. Expansion scientifique française, Paris, p 117–141
22. Dejour D, Kuhn A, Dejour H (1998) Ostéotomie tibiale de déflexion et laxité chronique antérieure, à propos de 22 cas. Rev Chir Orthop 84(SII): 28–29
23. Lerat JL (2000) Ostéotomies dans la gonarthrose. Cahiers d'Enseignement SOFCOT. Expansion scientifique française, Paris, p 165–201
24. Hulet C, Burdin G, Locker B, Vielpeau C (2004) Résultats et complications après reconstruction du ligament croisé antérieur. Conférence d'Enseignement SOFCOT. Expansion Scientifique Française, Paris, p 143–160
25. Ducat A, Sariali E, Lebel B, Mertl P, Hernigou P, Flecher X, Zayni R, Bonnin M, Jalil R, Amzallag J, Rosset P, Servien E, Gaudot F, Judet T, Catonne´ Y (2012) Posterior tibial slope changes after opening- and closing-wedge high tibial osteotomy: a comparative prospective multicenter study. Orthop Traumatol Surg Res 98(1):68–74
26. Elser F, Imhoff AB (2007) Combined high tibial osteotomy, anterior cruciate ligament reconstruction, and cartilage transplantation in young athletes. Oper Tech Orthop 17:46–50
27. Hulet C, Acquitter Y, Burdin G, Locker B, Vielpeau C (2003) Positionnement des greffes du LCA. Pathologie ligamentaire du genou. Springer, Paris, pp 307–320
28. Beaufils P, Cassard X, Charrois O (2004) Réparation méniscale. Rev Chir Orthop 90(Suppl 8):3S49–3S76
29. Bonnin M, Carret JP, Dimnet J, Dejour H (1996) The weight-bearing knee after anterior cruciate ligament rupture. An in vitro biomechanical study. Knee Surg Sports Traumatol Arthrosc 3:245–251
30. Dejour D, Bonin N, Schiavon M, Sanchez S (2003) Arthrose et laxité chronique antérieure. Les facteurs de l'arthrose et les options thérapeutiques. Pathologie ligamentaire du genou. Springer, Paris, p 549–565
31. Neyret P, Zuppi G, Aït Si Selmi T (2000) Tibial deflexion osteotomy. Oper Techn Sports Med 8: 61–66

Part XI
Intraoperative Complications

Intraoperative Complications: Solutions?

40

Mohsen Hussein

Contents

M. Hussein
Artros Center for Orthopaedic Surgery
and Sports Medicine, Tehnoloski Park 21,
1000 Ljubljana, Slovenia
e-mail: mhussein@artros.si

Reconstruction of the ACL has become a commonly performed procedure, and the number of reconstructions that are performed annually continues to increase. Overall good to excellent results have been reported. However, a critical review of the literature reveals that success rates vary between 69 and 95 % [1–3]. The increase in number of ACL reconstructions performed has subsequently led to an increase in ACL failure rates and the need for revision surgery. The most frequent reason for graft failure are improper surgical techniques (60 %), failure of graft incorporation (30 %), and trauma (10 %).

In this chapter the four most severe intraoperative complications are discussed.

40.1 Wrong Tunnel Placement: What to Do?

The most common error in ACL reconstruction is the nonanatomic placement of the tibial and/or femoral tunnel [4]. Therefore tunnel placement is the key to successful ACL reconstruction in primary and revision cases. Tunnel mismatch can result in abnormal knee kinematics, limited range of motion, unphysiologic graft tension, and, ultimately, graft failure. Biological healing of the graft-bone interface may also be affected [5].

R. Siebold et al. (eds.), *Anterior Cruciate Ligament Reconstruction*,
DOI 10.1007/978-3-642-45349-6_40, © ESSKA 2014

Research has shown, that if the femoral tunnel is placed too anteriorly, it will cause graft lengthening when the knee is flexed. Placing it too posteriorly will result in decreased length of the graft and laxity in flexion. A too medial or lateral position will cause graft impingement.

On the tibial side, a too anterior tunnel position will result in impingement of the ACL graft on the roof of the intercondylar notch (roof impingement) or on the PCL (PCL impingement). Too posterior tunnel position will put the PCL at risk during reaming. An excessive medial or lateral placement of the tibial tunnel will cause damage to the lateral meniscus, lateral femoral condyle, and the cartilage on the medial tibial plateau.

The first step to avoid wrong tunnel placement is to ensure good visualization of the tibial and femoral ACL insertion sites. A high anterolateral portal is very helpful to improve the visualization of the ACL tibial insertion site. The medial portal is essential to allow improved visualization of the ACL femoral insertion site and of the intercondylar notch. It also allows the surgeon to perform measurement of the ACL insertion sites on the tibia and femur. The accessory portal is essential to achieve correct placement of the femoral tunnel [6] (Fig. 40.1).

The second step is to ensure accurate guide pin placement at the ACL anatomic insertion site. In DB ACL reconstruction the PL tunnel should be placed at the center of the PL femoral insertion site. In most cases this site is clearly visible. If the PL bundle insertion site is not visible, the guide pin should be placed below the lateral intercondylar ridge and anterior to the bifurcate ridge with the knee flexed in 90°. This is approximately 6 mm arthroscopically posterior to the anterior articular cartilage border and 3 mm superior to the inferior border. Then, the AM femoral tunnel should be established in a similar way approximately 2 mm posterior to the posterior rim of the PL tunnel, in a horizontal or slightly superior position. On the tibia, an ACL tibial tunnel director guide set at 65° should be placed in the insertion site of the PL bundle, based on anatomic landmarks and previous marking. The position of the director guide

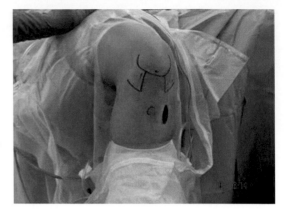

Fig. 40.1 Portals

on the tibial cortex is just anterior to the superficial fibers of the medial collateral ligament. Following PL guide pin placement, a second guide is set to 55° and positioned in the AM tibial footprint. The starting point of the AM tunnel on the tibial cortex is more anterior, central, and proximal than the starting point of the PL tunnel [6].

In SB ACL reconstruction the position of the femoral tunnel is between the target point of the AM and PL bundle. It is in the lower third of the medial wall of the lateral femoral condyle at the center of the femoral insertion site. On the tibial side an ACL tibial tunnel director guide is placed in the center of the ACL tibial insertion site, based on anatomic landmarks and previous marking.

We advise the use of transportal drilling technique as recent studies have shown that using transtibial drilling leads mostly to nonanatomic, femoral tunnel placement [7, 8]. For many years, the gold standard was to place the femoral tunnel in the posterior-superior corner of the lateral femoral condyle. For better reproducibility and simplification for the surgeon, the o'clock position was frequently used for orientation. However, using the "o'clock" method can often lead to misconceptions because of the 3-dimensional nature of the intercondylar notch, where the clock face can be put anywhere along the anterior-to-posterior axis [5].

To avoid wrong tunnel placement, the guide pin position should be carefully verified prior to tunnel drilling. It is helpful to start with a smaller

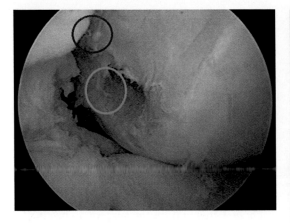

Fig. 40.2 View through medial portal: drilled femoral tunnel in anatomic position for ACL reconstruction. *Green circle*: femoral tunnel that interferes with the anatomically correct position. *Red circle*: The tunnel is placed too far and does not interfere correct tunnel

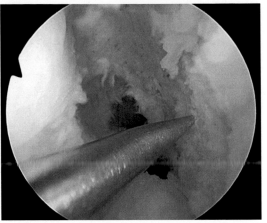

Fig. 40.3 Marking the femoral insertion site

reamer (e.g., 5 mm) so that there is still the possibility to redirect the pin guide ensuring accurate anatomic tunnel placement. In revision surgery, if the tunnels are not in the center of the anatomical insertion, they can be expanded for more accurate placement. Therefore, a larger graft has to be used if (e.g., additional allograft). For autograft ACL reconstruction, alternative fixation techniques such as stacked interference screws may be considered. Alternatively, the two incision techniques can be used [9]. If the tunnel is placed in a nonanatomic position, a new tunnel in the correct position could be established starting with small reamer and then gradually expanding the tunnel with dilatators. On the tibial side, the same principle can be applied. If the existing tunnel is slightly malpositioned, it can be expanded anteriorly or posteriorly. The exterior starting point of the tibial guide can be varied to allow better positionining of the bone tunnel [4]. In revision surgery, if the old tunnel positions interfere with the correct anatomic position of the femoral or tibial tunnel, a two-stage ACL revision should be considered (Fig. 40.2). In the first surgery, the tunnels should be filled with bone graft prior to later revision surgery. Close clinical follow-up is also very important postoperatively and should include candid communication with the patient and family.

Tricks and Pearls

In double-bundle ACL reconstruction, drill the AM femoral tunnel through the anteromedial portal to get more divergency between the femoral tunnels; this is helpful, especially when the intercondylar notch is narrow.

Individualize the surgery by measuring each tibial and femoral insertion sites, and calculating proper tunnel and graft size.

Pitfalls

Positioning the femoral tunnel too posterior: Viewing the medial wall of the lateral femoral condyle through the lateral portal, especially in knees with narrow intercondylar notch, may give a wrong impression of the target point for femoral tunnel. It may seem too anteriorly causing hypercorrection. To avoid this pitfall it is advised to mark this point with thermal device or microfracture pick with the arthroscope through the lateral portal and then switch it to the medial portal to check. After introducing the guide pin, introduce the proper reamer to contact the bone and check again; after that start drilling with smaller diameter reamer (Fig. 40.3).

Malpositioning of the tibial guide pin: To avoid this pitfall, obtain good visualization of the tibial insertion site, exact marking of the target point for the center of the tibial tunnel, and stop drilling of the guide wire before it hits the tip of the tibial guide. If the tibial guide is not at the target point, try again after changing the angle of the tibial guide and replace the exterior starting point a bit medially or laterally to eliminate the possibility of going through the first tunnel. If it happens again, introduce the smaller reamer, redirect the pin guide during dilatation up to the desired tunnel diameter.

40.2   Graft Too Short or Too Thin

Anterior cruciate ligament (ACL) reconstruction with hamstring tendons has gained widespread popularity. Clinical studies have revealed that autogenous semitendinosus (ST) and gracilis tendon (GT) grafts provide equal postoperative results but with decreased risk of anterior knee pain due to donor-site morbidity in comparison

with the bone–patellar tendon–bone autograft. In addition, improved fixation techniques have led to increased use of ST and GT as an alternative to the bone–patellar tendon–bone grafts [10].

Diameters and lengths of autogenous ST and GT grafts show clinically significant anatomic variation (Fig. 40.4). The difficulty in predicting the available diameters and lengths of these tendons may affect their use as ACL grafts. In addition, common fixation techniques require grafts of a certain diameter or length. Thus, it might be beneficial for the surgeon to be able to predict the size of a potential ST or GT autograft to avoid insufficient graft size or length. If the predictive factors indicated that the graft might be of insufficient graft size or length, alternative graft sources could be procured before surgery [10]. For graft length, height is the most significant predictor for both ST and GT length, which is consistent with the findings of Treme et al. [11]. It was observed that females and smaller patients show a greater risk of an ST and GT graft shorter than 240 and 220 mm, respectively.

Double-bundle anterior cruciate ligament reconstruction generally requires triple- or 4-stranded ST and GT grafts to reconstruct the

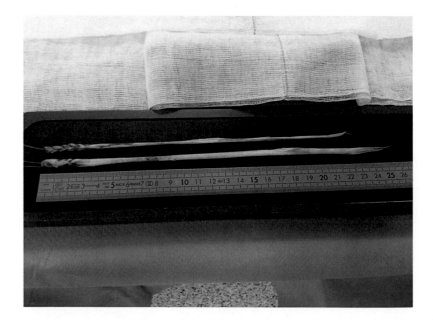

Fig. 40.4 Hamstring autografts

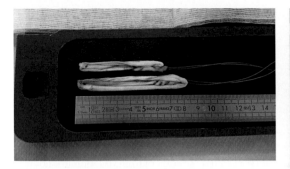

Fig. 40.5 Triple-stranded ST and GT grafts for double-bundle ACL reconstruction

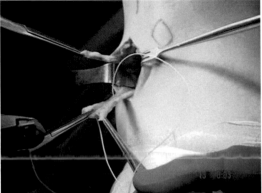

Fig. 40.6 Graft harvesting

antcromedial and postcrolateral bundle, respectively (Fig. 40.5).

For ST graft size, 7 mm should be considered as the minimum diameter for single-bundle ACL reconstruction [10–14]. A 4-stranded ST graft less than 6 mm and a 4-stranded GT graft less than 5.5 mm in diameter were considered too small for double-bundle ACL reconstruction.

For 4-stranded hamstring tendon grafts, a minimum length of 60 mm is recommended [12, 13]. An ST tendon with a length less than 24 cm and a GT tendon less than 22 cm were considered too short. For double-bundle ACL reconstruction with two 4-stranded hamstring grafts, the ST graft is used to reconstruct the AM bundle. The acceptable lengths of the ST graft in the femoral and tibial tunnels are both at least 15 mm. The GT graft is always used to reconstruct the PL bundle. The acceptable lengths of the GT graft in the femoral and tibial tunnels are both at least 15 mm. Complications with the use of hamstring tendons in ACL reconstruction are rare and in some cases associated with failure in graft harvest. The harvested grafts are inconsistent regarding the length and the size [15]. This will be due to anatomically small tendons, short tendons, or intraoperative complication with non-adequate harvesting techniques. In some cases one or both tendons may be absent. In these cases the surgeon should use another graft [16].

It is very important to pay great attention to the anatomy and anatomic variations of the hamstrings during the harvest. Patience and precise techniques are the key to grafts with good quality and sufficient length and size. The gracilis and semitendinosus tendons are easily identified on the undersurface (Fig. 40.6). It is important to identify and cut their expansions to the gastrocnemius prior to stripping because of consistent bands that run from both tendons. After that, this region can be palpated digitally to ensure that all bands had been resected.

If one or both tendons are too short to be doubled, another autograft or allograft can be used. Thus, additional availability of these grafts as well as increased morbidity has to be regarded.

Length can be added to the tendons by utilizing Dacron tape. Using it on the femoral side, less graft is needed on the tibial side and shorter graft can be used [15].

If the harvested tendons are too thin, each of them could be doubled, tripled, or quadrupled to get a graft with proper diameter. This is especially helpful during double-bundle ACL reconstruction.

Tricks and Pearls
Digital palpation is helpful to ensure that all bands had been resected.
Deflate the tourniquet just prior to stripping with open or closed stripper.
Add more knee extension before stripping.

Pitfalls
Understatement of graft measuring: If the graft is undersized, it will pass easily

> through the tunnel, but the healing surface is less. If the graft is oversized, then the surgeon could have problems with its passage. Sizing devices, reamers, and dilatators can be used with an accuracy of 0.5 mm.

40.3   Graft on the Floor: What To Do?

Contamination of the graft could be caused by skin contact or due to falling on the floor. In a survey of sports medicine physicians, 25 % of the surgeons reported a graft contamination during ACL reconstruction. In these cases, the contamination occurred with the graft falling on the floor [17]. There is no gold standard reported in such case. A survey of sports medicine specialists on how to manage an intraoperative graft contamination [18], the most frequent response (75 %) was to decontaminate the graft and continue with the operation. Other available options included harvesting another type of autograft (18 %) or switching to allograft tissue (7 %). Harvesting another graft exposes the patient to additional donor-site morbidity [18]. Utilizing allograft tissue adds considerable cost to the procedure [19] and increases the risk of disease transmission, delayed incorporation, risk of tunnel enlargement, question of availability, and possible compromise in functional outcomes [20, 21]. To minimize further patient morbidity, sterilization of the contaminated graft is usually the most suitable option [17].

Plante et al. evaluated bacterial contamination of hamstring autografts dropped on the floor and methods of graft decontamination; they found that a total of 75 isolates were identified by positive culture and the most common organisms were *Staphylococcus aureus* (44 %), *Propionibacterium acnes* (10.7 %), coagulase-negative *Staphylococcus* (9.3 %), and *Bacillus* (9.3 %) [21].

The time on the floor (5 sec versus 15 sec) does not seem to affect the rate of positive cultures. Longer and shorter times contamination exposures were not evaluated as those were not felt to be realistic in the operating room setting [21].

Unfortunately, there is not a gold standard reported in the literature regarding sterilization of intraoperative contaminated grafts. In the survey of sports medicine specialists, the most frequent response is that 13 of 43 (30 %) contaminated grafts that underwent cleansing were cleaned with Hibiclens (Regent Medical, Norcross, GA), or chlorhexidine gluconate. The cleansing protocols by which the grafts were treated with chlorhexidine gluconate varied among the respondents. The majority of respondents soaked the graft in chlorhexidine gluconate solution for time periods ranging from 90 s to 30 min. Chlorhexidine gluconate is a long-lasting, cationic bisbiguanide [17, 22, 23]. The compound is both bactericidal and fungicidal; however, it does not destroy spores or mycobacterial species. It has a low order of activity against viruses. At lower concentrations, chlorhexidine is a potent membrane-active agent against gram-positive and gram-negative organisms, causing intracellular release of potassium ions and pentose sugars. At higher concentrations, there is irreversible damage to the outer membrane of gram-negative bacteria and the cell wall of gram-positive bacteria. It is more effective against gram-positive than gram-negative organisms [17, 22, 23].

Several laboratory studies have investigated cleansing techniques for contaminated grafts. Molina et al. [24] reported late growth of a gram-negative rod in 1 of 50 (2 %) ACL specimens dropped on an operating room floor for 15 s and soaked in full-strength chlorhexidine gluconate solution for a minimum of 90 s. Goebel et al. [25] compared three separate solutions, 10 % povidone-iodine, a triple antibiotic solution (0.1 % gentamicin, 0.1 % clindamycin, 0.05 % polymyxin), and 4 %

chlorhexidine gluconate, to treat rabbit BPTB grafts contaminated with two separate organisms: 4 % chlorhexidine gluconate was the only solution effective in decontaminating all grafts. In the second part of their study, contaminated grafts with virulent organisms (*S. aureus*, *Enterococcus faecalis*, *Klebsiella pneumoniae*, *Escherichia coli*, and *Pseudomonas aeruginosa*) were treated with 4 % chlorhexidine gluconate solution alone, 4 % chlorhexidine gluconate solution followed by triple antibiotic solution, and 4 % chlorhexidine gluconate followed by 10 % povidone-iodine solution. The combination of 4 % chlorhexidine gluconate and triple antibiotic solution was successful in eliminating all of the organisms from the contaminated grafts. Thus, the authors recommended the use of both of these agents in cleansing contaminated BPTB grafts. Burd et al. [22] found that power irrigation with 3 L of 2 % chlorhexidine gluconate provided a shorter and equally effective measure for cleaning human Achilles allografts contaminated with four different organisms (*S. aureus*, *S. epidermidis*, *P. aeruginosa*, and *K. pneumoniae*). The total time needed to decontaminate the allograft was approximately 10–12 min, allowing a 1-min bacterial inoculation, 2–3 min to swish the graft in a normal saline bath while setting up irrigation equipment, and 7–8 min to irrigate the tissue with 3 L of 2 % chlorhexidine gluconate and 1 L of normal saline solution. They also noted that 2 and 4 % chlorhexidine gluconate irrigation decontaminated the grafts equally as well.

Although these studies demonstrate an effective ability to decontaminate the grafts, potential side effects of graft cleansing need to be considered; they include [1] increasing polymorphonuclear granulocyte toxicity and impairing phagocytic efficiency [2], causing intra-articular reactive synovitis and chondrolysis, and [3] increasing postoperative morbidity [17, 22].

Although several cleansing protocols were used successfully, basic science studies support a

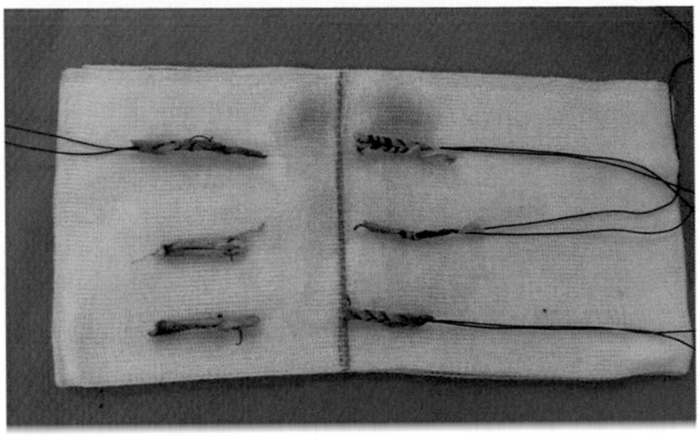

Fig. 40.7 Pieces of the graft before falling in the floor during our study

combination of chlorhexidine and triple antibiotic solution [17].

Also our ongoing study supports these results and conclusions (Fig. 40.7).

We recommend the following protocol:
- Sterile retrieving off the floor as soon as possible (within 15 s).
- Removing of all sutures and other foreign materials (e.g., loop).
- Bathing the graft in saline solution for 3 min.
- Cleansing the graft in 2 % chlorhexidine gluconate solution for 5 min.
- Cleansing the graft in triple antibiotic solution (0.1 % gentamicin, 0.1 % clindamycin, 0.05 % polymyxin) for 5 min.
- Washing the graft in saline solution for 3 min.
- New suturing and resizing of the graft.
- Additional intraoperative and postoperative antibiotics.
- Close clinical follow-up.

Tricks and Pearls
- Keep a management protocol for contaminated grafts in theatre.
- Remove all foreign materials from the graft (sutures, buttons, etc.).
- Use intra- and postoperative antibiotics.

40.4 Insufficient Tibial or Femoral Fixation

Graft fixation is the weak link in ACL reconstruction, representing the initial limiting factor in the early postoperative period [26–28] especially during the first 6–8 weeks. In this time, the graft pullout is more likely to occur at the fixation point. Fixation must be highly secured to prevent changes in graft position during its graft incorporation.

Many systems are available for the fixation of hamstring tendon grafts: sutures tied to a post or over buttons, screws and washers, staples, interference screws, and cross-pin techniques. Some surgeons suggested a combination of these methods [15]. Graft fixation on the femoral side may be achieved by either suspensory or aperture methods. Fixation of the graft on the tibial side can be achieved with sutures and post screws, interference screws, or staples. Most commonly all these fixation techniques give adequate fixation when properly used, but each of them has advantages and disadvantages. The advantage of suspensory techniques is a tight placing of the graft within the femoral tunnel so that the healing surface is larger. The disadvantage is that the fixation point is far from the tunnel and the joint. Also, fixation with staples has the same disadvantage, besides that it presents high risk of graft traumatization.

Graft constructs fixed to bone at the intraarticular apertures with interference screws have been shown to undergo less stretching and to be stiffer than either suspensory-fixed grafts or grafts fixed externally to the drilled tunnel. The shorter distance between the fixation points results in less stress and strain that can cause graft elongation and tunnel widening. The disadvantages are distortion of the graft and reduction of the healing surface [29]. There are many questions still unanswered about fixation: Which technique is the easiest to perform? Which gives the best results and reduces the chance of elongation and laxity? Which materials?

If there is any concern about fixation strength using these methods, secondary techniques should be employed. For example, post-, washer- and staple fixation can be easily added and used as secondary fixation [9, 28, 30]. It is imperative that the surgeon is familiar with different alternative techniques and the equipment is available. On the femoral side, supplemental fixation can include the Endobutton, screw over post technique or button technique using a second incision and securing the graft to the lateral cortex, and standard or soft tissue interference screws. On the tibial side increasing fixation strength by supplementary tibial fixation with a staple has been shown to be effective in decreasing the incidence of joint laxity after hamstring tendon reconstruction. Increasing fixation strength may be achieved by using other means such as longer screws, increased diameter thread, or both longer and increased diameter screws [29].

> **Tricks and Pearls**
> - The surgeon should be familiar with different fixation techniques and devices. These must be available in the operation room for switching from one technique to another.
> - The exact measurement of the tunnel and graft length and width is essential to avoid intraoperative complications with graft passage and fixation. Marking of the graft is very important especially in the femoral suspensory fixation.
> - Remove all bone debris from the joint and the femoral tunnel (Fig. 40.8).
> - Use intraoperative X-ray if you are in doubt about correct setting of the femoral fixation.

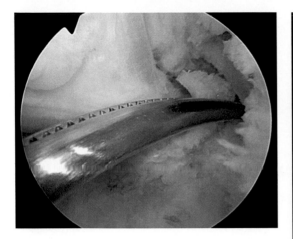

Fig. 40.8 Removing all bone debris from the joint and the femoral tunnel

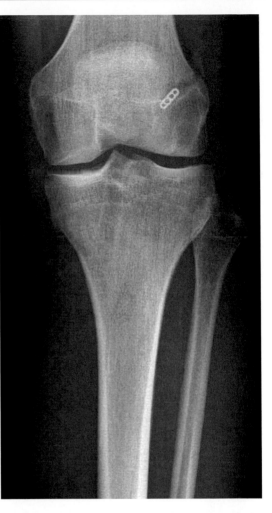

Pitfalls
- On the femoral side fixation placing the button within the soft tissue. To avoid this complication the femoral tunnel should not be drilled more than 10 mm deeper than the desired length of the graft.
- The button device retracts back in the femoral tunnel toward the joint (Fig. 40.9). To avoid this complication the femoral tunnel should be visualized through the medial portal (tunneloscopy) to ensure that the femoral cortex is not violated and blowed out during drilling with the reamer (you can see the bone ring at the end of the tunnel) (Fig. 40.10). In such a case use different fixation (e.g., screw).
- The screw can violate the graft if it is too large or not adequate directed. On the other hand, the fixation may be too loose if the screw is too small or the bone is very soft. To avoid these intraoperative complications, adequate screw size should be used regarding bone condition (hard bone, osteoporosis), tunnel and graft diameter.

Fig. 40.9 The Endobutton retracted back through the femoral tunnel

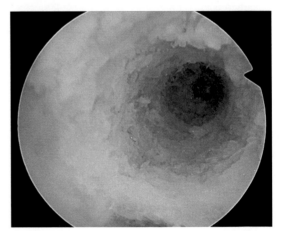

Fig. 40.10 Viewing the femoral tunnel through the medial portal

Memory

Non-anatomical tunnel position is one of the major reasons for failure of ACL reconstruction. It may result in abnormal knee kinematics, limited range of motion, unphysiologic graft tension, and ultimately graft failure. Proper matching of the graft to the intercondylar notch is an important aspect in ACL reconstruction too. Appropriate fixation is essential for postoperative stability and rehabilitation. Graft contamination during surgery is a rare intraopertaive incident. The surgeon should be ready to react in this situation.

References

1. Bach BR Jr, Levy ME, Bojchuk J, Tradonsky S, Bush-Joseph CA, Khan NH (1998) Single incision endoscopic anterior cruciate ligament reconstruction using patellar tendon autograft. Minimum two-year follow-up evaluation. Am J Sports Med 26:30–40
2. Freedman KB, D'Amato MJ, Nedeff DD et al (2003) Arthroscopic anterior cruciate ligament reconstruction: A meta-analysis comparing patellar tendon and hamstring tendon autografts. Am J Sports Med 31:2–11
3. Kamath GV, Redfern JC, Greis PE, Burks RT (2011) Revision anterior cruciate ligament reconstruction. Am J Sports Med 39:199–217
4. Miller MD, Harner CD (2001) Revision anterior cruciate ligament surgery. In: Chow JC (ed) Advanced arthroscopy. Springer, New York, pp 471–488
5. Kopf S, Forsythe B, Wong AK et al (2010) Nonanatomic tunnel position in traditional transtibial single-bundle anterior cruciate ligament reconstruction evaluated by three-dimensional computed tomography. J Bone Joint Surg Am 92: 1427–1431
6. Hussein M, van Eck CF, Cretnik A, Dinevski D, Fu FH (2012) Individualized anterior cruciate ligament surgery: a prospective study comparing anatomic single- and double-bundle reconstruction. Am J Sports Med 40(3):1781–1782
7. Aglietti P, Giron F, Losco M, Cuomo P, Ciardullo A, Mondanelli N (2009) Comparison between single- and double-bundle anterior cruciate ligament reconstruction: a prospective, randomized, single-blinded clinical trial. Am J Sports Med 38:25–34
8. Shen W, Forsythe B, Ingham SM, Honkamp NJ, Fu FH (2008) Application of the anatomic double-bundle reconstruction concept to revision and augmentation anterior cruciate ligament surgeries. J Bone Joint Surg Am 90(Suppl 4):20–34
9. Getelman MH, Friedman MJ (2000) Complication and pitfalls in anterior cruciate ligament reconstruction with synthetic grafts. In: Malek MM (ed) Knee surgery. Springer, New York, p 113–120
10. Xie G, Huangfu X, Zhao J (2012) Prediction of the graft size of 4-stranded semitendinosus tendon and 4-stranded gracilis tendon for anterior cruciate ligament reconstruction: a Chinese Han patient study. Am J Sports Med 40(5):1161–1166
11. Treme G, Diduch DR, Billante MJ, Miller MD, Hart JM (2008) Hamstring graft size prediction: a prospective clinical evaluation. Am J Sports Med 36(11): 2204–2209
12. Sastre S, Popescu D, Núñez M, Pomes J, Tomas X, Peidro L (2010) Double-bundle versus single-bundle ACL reconstruction using the horizontal femoral position: a prospective, randomized study. Knee Surg Sports Traumatol Arthrosc 18(1):32–36
13. Maeda A, Shino K, Horibe S, Nakata K, Buccafusca G (1996) Anterior cruciate ligament reconstruction with multistranded autogenous semitendinosus tendon. Am J Sports Med 24(4):504–509
14. Yasumoto M, Deie M, Sunagawa T, Adachi N, Kobayashi K, Ochi M (2006) Predictive value of preoperative 3-dimensional computer tomography measurement of semitendinosus tendon harvested for anterior cruciate ligament reconstruction. Arthroscopy 22(3):259–264
15. Larsen RV (2000) Complication and pitfalls in anterior cruciate ligament reconstruction with hamstring tendons. In: Malek MM (ed) Knee surgery. Springer, New York, p 77–88
16. Slapey GS, Frieman MJ (2001) Arthroscopic ACL reconstruction: semitendinosus. In: Chow JC (ed) Advanced arthroscopy. Springer, New York, pp 419–433
17. Izquierdo R Jr, Cadet ER, Bauer R et al (2005) A survey of sports medicine specialists investigating the preferred management of contaminated anterior cruciate ligament grafts. Arthroscopy 21(11): 1348–1353
18. Pasque CB, Geib TM (2007) Intraoperative anterior cruciate ligament graft contamination. Arthroscopy 23(3):329–331
19. Nagda SH, Altobelli GG, Bowdry KA et al (2009) Cost analysis of outpatient anterior cruciate ligament reconstruction: autograft versus allograft. Clin Orthop Relat Res 468:1418–1422
20. Marrale J, Morrissey MC, Haddad FS (2007) A literature review of autograft and allograft anterior cruciate ligament reconstruction. Knee Surg Sports Traumatol Arthrosc 15(6):690–704
21. Plante JM et al (2013) Evaluation of sterilization methods following contamination of hamstring autograft during anterior cruciate ligament reconstruction. Knee Surg Sports Traumatol Arthrosc 21:696–701
22. Burd T, Conroy BP, Meyer SC, Allen WC (2000) The effects of chlorhexidine irrigation solution on

contaminated bone-tendon allografts. Am J Sports Med 28:241–244

23. Russell AD, Day MJ (1993) Antibacterial activity of chlorhexidine. J Hosp Infect 25:229–238

24. Molina ME, Nonweiller DE, Evans JA, Delee JC (2000) Contaminated anterior cruciate ligament grafts: the efficacy of 3 sterilization agents. Arthroscopy 16:373–378

25. Goebel ME, Drez D Jr, Heck SB, Stoma MK (1994) Contaminated rabbit patellar tendon grafts. In vivo analysis of disinfecting methods. Am J Sports Med 22:387–391

26. Steiner ME, Hecker AT, Brown CH Jr et al (1994) Anterior cruciate ligament fixation: comparison of hamstring and patellar tendon grafts. Am J Sports Med 22:240–247

27. Kurosaka M, Yoshiya S, Andrish JT (1987) A biomechanical comparison of different surgical techniques of graft fixation in anterior cruciate ligament reconstruction. Am J Sports Med 15:225–229

28. Jones DG, Galland M, Fu FH (2000) Complications and pitfalls in anterior cruciate ligament revision reconstruction. In: Malek MM (ed) Knee surgery. Springer, New York, p 138–158

29. Hill PF, Russell VJ, Salmon LJ, Pinczewski LA (2005) The influence of supplementary tibial fixation on laxity measurements after anterior cruciate ligament reconstruction with hamstring tendons in female patients. Am J Sports Med 33(1):94–101

30. Pevny T, Hunter RE (2001) Anterior cruciate ligament reconstruction. In: Chow JC (ed) Advanced arthroscopy. Springer, New York, pp 419–433

Part XII

Postoperative Complications

Postoperative Complications: Solutions?

41

Jüri Kartus, Francis Fernandez, and Rainer Siebold

Contents

41.1 Postoperative Infection

Jüri Kartus

41.1.1 Background

Deep postoperative infection or septic arthritis is a rare but potentially devastating complication after ACL reconstruction. Where the agents origin from varies, probably the skin of the patient is one important source [24], but other sources such as contaminated graft preparation boards [30] and cannulated surgical instruments [25] have been reported.

Commonly somewhere between 0.5 and 1.8 % of the patients undergoing ACL reconstruction using autografts or allografts suffer septic arthritis [1, 2, 10, 21, 23, 41]. The most common microorganism involved in septic arthritis is some type of staphylococci, but also other agents

J. Kartus, MD, PhD (✉)
Department of Orthopedics, NU-Hospital Group,
Trollhättan/Uddevalla, Sweden
e-mail: juri.kartus@vgregion.se

F. Fernandez
HKF: Center for Specialised Hip-Knee-Foot Surgery,
ATOS Hospital Heidelberg, Bismarckstr. 9-15,
69115 Heidelberg, Germany

R. Siebold (✉)
Institute for Anatomy and Cell Biology,
Ruprecht-Karls University Heidelberg,
Im Neuenheimer Feld 307,
69120 Heidelberg, Germany

HKF: Center for Specialised Hip-Knee-Foot
Surgery, ATOS Hospital Heidelberg,
Bismarckstr. 9-15, 69115 Heidelberg, Germany
e-mail: rainer.siebold@atos.de

R. Siebold et al. (eds.), *Anterior Cruciate Ligament Reconstruction*,
DOI 10.1007/978-3-642-45349-6_41, © ESSKA 2014

like streptococcus and enterobacter species can be found [1, 21, 23, 24, 41].

If this condition is diagnosed early and properly treated, there is a high possibility that the patient will return to normal in terms of range of motion and laxity if the graft can be retained; furthermore, return to activity at the same or slightly lower level than uncomplicated cases can be expected [2, 10, 16, 22].

41.1.2 Suggested Preoperative Planning to Decrease the Risk in Septic Arthritis

To decrease the amount of patient suffering postoperative septic arthritis, it is important to identify and treat or at least consider risk factors before surgery.

If diabetes is a comorbidity, it should be well controlled before ACL reconstruction, as for all types of surgery [5]. Other comorbidities requiring medication with antibiotics, corticosteroids, or other immunosuppressive agents must also be considered.

Patients should strongly be advised to stop smoking since smoking is associated with increased risk in postoperative infections [36].

Patients should be informed to quit chronic nail biting [42] and treat their paronychias and blisters if present, as well as severe acne [26] before surgery, as these are risk factors which might increase bacteremia and subsequently cause postoperative joint infection.

Patients should be informed that piercings or tattoos should not be performed neither close before nor close after the operation since they have been reported to cause infections such as bacterial endocarditis [13]. All body art should be clean and dry without any edema or exudates present.

All loose metal or plastic foreign bodies such as piercings and artificial nails should be removed before surgery.

No shaving or waxing of legs should be performed by the patient close before surgery.

Proper preoperative whole body scrubbing with chlorhexidine soap should be started already at home the day before the operation and continued the morning of the day of surgery.

Prophylaxis should be given with cloxacillin, clindamycin, or cephalosporin directed toward staphylococci [24] at surgery, administered intravenously 15 min before skin incision and definitely before a tourniquet is applied. The author also prefers to administer one additional dose before admission from the outpatient clinic approximately 6–8 h after the first dose.

> **Tips and Tricks**
> - Never operate on a patient with other ongoing infections such as severe paronychia and dental infections or with conditions causing bacteremia such as fresh piercings or tattoos.
> - Do not be afraid of taking history in terms of smoking and body art.
> - Always check that proper preoperative antibiotic prophylaxis has been given before skin incision.
> - Better to be safe than sorry.

> **Pitfalls**
> - The patient does not give a true history in terms of smoking and not visible ongoing infections.
> - Administration of preoperative antibiotic prophylaxis is missed.
> - The patient did not scrub themselves with chlorhexidine soap before surgery. In that case let the patient shower and whole body scrub with chlorhexidine soap directly before surgery.

41.1.3 Suggested Precautions During Surgery to Decrease the Risk for Postoperative Septic Arthritis

Drape the knee with an iodine-treated plastic drape (Fig. 41.1).

Use large enough arthroscopic portals (1 cm) to avoid sharp instruments push skin debris into the joint (Pinczewski L, personal communication, 2000) (Fig. 41.2).

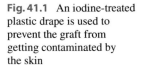
Fig. 41.1 An iodine-treated plastic drape is used to prevent the graft from getting contaminated by the skin

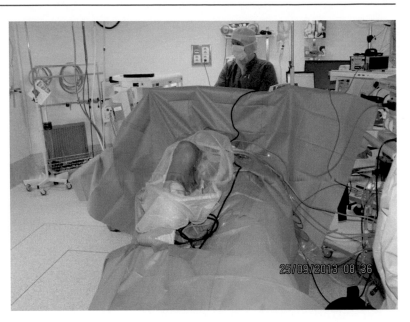

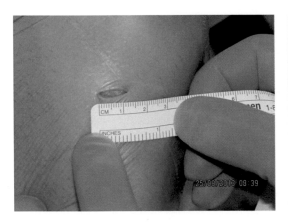
Fig. 41.2 One centimeter arthroscopic portals are made to avoid sharp instruments bring skin or plastic debris into the knee joint

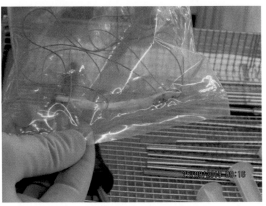
Fig. 41.3 The graft is kept in a plastic bag between preparation and implantation into the knee joint

Put the graft in a plastic bag between preparation and implantation into the knee to decrease the risk in contamination (Fig. 41.3).

Never let the graft touch the skin of the patient (Pinczewski L, personal communication, 2000), touch unnecessary surgical instruments or get soaked by leaking fluid from the arthroscopic portals.

Cut one limb of all threads short before removing them. Never pull one limb and let the other limb pass the skin with the risk of bringing skin debris into the bone tunnels when removing the threads (Pinczewski L, personal communication, 2000) (Fig. 41.5).

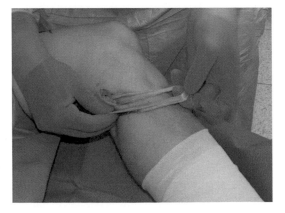
Fig. 41.4 The graft should not be in contact with the skin during preparation to avoid contamination with skin debris

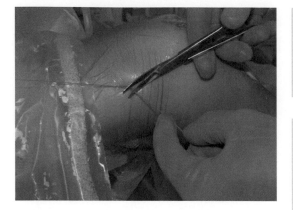

Fig. 41.5 Cut one limb of all threads short before removing them. This decreases the risk in bringing skin debris into the bone tunnels when removing the threads

> **Tips and Tricks**
> - In the rare event that the graft is dropped on the floor, the author suggests to rinse it with saline and then soak it in a 4 % chlorhexidine solution [27] before implantation.
> - If the graft touches the skin during surgery, consider to give 3 days of additional oral antibiotic prophylaxis.

41.1.4 Clinical Findings and Evaluation

The patients most often present at the clinic with pain, swelling, and fever usually after a 1–2-week interval of improvement after surgery [23]. The increased C-reactive protein (CRP), usually above 100 mg/L, is the best blood test to indicate septic arthritis. But CRP below 100 mg/L does not exclude septic arthritis [30]. The aspirate from the knee strongly indicates septic arthritis if it is nontransparent, reveals increased WBC to above 50–75,000/microL [15], and has a decrease in the synovial fluid glucose concentration below 50 % of the concentration in the blood as well as a synovial fluid lactate concentration above 7–10 mmol/L. The lactate analysis is also considered a most reliable indicator of septic arthritis [6] before cultures are available.

> **Tips and Tricks**
> - Always aspirate the knee and secure bacterial cultures before starting treatment with antibiotics.

> **Pitfalls**
> - Septic arthritis can present long time after surgery, even after 3 months or more, and must therefore be suspected and excluded if the patient presents with the above symptoms [31, 44].

41.1.5 Suggested Treatment of the Postoperative Septic Knee

As soon as possible after a postoperative septic knee is suspected and bacterial cultures have been secured, the patient should be started on intravenous antibiotics [23] such as cloxacillin (2 g×3) together with fusidic acid (0.5 g×3) orally or intravenous vancomycin (dose according to subsequent blood concentrations) until the cultures are available. These antibiotics aim at treating staphylococci species, which are the most probable agents causing the septic arthritis.

The patient should undergo arthroscopic lavage with massive amounts of saline (>10 L), in conjunction with removal of loose or visible intra-articular hardware, debridement, and arthroscopic synovectomy the same day they present with a suspected postoperative septic knee [16, 23]. At surgery, tissue samples should be obtained from the knee for additional cultures. The graft should be retained unless it is loose or lacerated.

The CRP should be checked daily as an indicator of how the knee responds to the treatment, and the antibiotics should be adjusted once the cultures are available [23].

If the CRP does not decrease the second postoperative day, the patient should undergo repeat arthroscopic lavage and debridement every second to third day until the CRP starts to decrease substantially, usually three to four arthroscopies altogether.

At every repeat arthroscopy new bacterial cultures should be obtained, because it could happen that the resistance pattern of the involved bacteria changes. At these repeat arthroscopic lavages, the graft is still retained if not loose or lacerated.

Once the CRP has substantially decreased and is below 50 mg/L, no fever is present, and the patient feels better, the treatment can be continued with two different oral antibiotics in line with the cultures and with outpatient controls of the CRP and the status of the knee.

The two different oral culture-specific antibiotics (e.g., flucloxacillin and fusidic acid) should be continued until 6 weeks after the postoperative septic knee was diagnosed, followed by one type of antibiotic (e.g., flucloxacillin) for another 6 weeks.

In terms of axial loading of the lower extremity, the patient should use crutches with toe-touch weight bearing until the CRP has normalized. Gentle physiotherapy with range of motion exercises should be started when the CRP has normalized.

If the graft was lacerated, underwent hypotrophy, or was excised during treatment of the septic knee, revision ACL surgery should not be performed before 6 months.

> **Tips and Tricks**
> - After the initial arthroscopic lavage, it is not uncommon that the CRP still increases on the first and second postoperative days, and this does not necessary indicate failure of treatment.
> - If fusidic acid and clindamycin are used, they can be given orally instead of intravenously because of their fast and thorough absorption from the gastrointestinal system.

> **Pitfalls**
> - If a patient presents at the clinic with minor swelling, pain, and discomfort from the knee close after ACL reconstruction, do not start treatment with oral antibiotics without securing cultures through aspiration.

> - In approximately 30 % of cases, no growth of bacteria is found in the cultures [31]. In that case treat the patient for staphylococci infection according to the same guidelines as if the cultures were positive.

> **Memory**
> - Septic knee after ACL reconstruction is a rare but potentially devastating complication after ACL reconstruction.
> - If this condition is diagnosed early and properly treated, there is a high possibility that the patient will return to normal in terms of range of motion and laxity if the graft can be retained.
> - Increase in CRP to 100 mg/L, synovial fluid glucose concentration below 50 % of the concentration in the blood, and synovial fluid lactate concentration above 7–10 mmol/L are strong indicators for septic arthritis.
> - As soon as possible after a postoperative septic knee is suspected and bacterial cultures have been secured, the patient should be started on intravenous antibiotics and undergo arthroscopic lavage and arthroscopic synovectomy.
> - If the CRP does not decrease the second postoperative day, the patient should undergo repeat arthroscopic lavage and debridement every second to third day until the CRP starts to decrease, usually three to four arthroscopies altogether.
> - When the patient is discharged from the hospital, two different oral culture-specific antibiotics should be continued until 6 weeks after the postoperative septic knee was diagnosed, followed by one type of antibiotic (e.g., flucloxacillin) for another 6 weeks.
> - If no growth of bacteria is found in the cultures and the laboratory tests and clinical findings indicate septic arthritis, then treat the patient for staphylococci infection according to the same guidelines as if the cultures were positive.

41.2   Restricted Range of Motion and Arthrofibrosis

Jüri Kartus

41.2.1   Background on the Importance of Regaining Full Range of Motion

There appears to be agreement in the literature that the restoration of full extension compared with the non-injured side after ACL reconstruction is essential in order to avoid postoperative discomfort in the anterior knee region. Irrgang and Harner [8] and Kartus et al. [11] have stated that the loss of extension contributes to anterior knee pain. Steadman et al. [40] reported that anterior scarring and flexion contracture after ACL reconstruction and other procedures caused anterior knee pain and could be successfully treated with arthroscopic release.

The influence of loss of flexion on anterior knee pain is controversial. Stapleton [39] and Kartus et al. [11] have stated that the loss of flexion causes significantly more anterior knee pain than the loss of extension. However, Irrgang and Harner [8] found that a loss of flexion rarely matters, unless the knee flexion is less than 110°.

Although these reports are all concerned with the use of patellar tendon autografts or allografts [8], we can generalize and state that the return of full range of motion (ROM) including full hyperextension is essential to reduce anterior knee problems after ACL reconstruction using any type of graft. However, the return of full range of motion might not always be possible even if no arthrofibrosis is present. Kartus et al. [12] reported more pain and loss of motion both in flexion and extension after ACL reconstruction using both patellar tendon and hamstring tendon autografts if the patients underwent concomitant meniscal resection than if the patients had intact menisci.

Loss of motion after injury or ACL reconstruction is often called arthrofibrosis. But true arthrofibrosis with severe intra-articular scar formation does not occur as often as benign postoperative loss of motion due to mechanical causes or due to minor scar formation such as an anterior nodula, the so-called cyclops syndrome [9]. The classification of Shelbourne et al. [35] is useful to diagnose the severity of arthrofibrosis based on the amount of loss of motion in extension, flexion, or both as well as the mobility of the patella.

41.2.2   Suggestions of How to Avoid and Treat Restricted Range of Motion and Arthrofibrosis

It has been a widespread algorithm to delay ACL reconstruction until the swelling has subsided and the ROM is restored [32, 34] even though it has been reported that early reconstruction does not result in loss of motion [3]. It is today also widespread to use an even more accelerated rehabilitation protocol than originally described by Shelbourne and Nitz [33], with immediate full weight bearing and without the use of cast or brace after the reconstruction.

The cause of arthrofibrosis is not fully understood. The most common causes are reported to be bad surgical technique and poor rehabilitation [7]. It has also been discussed that certain HLA types are more prone to develop arthrofibrosis [37].

The best treatment of loss of motion is to avoid it with proper postoperative rehabilitation involving early return to full range of motion [28].

In the event that early loss of motion occurs after ACL reconstruction, the author's recommendations are as follows:

- If the patient presents at 6 weeks postoperatively with more loss of extension than 5° and less than 110° of flexion [28], then infection should first be excluded. A prolonged period of physiotherapy together with the use of ice and NSAID medication to restore the motion and get the swelling to subside should then be prescribed [18].

- If this does not restore motion within 12 weeks after the index operation, it is the author's suggestion to undergo standard X-ray examination to assess the tunnel placements and to exclude loose bodies or loose hardware as a cause for lost motion. In case the X-ray examination reveals a mechanical cause, then arthroscopic surgery should be performed as soon as possible.
- If no mechanical cause is found at 12 weeks postoperatively and infection has been excluded, then one injection of intra-articular local anesthetics and cortisone or oral corticosteroids for a few days [29] followed by continued physiotherapy should be tried.
- If motion does not restore within another 4–6 weeks, the patient should be scheduled for arthroscopic debridement and manipulation under anesthesia without delay [19, 28]. During surgery the intercondylar notch and all knee compartments should be cleaned from scar tissue, and the graft should be checked during full range of motion for impingement toward the femoral condyles, and if necessary a notch-plasty should be performed.
- In rare cases repeat arthroscopic procedures are needed, and in the worst scenario even open debridement can be performed [14].

41.3 Cyclops Syndrome After Anterior Cruciate Ligament Reconstruction

Francis Fernandez and Rainer Siebold

41.3.1 Introduction

Anterior cruciate ligament (ACL) surgery is a highly successful surgery to regain full function and to return to previous activity. However, some patients are unable to achieve full extension after surgery despite proper graft placement. Studies have shown that a common finding in these patients is the development fibrous scar tissue in the intercondylar notch [9, 17].

41.3.2 Cyclops Syndrome

The "cyclops syndrome" was first described by Jackson and Schaefer in 1990. They reported a fibrovascular nodular lesion that caused diminished extension after ACL surgery [9]. The lesion was called a "cyclops syndrome" due to its arthroscopic appearance (Fig. 41.6a, b): it is a round fibrous nodule vascular infiltration resembling an eye [38]. It is usually found anterior or anterolateral to the ACL graft on MRI. The

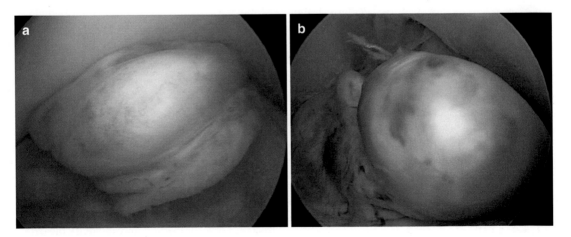

Fig. 41.6 Arthroscopic aspects of two cyclops syndroms. (**a**) Vascular infiltration of the cyclops. (**b**) The cyclops causing impingement on extension

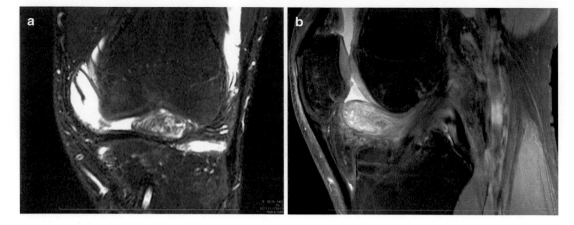

Fig. 41.7 Coronal (**a**) and sagittal (**b**) MRI views of a cyclops lesion located in the anterior portion of the intercondylar notch

reported frequency of cyclops syndrome varies from 2.2 to 21 % after ACL surgery [17, 38].

The incidence of cyclops lesions is high, but not all cause symptoms [17].

41.3.3 Pathophysiology

The pathophysiology of the cyclops lesion is uncertain, but there are many theories on how it develops. Jackson and Schaefer believed that formation of the nodule is caused by intra-articular debris from the drilling of the ACL tunnels [9, 38]. This remaining debris could be part of the fibroproliferative process of the cyclops lesion. Another theory states that the cyclops lesion forms during the reparative process of an injured anterior cruciate ligament, which explains the formation of cyclops lesions even before an ACL reconstruction [43]. There is also the impingement theory for the formation of this lesion. Grafts which are placed too anteriorly can cause injury to the graft by impingement to the intercondylar notch. The ventral fiber breakage initiates a fibro-inflammatory process which forms the cyclops lesion [43].

41.3.4 Clinical Diagnosis

The diagnosis of cyclops syndrome is based on clinical and MRI findings. Patients who develop a cyclops syndrome usually present 3–4 months after ACL reconstruction. They complain of pain in the infrapatellar area on terminal extension and inability to extend their knee. Some patients describe a catching with an audible "clunk" when walking or running. Physical therapy is not able to regain this extension loss [38].

MRI is reported to have a sensitivity of 85 % and a specificity of 84 % to diagnose a cyclops lesion. A lesion greater than 1 cm in at least 1 dimension increases specificity but does not increase sensitivity [4, 20]. On MRI, the lesion is most commonly found in the intercondylar notch anterior or anterolateral to the insertion of the ACL graft. It presents with an intermediate to low signal intensity on T1-weighted sequences or heterogeneous to intermediate signal intensity on T2-weighted sequences (Fig. 41.7a, b). On STIR images, the lesion in front of the notch has a heterogeneous signal intensity which can be differentiated from edema in the anterior portion of the notch.

41.3.5 Treatment

Asymptomatic cyclops lesions don't have to be treated. Physical therapy may decrease the extension loss, but full extension might not be possible since the main problem is the mechanical block. In case of a cyclops syndrome with persistent

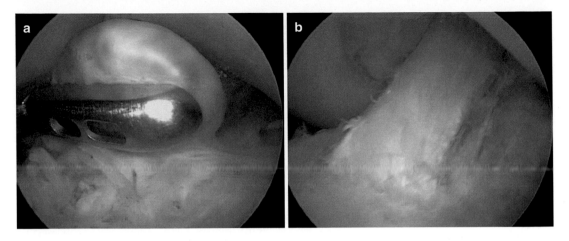

Fig. 41.8 Removal of cyclops lesion (**a**) and intact ACL reconstruction (**b**)

extension loss and pain, the treatment of choice is an arthroscopic debridement (Fig. 41.8a, b). After debridement of the lesion, most patients regain full extension and are symptom-free. In most studies, there has been no recorded recurrence of cyclops syndrome [17, 38].

Memory

Cyclops syndrome is a common cause of knee extension loss after ACL reconstruction. The histologic correlate is a fibrous nodule along the anterior portion of the ACL graft, which impinges on the intercondylar notch. In case of persistent symptoms the only treatment is debridement of this lesion to regain full range of motion.

References

1. Barker JU, Drakos MC, Maak TG, Warren RF, Williams RJ 3rd, Allen AA (2010) Effect of graft selection on the incidence of postoperative infection in anterior cruciate ligament reconstruction. Am J Sports Med 38(2):281–286. doi:10.1177/0363546509346414

2. Binnet MS, Basarir K (2007) Risk and outcome of infection after different arthroscopic anterior cruciate ligament reconstruction techniques. Arthroscopy 23(8):862–868. doi:10.1016/j.arthro.2007.02.008. S0749-8063(07)00163-6 [pii]

3. Bottoni CR, Liddell TR, Trainor TJ, Freccero DM, Lindell KK (2008) Postoperative range of motion following anterior cruciate ligament reconstruction using autograft hamstrings: a prospective, randomized clinical trial of early versus delayed reconstructions. Am J Sports Med 36(4):656–662. doi:10.1177/0363546507312164. 0363546507312164 [pii]

4. Bradley DM, Bergman AG, Dillingham MF (2000) MR imaging of cyclops lesions. AJR Am J Roentgenol 174(3):719–726

5. Capuano F, Roscitano A, Simon C, Sclafani G, Benedetto U, Comito C, Tonelli E, Sinatra R (2006) Intensive hyperglycemia control reduces postoperative infections after open heart surgery. Heart Int 2(1):49. doi:10.4081/hi.2006.49. hi.2006.49 [pii]

6. Carpenter CR, Schuur JD, Everett WW, Pines JM (2011) Evidence-based diagnostics: adult septic arthritis. Acad Emerg Med 18(8):781–796. doi:10.1111/j.1553-2712.2011.01121.x

7. Graf B, Uhr F (1988) Complications of intra-articular anterior cruciate reconstruction. Clin Sports Med 7(4):835–848

8. Irrgang JJ, Harner CD (1995) Loss of motion following knee ligament reconstruction. Sports Med 19(2): 150–159

9. Jackson DW, Schaefer RK (1990) Cyclops syndrome: loss of extension following intra-articular anterior cruciate ligament reconstruction. Arthroscopy 6(3):171–178

10. Judd D, Bottoni C, Kim D, Burke M, Hooker S (2006) Infections following arthroscopic anterior cruciate ligament reconstruction. Arthroscopy 22(4):375–384. doi:10.1016/j.arthro.2005.12.002. S0749-8063(05)01654-3 [pii]

11. Kartus J, Magnusson L, Stener S, Brandsson S, Eriksson BI, Karlsson J (1999) Complications following arthroscopic anterior cruciate ligament reconstruction. A 2-5-year follow-up of 604 patients with special emphasis on anterior knee pain. Knee Surg Sports Traumatol Arthrosc 7(1):2–8

12. Kartus JT, Russell VJ, Salmon LJ, Magnusson LC, Brandsson S, Pehrsson NG, Pinczewski LA (2002) Concomitant partial meniscectomy worsens outcome after arthroscopic anterior cruciate ligament reconstruction. Acta Orthop Scand 73(2):179–185

13. Kluger N (2009) Bacterial endocarditis and body art: suggestions for an active prevention. Int J Cardiol 136(1):112–113. doi:10.1016/j.ijcard.2008.03.083. S0167-5273(08)00558-5 [pii]

14. Magit D, Wolff A, Sutton K, Medvecky MJ (2007) Arthrofibrosis of the knee. J Am Acad Orthop Surg 15(11):682–694. 15/11/682 [pii]

15. Martinez-Castillo A, Nunez C, Cabiedes J (2010) Synovial fluid analysis. Rheumatol Clin 6(6):316–321. doi:10.1016/j.reuma.2009.12.010. S1699-258X(10)00064-1 [pii]

16. McAllister DR, Parker RD, Cooper AE, Recht MP, Abate J (1999) Outcomes of postoperative septic arthritis after anterior cruciate ligament reconstruction. Am J Sports Med 27(5):562–570

17. McMahon PJ, Dettling JR, Yocum LA et al (1999) The cyclops lesion: a cause of diminished knee extension after rupture of the anterior cruciate ligament. Arthroscopy 15(7):757–761

18. Millett PJ, Wickiewicz TL, Warren RF (2001) Motion loss after ligament injuries to the knee. Part I: causes. Am J Sports Med 29(5):664–675

19. Millett PJ, Wickiewicz TL, Warren RF (2001) Motion loss after ligament injuries to the knee. Part II: prevention and treatment. Am J Sports Med 29(6):822–828

20. Minné C, Velleman M, Suleman F (2012) MRI findings of cyclops lesions of the knee. SA Orthop J 11:56–60

21. Monaco E, Maestri B, Labianca L, Speranza A, Vadala A, Iorio R, Ferretti A (2010) Clinical and radiological outcomes of postoperative septic arthritis after anterior cruciate ligament reconstruction. J Orthop Sci 15(2): 198–203. doi:10.1007/s00776-009-1447-3

22. Monaco E, Maestri B, Vadala A, Iorio R, Ferretti A (2010) Return to sports activity after postoperative septic arthritis in ACL reconstruction. Phys Sportsmed 38(3):69–76. doi:10.3810/psm.2010.10.1810

23. Mouzopoulos G, Fotopoulos VC, Tzurbakis M (2009) Septic knee arthritis following ACL reconstruction: a systematic review. Knee Surg Sports Traumatol Arthrosc 17(9):1033–1042. doi:10.1007/s00167-009-0793-1

24. Nakayama H, Yagi M, Yoshiya S, Takesue Y (2012) Micro-organism colonization and intraoperative contamination in patients undergoing arthroscopic anterior cruciate ligament reconstruction. Arthroscopy 28(5):667–671. doi:10.1016/j.arthro.2011.10.023. S0749-8063(11)01250-3 [pii]

25. Parada SA, Grassbaugh JA, Devine JG, Arrington ED (2009) Instrumentation-specific infection after anterior cruciate ligament reconstruction. Sports Health 1(6):481–485. doi:10.1177/1941738109347975. 10.1177_1941738109347975 [pii]

26. Perry A, Lambert P (2011) Propionibacterium acnes: infection beyond the skin. Expert Rev Anti Infect Ther 9(12):1149–1156. doi:10.1586/eri.11.137

27. Plante MJ, Li X, Scully G, Brown MA, Busconi BD, DeAngelis NA (2013) Evaluation of sterilization methods following contamination of hamstring autograft during anterior cruciate ligament reconstruction. Knee Surg Sports Traumatol Arthrosc 21(3):696–701. doi:10.1007/s00167-012-2049-8

28. Robertson GA, Coleman SG, Keating JF (2009) Knee stiffness following anterior cruciate ligament reconstruction: the incidence and associated factors of knee stiffness following anterior cruciate ligament reconstruction. Knee 16(4):245–247. doi:10.1016/j.knee.2008.12.014. S0968-0160(08)00246-9 [pii]

29. Rue JP, Ferry AT, Lewis PB, Bach BR Jr (2008) Oral corticosteroid use for loss of flexion after primary anterior cruciate ligament reconstruction. Arthroscopy 24(5):554–559 e551. doi:10.1016/j.arthro.2007.10.013. S0749-8063(07)01042-0 [pii]

30. Schollin-Borg M, Michaelsson K, Rahme H (2003) Presentation, outcome, and cause of septic arthritis after anterior cruciate ligament reconstruction: a case control study. Arthroscopy 19(9):941–947. aS0749806303008119 [pii]

31. Scully WF, Fisher SG, Parada SA, Arrington EA (2013) Septic arthritis following anterior cruciate ligament reconstruction: a comprehensive review of the literature. J Surg orthop adv 22(2):127–133

32. Shelbourne KD, Foulk DA (1995) Timing of surgery in acute anterior cruciate ligament tears on the return of quadriceps muscle strength after reconstruction using an autogenous patellar tendon graft. Am J Sports Med 23(6):686–689

33. Shelbourne KD, Nitz P (1990) Accelerated rehabilitation after anterior cruciate ligament reconstruction. Am J Sports Med 18(3):292–299

34. Shelbourne KD, Wilckens JH, Mollabashy A, DeCarlo M (1991) Arthrofibrosis in acute anterior cruciate ligament reconstruction. The effect of timing of reconstruction and rehabilitation. Am J Sports Med 19(4):332–336

35. Shelbourne KD, Patel DV, Martini DJ (1996) Classification and management of arthrofibrosis of the knee after anterior cruciate ligament reconstruction. Am J Sports Med 24(6):857–862

36. Singh JA (2011) Smoking and outcomes after knee and hip arthroplasty: a systematic review. J Rheumatol 38(9):1824–1834. doi:10.3899/jrheum.101221. jrheum. 101221 [pii]

37. Skutek M, Elsner HA, Slateva K, Mayr HO, Weig TG, van Griensven M, Krettek C, Bosch U (2004) Screening for arthrofibrosis after anterior cruciate ligament reconstruction: analysis of association with human leukocyte antigen. Arthroscopy 20(5):469–473. doi:10.1016/j.arthro.2004.03.003. S0749806304003068 [pii]

38. Sonnery-Cottet B, Lavoie F, Ogassawara R et al (2010) Clinical and operative characteristics of cyclops syndrome after double-bundle anterior cruciate ligament reconstruction. Arthroscopy 26(11):1483–1488

39. Stapleton TR (1997) Complications in anterior cruciate ligament reconstructions with patellar tendon grafts. Sports Med Arthrosc Rev 5:156–162

40. Steadman JR, Dragoo JL, Hines SL, Briggs KK (2008) Arthroscopic release for symptomatic scarring of the anterior interval of the knee. Am J Sports Med 36(9):1763–1769

41. Torres-Claramunt R, Pelfort X, Erquicia J, Gil-Gonzalez S, Gelber PE, Puig L, Monllau JC (2012) Knee joint infection after ACL reconstruction: prevalence, management and functional outcomes. Knee Surg Sports Traumatol Arthrosc. doi:10.1007/s00167-012-2264-3

42. Tosti A, Peluso AM, Bardazzi F, Morelli R, Bassi F (1994) Phalangeal osteomyelitis due to nail biting. Acta Derm Venereol 74(3):206–207

43. Wang J, Ao Y (2009) Analysis of different kinds of cyclops lesions with or without extension loss. Arthroscopy 25(6):626–631

44. Williams RJ 3rd, Laurencin CT, Warren RF, Speciale AC, Brause BD, O'Brien S (1997) Septic arthritis after arthroscopic anterior cruciate ligament reconstruction. Diagnosis and management. Am J Sports Med 25(2):261–267

Rehabilitation and Return to Sports

42

Amelie Stoehr, Hermann Mayr,
Barbara Wondrasch, and Christian Fink

Contents

A. Stoehr, MD (✉)
Knee Surgery and Sports Traumatology,
OCM-Clinic, Steiner Str. 6, 81369 Munich, Germany
e-mail: ameliestoehr@hotmail.de

H. Mayr, MD, PhD
Department of Orthopedic Surgery, OCM-Clinic,
Steiner Str. 6, 81369 Munich, Germany

B. Wondrasch, PT, MSc
Department of Health and Social Sciences,
University of Applied Sciences St. Poelten,
Matthias Corvinus-Strasse 15,
3100 St. Poelten, Austria

C. Fink, MD, PhD
Research – Knee/Sports Medicine,
Sportsclinic Austria GmbH,
Olympiastrasse 39, 6020 Innsbruck, Austria

The successful and fast return of an athlete to his pre-injury level of sports strongly depends on the rehabilitation protocol [3]. From animal trials, we got information on the remodeling process and the mechanical strength of various ligament grafts after ACL reconstruction during the healing period. The stability of synovialized ligament grafts seems to be significantly lower than that of non-synovialized patellar tendon grafts after 12 weeks but is similar again after 24 weeks [11]. These findings may be relevant for the follow-up treatment of ACL grafts in humans as the biological healing behavior of the graft can hardly be influenced. In recent decades there was little agreement among surgeons and little evidence regarding the postoperative treatment after ACL reconstruction. In order to reduce costs and complications and fasten return to sports and graft healing as well as knee function and muscle strength, extensive literature searches for evidence-based recommendations have shown certain consensus nowadays [10, 22].

42.1 Initial and Early Phase (0–6 Weeks)

In the early phase of rehabilitation after ACL reconstruction pain reduction, decongestant, and anti-inflammatory actions, the restoration of free knee joint mobility and neuromuscular control are especially important [23].

R. Siebold et al. (eds.), *Anterior Cruciate Ligament Reconstruction*,
DOI 10.1007/978-3-642-45349-6_42, © ESSKA 2014

Literature shows no significant association of postoperative brace treatment with a better outcome, rated subjectively or objectively, after ACL reconstruction [25].

In case of relevant effusion, puncturing of the knee is recommended to reduce the capsular distension and the associated arthrogenic muscle inhibition [1, 9].

Cryotherapy helps controlling pain and inflammation as well as NSAID ingestion [13, 16].

> **Tricks and Pearls**
> Cold application up to three times a day for maximal 10 min at 5–6 °C temperature of the cooling unit is useful against swelling. Application of cold packs in the back of the knee should be avoided.

Leg elevation in supine position prevents increased soft tissue swelling. Active foot movement and knee flexor tensioning can even start on operation day. In the first 2 weeks, knee extensor muscle training should be performed with isometric closed kinetic chain (safe range 0–50°) exercises only, in order to avoid increased translation and to harm the graft.

> **Tricks and Pearls**
> Active stretch exercises at home with a soft ball in the back of the knee improve lymph flow. Closed chain exercises sitting on a chair with a skateboard under the sole facilitate movement of the hip, knee, and ankle.

Open chain exercises are safe from week 2 in a range of 100–50° without additional weight. Recent studies suggest that both open and closed kinetic chain exercises are beneficial in the early rehabilitation phase after ACL reconstruction and show similar loads on the graft and comparable effects on the healing response [4, 8, 19, 22].

Lymphatic drainage and patella mobilization should be applied to reduce the inflammatory irritation of the knee and retropatellar overload

due to reparative fibrotic changes in the early phase after the operation in order to prevent arthrofibrosis and quadriceps inhibition [15].

> **Avoid Pitfalls**
> Exercises with pain and early strength training increase the risk of arthrofibrosis.

An early start with active and passive range of motion (ROM) training with an emphasis on full extension is necessary to reduce pain and prevent patellofemoral disorders, alterations in gait pattern, and quadriceps atrophy [1, 4, 23]. In addition, the load on the cartilage will reduce degeneration by immobilization. Immediate exercise with a CPM (continuous passive motion) machine (Fig. 42.1) leads to physiological cartilage nutrition and can prevent early adhesions in the joint, but the use is not evidence based.

Partial weight-bearing on crutches might be useful to normalize the joint milieu during the first postoperative days. Literature supports immediate weight-bearing after ACL reconstruction due to reduced anterior knee pain and lacking effects to knee joint stability [4, 19]. Early postoperative weight-bearing advantages are cartilage nutrition, facilitation of collagen reorganization during healing, and allowing osseous and soft tissues of the knee to respond to normal

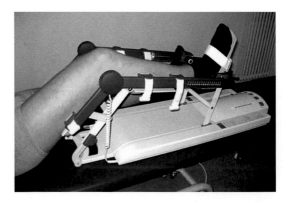

Fig. 42.1 Immediate exercise with a CPM (continuous passive motion) machine leads to physiological cartilage nutrition and can prevent early adhesions in the joint (© Amelie Stoehr)

physiological loading [6]. Most patients return to full weight-bearing between the 7th and 14th postoperative days. Sufficient neuromuscular control and a non-limping gait pattern are criteria for walking without crutches [22].

> **Tricks and Pearls**
> During the first 4 postoperative weeks, stair climbing is recommended with the healthy leg up first and with the operated leg down first to avoid overload of the graft and a possible pivoting during this period of neuromuscular deficits.

> **Avoid Pitfalls**
> In case of meniscus sutures and cartilage surgery, a much longer discharge on crutches may be required.

The "how" of the most effective quadriceps and hamstring muscle strength training programs after ACL reconstruction in terms of protecting the healing graft and gaining as much as muscle strength at once has been addressed in numerous studies [5, 7, 20]. Both open kinetic chain (OKC) and closed kinetic chain (CKC) exercises have been described in rehabilitation programs used for patients after ACL reconstruction [5, 20]. Exercises in a closed kinetic chain are so-called functional movements with the distal segment secured on a fixed base. It produces co-contraction of the muscles surrounding the joint and compression within the joint and therefore causes more joint stability. Exercises performed with the distal segment of the limb moved are referred to as OKC exercises. Quadriceps muscle strengthening exercises in an OKC were thought to increase strain in the ACL graft and were therefore eclipsed in the last years. However, knee extensor strengthening in OKC is essential in the rehabilitation after ACL reconstruction as this exercise considerably addresses the quadriceps muscle [20].

> **Tricks and Pearls**
> Early training of fine motor skills of the entire body is helpful to avoid imbalances.

A recent published review presented that ACL loading is generally greater during OKC exercises compared with exercises in a CKC system. Furthermore, it was demonstrated that both in the OKC and in the CKC system exercises in a range of 10–50° flexion produce more load on the ACL than in a range of 50–100° of knee flexion. The exercise technique itself (trunk position, feet position, etc.) might also influence the extent of ACL load [5].

Therefore, both OKC and CKC exercises with variations of the exercise technique are recommended to improve quadriceps muscle strength.

Leg press exercises with a maximum load of one third of body weight and ROM E/F 0–40–90° can start in week 2. In addition, the muscles of the foot and ankle should be trained to be stabilized. Stretching under the guidance of the therapist is helpful to prevent muscular imbalance. Neuromuscular training should start as soon as full weight-bearing is possible [4, 19, 23]. Between weeks 3 and 6, previous physiotherapy will continue under appropriate guidance for self-therapy.

> **Tricks and Pearls**
> The patient is allowed to start with cycling on an ergometer with low resistance when reaching a knee flexion of 100°. This facilitates the flexion by continuous motion.

Coordination exercises, aqua jogging, stepping on a stair-stepping machine, and one-legged stabilization exercises will improve knee function.

> **Tricks and Pearls**
> Training on seesaw (Fig. 42.2) and mini trampoline (Fig. 42.3) encourages the sense of body balance.

Fig. 42.2 Training on seesaw encourages the sense of body balance (© Cornelia Jungfer-Mayr)

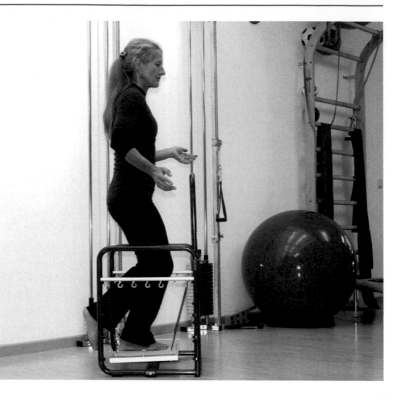

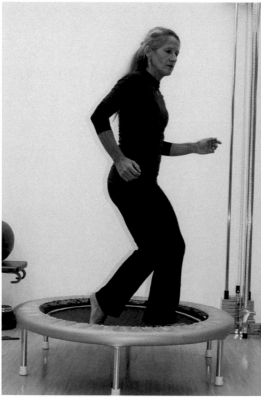

Fig. 42.3 Training on mini trampoline encourages the sense of body balance (© Cornelia Jungfer-Mayr)

Avoid Pitfalls
Jumping exercises should not be performed during the first 6 postoperative weeks because of the missing proprioception of the transplant. Stability tests, isokinetic testing, and leg curl for quadriceps training are not advisable during the first 8 weeks after surgery [19, 22]. Constant pain, inflammation, and limited ROM during the postoperative rehabilitation after ACL reconstruction increase the risk of a developing arthrofibrosis [1, 12, 15] and should be taken care of.

42.2 Intermediate Phase (6–12 Weeks)

This phase includes resolving impairments such as swelling, pain, and lack of range of motion (ROM) and normalizing lower extremity muscle strength for performing activities of daily living (ADLs) without interference in the healing process of the graft. At the end of this phase, walking with a normal gait pattern and low-level sport

Fig. 42.4 Leg press
(© Sporttherapie Mag.
Huber GmbH)

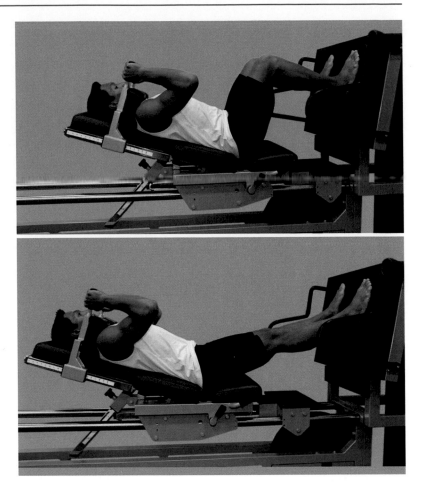

activities (meaning no pivoting sport activities) should be possible.

Pain and swelling can be addressed by the use of cryotherapy and different taping techniques. ROM should be restored with emphasis on full extension. Manual therapy techniques such as patella mobilizations and glide movements of the tibia are beneficial to increase ROM and therefore to prevent postsurgical complications like arthrofibrosis. Loss of full knee extension is one of the most common complications and can influence the postoperative outcome [22]. Full active and passive extension (even hyperextension) should therefore be emphasized. Furthermore, muscle stretching of the gastrocnemius, the hamstring, and the quadriceps muscles should be performed to prevent muscular disbalances. Quadriceps and hamstring strengthening exercises are essential to

restore lower extremity muscle strength and to actively stabilize the knee joint. Furthermore, the hip abductors should be addressed to normalize gait pattern.

In the intermediate phase, CKC exercises are emphasized to increase joint stability and to minimize loading on the healing graft. For example, the leg press (Fig. 42.4) is an effective machine for lower extremity strengthening with low load on the ACL graft. At the beginning of this phase, a light resistance between 0° and 50° knee flexion angles should be used. Since the pain and swelling decreases, the knee flexion angles and resistance can be increased. Another CKC exercise is the double-leg squat (Fig. 42.5) which also results in minimal strain on the ACL graft. The strengthening program after ACL reconstruction should start with double-leg squats before progressing to single-leg

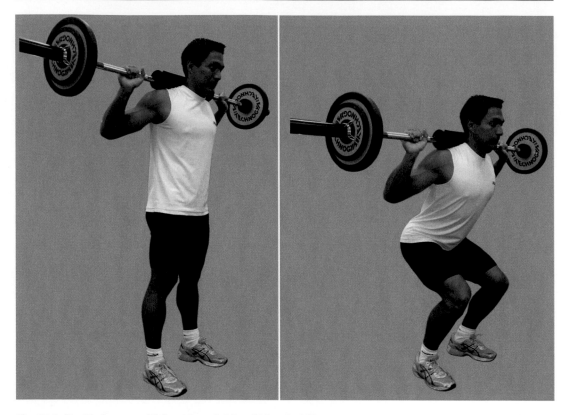

Fig. 42.5 Double-leg squat (© Sporttherapie Mag. Huber GmbH)

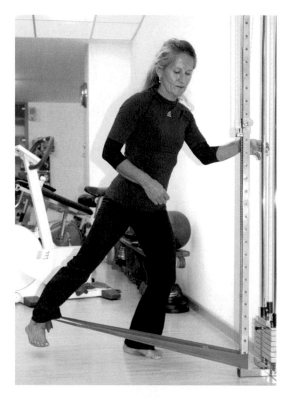

squats. Though the single-leg squats produce low strain on the ACL graft as well, more neuromuscular control is needed which might be too challenging for patients in this phase. Hip muscles, in particular the abductors and the external rotators, are very important to counteract with the knee valgus movement and the muscular malalignment of the lower limb. Both knee valgus movement and muscular malalignment are factors increasing the chance of a reinjury of the ACL and should therefore be addressed in postoperative rehabilitation after ACL reconstruction [14]. Hip muscle strengthening can be performed both in weight-bearing and non-weight-bearing positions. Figures 42.6 and 42.7 show some examples of hip muscle strengthening exercises.

Fig. 42.6 Dynamic hip abduction with the contralateral leg produces functional activation of the abductors on the standing leg (© Cornelia Jungfer-Mayr)

Fig. 42.7 Seated hip abduction (© Barbara Wondrasch)

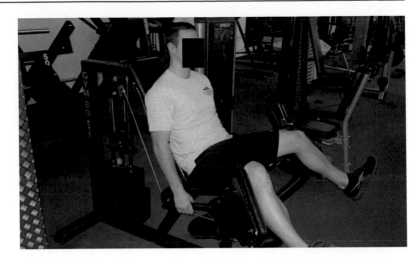

Tricks and Pearls
Enhance functional lower extremity alignment before starting one leg strengthening exercise intensely.

Avoid Pitfalls
Avoid pain and effusion during and after strength training to prevent optimal joint homeostasis.

Neuromuscular training is very essential for functional recovery and to prevent reinjury of the ACL. It has been demonstrated that simply restoring mechanical restraints will not lead to a satisfactory outcome [17]. Neuromuscular training can optimize muscle activation pattern and can therefore control abnormal joint translation during functional activities [16, 18, 22].

The neuromuscular training in the intermediate phase consists of static and dynamic balance exercises. Static balance exercises can include single- and double-leg stance on flat surfaces with progression to unstable surfaces (e.g., mat, wobble board, and Bosu). Dynamic balance exercises comprise stepping movements in different directions (forward–backward, right–left) on flat surfaces or unstable surfaces with the aim to keep the knee stable during the landing phase. Figures 42.8 and 42.9 demonstrate some of these exercises.

Furthermore, the neuromuscular training should include more complex exercises simulating functional movement patterns. These kinds of exercises might improve the interaction between stabilizing structures of the kinetic chain of the lower limb which includes the trunk, the hip, the knee, and the ankle.

42.3   Late Phase

The late phase of rehabilitation focuses on regaining dynamic joint stability to allow functional movement patterns, which are needed both for low-level and high-level sport activities. Dynamic knee stability is defined as the ability of the knee joint to remain stable during rapidly changing loads occurring during activities such as running, jumping, and cutting maneuvers and is provided by the neuromuscular system [22]. The neuromuscular system is based on muscle strength neuromuscular control [2, 18, 22]. However, both a loss of neuromuscular control and a loss of muscle strength of the lower extremity are reported to be two of the main impairments after ACL reconstruction [4].

Muscle strength training and neuromuscular training should be continued in this phase with special emphasis on the individual's deficits, which have to be identified.

As the tensile strength of the graft increases in this phase, strength exercises in the OKC can be implemented in this phase to target the quadriceps muscle strength [5]. Furthermore,

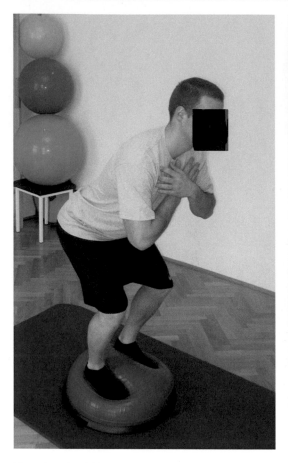

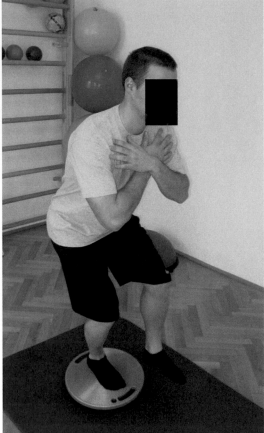

Fig. 42.8 Double-leg stance on a Bosu (© Barbara Wondrasch)

Fig. 42.9 One-leg stance on a wobble board (© Barbara Wondrasch)

additional weight and more resistance can be used for the muscle strength training.

In this phase the neuromuscular training is more focused on dynamic joint stability which can be achieved by dynamic tasks, agility training, and plyometric exercises. During these exercises it is important that the patients are able to maintain the knee and the hip in an upright position and to maintain the position of the center of the mass along a vertical axis to avoid deleterious loading pattern in the knee joint [12]. Furthermore, sports-specific agility training with cutting maneuvers, acceleration and deceleration, and variations in running has been reported to improve arthrokinetic reflexes and to reduce the risk of reinjury.

> **Tricks and Pearls**
> Try to diversify the training and adapt it to the individual's demands to increase compliance.

A big issue and concern is the athlete's question: "When can I play again?" Typically athletes are permitted to return to sports around 3–9 months after ACL reconstruction [19]. However, Ardern et al. showed that only 33 % of participants had attempted competitive sports at their pre-injury level by 12 months after ACL reconstruction. The authors recommend that there should be a longer postoperative rehabilitation period to facilitate a

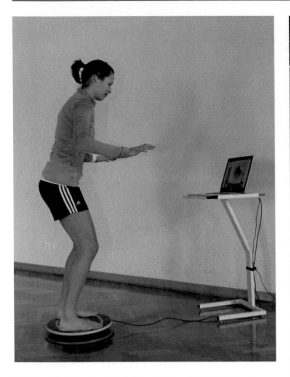

Fig. 42.10 Two-leg Stability Test on the MFT Challenge Disc(© Barbara Zisch)

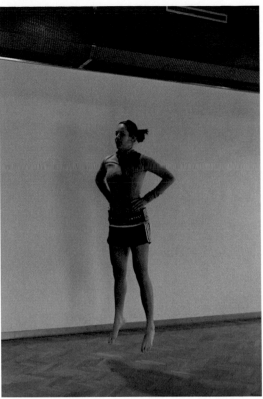

Fig. 42.11 Counter Movement Jump (© Barbara Zisch)

successful return to sports after ACL reconstruction [2]. However, time should not be the only factor influencing the decision of when returning to sports. Restored lower limb muscle function, such as knee muscle strength and jumping ability, is considered to be important after ACL reconstruction to determine the optimal time point of return to sports [21]. Lots of test batteries have been established, including tests for lower extremity muscle strength and one-leg hop tests, to assess functional performance after ACL reconstruction [19, 24].

Zisch et al. from the Sportsclinic Austria developed a test battery combining various tests for an objective evaluation of the patient's performance through the end of rehabilitation. The test battery concludes eight different functional tests: (1) two-leg Stability Test (Fig. 42.10), (2) one-leg Stability Test, (3) two-leg Counter Movement Jump (CMJ) (Fig. 42.11), (4) one-leg CMJ, (5) Plyometric Jumps, (6) Speedy Test, (7) Quick Feet Test (Fig. 42.12), and (8) Standing Heel-Raise Test.

A study with healthy subjects was performed to test the reliability of this test battery. The study sample included 100 healthy subjects (50 women, 50 men) with a mean age of 24.8 ± 3.6. Since July 2011 the protocol is routinely used for patients following ACL reconstruction. Until September 2011 ten professional athletes (Alpine ski racing, Nordic ski jumping) have been evaluated. In these athletes, an isokinetic assessment of flexor and extensor torque values (Contrex Inc.) was added. The results show that all tests documented good reliability (ICC 0.76–0.92). Standards were created for both genders for all eight tests, so that the result of patients can be classified from "excellent" to "good," "fair," "bad," and "very bad" in each test. Significant differences between males and females were found in almost every functional test ($p < 0.001$ to $p = 0.003$), except for the Standing Heel-Raise Test (dominant leg $p = 0.555$, nondominant leg $p = 0.198$).

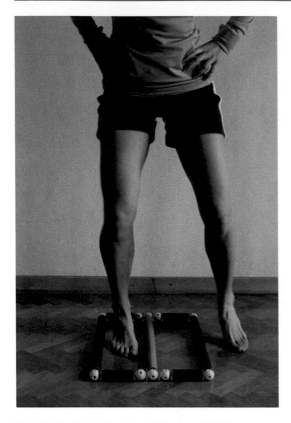

Fig. 42.12 Quick Feet Test (© Barbara Zisch)

The first assessment was performed 4 months following ACL reconstruction. Based on the results, specific advice could be given in order to selectively address the deficits. A retest was performed at 6 months postoperatively. Based on these results, return to sports was allowed or delayed. The conclusion was that each test in the protocol has been found to be reliable and easy to assess. The protocol seems to be extremely helpful in the objective evaluation of patients following ACL reconstruction. It was found to be a good tool in the decision when to allow return to sports at a certain level. If this will result in a reduced reinjury, risk has to be seen in the future.

Avoid Pitfalls

Early resumption of high-level sport activities may result in a re-rupture of the ACL graft.

Memory

Initial and Early Phase (0–6 Weeks)

Immediately after surgery and up to 6 weeks postoperatively, it is important to relieve soft tissue and joint irritation and to achieve full knee extension and a flexion of at least 90–120°. Pain should be avoided throughout the treatment. Lymphatic drainage is useful. In the early phase, attention should be paid to patella mobility and fine motor skills.

Intermediate Phase (6–12 Weeks)

This phase includes resolving impairments such as swelling, pain, and lack of range of motion (ROM) and normalizing lower extremity muscle strength for performing activities of daily living (ADLs) without interference in the healing process of the graft. At the end of this phase, walking with a normal gait pattern and low-level sport activities (meaning no pivoting sport activities) should be possible.

Late Phase

The late phase of rehabilitation focuses on regaining dynamic joint stability to allow functional movement patterns, which are needed both for low-level and high-level sport activities. The main focus of strength and neuromuscular training should be put on dynamic tasks and sports-specific tasks.

References

1. Allum R (2003) Aspects of current management, complications of arthroscopic reconstruction of the anterior cruciate ligament. J Bone Joint Surg Br 85-B:12–16
2. Ardern CL, Webster KE, Taylor NF, Feller JA (2011) Return to the preinjury level of competitive sport after anterior cruciate ligament reconstruction surgery: two-thirds of patients have not returned by 12 months after surgery. Am J Sports Med 39:538–543
3. Beynnon B, Johnson R, Fleming B (2002) The science of anterior cruciate ligament rehabilitation. Clin Orthop 402:9–20

4. Beynnon B, Johnson R, Abate J, Fleming B, Nichols C (2005) Treatment of anterior cruciate ligament injuries, Part 2. Am J Sports Med 33:1751–1767

5. Chmielewski TL, Rudolph KS, Snyder-Mackler L (2002) Development of dynamic knee stability after acute ACL injury. J Electromyogr Kinesiol 12:267–274

6. Escamilla RF, Macleod TD, Wilk KE, Paulos L, Andrews JR (2012) Anterior cruciate ligament strain and tensile forces for weight-bearing and non-weight-bearing exercises: a guide to exercise selection. J Orthop Sports Phys Ther 42:208–220

7. Escamilla RF, Macleod TD, Wilk KE, Paulos L, Andrews JR (2012) Cruciate ligament loading during common knee rehabilitation exercises. Proc Inst Mech Eng H 226:670–680

8. Fleming B, Oksendahl H, Beynnon B (2005) Open- or closed kinetic chain exercises after anterior cruciate ligament reconstruction. Exerc Sport Sci Rev 33:134–140

9. Hopkins JT, Ingersoll CD (2000) Arthrogenic muscle inhibition: a limiting factor in joint rehabilitation. J Sport Rehabil 9:135–159

10. Kruse LM, Gray B, Wright RW (2012) Rehabilitation after anterior cruciate ligament reconstruction: a systematic review. J Bone Joint Surg Am 94(19):1737–1748

11. Mayr HO, Stoehr A, Dietrich M, von Eisenhart-Rothe R, Hube R, Senger S, Suedkamp NP, Bernstein A (2012) Graft-dependent differences in the ligamentization process of anterior cruciate ligament grafts in a sheep trial. Knee Surg Sports Traumatol Arthrosc 20(5):947–956

12. Mayr HO, Weig TG, Plitz W (2004) Arthrofibrosis following ACL reconstruction–reasons and outcome. Arch Orthop Trauma Surg 124(8):518–522

13. Mc Carty L, Bach B (2005) Rehabilitation after patellar tendon autograft anterior cruciate ligament reconstruction. Tech Orthop 20:439–451

14. Myer GD, Paterno MV, Ford KR, Quatman CE, Hewett TE (2006) Rehabilitation after anterior cruciate ligament reconstruction: criteria-based progression through the return-to-sport phase. J Orthop Sports Phys Ther 36:385–402

15. Potter N (2006) Complications and treatment during rehabilitation after anterior cruciate ligament reconstruction. Oper Tech Sports Med 14:50–58

16. Raynor M, Pietrobon R, Guller U, Higgins L (2005) Cryotherapy after ACL reconstruction. J Knee Surg 18:123–129

17. Risberg MA, Holm I, Myklebust G, Engebretsen L (2007) Neuromuscular training versus strength training during first 6 months after anterior cruciate ligament reconstruction: a randomized clinical trial. Phys Ther 87:737–750

18. Risberg MA, Mork M, Jenssen HK, Holm I (2001) Design and implementation of a neuromuscular training program following anterior cruciate ligament reconstruction. J Orthop Sports Phys Ther 31:620–631

19. Risberg M, Lewek M, Snyder-Mackler L (2004) A systematic review of evidence for anterior cruciate ligament rehabilitation, how much and what type. Phys Ther Sport 5:125–145

20. Tagesson S, Oberg B, Good L, Kvist J (2008) A comprehensive rehabilitation program with quadriceps strengthening in closed versus open kinetic chain exercise in patients with anterior cruciate ligament deficiency: a randomized clinical trial evaluating dynamic tibial translation and muscle function. Am J Sports Med 36:298–307

21. Thomee R, Kaplan Y, Kvist J et al (2011) Muscle strength and hop performance criteria prior to return to sports after ACL reconstruction. Knee Surg Sports Traumatol Arthrosc 19:1798–1805

22. van Grinsven S, van Cingel RE, Holla CJ, van Loon CJ (2010) Evidence-based rehabilitation following anterior cruciate ligament reconstruction. Knee Surg Sports Traumatol Arthrosc 18:1128–1144

23. Wilk K, Reinold M, Hooks T (2003) Recent advances in the rehabilitation of isolated and combined anterior cruciate ligament injuries. Orthop Clin North Am 34:107–137

24. Williams GN, Chmielewski T, Rudolph K, Buchanan TS, Snyder-Mackler L (2001) Dynamic knee stability: current theory and implications for clinicians and scientists. J Orthop Sports Phys Ther 31:546–566

25. Wright RW, Fetzer GB (2007) Bracing after ACL Reconstruction- A systematic review. Clin Orthop Relat Res 455:162–168

Prevention of ACL Tear and Rerupture

43

Amelie Stoehr, Barbara Wondrasch, and Hermann Mayr

Contents

A. Stoehr, MD (✉)
Knee Surgery and Sports Traumatology,
OCM-Clinic, Steiner Str. 6, 81369 Munich, Germany
e-mail: ameliestoehr@hotmail.de

B. Wondrasch, PT, MSc
Department of Health and Social Sciences,
University of Applied Sciences St. Poelten,
Matthias Corvinus-Strasse 15,
3100 St. Poelten, Austria

H. Mayr, MD, PhD
Orthopedic Surgery, OCM-Clinic, Steiner Str. 6,
81369 Munich, Germany

Anterior cruciate ligament (ACL) rupture is an injury that puts an athlete at high risk of future osteoarthritis. Identification of potential risk factors and development of ACL prevention programs may decrease the risk of injury [35].

Almost 80 % of ACL injuries are noncontact injuries [2, 29]. The reinjury rate after ACL reconstruction can be up to 35 % [2, 15]. Literature on sport-specific outcomes from ACL reconstruction is limited with minimal data [38]. Different methodological approaches were used to determine the exact injury mechanisms. Movement patterns, such as change of direction, cutting maneuvers with deceleration, landing from a jump near to extension, or hyperextension and hyperflexion, as well as maximal quadriceps contraction at forced flexion, have been reported to be responsible for ACL tears [1, 11, 12]. These movement patterns involve knee valgus, varus, internal, and external rotation moments and anterior translation of the tibia. Literature shows that anterior translation force is most detrimental for isolated ACL ruptures, especially when the knee is flexed at about 20–30° [2, 22, 25, 26, 23], but that sagittal and transverse plane loading mechanisms may as well contribute to noncontact ACL injuries [35]. Understanding the mechanism of ACL injuries is beneficial to develop specific prevention strategies [2, 4, 23].

R. Siebold et al. (eds.), *Anterior Cruciate Ligament Reconstruction*,
DOI 10.1007/978-3-642-45349-6_43, © ESSKA 2014

43.1 Risk Factors and Gender Differences

43.1.1 Risk Factors

It is important to note that ACL injuries are not random events but often occur due to underlying causes or risk factors. To develop a prevention program, it is necessary to know and understand these risk factors as they may have individual reasons such as anatomical, hormonal, and neuromuscular differences or are dependent on environmental conditions and type of competition [29].

Abnormal lower extremity alignment, e.g., valgus alignment (Fig. 43.1), can increase ACL strain values and is, therefore, a predisposing factor for ACL injury. The position of the hip and foot, in particular, influences secondary knee position and kinematics [29]. An anterior tilt of the pelvis will lead to an internally rotated, anteverted, and flexed position of the hip, which changes the moment vector of the gluteal muscles and weakens hamstrings. Whereas the gluteal muscles are important in preventing a dynamic

valgus collapse, the hamstrings are important in preventing static and dynamic genu recurvatum and anterior tibial displacement [2, 29].

If the difference between the passive and active Q-angle, the angle formed by a line drawn from the anterior-superior iliac spine to the central patella and a second line drawn from the central patella to the tibial tubercle, is too high, the lower limb biomechanics may be altered and, thus, are at increased risk from static and dynamic valgus stress. An increased body mass index, general joint laxity, and genetic predisposition are other intrinsic risk factors [2, 36].

An intercondylar notch (Fig. 43.2) shaped like a Gothic arch has been related to a higher risk of ACL rupture [2, 37], and a significant correlation of the ACL cross-sectional area size to the notch surface area was seen. As the mechanism of ACL tears in subjects with a small intercondylar notch is not fully understood, it has been suggested that an impingement of the ACL at the anterior and posterior roof of the notch may occur during tibial external rotation and abduction [8, 32].

The neuromuscular control system is primarily responsible for unconscious activation of the dynamic restraints surrounding the joint, generates movements, and determines the biomechanics of actions. This requires complex interactions in the motor sensory system, which consists of the physiologic systems of the complex neurosensory and neuromuscular processes [33]. Sensory

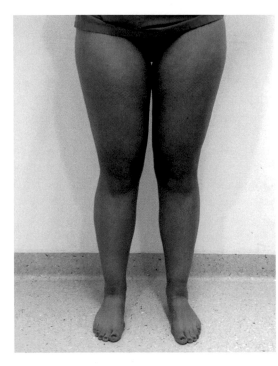

Fig. 43.1 Valgus alignment is a predisposing factor for ACL injury (© Amelic Stoehr)

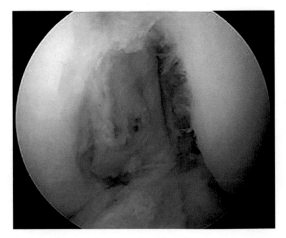

Fig. 43.2 Intercondylar notch shaped like a Gothic arch is related to higher risk for ACL injury (© Amelic Stoehr)

receptors, which are located in joints and muscles, send peripheral afferent signals to the central nervous system (CNS) [5]. The CNS processes these signals into motor responses, resulting in muscle activation for locomotion, functional tasks, and joint stabilization. In this way, both muscle actions are coordinated, especially antagonist-agonist relationships, which are crucial for joint stability and balance. Balance is determined by the ability to maintain a position, the ability to voluntary move, and the ability to react to perturbation. To prevent and reduce knee kinetics that increase the risk of ACL injury, the co-activation of hamstrings and quadriceps, as well as good balance, is extremely important. A poor motor sensory system will lead to inefficient balance strategies and uncoordinated muscle activation patterns, both of which result in a greater risk of injury [30].

Muscular fatigue may increase the risk of noncontact and contact ACL injuries by altering the neuromuscular control. Skill level and physical fitness as well as protective and sports equipment are other factors [2].

Studies show that athletes generally have a higher risk for an ACL injury during competition than during practice and training [27, 29].

43.1.2 Gender Differences

The incidence of anterior cruciate ligament (ACL) tear is much higher in female than in male athletes. Intrinsic factors such as increased quadriceps angle and posterior tibial slope may predispose females to ACL rupture. Compared with males, females are more likely to have a smaller intercondylar notch widths and ACL cross-sectional area; however, no conclusive correlation between ACL size and notch dimension exists, especially in relation to risk of ACL injury [32]. Female athletes who land with the knees in inadequate flexion and in greater valgus and external rotation are at increased risk of ACL injury [11]. According to literature, a relationship between the menstrual cycle and the time of ACL injury is obvious [2, 9, 20].

The menstrual cycle of females, especially the preovulatory phase, seems to be a risk factor for noncontact ACL injuries that are consistent with the estrogen surge seen during this phase of the cycle [20]. The use of oral contraceptives may decrease this injury risk, but further evidence is needed. Sex hormones can reduce motor coordination in female athletes and may play a role in noncontact ACL injuries [2, 9, 36].

Neuromuscular intervention protocols have been shown to reduce the rate of injury in girls and women [18, 19, 21]. Following ACL reconstruction, female athletes are more likely than male athletes to rupture the contralateral ACL; however, males and females are equally likely to rupture the reconstructed knee. Long-term studies demonstrate no difference between males and females [36, 38].

A multifactorial etiology seems to be responsible for noncontact ACL tears in female athletes. Prior epidemiological data demonstrate that neuromuscular and biomechanical risk factors may contribute in isolation or combination with intrinsic factors, to increase relative noncontact ACL injury rates in female athletes [2].

43.2   Pivoting and Non-Pivoting Sports

Patients usually return to pivoting and contact sports between 6 months and 1 year after ACL reconstruction. Non-pivoting sports with guided movements and without significant injury potential, e.g., cycling or jogging, are an early option during rehabilitation. Prevention of ACL injuries is a challenging task and often sport-specific.

> **Tricks and Pearls**
> Prevention strategies should consider the risk factors for an ACL injury and should eliminate them as much as possible.

Pivoting sports such as contact sports, indoor ball games, and Alpine skiing are combined with a high risk of an ACL injury. Therefore, special sport-specific training programs may lead to a reduction in this risk of injury. Training should always reach the individual physical limit but not take place in the physical fatigue. Anticipation of accident mechanisms in contact and ball sports seems very important. The aim should be to avoid severe collisions with an opponent such as a pressing impact in soccer or to care for the positioning of team players in volleyball. Neuromuscular and biomechanical risk factors can be reduced by specific sports technique modifications or by neuromuscular and balance training, strength training of the lower extremity, and core stability training [3, 7, 13, 16, 29, 36]. These training components should be combined within a prevention program and should be individualized and adapted to each patient's or athlete's requirements.

> **Avoid Pitfalls**
> As most noncontact ACL ruptures happen during landing or deceleration movements, both these tasks could be modified and adapted.

Landing maneuvers with extended hip and knee joint posture at the initial contact increase load on the ACL, decrease muscular stability, and should, therefore, be avoided [2, 29]. Landing techniques with initial contact at the forefoot, with hip flexion and knee, reportedly decrease the risk of an ACL injury [13, 16, 24, 27]. Thus, new landing strategies should be implemented and practiced until these tasks can be performed automatically.

Deceleration movements produce high anterior shear forces, which are absorbed by muscles surrounding the joint. However, deceleration rapidly leads to muscle fatigue and then the forces are directly applied to the ACL. To reduce these shear forces and to greater dissipate these forces, the use of a three-step deceleration technique has been recommended [3, 5, 6].

> **Tricks and Pearls**
> Neuromuscular training emphasizes on dynamic stability and proprioception, rather than altering strength and aims, to improve balance strategies and muscle activation patterns.

The focus of neuromuscular training is appropriate body positioning and posture, and the awareness of positioning and posture, to promote proper dynamic muscular stabilization during functional activities (Fig. 43.3). These activities are designed to emphasize quality of movement rather than quantity of movement. If the neuromuscular control of the lower limbs is inefficient or too slow, large forces are placed on the lower extremity and can jeopardize the functionality of capsule-ligamentous structures and joints.

Neuromuscular training should be performed in both a static and dynamic manner and should include balance training that focuses on sensory (visual, vestibular, somatosensory), motor (coordinated stabilizing neuromuscular strategies), and biomechanical components (body segment alignment against gravity) (Fig. 43.4) [16, 17].

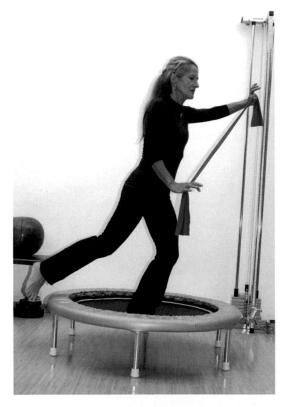

Fig. 43.3 Neuromuscular training emphasizes improving balance strategies and muscle activation patterns to promote proper dynamic muscular stabilization during functional activities (© Cornelia Jungter-Mayr)

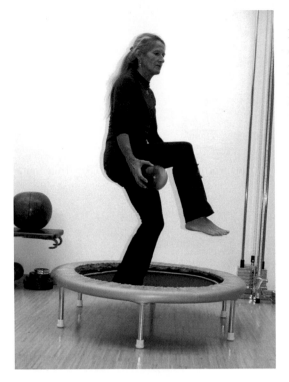

Fig. 43.4 Balance training that focuses on sensory, motor, and biomechanical components (© Cornelia Jungter-Mayr)

Tricks and Pearls
Strength training includes strength endurance training, as well as bodybuilding training (muscle hypertrophy), recruitment training, power training, explosive power training, and plyometrics.

Strength endurance training seems to have a protective effect on the ACL, as strength endurance delays muscle fatigue, which leads to lessened muscular stability in a joint. It was demonstrated that hamstring fatigue will produce transverse plane, dynamic knee-control deficits [19, 33]. Bodybuilding training and recruitment training are important for stabilizing the joint and form the basis for explosive power training and plyometrics. The literature shows that plyometric training has practically the greatest influence in reducing noncontact ACL injuries [3, 19].

Core stability is the ability of the lumbopelvic hip complex to prevent buckling and to hold and control the position and movement of the central portion of the body (Fig. 43.5). The core consists of many different muscles that stabilize the abdomen, spine, pelvis, and shoulders and enables us to stand upright and move on two feet. The core also provides the foundation for all arm and leg movements. Thus, these muscles help to control movements, transfer energy, shift body weight, and move in any direction. Power is derived and controlled by the trunk, allowing more efficient and better-coordinated movement of the limbs. Current evidence suggests that decreased core stability may predispose one to injury and that appropriate training may reduce injury [2, 3].

Core stability training includes the rectus abdominis, erector spinae, external and internal obliques, transverses abdominis, as well as the hip flexors, hip adductors, and hip abductors. The training should include exercises with body weight, with additional weight and resistance, and with the use of balance tools (Fig. 43.6).

The current literature reveals that multicomponent programs decrease the risk and incidence of ACL injuries [3, 10, 13, 18, 24, 28].

Tricks and Pearls
In particular, lower extremity plyometrics, dynamic balance, strength, and body awareness seem to be the most successful training components in reducing ACL injuries.

Programs that aim on reduction of high-risk valgus and sagittal plane movements will probably prove to be superior for ACL injury prevention [28].

In terms of an exogenous prevention measure to avoid ACL ruptures, protection ortheses have long been used in American football, motocross, and ice hockey. Bracing decreases the excessive tibial rotation in ACL-deficient patients during high-demand activities and may prevent further severe knee injuries [14, 34]. Custom-fit functional braces show superior results over general prophylactic knee braces

Fig. 43.5 Core stability training to improve the lumbopelvic hip complex (© Cornelia Jungter-Mayr)

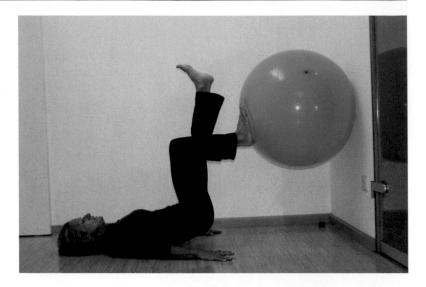

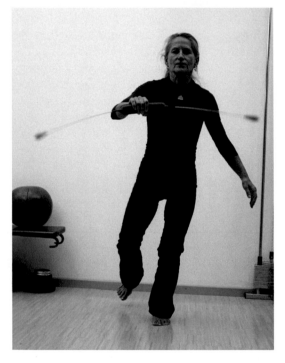

Fig. 43.6 Body weight exercises with additional weight and resistance and the use of balance tools (© Cornelia Jungter-Mayr)

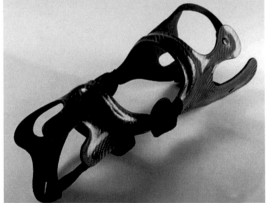

Fig. 43.7 A newly released custom-fit model is now to be used in skiing (EXOSPrevenThesis with courtesy of ORTEMA)

due to improved sizing and fitting of the thigh and tibial cuffs. On the negative side, the presence of a brace may slow an athlete's straight-ahead sprint speed, reduces its sensorimotor skills, and causes early fatigue to its wearer [1]. A newly released custom-fit model (Fig. 43.7) is now to be used in skiing.

Memory

Valgus morphotype, female gender, functional genu recurvatum, and the so-called Gothic notch are significant risk factors for anterior cruciate ligament rupture. Most noncontact ACL ruptures happen during landing or deceleration. Lower extremity plyometrics, dynamic balance, strength, and body awareness seem to be the most successful preventive components in reducing ACL injuries. Neuromuscular training regarding body positioning and posture promotes proper dynamic muscular stabilization during sports activities.

References

1. Albright JP, Saterbak A, Stokes J (1995) Use of knee braces in sport. Current Recommendations. Sports Med 20(5):281–301. Review
2. Alentorn-Geli E, Myer GD, Silvers HJ et al (2009) Prevention of non-contact anterior cruciate ligament injuries in soccer players. Part 1: Mechanisms of injury and underlying risk factors. Knee Surg Sports Traumatol Arthrosc 17(7):705–729
3. Alentorn-Geli E, Myer GD, Silvers HJ et al (2009) Prevention of non-contact anterior cruciate ligament injuries in soccer players. Part 2: A review of prevention programs aimed to modify risk factors and to reduce injury rates. Knee Surg Sports Traumatol Arthrosc 17(8):859–879
4. Bahr R, Krosshaug T (2005) Understanding injury mechanisms: a key component of preventing injuries in sport. Br J Sports Med 39(6):324–329
5. Besier TF, Lloyd DG, Ackland TR, Cochrane JL (2001) Anticipatory effects on knee joint loading during running and cutting maneuvers. Med Sci Sports Exerc 33(7):1176–1181
6. Besier TF, Lloyd DG, Cochrane JL, Ackland TR (2001) External loading of the knee joint during running and cutting maneuvers. Med Sci Sports Exerc 33(7):1168–1175
7. Chappell JD, Limpisvasti O (2008) Effect of a neuromuscular training program on the kinetics and kinematics of jumping tasks. Am J Sports Med 36(6):1081–1086
8. Dienst M, Schneider G, Altmeyer K, Voelkering K, Georg T, Kramann B, Kohn D (2007) Correlation of intercondylar notch cross sections to the ACL size: a high resolution MR tomographic in vivo analysis. Arch Orthop Trauma Surg 127:253–260
9. DiStefano LJ, Padua DA, DiStefano MJ, Marshall SW (2009) Influence of age, sex, technique, and exercise program on movement patterns after an anterior cruciate ligament injury prevention program in youth soccer players. Am J Sports Med 37(3):495–505
10. Engebretsen AH, Myklebust G, Holme I, Engebretsen L, Bahr R (2008) Prevention of injuries among male soccer players: a prospective, randomized intervention study targeting players with previous injuries or reduced function. Am J Sports Med 36(6):1052–1060
11. Fauno P, Wulff Jakobsen B (2006) Mechanism of anterior cruciate ligament injuries in soccer. Int J Sports Med 27(1):75–79
12. Feagin JA Jr, Lambert KL (1985) Mechanism of injury and pathology of anterior cruciate ligament injuries. Orthop Clin North Am 16(1):41–45
13. Gilchrist J, Mandelbaum BR, Melancon H et al (2008) A randomized controlled trial to prevent noncontact anterior cruciate ligament injury in female collegiate soccer players. Am J Sports Med 36(8):1476–1483
14. Giotis D, Zampeli F, Pappas E, Mitsionis G, Papadopoulos P, Georgoulis AD (2013) The effect of knee braces on tibial rotation in anterior cruciate ligament-deficient knees during high-demand athletic activities. Clin J Sport Med 23(4):287–292
15. Granan LP, Bahr R, Steindal K, Furnes O, Engebretsen L (2008) Development of a national cruciate ligament surgery registry: the Norwegian National Knee Ligament Registry. Am J Sports Med 36(2):308–315
16. Guskiewicz KM, Perrin DH (1996) Effect of orthotics on postural sway following inversion ankle sprain. J Orthop Sports Phys Ther 23(5):326–331
17. Guskiewicz KM, Perrin DH, Gansneder BM (1996) Effect of Mild Head Injury on Postural Stability in Athletes. J Athl Train 31(4):300–306
18. Hewett TE, Lindenfield TN, Riccobene J V, Noyes FR (1999) The effect of neuromuscular training on the incidence of knee injury in female athletes. A prospective study. Am J Sports Med 27(6):699–706
19. Hewett TE, Stroupe AL, Nance TA, Noyes FR (1996) Plyometric training in female athletes. Decreased impact forces and increased hamstring torques. Am J Sports Med 24(6):765–773
20. Hewett TE, Zazulak BT, Myer GD (2007) Effects of the menstrual cycle on anterior cruciate ligament injury risk: a systematic review. Am J Sports Med 35(4):659–668
21. Kerson GB, Colston MA, Short NI, Neal KL, Hoewischer PE, Pixley JJ (2004) Neuromuscular changes in female collegiate athletes resulting from a plyometric jump-training program. J Athl Train 39(1):17–23
22. Koga H, Nakamae A, Shima Y et al (2010) Mechanisms for noncontact anterior cruciate ligament injuries: knee joint kinematics in 10 injury situations from female team handball and basketball. Am J Sports Med 38:2218–2225
23. Krosshaug T, Andersen TE, Olsen OE, Myklebust G, Bahr R (2005) Research approaches to describe the mechanisms of injuries in sport: limitations and possibilities. Br J Sports Med 39(6):330–339
24. Mandelbaum BR, Silvers HJ, Watanabe DS et al (2005) Effectiveness of a neuromuscular and proprioceptive training program in preventing anterior cruciate ligament injuries in female athletes: 2-year follow-up. Am J Sports Med 33(7):1003–1010
25. Markolf KL, Burchfield DM, Shapiro MM, Shepard MF, Finerman GA, Slauterbeck JL (1995) Combined knee loading states that generate high anterior cruciate ligament forces. J Orthop Res 13(6):930–935
26. Markolf KL, Gorek JF, Kabo JM, Shapiro MS (1990) Direct measurement of resultant forces in the anterior cruciate ligament. An in vitro study performed with a new experimental technique. J Bone Joint Surg Am 72(4):557–567
27. Myklebust G, Engebretsen L, Braekken IH, Skjolberg A, Olsen OE, Bahr R (2003) Prevention of anterior cruciate ligament injuries in female team handball players: a prospective intervention study over three seasons. Clin J Sport Med 13(2):71–78
28. Quatman CE, Hewett TE (2009) The anterior cruciate ligament injury controversy: is "valgus collapse" a sex-specific mechanism? Br J Sports Med 43:328–335

29. Renstrom P, Ljungqvist A, Arendt E et al (2008) Non-contact ACL injuries in female athletes: an International Olympic Committee current concepts statement. Br J Sports Med 42(6):394–412
30. Riemann BL, Lephart SM (2002) The sensorimotor system, part II: the role of proprioception in motor control and functional joint stability. J Athl Train 37(1):80–84
31. Risberg MA, Holm I, Myklebust G, Engebretsen L (2007) Neuromuscular training versus strength training during first 6 months after anterior cruciate ligament reconstruction: a randomized clinical trial. Phys Ther 87(6):737–750
32. Rizzo M, Holler SB, Bassett FH 3rd (2001) Comparison of males' and females' ratios of anterior-cruciate-ligament width to femoral-intercondylar-notch width: a cadaveric study. Am J Orthop 30(8): 660–664
33. Rudolph KS, Snyder-Mackler L (2004) Effect of dynamic stability on a step task in ACL deficient individuals. J Electromyogr Kinesiol 14(5):565–575
34. Sanders MS, Cates RA, Baker MD, Barber-Westin SD, Gladin WM, Levy MS (2011) Knee injuries and the use of prophylactic knee bracing in off-road motorcycling:results of a large-scale epidemiological study. Am J Sports Med 39(7):1395–1400
35. Soligard T, Myklebust G, Steffen K et al (2008) Comprehensive warm-up programme to prevent injuries in young female footballers: cluster randomised controlled trial. BMJ 337:a2469
36. Sutton KM, Bullock JM (2013) Anterior cruciate ligament rupture: differences between males and females. J Am Acad Orthop Surg 21(1):41–50
37. Uhorchak JM, Scoville CR, Williams GN, Arciero RA, St Pierre P, Taylor DC (2003) Risk factors associated with noncontact injury of the anterior cruciate ligament: a prospective four-year evaluation of 859 West Point cadets. Am J Sports Med 31:831–842
38. Warner SJ, Smith MV, Wright RW, Matava MJ, Brophy RH (2011) Sport-specific outcomes after anterior cruciate ligament reconstruction. Arthroscopy 27(8):1129–1134

Index

R. Siebold et al. (eds.), *Anterior Cruciate Ligament Reconstruction*,
DOI 10.1007/978-3-642-45349-6, © ESSKA 2014

Printed in the United States
By Bookmasters